Biochemistry Review

SAUNDERS TEXT AND REVIEW SERIES

BIOCHEMISTRY REVIEW

ROBERT ROSKOSKI, JR., M.D., Ph.D.
Fred G. Brazda Professor of Biochemistry and Molecular Biology
Louisiana State University Medical Center
New Orleans, Louisiana

JACK D. HERBERT, Ph.D.
Associate Professor of Biochemistry and Molecular Biology
Louisiana State University Medical Center
New Orleans, Louisiana

W.B. SAUNDERS COMPANY
A Division of Harcourt Brace & Company
Philadelphia London Toronto Montreal Sydney Tokyo

W.B. SAUNDERS COMPANY
A Division of Harcourt Brace & Company

The Curtis Center
Independence Square West
Philadelphia, Pennsylvania 19106

Library of Congress Cataloging-in-Publication Data

Roskoski, Robert.
Biochemistry review / Robert Roskoski and Jack D. Herbert.

p. cm.

ISBN 0–7216–5175–5

1. Biochemistry. I. Herbert, Jack D. II. Title.
[DNLM: 1. Biochemistry. QU 4 R821b 1996]

QP514.2.R665 1996 612′.015′076—dc20

DNLM/DLC 95-41655

BIOCHEMISTRY REVIEW ISBN 0–7216–5175–5

Printed in the United States of America.

Last digit is the print number: 9 8 7 6 5 4 3 2 1

To those generations of students who
forced us to reexamine and then, chastened, to clarify
our own cloudy understanding of so much that we thought we knew.

PREFACE

This book provides a succinct outline review of the essentials of biochemistry and molecular biology, and each chapter contains review questions and explanations. Chapters 1 to 6 cover the fundamentals, Chapters 7 to 14 consider intermediary metabolism, Chapters 15 to 18 cover the area of molecular biology, and Chapters 19 to 24 cover specialized topics of cell biology. Chapter 25, on the integration of energy metabolism, considers metabolic regulation, feeding and fasting, and diabetes. Following Chapter 25, the comprehensive examination contains a randomized selection of biochemical items similar to those encountered in standardized examinations. The appendix consists of a glossary of selected biochemical and medical terms for students. We believe that instructors also will find the medical definitions helpful. The appendix additionally contains helpful hints for studying biochemistry and a list of items that students should master. The order of topics in this review parallels that found in *Biochemistry* (1996) by Robert Roskoski, Jr., also published by the W.B. Saunders Company.

On the inside of the front cover are printed lists of some general principles of biochemistry and general principles of bioenergetics. These principles are guidelines for understanding and analyzing reactions and metabolic pathways. Although the principles are numbered for reference, it is the concept and not the arbitrary number that is important. These concepts help make sense out of what is sometimes regarded as a tangled mass of interconnected metabolic reactions. Learning is facilitated by relating new material to the familiar. Once the concept behind each principle is mastered, it is easier for the student to relate the unfamiliar to these principles and to prototypical reactions and processes.

ORGANIZATION

The questions at the end of each chapter and in the comprehensive examination appear in the formats used on the United States Medical Licensing Examination. Some questions are based upon recall, enabling readers to assess the depth and extent of their knowledge. Other questions require the application of the fundamentals of biochemistry to understand clinical situations. Besides common clinical conditions such as diabetes, atherosclerosis, infectious diseases, and cancer, many questions are based upon metabolic abnormalities that accompany both common and rare inborn errors of metabolism. The emphasis, however, is not so much on rare diseases as on understanding and explaining the metabolic aberration that results from the metabolic disease.

CLINICAL CASES

The self-evaluation at the end of each chapter concludes with a narrative concerning a clinical situation and approximately four questions. These case presentations, which are something extra (*lagniappe*), are designed to illustrate the importance of biochemistry in understanding the pathogenesis of disease. Because biochemistry is generally taught early in the course of study, care was taken not to make the cases too arcane. The specialized medical descriptions are explained where they are used, and the normal values for the clinical studies are noted directly in the text. The standard laboratory values are listed in *Cecil Textbook of Medicine* (1992), published by the W.B. Saunders Company. These narratives are longer and more intricate than are generally used in standard examinations. The approach and potential insight gained from considering these cases are designed to solidify biochemical and medical principles and approaches. These cases can also be used for practice- or problem-based learning.

CONVENTIONS

The tricarboxylic acid cycle, or citric acid cycle, is called the Krebs cycle in honor of its discoverer and because clinicians rarely use the former terms. The nonsystematic name glyceride is used for acylglycerol, again because clinicians prefer the term glyceride. The calorie is used as the nutritional unit of energy owing to its widespread use in the United States. Extensive use is made of the International System of units, however, and the joule is used as the unit of energy for all calculations involving bioenergetics.

ACKNOWLEDGMENTS

We thank Carol Vartanian for editing this book and for providing balanced feedback in a gracious and cordial manner. We are grateful to Dr. Ab Sadeghi-Nejad of Tufts University and the New England Medical Center for his valuable comments on the 25 clinical cases. We thank Martha Gay for editing the questions and answers. Finally, we credit Risa Clow, illustrator at the W.B. Saunders Company, for overseeing the art work, and William R. Schmitt, Editorial Manager at the W.B. Saunders Company, who served as acquisitions editor.

TO THE STUDENT

One principle not listed on the cover, but which is given in all of our classes, is that *biochemistry is fun!*

ROBERT ROSKOSKI, JR., M.D., Ph.D.
JACK D. HERBERT, Ph.D.

COMPANION TEXT

The material in this book complements that in *Biochemistry* (1996) by Robert Roskoski, Jr., published by the W.B. Saunders Company. The 25 chapters in this review parallel those of *Biochemistry.* The illustrations, explanations, and topics in the companion text are more comprehensive than those in this review. The companion text, however, lacks questions and answers, case studies, a comprehensive examination, study hints, and a biochemistry and medical glossary.

CONTENTS

CHAPTER TWENTY-TWO

CHAPTER TWENTY-THREE

CHAPTER TWENTY-FOUR

CHAPTER TWENTY-FIVE

CHAPTER ONE

CELLS: THE UNITS OF LIFE

SYNOPSIS

OBJECTIVES

1. To define biochemistry and describe the chemical composition of humans.
2. To define the salient features of metabolism.
3. To compare eukaryotic and prokaryotic cells.
4. To classify bacteria as gram positive and gram negative.
5. To compare DNA- and RNA-containing viruses.

Objective 1: To define biochemistry and describe the chemical composition of humans.

I. Definition of biochemistry
- A. Biochemistry includes the study of the molecular composition of living cells
  - 1. *All forms of life are constructed from fundamental units called cells* (PRINCIPLE 2 OF BIOCHEMISTRY)
    - a. The molecules that make up cells and tissues of the body perform specific functions
      - (1) **DNA** serves as the genetic repository
      - (2) **RNA** transfers genetic information from DNA into protein
      - (3) **Proteins** serve structural, catalytic, regulatory, and defensive roles
      - (4) **Carbohydrates** play a structural role in cells and tissues and serve as a storage form of energy
      - (5) **Lipids** play structural and regulatory roles in cells and serve as the main storage form of energy
    - b. *Cells obey the laws of chemistry and physics* (PRINCIPLE 3 OF BIOCHEMISTRY)
  - 2. Membranes occur in all cells
    - a. Biological membranes are made up of lipid bilayers and associated proteins
      - (1) Proteins that are embedded in the lipid are called **integral** membrane proteins
      - (2) Proteins bound at the surface of a membrane are called **peripheral** proteins
    - b. Lipids and proteins can readily diffuse laterally in membranes, but they cannot easily go from one leaflet of the bilayer to the other (i.e., flip-flop is disallowed)
- B. Biochemistry also includes the study of the chemical reactions that biological compounds undergo and the regulation of these reactions

II. Composition of average human adults
- A. 55% Water
- B. 19% Protein
- C. 19% Fat
- D. 7% Mineral
- E. $<$ 1% carbohydrate
- F. $<$ 1% nucleic acid

Objective 2: To define the salient features of metabolism.

III. Metabolism
- A. Definitions
  - 1. **Metabolism** refers to all of the chemical reactions of an organism
  - 2. **Catabolism** refers to the degradation of large, complex molecules into smaller simple metabolites
  - 3. **Anabolism** refers to the biosynthetic conversion of smaller into larger molecules
  - 4. A **chemical reaction** is the process that converts one or more chemical compounds to other chemical compounds
  - 5. **Enzymes** are proteins that catalyze nearly all biochemical reactions (PRINCIPLE 5 OF BIOCHEMISTRY)
  - 6. **Ribozymes** are RNA molecules that catalyze a few reactions in non-humans
- B. Three stages of catabolism (Krebs's classification)
  - 1. Stage I is the hydrolytic breakdown of complex molecules into their building blocks
  - 2. Stage II is the conversion of the building blocks to acetyl coenzyme A
  - 3. Stage III is the oxidation of acetyl coenzyme A to carbon dioxide by the Krebs cycle and the synthesis of ATP by oxidative phosphorylation

C. Bioenergetics
1. Each step of metabolism is accompanied by an energy change
2. *Lipmann's law states that ATP serves as the common currency of energy exchange in all living systems* (PRINCIPLE 10 OF BIOCHEMISTRY)

Objective 3: To compare eukaryotic and prokaryotic cells.

IV. Eukaryotes
A. General properties
1. Structure
a. Eukaryotes have a well-defined **nucleus** surrounded by a nuclear membrane, and the cells are divided into several membrane-bounded compartments (Fig. 1–1)
(1) The nuclei of human somatic cells contain 23 pairs (46 total) of chromosomes
(2) Of these, 22 pairs are alike in males and females and are called autosomes
(3) The remaining pair are the sex chromosomes, denoted XX in females and XY in males
b. Human cells consist of a variety of subcellular components (Table 1–1)
(1) **Lysosomes,** which participate in the hydrolytic degradation of cellular macromolecules, contain **hexosaminidase A** (which is deficient in Tay-Sachs disease), **β-glucosidase** (which is deficient in Gaucher disease), and many other hydrolases
(2) The **endoplasmic reticulum** consists of rough and smooth components based on the presence or absence of ribosomes, respectively
(3) The **cytoskeleton,** which is responsible for the structural framework of the cell, is composed of microfilaments, intermediate filaments, and microtubules
(a) **Microfilaments** are made of actin and myosin
(b) Major classes of **intermediate filaments** include keratins, desmin, vimentin, neurofilaments, and glial filaments
(c) Tubulin makes up **microtubules,** flagella, and centrioles (centrioles function as organizing centers for the mitotic spindle during cell division)
2. Size
a. Most human cells are about (20 μm)^3, although there is a considerable range in size
b. The mature red blood cell has a diameter of 7 μm (this value can be used to measure relative sizes by microscopy)

B. Cell division
1. Mitosis
a. Mitosis, which occurs in somatic cells, involves the production of daughter cells containing the diploid genome
b. Mitosis (M), which lasts for 1–2 hours, is the shortest phase of the cell cycle; the other phases are G_1, S, and G_2
(1) G_1 and G_2 are gaps, and S refers to the DNA synthesis phase; these three stages make up interphase

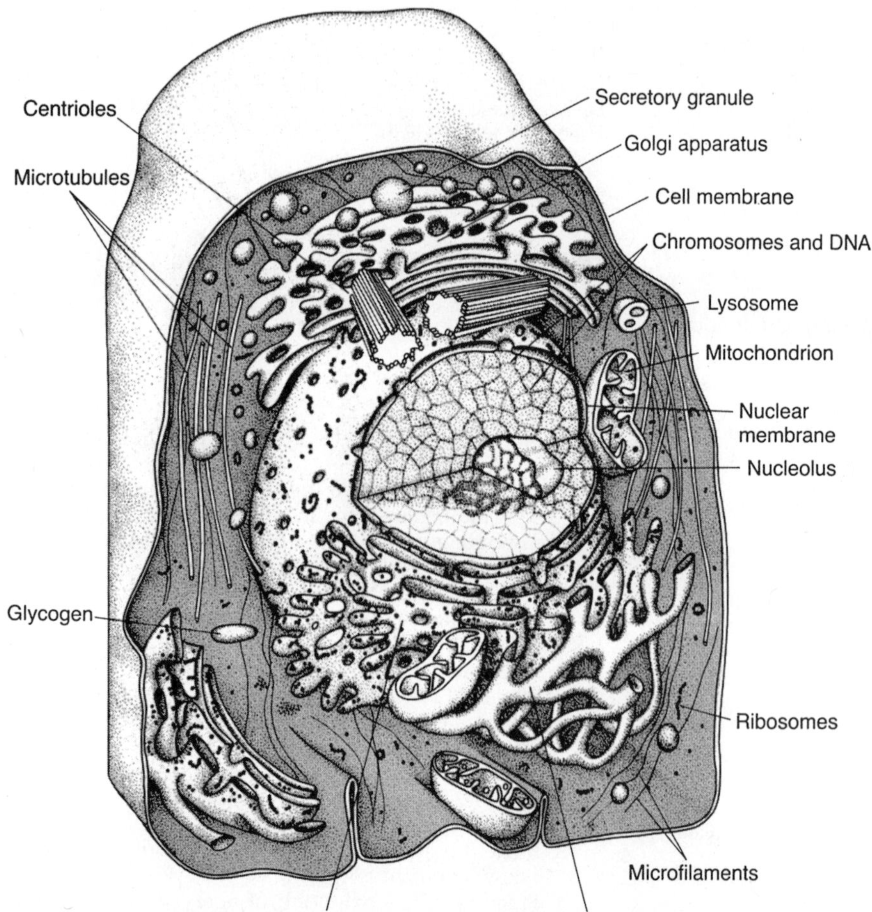

FIGURE 1–1. Diagram of a typical cell. Reproduced, with permission, from A. C. Guyton. *Textbook of Medical Physiology,* 8th ed. Philadelphia, W.B. Saunders Company, 1991, p. 10.

TABLE 1–1. Metabolic Properties of Animal Cell Components

Component	General Properties	Associated Biochemical Processes
Cytosol	Nonsedimentable	Glycolysis, gluconeogenesis, glycogenesis, glycogenolysis, pentose phosphate pathway; fatty acid, steroid, purine, pyrimidine synthesis; copper-zinc superoxide dismutase.
Lysosome	"Wastebasket" of the cell	Acidic compartment containing cathepsins (which degrade several classes of proteins), DNAse, RNAse, hexosaminidase A, β-glucosidase, and sphingomyelinase.
Mitochondrion	"Powerhouse" of the cell, major site of ATP formation	Krebs cycle, β-oxidation of fatty acids, oxidative phosphorylation, and pyruvate dehydrogenase activity; manganese superoxide dismutase.
Nucleus	Repository and expression of genes	DNA replication, RNA synthesis and processing.
Peroxisome	Hydrogen peroxide metabolism	Catalase, D- and L-amino acid oxidase.
Plasma membrane	Boundary between cell exterior and interior	Sodium-potassium ATPase, insulin and glucagon receptors, glucose translocases, LDL receptors, and γ-glutamyl transpeptidase.
Smooth endoplasmic reticulum	Complex lipid biosynthesis	Phospholipid synthesis, steroid hydroxylation, and cytochrome P-450 activity.
Rough endoplasmic reticulum and Golgi	Synthesis of membrane proteins and proteins for export	Protein synthesis and processing.

(2) The stages of mitosis include prophase, metaphase, anaphase, and telophase
(3) Chromosomes form discrete and identifiable bodies during metaphase

2. Meiosis
   a. Meiosis is the type of cell division that reduces the diploid number (2N) of chromosomes to the haploid number (1N) of the gamete (egg or sperm)
   b. The possession of three copies of human chromosome 21 (trisomy 21) results in Down syndrome and is the most common abnormality of the number of autosomes in live-born infants
   c. Trisomy results from meiotic nondisjunction
      (1) **Nondisjunction** is the failure of two members of a chromosome pair to disjoin during meiosis I, or of two chromatids of a chromosome to disjoin during meiosis II
      (2) Both chromosomes pass to one daughter cell and the other daughter cell receives neither

V. Prokaryotes
   A. General properties
      1. Structure
         a. Prokaryotes, including bacteria, lack a well-defined nucleus
         b. Bacterial cells are surrounded by a plasma membrane and cell wall
         c. Bacteria lack an intracellular membrane network, and they lack intracellular organelles
      2. Size
         a. Bacterial cells are much smaller than human cells
         b. The size of a typical bacterium is about 1 μm (diameter) by 2 μm (length)—about the size of a mitochondrion
   B. Cell division
      1. Under optimal nutritional conditions, prokaryotes can divide every 20 minutes
      2. Prokaryotes divide by binary fission

Objective 4: To classify bacteria as gram positive and gram negative.

VI. Bacteria
   A. Gram-positive bacteria
      1. The gram-positive bacteria have a thick cell wall that retains crystal violet
      2. Many common pathogens are gram-positive bacteria
         a. *Staphylococcus aureus* is a common cause of boils, wound infections, and pneumonia
         b. *Streptococcus pneumoniae,* which is a common cause of middle ear infection and meningitis, is the most common cause of gram-positive pneumonia
         c. *Streptococcus mutans* can produce dental caries
   B. Gram-negative bacteria
      1. The gram-negative bacteria have a thin outer membrane, a peptidoglycan layer, and an intermembrane space; lacking the thick cell wall, gram-negative organisms are unable to retain crystal violet
      2. Many common pathogens are gram-negative bacteria
         a. *Escherichia coli* can cause diarrhea, urinary tract infection, and peritonitis
         b. *Helicobacter pylori* is associated with gastritis and peptic ulcer
         c. *Haemophilus influenzae* is a common cause of meningitis, middle ear infection, pharyngitis, and pneumonia
         d. *Salmonella typhi* is the causative agent of typhoid fever
         e. *Chlamydia pneumoniae* can produce atypical pneumonia

Objective 5: To compare DNA- and RNA-containing viruses.

VII. Viruses
   A. All viruses are incapable of independent existence and are obligate cellular parasites
   B. **DNA viruses** have DNA as their genome
      1. Adenovirus is a common cause of upper respiratory and lower respiratory infections
      2. Hepatitis B virus is the causative agent of hepatitis B, which is common throughout the world
   C. **RNA viruses** have RNA as their genome
      1. Retroviruses, including HIV (the causative agent of AIDS), have an RNA genome and a DNA intermediate in their replication cycle
      2. Poliovirus is an RNA virus, but it lacks a DNA intermediate in its replication cycle

QUESTIONS

DIRECTIONS. (Items 1–7): Each of the numbered items or incomplete statements in this section is followed by answers or by completions of the statement. Select the ONE lettered answer or completion that is BEST in each case. Correct answers and explanations are given at the end of the chapter.

1. An individual with cholera can die within 24 hours because of the loss of which of the following body components?

   (A) Carbohydrate
   (B) Nucleic acid
   (C) Protein
   (D) Water
   (E) Lipid

2. Lipmann's law states that the common currency of energy exchange is

   (A) acetyl-CoA
   (B) ATP
   (C) glucose
   (D) heat
   (E) oxygen

3. Which of the following virus particles contains RNA?

   (A) Adenovirus
   (B) Hepatitis B virus
   (C) Herpes simplex
   (D) Human immunodeficiency virus (HIV)
   (E) Variola virus

4. Which of the following is a true statement regarding a composite virus containing the DNA from Epstein-Barr virus and the protein envelope of the varicella virus?

   (A) The progeny would be Epstein-Barr virus
   (B) The progeny would be varicella virus
   (C) The progeny would be a composite virus
   (D) The host-cell range of the composite virus would be the same as that of Epstein-Barr virus
   (E) Mutant forms of varicella virus would be formed

5. A 19-year-old woman in the third trimester of pregnancy develops pyuria, dysuria, and flank pain. The organism most likely to be isolated on urine culture is

   (A) *Escherichia coli*
   (B) *Neisseria gonorrhoeae*
   (C) *Staphylococcus aureus*
   (D) *Streptococcus mutans*
   (E) *Streptococcus pyogenes*

6. Which one of the following cellular mechanisms causes the production of cells with the karyotype illustrated at the top of the next column?

   (A) Cytokinesis (cell division) without karyokinesis (nuclear division)
   (B) Crossing-over of chromatids during mitosis
   (C) Nondisjunction during meiosis
   (D) Chromosomal translocation
   (E) Normal mitosis and meiosis

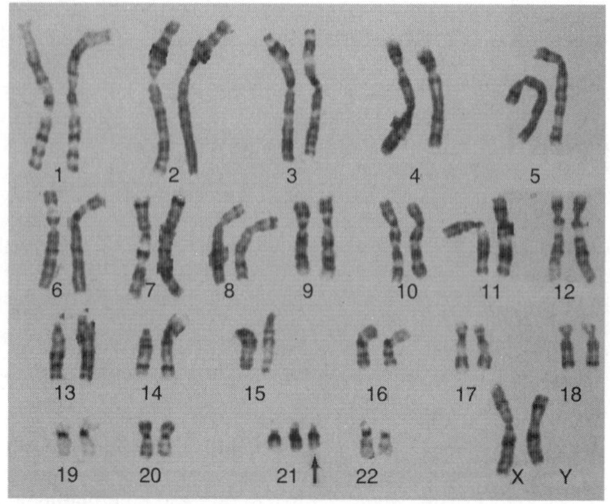

7. At the time when these chromosomes were harvested, the cell from which they were taken was in which of the following phases?

   (A) S phase
   (B) G_1 phase
   (C) G_2 phase
   (D) interphase
   (E) metaphase

DIRECTIONS. (Items 8–15): Each set of matching questions in this section consists of a list of lettered options followed by several numbered items. For each numbered item, select the ONE lettered option that is most closely associated with it. Each lettered option may be selected once, more than once, or not at all.

Items 8–12

(A) Cytosol
(B) Lysosome
(C) Mitochondrion
(D) Nucleus
(E) Peroxisome
(F) Plasma membrane
(G) Rough endoplasmic reticulum and Golgi
(H) Smooth endoplasmic reticulum

For each description of a biochemical process, select the most appropriate cellular component.

8. Major site of ATP production and the target of cyanide poisoning
9. Site of functional LDL receptor, which is missing or defective in familial hypercholesterolemia
10. Major site of catalase activity
11. Site of complex lipid biosynthesis and cytochrome P-450
12. Site of action of sphingomyelinase (defective in Niemann-Pick disease), a hydrolase with an acid pH optimum

Items 13–15

(A) *Bordetella pertussis*
(B) *Campylobacter jejuni*
(C) *Helicobacter pylori*
(D) *Legionella pneumophila*
(E) *Neisseria gonorrhoeae*
(F) *Staphylococcus aureus*
(G) *Streptococcus mutans*
(H) *Streptococcus pyogenes*

For each description, select the most appropriate bacterium.

13. Gram-positive bacterium that can cause dental caries
14. Gram-negative bacterium that can cause peptic ulcers
15. Gram-negative bacterium that can cause whooping cough

Items 16–18

History

The patient is a 54-old accountant who was in excellent health until 2 days ago when he noticed the onset of myalgias (muscle pain) and fever. He awoke on the second day with marked left anterior chest pain. The pain was greatest during inspiration. He recorded his temperature at 39.7 °C (103.5 °F).

Physical Examination

Temperature, 39.4 °C (103 °F); pulse, 95/min and regular; respirations, 22/min and shallow; blood pressure, 122/82 mm Hg. The patient appeared moderately ill and uncomfortable because of pain. The lungs were clear to percussion, but rales (abnormal sounds heard through a stethoscope) were heard over the left anterior chest.

Laboratory

Chest x-ray, left upper lobar infiltration
Electrocardiogram, normal
White blood cell count, 25,200/μL (normal, 4500–11,000/μL)
Neutrophils, 85% (normal, 54–62%)
Lymphocytes, 11% (normal, 23–33%)
Monocytes, 4% (normal, 3–7%)
Red blood count, 5.1 million/μL (normal ♂, 4.3–5.7 million/μL)
Hematocrit, 44% (normal ♂, 39–49%)
Arterial oxygen saturation, 96% (normal, 95–100%)
Lactate dehydrogenase (LDH), 260 U/L (normal, 210–380 U/L)
Creatine phosphokinase (CPK), 56 U/L (normal ♂, 40–175 U/L)
Aspartate aminotransferase (AST, SGOT), 18 U/L (normal, 10–30 U/L)
Serum glucose, 82 mg/dL (normal, 70–105 mg/dL)
Sputum yielded scant material that was taken for a Gram stain.
Blood cultures were also taken.

16. Which one of the following findings helps exclude diagnoses other than bacterial pneumonia that might be responsible for left anterior chest pain?
    (A) Chest x-ray
    (B) Creatine phosphokinase
    (C) Temperature
    (D) White blood cell count
    (E) Serum glucose

Items 17–18

(A) Adenovirus
(B) *Chlamydia pneumoniae*
(C) *Haemophilus influenzae*
(D) *Mycobacterium tuberculosis*
(E) *Streptococcus pneumoniae*

Correlate the most likely cause of typical bacterial pneumonia in this patient with the Gram stain finding.

17. Lancet-shaped gram-positive diplococci
18. Gram-negative organism

ANSWERS AND EXPLANATIONS

1. The answer is D: water. Death from cholera is a result of dehydration and circulatory collapse. Nearly all biochemical reactions occur in water, the most abundant constituent in the body (55% by mass). Protein (19%) and lipid are the most abundant organic constituents. The percentage of fat varies considerably in human populations with an average value of about 19%. Well-trained athletes have a body composition that is only 10% fat. The amount of carbohydrate and nucleic acid is small ($\approx$1%). Of the inorganic minerals, calcium (a constituent of bones and teeth) is the most abundant. *Biochemistry,* p. 2.
2. The answer is B: ATP. ATP is the common currency of energy exchange for all organisms (Lipmann's law). Life is concerned with the production and utilization of ATP. Acetyl-CoA is the substrate for the Krebs cycle, and its oxidative metabolism provides reducing substrates for oxidative phosphorylation and ATP formation. Glucose and fats are fuels for oxidative metabolism, which generates ATP. Humans and other organisms are unable to use heat as a source of metabolic energy. The reaction of oxygen with reductants yields ATP, the biological unit of energy, but oxygen *per se* does not energize muscle contraction, ion transport, or anabolic reactions. *Biochemistry,* p. 3.
3. The answer is D: HIV. Although adenovirus, hepatitis B virus, herpes simplex, and variola virus (a poxvirus) contain DNA as their genetic material, a few viruses, such as human immunodeficiency virus (HIV) and poliovirus, contain RNA. HIV is replicated via a DNA intermediate. Because information is transferred from RNA to DNA

(opposite to the usual direction of information flow), HIV and related viruses are called retroviruses. Poliovirus is an RNA virus that does not go through a DNA intermediate, hence poliovirus is not a retrovirus. Hepatitis B virus is a DNA virus whose replication involves an RNA intermediate that serves as a template for DNA synthesis. *Biochemistry,* p. 12.

4. The answer is A: the progeny will be Epstein-Barr virus. It is possible to package viral nucleic acids in the protein coats of different viruses in favorable cases. It is the genetic material or nucleic acid that codes for the proteins required for replication; thus, it is the Epstein-Barr viral DNA that determines the progeny. Crick's law states that information cannot go from protein to nucleic acid (PRINCIPLE 25 OF BIOCHEMISTRY). The protein coat of a virus is recognized by plasma membrane receptors, and it is the coat protein that determines the host range that a viral particle can infect. *Biochemistry,* p. 270.
5. The answer is A: *Escherichia coli.* This bacterium, although a physiological inhabitant of the large bowel, can also cause disease, one of the most common of which is urinary tract infection, especially in women. The other bacteria listed are not common causes of urinary tract infection. *Pseudomonas aeruginosa* is another gram-negative organism that often causes urinary tract infection. *Biochemistry,* p. 11.
6. The answer is C: nondisjunction during meiosis. The most common mechanism for producing trisomy is the failure of sister chromatids to separate during meiosis (nondisjunction). Cytokinesis refers to the division of one cell into two cells, and karyokinesis is nuclear division. Crossing-over is the exchange of part of one homologous chromosome with another during meiosis. Translocation refers to the joining of a part of one chromosome to another, as occurs frequently in chronic myelogenous leukemia with the formation of the Philadelphia chromosome by reciprocal translocation of chromosomes 9 and 22. *Biochemistry,* p. 9.
7. The answer is E: metaphase. Prophase, metaphase, anaphase, and telophase are the subdivisions of mitosis when individual chromosomes are visible. Individual chromosomes are not visible during interphase. The subdivisions of interphase are G_1, S, and G_2. *Biochemistry,* p. 9.
8. The answer is C: mitochondrion. This is the location of the enzymes of the Krebs cycle, β-oxidation of fatty acids, and oxidative phosphorylation. The mitochondrion is the powerhouse of the cell. Cyanide is a potent inhibitor of cytochrome oxidase, a component of the mitochondrial electron transport chain. *Biochemistry,* p. 6.
9. The answer is F: plasma membrane. Familial hypercholesterolemia results from defects in the LDL receptor that is localized in the plasma membrane, and more than 20 separate mutations have been described. As a result of impaired uptake, affected individuals have elevated LDL in plasma. These patients have xanthomas (nodular swellings of various tendons due to cholesteryl ester deposition in macrophages) and premature atherosclerosis. The disease is autosomal dominant, and most patients are heterozygotes with about half the normal amount of functional receptors. *Biochemistry,* p. 200; *Nelson,* p. 355.
10. The answer is E: peroxisome. The peroxisome is an organelle that is active in hydrogen peroxide generation and metabolism. It contains D-amino acid oxidase and L-amino acid oxidase, which produce hydrogen peroxide, and the peroxisome contains catalase, the enzyme that converts hydrogen peroxide to oxygen and water. *Biochemistry,* p. 6.
11. The answer is H: smooth endoplasmic reticulum. This organelle is the membrane network inside the cell that does not have attached ribosomes. Many aspects of lipid metabolism involve this organelle because of the poor solubility of lipids in the hydrophilic cytosol and their greater solubility in the membrane. Cytochrome P-450, which is a family of more than 30 molecular entities, forms an electron transport chain that participates in the desaturation of fatty acids; steroid hormone hydroxylation; and barbiturate, drug, and ethanol metabolism. *Biochemistry,* p. 6.
12. The answer is B: lysosome. The lysosome contains the enzyme that is defective in Niemann-Pick and a wide variety of other lipid storage diseases. Because of the inability to degrade sphingolipid substrate, the lysosomes and cells become engorged and dysfunctional. Lysosomes are intracellular organelles that contain a variety of hydrolases (cathepsins or proteases, DNAse, RNAse, lipases, and glycosidases) that function at slightly acidic pH ($\approx$5). These enzymes catalyze the degradation of a variety of molecules and have gained the distinction of being the "wastebasket" of the cell because of their role in degrading cellular molecules. *Biochemistry,* p. 6.
13. The answer is G: *Streptococcus mutans.* This is a gram-positive organism, lacking an electron transport chain, that derives its energy by converting glucose to lactic acid by anaerobic glycolysis. Lactic acid dissolves enamel, producing dental caries. *Biochemistry,* p. 10.
14. The answer is C: *Helicobacter pylori.* Researchers recognized in the 1990s that this organism is a causative agent in some forms of peptic ulcer. The necessity of treating peptic ulcer with antibiotics in addition to histamine receptor blockers or proton pump inhibitors is undergoing evaluation. *Biochemistry,* p. 11.
15. The answer is A: *Bordetella pertussis.* DPT (diphtheria, pertussis, and tetanus) form the classical triad used in childhood immunization. Vaccines for polio and measles have been added to the triad. Pertussis toxin is a protein that catalyzes the ADP ribosylation and inactivation of the α-subunit of G_i, a G-protein involved in signal transduction. *Biochemistry,* p. 11.
16. The answer is B: creatine phosphokinase. Elevation of serum creatine phosphokinase occurs 6–12 hours after a myocardial infarction, and the enzyme remains elevated for a few days after the initial insult. Creatine phosphokinase is not present in lungs and is not elevated because of bacterial pneumonia. A normal electrocardiogram and normal creatine phosphokinase rule cardiac problems unlikely in this patient. An elevated white blood cell count with an increased percentage of polymorphonuclear leukocytes and fever occur with most systemic bacterial infections. The chest x-ray points to a pulmonary infection (pneumonia). Left anterior chest pain can also result from a myocardial infarction (heart attack), but such pain does not vary with respiration. A normal blood glucose does not aid in the diagnosis of bacterial pneumonia. Sometimes systemic infections will aggravate latent diabetes mellitus and produce an elevated serum glucose. *Biochemistry,* p. 64.
17. The answer is E: *Streptococcus pneumoniae.* This organism is a gram-positive agent that can cause pneumonia. Typical pneumonia is characterized by sudden onset, high fever, often accompanied by chills and rigors, ill appearance, and few or no upper respiratory symptoms. The elevated white blood count with an increase in the

proportion of segmented neutrophils is indicative of an acute inflammatory disease. *Biochemistry,* p. 11; *Cecil,* pp. 409 and 1608.

18. The answer is C: *Haemophilus influenzae.* This organism is gram negative and frequently causes typical pneumonia. Both gram-negative and gram-positive organisms can produce bacterial pneumonia as seen in this patient, and a Gram stain of the sputum, sputum culture, or blood cultures is performed to make the diagnosis. *Mycobacterium tuberculosis,* which gives a characteristic acid-fast stain, produces a pulmonary infection that is more chronic in its course and is not accompanied by high fever and a markedly elevated white blood cell count. The chest x-ray in tuberculosis characteristically reveals cavitary lesions, and these were not observed in this patient. *Chlamydia pneumoniae,* a gram-negative bacterium, and adenovirus (not a bacterium) can produce atypical pneumonia, a disease in which the signs and symptoms are less severe than described in this patient. *Biochemistry,* p. 11.

REFERENCES

Behrman, R. E. *Nelson Textbook of Pediatrics,* 14th ed. Philadelphia, W. B. Saunders Company, 1992.

Roskoski, R., Jr. *Biochemistry.* Philadelphia, W. B. Saunders Company, 1996.

Wyngaarden, J. B., L. H. Smith, Jr., and J. C. Bennett (eds.). *Cecil Textbook of Medicine,* 19th ed. Philadelphia, W. B. Saunders Company, 1992.

CHAPTER TWO

VITAMINS, MINERALS, AND NUTRITION

SYNOPSIS

OBJECTIVES

1. To describe the elements and compounds found in humans.
2. To describe the functions of vitamins.
3. To identify essential dietary components and to calculate daily caloric requirements.

Objective 1: To describe the elements and compounds found in humans.

I. Minerals found in humans
  A. Abundant minerals
    1. **Calcium** is the most plentiful mineral (≈1 kg/70-kg human)
    2. **Potassium** is the chief intracellular cation
    3. **Sodium** is the chief extracellular cation
    4. **Chloride** is the chief extracellular anion
  B. Trace minerals
    1. **Iron** is involved in oxygen transport (as hemoglobin) and in oxygen metabolism
      a. Iron-binding proteins
        (1) **Transferrin** is the plasma iron transport protein, and serum transferrin level represents the iron-binding capacity
        (2) **Ferritin** is a cellular iron storage protein
        (3) **Hemosiderin** is an insoluble aggregate of ferritin
      b. Abnormalities of iron metabolism
        (1) **Iron deficiency anemia** is a prevalent disorder in women and children; erythrocytes are hypochromic (containing less hemoglobin) and microcytic (small)
        (2) **Hemochromatosis** is the condition that results from excess iron
    2. **Cobalt** is a constituent of vitamin B_{12}
    3. **Iodine,** which is a component of thyroid hormone, is required for growth, development, and maintenance of normal cells and tissues
      a. Iodine deficiency results in a goiter (enlarged thyroid)
      b. Hypothyroidism in children produces cretinism, and in adults results in myxedema
      c. Graves disease consists of hyperthyroidism, goiter, and an oculopathy, and this disorder is often treated with radioiodine (^{131}I), which is concentrated by the thyroid cells and destroys them with x-rays and γ-rays
    4. **Manganese** occurs in mitochondrial superoxide dismutase, and **copper** and **zinc** occur in cytosolic superoxide dismutase
  C. Toxic elements
    1. **Lead** poisoning (plumbism) in children is most commonly the result of eating lead-based paint
    2. **Radon,** a radioactive gas produced via the radioactive decay of uranium, seeps from the earth into homes and is implicated in the production of lung cancer
    3. **Mercury** poisoning can result from exposure to contaminated food, water, or air
      a. Mercuric salts are commonly used in industry
      b. Elemental mercury vapor can be released during the preparation of silver-amalgam dental restorations

II. Biological molecules
  A. Five types of chemical bonds are important in determining the structure of biological molecules including (1) covalent bonds, (2) ionic bonds (salt bridges), (3) hydrogen bonds, (4) hydrophobic bonds, and (5) van der Waals bonds
  B. A large number of functional groups occur in biological molecules (Table 2–1)
    1. Among the more important are the amino, hydroxyl, thiol, carboxyl, and phosphate groups
    2. Many biological molecules contain carbon atoms with four different substituents; such chiral molecules can exist in two different configurations that are nonsuperimposable mirror images
      a. The reference carbon atoms of amino acids in proteins correspond to L-glyceraldehyde and have the L-configuration
      b. The reference carbon atoms of most sugars correspond to D-glyceraldehyde and have the D-configuration

TABLE 2–1. Selected Functional Groups in Biochemicals

Group	Structure	Group	Structure
Alcohol	$R-OH$	**Phosphate groups**	
Amine	$R-NH_2$	Acylphosphate	$R-C(=O)-OPO_3^{2-}$
Carbonyl groups		Diphosphate	$RO-P(=O)(O^-)-O-P(=O)(O^-)-O^-$
Aldehyde	$R-C(=O)-H$	Ester	$RO-PO_3^{2-}$
Ketone	$R-C(=O)-R'$	Phosphate	$HO-P(=O)(O^-)-O^-$
Carboxyl groups		Phosphoramidate	$R-N(H)-PO_3^{2-}$
Acid	$R-C(=O)-OH$	Triphosphate	$RO-P(=O)(O^-)-O-P(=O)(O^-)-O-P(=O)(O^-)-O^-$
Amide	$R-C(=O)-NH_2$	**Sulfur**	
Ester	$R-C(=O)-OR'$	Disulfide	$R-S-S-R'$
		Ester	$RO-SO_3^-$
		Sulfonate	$R-SO_3^-$
Thioester	$R-C(=O)-SR'$	Thiol	$R-SH$
		Thioether	$R-S-R'$

C. Biochemical reactions involve the conversions of one or more biological molecules into one or more different compounds
   1. Biochemical reactions, like those in organic chemistry, involve discrete functional groups such as alcohols and amines
   2. A cardinal feature of biochemistry is the prominence of phosphorus, oxygen, nitrogen, and carbon in bond making and bond breaking

Objective 2: To describe the functions of vitamins.

III. Water-soluble vitamins (B complex and C)
   A. Properties
      1. Water-soluble vitamins are hydrophilic low-molecular-weight organic compounds ($<$ 1500 Da) that either cannot be synthesized by humans or are synthesized in inadequate amounts
      2. Water-soluble vitamins can be excreted by the kidneys and, with rare exceptions, are considered nontoxic
   B. Functions
      1. **Thiamine pyrophosphate** forms reaction intermediates with carbonyl groups
         a. Thiamine (B_1) participates in pyruvate dehydrogenase and α-ketoglutarate dehydrogenase reactions and in the transketolase reaction
         b. Thiamine deficiency, or beriberi, is prone to occur in individuals with high-carbohydrate diets
            (1) **Wet beriberi** results in edema because of abnormal cardiac function
            (2) **Dry beriberi** is due to nervous system dysfunction and can result in Wernicke-Korsakoff syndrome
               (a) **Wernicke syndrome** consists of ataxia, tremors, and disturbances in ocular motility
               (b) **Korsakoff syndrome** consists of confusion and memory impairment for recent events for which the patient compensates by confabulation (making up tales to give a fluent answer without regard to facts); affected individuals are usually disoriented for place and time
      2. **Riboflavin** (B_2) participates in oxidation-reduction reactions
      3. **Niacin** (B_3) participates in oxidation-reduction reactions
         b. Niacin deficiency, which produces the three D's of dermatitis, diarrhea, and dementia, results in **pellagra**

b. NAD^+, which contains niacin, can be formed during the metabolism of the amino acid tryptophan by an intricate series of reactions

4. **Pantothenate** (B_5) forms part of coenzyme A, which participates in acyl transfer reactions
5. **Pyridoxal phosphate** (a B_6 derivative) forms aldimine, or Schiff-base, linkages with proteins; this vitamin plays a pivotal role in nitrogen metabolism
   a. Pyridoxal phosphate is a cofactor in all human transaminases and selected dehydratases and decarboxylases
   b. Deficiency of vitamin B_6 in infants produces seizures; this is postulated to be due to a deficiency of GABA (γ-aminobutyric acid) biosynthesis as catalyzed by glutamate decarboxylase, a pyridoxal phosphate–containing enzyme
   c. Excess B_6 can cause a sensory neuropathy
6. **Folate** plays a key role in one-carbon metabolism
   a. Folate participates in the biosynthesis of purine nucleotides that occur in DNA and RNA
   b. Folate is required for the conversion of deoxyuridylate to deoxythymidylate, a component of DNA
   c. Antifolates are commonly used in the treatment of neoplasms
   d. Folate deficiency produces a megaloblastic anemia without central or peripheral nervous system deficits
7. **Cobalamin** (B_{12}), which contains cobalt, plays a role in carbon-transfer reactions
   a. Intrinsic factor, produced in the stomach, is required for B_{12} absorption in the ileum
   b. B_{12} deficiency can result from inadequate absorption (common) or inadequate intake (rare)
      (1) Cobalamin deficiency results in pernicious anemia, a megaloblastic anemia
         (a) White cells in pernicious anemia contain nuclei that are hypersegmented; red blood cells are large
         (b) The anemia can be corrected by folate administration
      (2) Cobalamin deficiency results in central and peripheral nervous system lesions
         (a) A sensory deficit can result
         (b) The nervous system lesions cannot be corrected by folate administration
   c. Vitamin B_{12} is a participant in two enzyme-catalyzed reactions in humans
      (1) Adenosylcobalamin is a cofactor in the **methylmalonyl-CoA mutase** reaction that yields succinyl-CoA
      (2) Methylcobalamin is a cofactor in the **methyl-tetrahydrofolate-homocysteine methyltransferase** reaction that yields methionine
8. **Ascorbate** (C) participates in enzymatic and nonenzymatic oxidation-reduction reactions
   a. Vitamin C is required for collagen and dopamine hydroxylation
   b. Scurvy results from inadequate vitamin C intake
      (1) The skeletal abnormalities seen in youths with scurvy are likely due to a deficiency of collagen hydroxylation
      (2) Ecchymosis and perifollicular petechiae (subcutaneous hemorrhaging) are related to connective tissue fragility
9. **Biotin** participates in ATP-dependent carbon dioxide fixation reactions

IV. Fat-soluble vitamins (A, D, E, and K)

A. **Vitamin A** has multiple functions
   1. **Retinal,** a vitamin A derivative, participates in the visual cycle, and a deficiency of vitamin A produces night blindness
   2. Vitamin A is formed from **β-carotene,** a plant-derived and lipid-soluble compound that also acts as an antioxidant in membranes

B. **Vitamin D** functions in calcium metabolism
   1. Vitamin D deficiency in children produces rickets
   2. Vitamin D deficiency in adults produces osteomalacia
      a. Osteoid in osteomalacia is normal
      b. Osteoid in osteoporosis is lacking, which differs from vitamin D deficiency
      c. Osteomalacia is rare, whereas osteoporosis is common in the elderly, especially in women

C. **Vitamin E** is an antioxidant
   1. Vitamin E plays a role in protecting membranes from reaction with reactive oxygen compounds
   2. Vitamin E deficiency results in the degeneration of the posterior columns of the spinal cord and nerve cells of the dorsal root ganglia

D. **Vitamin K** is required for the biosynthesis of blood clotting factors
   1. Vitamin K is required for the formation of γ-carboxyglutamate in proteins involved in blood clotting
   2. Vitamin K antagonists inhibit protein γ-carboxyglutamate synthesis
      a. Dicumarol is a vitamin K antagonist that is used therapeutically as an anticoagulant
      b. The action of vitamin K and dicumarol can be monitored by the prothrombin time

Objective 3: To identify essential dietary components and to calculate daily caloric requirements.

V. Essential dietary components

A. Essential dietary components cannot be synthesized in adequate amounts and must be included in the diet

B. The essential amino acids in humans include those in the acronym "PVT TIM HALL": **phenylalanine, valine, threonine, tryptophan, isoleucine, methionine, histidine, arginine, leucine,** and **lysine**
   1. Protein-calorie malnutrition in children produces **marasmus**
   2. Deficient protein but adequate calorie intake in children produces **kwashiorkor**

C. The essential fatty acids include **linoleate** and **linolenate**

D. After oxygen, water is the second most essential substance required for human life, and water is the most abundant compound in humans, accounting for about 55% of the lean body mass

VI. Energy

A. The basal metabolic rate (BMR) in humans requires about 25 kcal (100 kJ) of energy per kilogram (2.2 lb) per day; to calculate the total daily caloric energy requirement,
   1. Add 30% of the BMR for sedentary activity
   2. Add 40% of the BMR for moderate activity
   3. Add 50% of the BMR for heavy activity

B. Food is the source of metabolic fuel
   1. *Carbohydrate yields 4 kcal/g*
   2. *Protein yields 4 kcal/g*

3. *Fat yields 9 kcal/g*
4. Ethanol yields 7 kcal/g

C. Adipose tissue is the chief reservoir of metabolic energy
1. The energy content of 1 lb of adipose tissue is about 3500 kcal
2. The expenditure of 3500 kcal in excess of energy intake results in the loss of about 1 lb of adipose tissue

QUESTIONS

DIRECTIONS. (Items 1–4): Each of the numbered items or incomplete statements in this section is followed by answers or by completions of the statement. Select the ONE lettered answer or completion that is BEST in each case. Correct answers and explanations are given at the end of the chapter.

1. Type III glycogen storage disease results in the accumulation of glycogen in liver cells. Which type of chemical bond is responsible for the inability of glycogen to decompose spontaneously?

(A) Covalent
(B) Hydrogen
(C) Hydrophobic
(D) Ionic
(E) van der Waals

2. Examination of the peripheral blood smear of a 24-year-old woman who had previously been in good health reveals hypochromic microcytic red cells. A deficiency of which one of the following nutrients is the most likely cause of this finding?

(A) Vitamin A
(B) Vitamin B_{12}
(C) Vitamin E
(D) Folate
(E) Iron

3. A cheeseburger has the following composition: 42 g carbohydrate, 28 g fat, and 50 g protein. This corresponds to which one of the following energy values in humans?

(A) 140 kcal
(B) 480 kcal
(C) 620 kcal
(D) 1060 kcal
(E) 1260 kcal

4. A newly diagnosed patient with type II diabetes mellitus, whose actual weight is 86 kg, has an ideal weight of 70 kg. This patient, whose activity is sedentary, was referred to a dietician for planning a diet corresponding to his activity and IDEAL weight. This patient's daily energy requirement is about

(A) 1750 kcal
(B) 2100 kcal
(C) 2275 kcal
(D) 2450 kcal
(E) 2625 kcal

DIRECTIONS. (Items 5–13): Each set of matching questions in this section consists of a list of several lettered options followed by several numbered items. For each numbered item, select the ONE lettered option that is most closely associated with it. To avoid spending too much time on matching sets with large numbers of options, it is generally advisable to begin each set by reading the list of options. Then, for each item in the list, try to generate the correct answer and locate it in the option list, rather than evaluating each option individually. Each lettered option may be selected once, more than once, or not at all.

Items 5–7

(A) Calcium
(B) Chloride
(C) Cobalt
(D) Copper
(E) Fluoride
(F) Iodide
(G) Iron
(H) Magnesium
(I) Phosphorus
(J) Potassium
(K) Radon
(L) Sodium

For each characteristic listed below, select the most appropriate element.

5. The transport of this substance from the inside to the outside of heart cells is inhibited by digitalis.
6. A pregnant woman who developed hypertension and seizures was treated with the sulfate salt of this substance.
7. The radioactive form of this element is used in treating Graves disease.

Items 8–11

(A) Beriberi
(B) Bleeding disorders
(C) Kwashiorkor
(D) Marasmus
(E) Night blindness
(F) Pellagra
(G) Pernicious anemia
(H) Rickets
(I) Scurvy

For each characteristic listed below, select the most appropriate disease.

8. Vitamin D deficiency produces this malady.
9. Symptoms of this disease include dermatitis, dementia, and diarrhea.
10. Deficient prolyl and lysyl hydroxylase activity in collagen production result in this ailment.
11. Deficient transketolase activity observed frequently in individuals with chronic intake of excess ethanol occurs with this disorder.

Items 12–13

For each clinical syndrome listed below, select the corresponding chemical structure in the diagram at the bottom of the page.

12. Deficiency produces seizures in infants.
13. Deficiency produces beriberi.

DIRECTIONS. (Items 14–18): Each of the numbered items or incomplete statements in this section is followed by answers or by completions of the statement. Select the ONE lettered answer or completion that is BEST in each case.

Items 14–18

History

A 67-year-old female has a chief complaint of progressive generalized fatigue. She has been unable to negotiate stairs or walk long distances without becoming fatigued and short of breath, and these symptoms have increased during the last 3 months. The patient complained of tingling in her legs and a feeling of coldness that she attributed to "poor circulation." Her dietary history including intake of fresh fruits and leafy vegetables was more than adequate, and there was no weight loss.

Physical Examination

Blood pressure, 126/82 mm Hg; temperature, 37 °C (98.6 °F); pulse, 80/min; respiratory rate, 14/min. The patient is a pale-appearing female in no acute distress, and she is oriented to time, place, and person. She exhibits decreased vibratory sensation distal to the midleg bilaterally. Peripheral pulses are normal and palpable in all extremities, and her motor strength is good. There are no skin lesions, but the patient is pale.

Laboratory

Hematocrit, 21% (normal ♀, 36–46%)
White blood count, 6600/μL (normal, 4500–11,000/μL)
Red blood cell count, 2.7 million/μL (normal ♀, 3.8–5.1 million/μL)

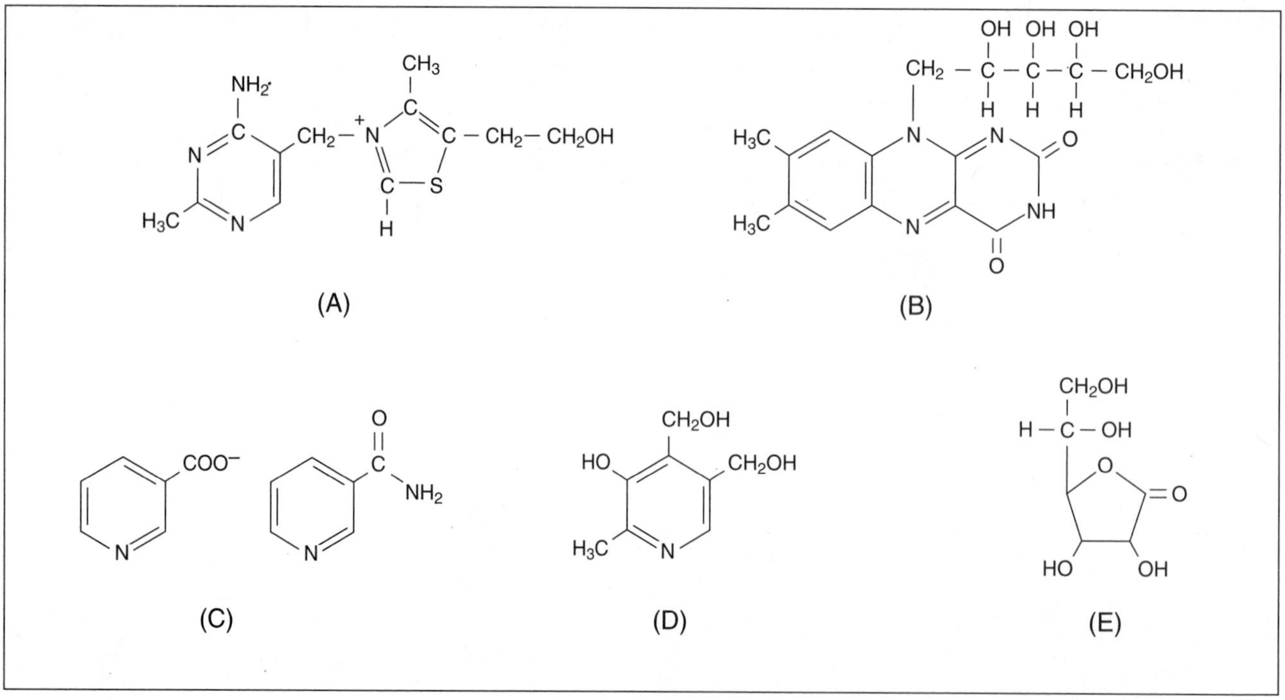

(A)

(B)

(C)

(D)

(E)

Total bilirubin/direct, 2.3/0.7 mg/dL (normal, 0.2–1.0/0.0–0.2 mg/dL)
Hemoglobin, 8.1 g/dL (normal, 12–16 g/dL)
Serum iron, 97 μg/dL (normal, 50–170 μg/dL)
Mean red blood cell volume, 118 fL (normal, 80–100 fL)
Corrected reticulocyte count, 1 (normal, 1)
Mean corpuscular hemoglobin concentration (MCHC), 33% Hb/cell (normal, 31–37% Hb/cell)
Lactate dehydrogenase (LDH), 4700 U/L (normal, 210–380 U/L)
Serum folate, 1.2 μg/dL (normal, 0.3–1.6 μg/dL)
Serum B_{12}, 8 ng/dL (normal, 10–70 ng/dL)
Serum methylmalonate, 3900 nM (normal, 70–270 nM)
Serum homocysteine, 80 μM (normal, 5–16 μM)
Thyroid-stimulating hormone (TSH), 2.0 μU/mL (normal, 2–10 μU/mL)
T_4, 7 μg/dL (normal, 5–12 μg/dL)
Cholesterol, 188 mg/dL (recommended, <200 mg/dL)
Serum glucose, 96 mg/dL (normal, 70–105 mg/dL)
Blood urea nitrogen (BUN), 12 mg/dL (normal, 7–18 mg/dL)
Creatinine, 0.9 mg/dL (normal ♀, 0.6–1.1 mg/dL)
Serum electrolytes, normal
Peripheral blood smear, macrocytosis, and hypersegmented neutrophils

14. The hematology determinations indicate that the patient has a
    (A) normochromic anemia
    (B) microcytic anemia
    (C) megaloblastic anemia
    (D) hypochromic anemia

15. The peripheral neuropathy (decreased sensation to vibration) and feeling of coldness in this patient are most likely due to a deficiency of
    (A) vitamin A
    (B) vitamin B_{12}
    (C) vitamin C
    (D) vitamin D
    (E) insulin

16. The elevated serum methylmalonate in this patient could be due to a deficiency of
    (A) ascorbate
    (B) biotin
    (C) folate
    (D) homocysteine methyltransferase
    (E) vitamin B_{12}

17. One cause of elevated serum homocysteine is a deficiency of
    (A) folate
    (B) ascorbate
    (C) niacin
    (D) thiamine
    (E) methionine

18. What is the most likely diagnosis based on the total picture?
    (A) Diabetes mellitus
    (B) Renal disease
    (C) Iron-deficiency anemia
    (D) Hypothyroidism
    (E) Pernicious anemia

ANSWERS AND EXPLANATIONS

1. The answer is A: covalent. Covalent bonds in biomolecules including glycogen are stable at room temperature with a bond energy on the order of 400 kJ/mol. The stability of other types of bonds (hydrogen, hydrophobic, ionic, van der Waals) is on the order of 10 kJ/mol and these bonds can break and re-form at physiological temperatures. Type III glycogen storage disease is due to a deficiency of the debranching enzyme that catalyzes the cleavage of α-1,6 covalent glycosidic bonds. Without this enzyme, the inability to degrade glycogen results in its excessive accumulation. *Biochemistry,* p. 17.
2. The answer is E: iron. Iron deficiency results in a hypochromic, microcytic anemia. Deficiency of vitamin B_{12} and folate both produce macrocytic anemias. Vitamin A deficiency produces night blindness. Vitamin E deficiency is associated with a central and peripheral neuropathy and muscle weakness. Neurologic symptoms begin with a loss of deep tendon reflexes and a mild loss in vibratory sensation. Ophthalmoplegia, impaired visual acuity and vision in dim lights may occur in later stages. *Biochemistry,* p. 16; *Cecil,* p. 2127.
3. The answer is C: 620 kcal. The caloric content of 1 g of carbohydrate or protein is 4 kcal, and that for fat is 9 kcal. The metabolic energy that humans can derive from the cheeseburger is [42 g carbohydrate × (4 kcal/g carbohydrate)] + [28 g fat × (9 kcal/g fat)] + [50 g protein × (4 kcal/g protein)] = 168 kcal + 252 kcal + 200 kcal = 620 kcal. *Biochemistry,* p. 34.
4. The answer is C: 2275 kcal. The basal metabolic rate (BMR) corresponds to the weight in kilograms times 25 kcal. For a sedentary individual, 0.3 times the BMR is added. For a moderately active person, 0.4 times the BMR is added. For a very active person, 0.5 times the BMR is added. In this case, the requirements are 70 kg × 25 kcal/kg + 0.3 × (70 kg × 25 kcal/kg) = 1750 kcal + 525 kcal = 2275 kcal. Note that the kilocalorie of the biochemist is equivalent to the Calorie of the nutritionist. *Biochemistry,* p. 34.
5. The answer is L: sodium. Digitalis and other cardiac glycosides inhibit the sodium/potassium ATPase of the plasma membrane. This enzyme transports three sodium ions from inside to outside the cell and two potassium ions from outside to inside the cell for each ATP used. *Biochemistry,* pp. 15, 460–461.
6. The answer is H: magnesium. Magnesium (as the sulfate salt) is given parenterally in the treatment of eclampsia. Magnesium ion is a calcium antagonist and decreases the activity of excitable cells. *Biochemistry,* p. 15.
7. The answer is F: iodide. Graves disease, or hyperthyroidism, is treated with radioiodine. This element is concentrated in the thyroid gland and destroys cells by

high-energy radiation. This sometimes leads to hypothyroidism, which is easily treated with oral thyroid hormone. It is easier to treat hypothyroidism than hyperthyroidism. *Biochemistry,* p. 16.

8. The answer is H: rickets. Vitamin D deficiency, due to inadequate exposure to sunlight (which converts 7-dehydrocholesterol to vitamin D) or to inadequate intake, results in skeletal deformities and rickets in children. Vitamin D deficiency in adults produces osteomalacia. The osteoid (organic matrix on which mineralization occurs) is normal in vitamin D deficiency but is lacking in osteoporosis. *Biochemistry,* p. 30.
9. The answer is F: pellagra. Pellagra is due to a deficiency of niacin. This compound participates in a multitude of oxidation-reduction reactions as $NAD(P)^+$, and it is surprising that deficiency of niacin is not accompanied by more symptoms. In addition to the three D's of dermatitis, dementia, and diarrhea, a fourth D, death, is sometimes added to the list. Pharmacologic doses (1 g three times daily) of niacin have been used in the treatment of hypercholesterolemia. The pharmacologic mechanism of the cholesterol lowering effect is unclear; these large doses of niacin are often accompanied by unwanted side effects such as cutaneous flushing and pruritus (itching). *Biochemistry,* p. 26.
10. The answer is I: scurvy. Ascorbate, which is deficient in scurvy, participates in the prolyl and lysyl hydroxylase reactions in collagen formation, accounting in part for the skeletal and connective tissue abnormalities. *Biochemistry,* p. 28.
11. The answer is A: beriberi. Thiamine pyrophosphate is a cofactor in the transketolase reaction; in this reaction, thiamine pyrophosphate reacts with and transfers two-carbon fragments. Beriberi often occurs in people with alcoholism, and the activity of transketolase in such individuals has been studied extensively. *Biochemistry,* p. 24.
12. The answer is D: pyridoxine. The active form of this vitamin is pyridoxal phosphate. Pyridoxal phosphate is a cofactor for all human transaminase reactions, certain dehydratases, and certain decarboxylases. The chief inhibitory neurotransmitter in brain is GABA (γ-aminobutyric acid), and this is synthesized from glutamate in a reaction catalyzed by glutamate decarboxylase, a pyridoxal phosphate-requiring enzyme. A deficiency of this activity is thought to be responsible for the development of seizures. *Biochemistry,* p. 26.
13. The answer is A: thiamine. This vitamin is converted to thiamine pyrophosphate, the active cofactor. This cofactor participates in a variety of oxidative decarboxylation reactions including pyruvate dehydrogenase, α-ketoglutarate dehydrogenase, and branched-chain keto acid dehydrogenase. These reactions are on mainstream metabolic pathways, and it is not surprising that cardiac muscle or nervous system symptoms develop as a result of a deficiency of this vitamin. Riboflavin (B) and niacin (C) are important participants in energy-yielding oxidation-reduction reactions. Niacin deficiency produces pellagra that is accompanied by the three D's of dermatitis, dementia, and diarrhea. Pyridoxine (D) deficiency as an isolated disorder is rare. Infants fed formulas lacking pyridoxine develop seizures. Ascorbate (E) deficiency produces scurvy with attendant connective tissue pathology that leads to skeletal defects in the young and easy bruising and bleeding in adults owing to connective tissue fragility. *Biochemistry,* p. 24.
14. The answer is C: megaloblastic anemia. The term megaloblastic anemia indicates that red cells are larger than normal, and this is indicated by the increased mean cell volume. Normocytic anemia, such as sickle cell anemia, indicates that red cells are normal in size. Microcytic anemia, such as iron deficiency anemia, indicates that red cells have decreased mean cell volume. Hypochromic anemia, also produced by iron deficiency, indicates that red cells have subnormal hemoglobin concentration. *Biochemistry,* p. 28.
15. The answer is B: vitamin B_{12}. Peripheral neuropathies with decreased vibratory sensation are common in pernicious anemia. Pathologic studies can show loss of myelin and axonal degeneration of the peripheral and cranial nerves, cerebral cortex, and dorsal and lateral columns of the spinal cord. Peripheral neuropathies also occur with niacin deficiency (pellagra), thiamine deficiency (beriberi), vitamin E deficiency, and excessive intake of vitamin B_6. Diabetes mellitus, which results from insulin deficiency and is a common cause of peripheral neuropathy, is characterized by hyperglycemia (not observed in this patient). Peripheral neuropathies are not associated with deficiencies of vitamins A, C, or D. *Biochemistry,* p. 27; *Cecil,* p. 2125.
16. The answer is E: vitamin B_{12}. A vitamin B_{12} derivative, adenosylcobalamin, is a cofactor for the methylmalonyl-CoA mutase reaction. This reaction is responsible for the conversion of methylmalonyl-CoA to succinyl-CoA. In the absence of adequate cofactor, methylmalonyl-CoA accumulates and undergoes hydrolysis to form methylmalonate, which escapes into the circulation and is excreted in the urine. Homocysteine methyltransferase also requires a vitamin B_{12} derivative (methylcobalamin), but a deficiency of this enzyme activity would not affect serum methylmalonate levels. The mutase reaction is not affected by ascorbate, folate, or biotin deficiency. *Biochemistry,* p. 24.
17. The answer is A: folate. The substrates for the homocysteine methyltransferase reaction include methyltetrahydrofolate and homocysteine, and the products include methionine and tetrahydrofolate. Dietary folate is reduced first to dihydrofolate and then tetrahydrofolate. Tetrahydrofolate reacts with a one-carbon donor such as serine to produce methylenetetrahydrofolate and glycine. Methylenetetrahydrofolate is reduced by NADH in a unidirectional reaction to form methyltetrahydrofolate. A deficiency of tetrahydrofolate can cause homocystinuria. Methylcobalamin is a cofactor for homocysteine methyltransferase, and B_{12} deficiency can also produce homocystinuria. Folate deficiency, vitamin B_{12} deficiency, or both deficiencies could result in an elevation of serum homocysteine. In this patient, folate levels are normal, and homocystinemia is the result of B_{12} deficiency. Normal serum levels of creatine and urea are not consistent with renal disease in the pathogenesis of this case. Ascorbate, niacin, and thiamine are not directly involved in homocysteine metabolism. A deficiency of methionine, a precursor, can result in a decrease and not an increase in serum homocysteine. *Biochemistry,* p. 242.
18. The answer is E: pernicious anemia. The rapid pulse and fatigue are a sign and symptom of anemia. Laboratory tests confirm the presence of a megaloblastic anemia. The two most common forms of megaloblastic anemia with attendant hypersegmentation of white cell nuclei are due to a deficiency of vitamin B_{12} or folate. The peripheral neuropathy is characteristic of vitamin B_{12} but not folate deficiency. Elevated serum homocyste-

ine can result from either vitamin B_{12} or folate deficiency, or a deficiency of both. Elevated methylmalonate, as observed in this patient, is not a result of folate deficiency. This diagnosis is confirmed by normal serum folate but depressed B_{12} levels. Causes of B_{12} deficiency include pernicious anemia, complete or partial gastrectomy, and small bowel disease. Vitamin B_{12} is synthesized by some microorganisms and is taken in the human diet from animal and dairy products. Strict vegans may develop vitamin B_{12} deficiency. Folate is present in leafy vegetables, but is destroyed by prolonged cooking. B_{12} is heat stable. Vitamin B_{12} and folate participate in one-carbon metabolism, and this metabolism involves purine and thymidylate biosynthesis. Deficient nucleotide metabolism results in decreased red cell production and hemolysis of immature cells (with elevated lactate dehydrogenase activity and elevated serum bilirubin, depending upon the severity of the disease, as observed in this patient). Megaloblastic anemias can also result from treatment of neoplasms with antifolates and other antimetabolites. Iron deficiency produces a microcytic anemia with depressed serum iron levels, not observed in this patient. Hypothyroidism is associated with fatigue; it is also accompanied by depressed thyroid hormone levels and hypercholesterolemia (not observed in this patient). *Biochemistry,* p. 27.

REFERENCES

Roskoski, R., Jr. *Biochemistry.* Philadelphia, W. B. Saunders Company, 1996.

Wyngaarden, J. B., L. H. Smith, Jr., and J. C. Bennett (eds.). *Cecil Textbook of Medicine,* 19th ed. Philadelphia, W. B. Saunders Company, 1992.

CHAPTER THREE

AMINO ACIDS AND PROTEINS

SYNOPSIS

OBJECTIVES

1. To outline protein structure and function.
2. To analyze acid-base problems by means of the Henderson-Hasselbalch equation.
3. To describe how amino acids determine the structure of proteins.
4. To describe the hierarchal structure of proteins and Anfinsen's law.

Objective 1: To outline protein structure and function.

I. Overview of protein structure and function
   A. The name protein is derived from Greek *protos* meaning "first" or "primary"
   B. The functions of proteins are diverse
      1. Proteins function as catalysts, receptor and effector molecules, contractile elements, transport molecules in the plasma and in cellular membranes, antibodies, and hormones
      2. Proteins play a structural role within the cell as the cytoskeleton where they make up microfilaments, intermediate filaments, and microtubules
      3. Collagen, a triple helical protein, plays a pivotal structural role in the extracellular space
         a. Collagen provides the matrix for bone, connective tissue, muscle, and the dentine of teeth
         b. *Collagen, the most prevalent protein in humans, makes up about one-third of total body protein by mass*

Objective 2: To analyze acid-base problems by means of the Henderson-Hasselbalch equation.

II. Acids, bases, and buffers
   A. Properties of pH
      1. Water dissociates into a proton and hydroxyl group as follows:

$$H_2O \rightleftharpoons H^+ + OH^-$$

      2. In pure water, $[H^+] = [OH^-] = 10^{-7}$ M
      3. The numerical product of their molar concentrations is 1×10^{-14}: $[H^+] \times [OH^-] = 1 \times 10^{-14}$
      4. The pH is defined by the following expression: **pH = $-\log_{10}$ [H$^+$]**
      5. At neutrality (when $[H^+] = [OH^-]$), pH = $-\log[10^{-7}]$ and pH = $-(-7) = +7$
      6. **Acids** are proton donors, and **bases** are proton acceptors; some alkalis are hydroxyl ion donors (hydroxyl ions are proton acceptors)
   B. Buffers and pH changes
      1. **Buffers** are substances that diminish the change in pH when acid or alkali is added
      2. Buffers are composed of weak acids and their salts or weak bases and their acids
      3. The physiologically important buffers in blood, saliva, and other body fluids, in order of their effectiveness as buffers, are (1) H_2CO_3–HCO_3^-, (2) $H_2PO_4^-$–HPO_4^{2-}, and (3) protein-protein$^-$
      4. Cells constantly generate acid as carbon dioxide (which forms carbonic acid) and lactic acid, and buffers of the cell and blood help to maintain physiological pH around 7.4
      5. The pH in saliva varies more than that of blood
         a. The pH of saliva varies physiologically from about 6 to 7.6
         b. The pH of saliva varies with the flow rate
            (1) The greater the rate, the higher is the pH
            (2) At high flow rates, the pH reaches 7.6
         c. Oral bacteria can generate lactic acid and decrease the local pH to 5.5 or less
            (1) Lactic acid dissolves tooth enamel and leads to caries
            (2) Saliva plays an important role in reestablishing and maintaining physiological pH to counteract the effects of oral microbes
   C. Henderson-Hasselbalch equation and physiological buffers
      1. **pH = pK_a + log [proton acceptor]/[proton donor],** where the pK_a of a compound is the pH value at which the concentration of the protonated compound equals that of the unprotonated compound
      2. The CO_2 system can be expressed as follows, where equations (a) and (b) are coupled:
         a. $CO_2 + H_2O \rightleftharpoons H_2CO_3$

b. $H_2CO_3 \rightleftharpoons H^+ + HCO_3^-$
c. $pH = 6.1 + \log [HCO_3^-]/[CO_2 + H_2CO_3]$
d. At pH 7.4, the ratio of salt to acid or $[HCO_3^-]/[CO_2 + H_2CO_3] \approx 20$

3. For the phosphate buffer system near physiological pH ($\approx$7),

$$H_2PO_4^- \rightleftharpoons H^+ + HPO_4^{2-} \text{ and}$$
$$pH = pK_a + \log [HPO_4^{2-}]/[H_2PO_4^-]$$

III. Acidosis and alkalosis (Table 3–1)

A. **Acidosis** (pH <7.35), which is common, is the condition associated with the production of excessive body acid or the inability to rid the body of acid

1. **Respiratory acidosis,** which occurs in chronic obstructive lung disease (emphysema), is associated with the inability to expel carbon dioxide
2. **Metabolic acidosis,** such as diabetic ketoacidosis, is produced by the excessive production of nonvolatile acid (not carbon dioxide), and the decrease in pH is accompanied by a decrease in plasma bicarbonate as required by the Henderson-Hasselbalch equation:

$$pH = 6.1 + \log [HCO_3^-]/[CO_2 + H_2CO_3]$$

B. **Alkalosis** (pH >7.45), which is uncommon, is the condition associated with the excessive elimination of acid or the intake of excessive alkali

1. **Respiratory alkalosis** is produced by the excessive expiration of carbon dioxide because of anxiety or because of meningitis
2. **Metabolic alkalosis** can be produced by emesis (excessive elimination of body acid) or by the intake of alkali such as sodium bicarbonate (an antacid)

C. We can use the Henderson-Hasselbalch equation,

$$pH = 6.1 + \log [HCO_3^-]/[CO_2 + H_2CO_3],$$

to evaluate the mechanisms for the production of acid-base defects and their correction

1. Respiratory acidosis
   a. The pH is decreased because the total acid, $[CO_2 + H_2CO_3]$, increases
   b. By excretion of excess acid in the urine and retention of bicarbonate, the body normalizes the pH
2. Respiratory alkalosis
   a. The pH is increased because the total acid, $[CO_2 + H_2CO_3]$, decreases
   b. By excretion of less acid in the urine and retention of less bicarbonate, the body normalizes the pH
3. Metabolic acidosis
   a. The pH is decreased because the bicarbonate is decreased
   b. To regain a normal pH, the body secretes an acid urine (NH_4^+ and $H_2PO_4^-$), retains bicarbonate, and increases pulmonary carbon dioxide expiration
   c. An increase in bicarbonate (the numerator) and a decrease in carbon dioxide (part of the denominator) increases the pH toward normal
4. Metabolic alkalosis
   a. The pH is increased because the bicarbonate is increased
   b. Decreased acid secretion in the urine leads to an increase in total acid, $[CO_2 + H_2CO_3]$, the denominator of the Henderson-Hasselbalch equation, and decreases the pH toward normal

TABLE 3–1. Classes of Acidosis and Alkalosis

Acid-base State	Plasma Bicarbonate	Plasma Carbonic Acid	Urinary pH
Normal	25	1.25	6–7
Metabolic acidosis	Decrease*	Decrease†	Decrease
Metabolic alkalosis	Increase*	Increase†	Increase
Respiratory acidosis	Increase†	Increase*	Decrease
Respiratory alkalosis	Decrease†	Decrease*	Increase

* Generally the primary defect.
† Generally a compensatory or corrective change.

Objective 3: To describe how amino acids determine the structure of proteins.

IV. Amino acid structures and properties

A. Standard, or coded, amino acids (Fig. 3–1)

1. The amino acids that are found in proteins are α-amino acids, and the 20 amino acids that are added during biosynthesis of proteins are called the standard, or coded, amino acids
2. Except for glycine, which lacks an asymmetric or chiral carbon atom (a carbon atom with four different substituents), the amino acids found in proteins possess the L-configuration (the absolute form corresponds to L-glyceraldehyde)
3. The four different substituents include a carboxyl group, an amino group, hydrogen, and a characteristic side chain called the R group

B. Families of amino acids

1. Amino acids with aliphatic (carbon and hydrogen) side chains: glycine (C_2), alanine (C_3), valine (C_5), leucine (C_6), and isoleucine (C_6)
2. Aromatic amino acids: phenylalanine, tyrosine, tryptophan
3. Sulfur-containing amino acids: methionine and cysteine (which can be oxidized to cystine)
4. Dicarboxylates and their derivatives: aspartate and asparagine (C_4); glutamate and glutamine (C_5)
5. Basic amino acids: lysine and arginine, which have positively charged R groups at pH 7.0, and histidine, with a pK_a of about 7
6. Amino acids with an alcohol side chain: serine (C_3) and threonine (C_4)
7. Proline (C_5), a cyclic amino acid

C. Distinctive properties of amino acids

1. Glycine lacks an asymmetric carbon atom
2. Threonine and isoleucine contain two asymmetric carbon atoms
3. Glycine and proline often occur at bends in proteins
4. Glycine occurs at every third residue in the collagen triple helix
5. Serine, threonine, and tyrosine in proteins can be phosphorylated
6. Methionine is the initiating amino acid in proteins
7. Methionine and tryptophan, which occur least frequently in proteins, have a single codon (the remainder have two or more)
8. Aspartate and glutamate bear negatively charged R groups at physiological pH
9. Glutamate is the predominant excitatory neurotransmitter in human brain

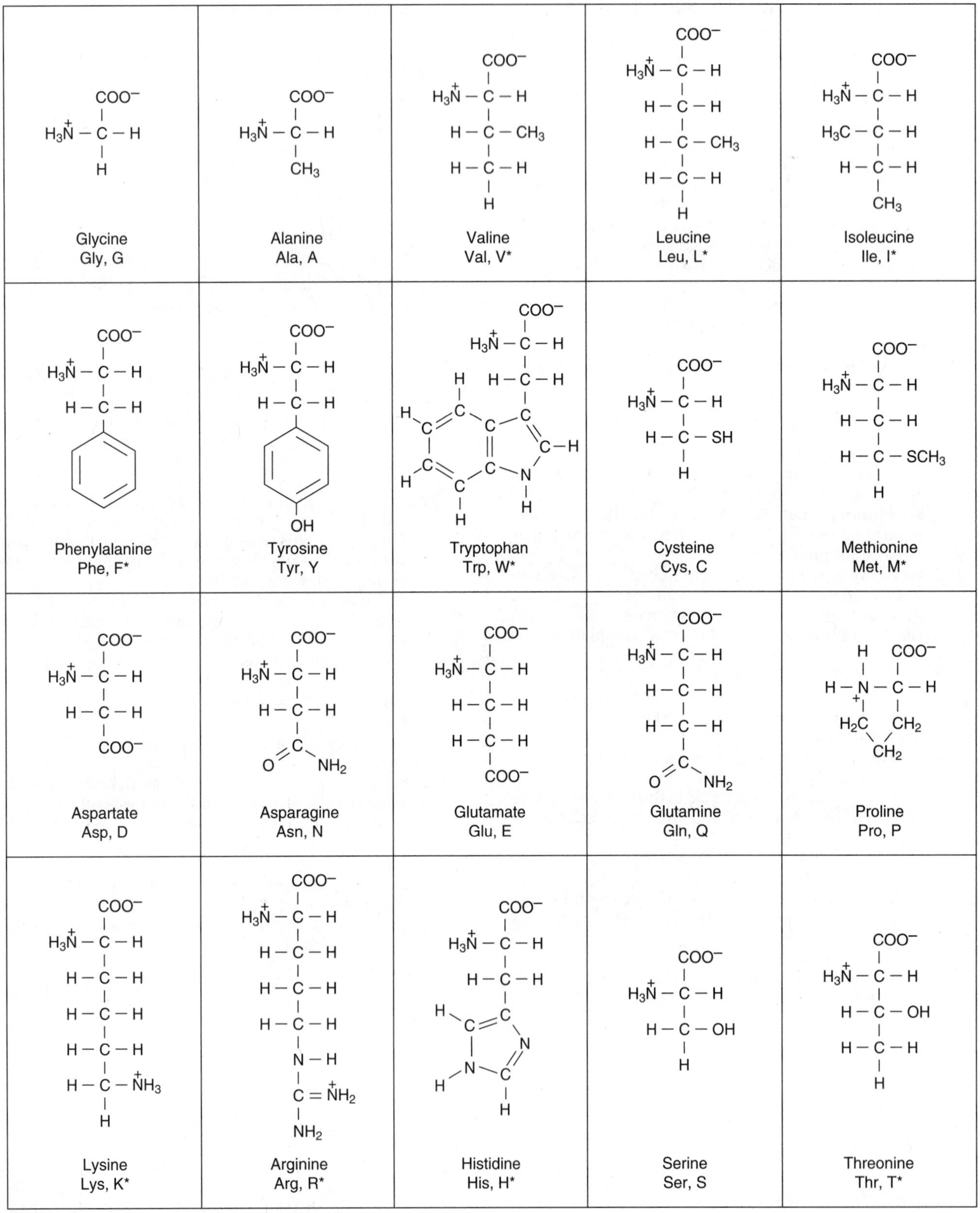

Glycine Gly, G	Alanine Ala, A	Valine Val, V*	Leucine Leu, L*	Isoleucine Ile, I*
Phenylalanine Phe, F*	Tyrosine Tyr, Y	Tryptophan Trp, W*	Cysteine Cys, C	Methionine Met, M*
Aspartate Asp, D	Asparagine Asn, N	Glutamate Glu, E	Glutamine Gln, Q	Proline Pro, P
Lysine Lys, K*	Arginine Arg, R*	Histidine His, H*	Serine Ser, S	Threonine Thr, T*

FIGURE 3-1. Standard amino acids. The three-letter and one-letter abbreviations are given. Amino acids essential in humans are denoted with an asterisk (*).

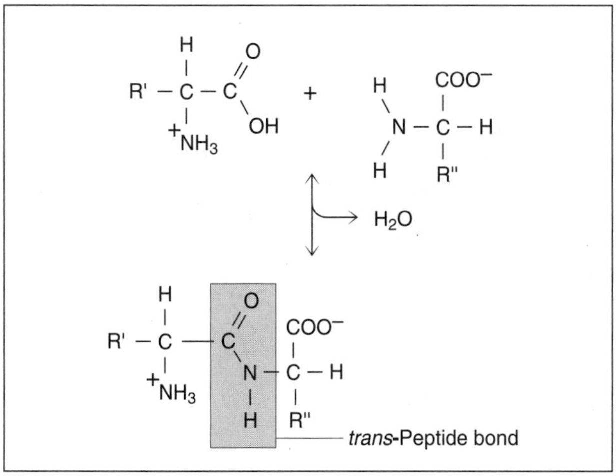

$$\text{R}'-\underset{\underset{^{+}\text{NH}_3}{|}}{\overset{\overset{\text{H}}{|}}{\text{C}}}-\text{C}\begin{matrix}\nearrow\!\!\!/\;\text{O}\\ \searrow\text{OH}\end{matrix} \; + \; \begin{matrix}\text{H}\\ \text{H}\end{matrix}\!\!>\!\text{N}-\underset{\underset{\text{R}''}{|}}{\overset{\overset{\text{COO}^-}{|}}{\text{C}}}-\text{H} \;\rightleftharpoons\; \text{R}'-\underset{\underset{^{+}\text{NH}_3}{|}}{\overset{\overset{\text{H}}{|}}{\text{C}}}-\overset{\overset{\text{O}}{\|}}{\text{C}}-\underset{\underset{\text{H}}{|}}{\text{N}}-\underset{\underset{\text{R}''}{|}}{\overset{\overset{\text{COO}^-}{|}}{\text{C}}}-\text{H} + \text{H}_2\text{O}$$

trans-Peptide bond

FIGURE 3-2. The peptide bond.

10. Arginine and lysine bear positively charged R groups at physiological pH
11. A fraction of the imidazole groups of histidine are positively charged at physiological pH, and the remainder are neutral

V. Peptides and peptide bonds (Fig. 3–2)
 A. The combination of an α-amino group of one amino acid with the carboxyl group of a second amino acid, with the elimination of water, results in the formation of a peptide bond
 B. The peptide bond is planar, and rotation about the C—N bond is prohibited
 C. Polypeptides and proteins are condensation polymers of amino acids
  1. An average polypeptide chain in a protein contains about 500 amino acid residues; a few contain more than 2000 amino acid residues
  2. The molecular masses of single polypeptide chains range from about 5000 to 300,000 Da
   a. To determine the approximate number of amino acids in a protein, divide the molecular mass by 110 (or 100 for a less accurate estimate)
   b. The 110-Da value approximates the average molecular mass of an amino acid residue in an average protein

Objective 4: To describe the hierarchal structure of proteins and Anfinsen's law.

VI. Protein structure
 A. All proteins exhibit primary, secondary, and tertiary structures; multimeric proteins also exhibit quaternary structure
 B. **Primary structure** refers to the sequence of amino acids and the nature and position of any covalently attached derivatives; *by convention, structures are written with the amino terminus on the left and carboxyl terminus on the right*
 C. **Secondary structure,** of which there are two major classes, refers to motifs of hydrogen bonding
  1. The first to be described, the **α-helix,** refers to a helix stabilized by hydrogen bonding between the carbonyl group (C=O) of one peptide bond (residue n) and the amide group (N—H) of the peptide bond of residue n + 4 with 3.6 residues per turn
  2. The second class of secondary structure to be described is called the **β-pleated sheet**
   a. Here, N—H and C=O groups from residues very far apart on the polypeptide chain or even residues on different polypeptide chains form hydrogen bonds
   b. Two varieties of β-pleated sheet are recognized based on the polarity of the polypeptide chains: parallel and antiparallel
    (1) When the chains are going in the same direction from the amino to carboxyl end of the molecule, the structure is a **parallel** β-pleated sheet
    (2) When the participating chains are going in opposite directions with respect to the amino and carboxyl termini, the structure is an **antiparallel** β-pleated sheet
 D. **Tertiary structure** of a protein, which is irregular, refers to the three-dimensional arrangement of the atoms of the molecule in space
 E. **Quaternary structure** refers to the manner in which subunits of a multimeric protein interact
  1. Most proteins consist of more than one subunit and exhibit quaternary structure
  2. Myoglobin is a monomeric protein, which is released from necrotic myocardial cells, that does *not* exhibit a quaternary structure

VII. Anfinsen's law and protein folding
 A. **Anfinsen's law** states that the secondary, tertiary, and quaternary structures are determined by the primary structure (PRINCIPLE 4 OF BIOCHEMISTRY)
 B. Chaperones are proteins that aid in protein folding during synthesis, but they are not responsible for the stability of the final product

VIII. Zinc finger and leucine zipper proteins
 A. **Zinc finger** domains each contain about 30 residues, including **two cysteines, two histidines,** and several hydrophobic amino acid residues
  1. The zinc atom is bound to the two cysteine and two histidine residues
  2. Many zinc finger proteins, such as transcription factor IIIA, bind to DNA
 B. **Leucine zipper** domains have leucine repeats at every *seventh* residue for 28 to 35 residues
  1. The leucine residues occur at the same relative position of an α-helix (3.6 residues per turn, or about 7 residues per two turns, of the helix)
  2. It is postulated that proteins containing such domains form an interdigitated connection that binds two such proteins together

QUESTIONS

DIRECTIONS. (Items 1–5): Each of the numbered items or incomplete statements in this section is followed by answers or by completions of the statement. Select the ONE lettered answer or completion that is BEST in each case. Correct answers and explanations are given at the end of the chapter.

1. What is the hydrogen ion concentration of a urine specimen with a pH of 5.0?

(A) 1×10^{-1} M
(B) 1×10^{-5} M
(C) 1×10^{-7} M
(D) 1×10^{-9} M
(E) 1×10^{-11} M

2. A patient presents in the emergency clinic with an arterial pH of 7.2, a total carbon dioxide concentration (HCO_3^- + CO_2 + H_2CO_3) of 15 mM, and a β-hydroxybutyrate concentration of 5 mM. This person has which one of the following disorders?

(A) Metabolic acidosis
(B) Metabolic alkalosis
(C) Respiratory acidosis
(D) Respiratory alkalosis

3. What is the [$H_2PO_4^-$] of a urine sample if the pH is 5.8 and the [HPO_4^{2-}] is 2 mM? (For the phosphate buffer system,

$H_2PO_4^- \rightleftarrows H^+ + HPO_4^{2-}$ with a pK_a of 6.8 and
$pH = pK_a + \log [HPO_4^{2-}]/[H_2PO_4^-]$).

(A) 0.2 mM
(B) 2.0 mM
(C) 12 mM
(D) 20 mM
(E) 200 mM

4. Glucose-6-phosphate dehydrogenase, an enzyme, has an altered electrophoretic mobility at pH 8.6 caused by the mutation of a valine residue to which one of the following amino acids?

(A) Asparagine
(B) Glutamate
(C) Isoleucine
(D) Methionine
(E) Serine

5. Myoglobin, a protein with a molecular mass of about 16,500, is released from cardiac muscle into the circulation following a myocardial infarction (heart attack). About how many amino acids does myoglobin contain?

(A) 50
(B) 100
(C) 150
(D) 200
(E) 250

DIRECTIONS. (Items 6–11): Each set of matching questions in this section consists of a list of lettered options followed by several numbered items. For each numbered item, select the ONE lettered option that is most closely associated with it. To avoid spending too much time on matching sets with large numbers of options, it is generally advisable to begin each set by reading the list of options. Then, for each item in the list, try to generate the correct answer and locate it in the option list, rather than evaluating each option individually. Each lettered option may be selected once, more than once, or not at all.

Items 6–8

(A) Asparagine
(B) Aspartate
(C) Cysteine
(D) Glycine
(E) Isoleucine
(F) Leucine
(G) Lysine
(H) Proline
(I) Serine
(J) Tryptophan

For each biochemical feature, select the most appropriate amino acid.

6. An imino or cyclic acid
7. Contains sulfur
8. Occurs at every third position in the collagen triple helix, and mutations that alter this residue can produce Ehlers-Danlos syndrome

Items 9–11

For each biochemical feature, select the most appropriate amino acid as shown in the illustration on page 21.

9. Most commonly phosphorylated amino acid residue in proteins
10. The initiating amino acid in protein synthesis
11. Contains two chiral carbon atoms

DIRECTIONS. (Items 12–15): Each of the numbered items or incomplete statements in this section is followed by answers or by completions of the statement. Select the ONE lettered answer or completion that is BEST in each case.

Items 12–15

History

A 14-year-old girl was brought to the emergency room by her mother because of vomiting, listlessness, and general malaise. The patient complains of easy fatigability. She is constantly hungry and, despite a large appetite and food intake consisting of 5 or 6 meals daily, she lost about 2.7 kg (6 lb) during the past 3 weeks. She says that her clothes have become baggy and loose fitting. She gives a history of polydipsia and polyuria. The patient's paternal grandmother died of renal disease and had poor circulation that required a leg amputation.

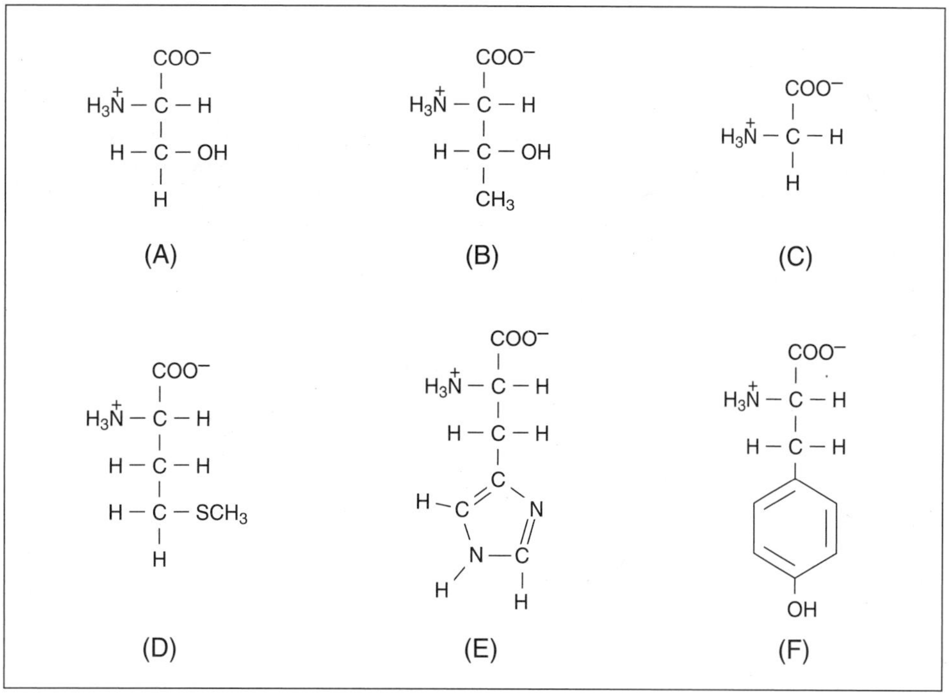

(A)
COO^-
$H_3\overset{+}{N} - C - H$
$H - C - OH$
H

(B)
COO^-
$H_3\overset{+}{N} - C - H$
$H - C - OH$
CH_3

(C)
COO^-
$H_3\overset{+}{N} - C - H$
H

(D)
COO^-
$H_3\overset{+}{N} - C - H$
$H - C - H$
$H - C - SCH_3$
H

(E)
COO^-
$H_3\overset{+}{N} - C - H$
$H - C - H$
C
H—C N
N—C
H H

(F)
COO^-
$H_3\overset{+}{N} - C - H$
$H - C - H$
OH

Physical Examination

Physical examination reveals a temperature of 36.3 °C (97.3 °F), a pulse rate of 132/min, respirations 26/min and labored, a blood pressure of 80/55 mm Hg, a height of 157 cm (5 ft, 2 in), and weight of 40 kg (87 lb). Her breath has a fruity odor.

Laboratory

Serum glucose, 642 mg/dL (normal, 70–105 mg/dL)
Sodium, 140 mEq/L (normal, 135–145 mEq/L)
Potassium, 6.2 mEq/L (normal, 3.5–5.1 mEq/L)
Chloride, 97 mEq/L (normal, 98–105 mEq/L)
Bicarbonate, 12 mEq/L (normal, 18–23 mEq/L)
Acetoacetate, 1.2 mM (normal, <0.1 mM)
β-Hydroxybutyrate, 6.4 mM (normal, <0.3 mM)
Venous serum pH, 7.1 (normal, 7.35–7.45)
White blood cell count, 8700/μL (normal, 4500–11,000/μL)
Urinalysis
 Specific gravity, 1.037 (normal, 1.003–1.035)
 Glucose, 4+ (normal, 0)
 Ketone bodies, 3+ (normal, 0)
 Microscopic examination, normal

12. The blood glucose and urinalysis are consistent with a diagnosis of
 (A) diabetes insipidus
 (B) diabetes mellitus
 (C) hypoglycemia
 (D) starvation
 (E) malabsorption

13. The acid-base abnormality exhibited by this patient is
 (A) metabolic acidosis
 (B) metabolic alkalosis
 (C) respiratory acidosis
 (D) respiratory alkalosis

14. Which one of the following compensatory mechanisms ameliorates the primary acid-base imbalance?
 (A) Increased urinary excretion of bicarbonate
 (B) Decreased urinary excretion of ammonium ion
 (C) Decreased urinary excretion of hydrogen ions
 (D) Decreased urinary excretion of phosphate as $H_2PO_4^-$
 (E) Increased respiratory rate

15. What should be the primary treatment for this patient?
 (A) Intranasal antidiuretic hormone
 (B) Parenteral insulin
 (C) Ammonium chloride
 (D) Food
 (E) Tolbutamide (a sulfonylurea)

SUPPLEMENTARY EXERCISES

16. Draw the structures of the ionized forms (zwitterions) of (a) alanine, (b) isoleucine, (c) tyrosine, (d) arginine, (e) histidine, (f) threonine, (g) methionine, and (h) cysteine.
17. What are the pH values of solutions with hydrogen ion concentrations of (a) 4.6×10^{-5} M and (b) 7.9×10^{-9} M?
18. What is the hydrogen ion concentration of a solution at pH 7.4?

Use the Following for Items 19–21.

For the phosphate buffer system:

$$H_2PO_4^- \rightleftharpoons H^+ + HPO_4^{2-},$$
$$pH = pK_a + \log [HPO_4^{2-}]/[H_2PO_4^-],$$

and

the pK_a at physiological ionic strength is 6.8.

19. Calculate the ratio of $[HPO_4^{2-}]/[H_2PO_4^-]$ at pH 7.4.
20. If the concentration of $[HPO_4^{2-}] + [H_2PO_4^-]$ is 5.00 mM, calculate the concentrations of $[HPO_4^{2-}]$ and $[H_2PO_4^-]$ at pH 7.4.
21. If the ratio of $[HPO_4^{2-}]/[H_2PO_4^-]$ is 0.32, calculate the pH.

Use the Following for Items 22–24.

For the carbon dioxide buffer system,

$$pH = pK_a + \log [HCO_3^-]/[CO_2 + H_2CO_3] \text{ and the } pK_a = 6.1.$$

22. Calculate the ratio of $[HCO_3^-]/[CO_2 + H_2CO_3]$ at pH 7.4.
23. If the concentration of total carbon dioxide ($[HCO_3^-] + [CO_2 + H_2CO_3]$) is 24 mM, calculate the concentration of $[HCO_3^-]$ and $[CO_2 + H_2CO_3]$ at pH 7.4.
24. Analysis of a patient's blood reveals the following: total carbon dioxide = 16 mM, and $[HCO_3^-]$ = 15 mM. Calculate the pH.

ANSWERS AND EXPLANATIONS

1. The answer is B: 1×10^{-5} M. $pH = -\log[H^+]$; $5.0 = -\log[H^+]$; $-5.0 = \log[H^+]$; $[H^+] = 1 \times 10^{-5}$ M.
2. The answer is A: metabolic acidosis. The primary diagnosis is acidosis based upon the pH. The two possibilities are metabolic and respiratory. In respiratory acidosis, there is an increase in total carbon dioxide and not a decrease. That there is an appreciable concentration of β-hydroxybutyrate confirms the impression that this is a metabolic acidosis. Elevation of serum lactic acid occurs in some forms of metabolic acidosis.
3. The answer is D: 20 mM. $pH = 6.8 + \log [HPO_4^{2-}]/[H_2PO_4^-]$;
$$5.8 = 6.8 + \log [HPO_4^{2-}]/[H_2PO_4^-];$$
$$-1.0 = \log [HPO_4^{2-}]/[H_2PO_4^-];$$
$$[HPO_4^{2-}]/[H_2PO_4^-] = 0.1;$$
$$2 \text{ mM}/[H_2PO_4^-] = 0.1;$$
$$0.1\ [H_2PO_4^-] = 2 \text{ mM};$$
$$[H_2PO_4^-] = 20 \text{ mM}.$$
4. The answer is B: glutamate. The R group of valine is uncharged at pH 8.6, but that of glutamate bears a negative charge. A mutation of valine to glutamate would alter the charge and electrophoretic mobility of a protein at pH 8.6. Although the R groups of asparagine and serine are polar, they are uncharged. The R groups of isoleucine and methionine are nonpolar and uncharged. More than 300 variants involving glucose-6-phosphate dehydrogenase have been described, and these affect 400 million people worldwide. Glucose-6-phosphate dehydrogenase deficiency can result in hemolytic anemias after the administration of antimalarials and other drugs. Some of these mutations result in a protein that is electrophoretically normal, and other mutations can increase or decrease the electrophoretic mobility. *Biochemistry,* p. 43.
5. The answer is C: 150. The average molecular mass of an amino acid residue in proteins is about 110 ($\approx$100). Dividing 16,500 by 110 yields 150.
6. The answer is H: proline. Proline is a cyclic amino acid because the α-carbon and the δ-carbon are linked to the amino group to form a five-membered ring. Ring formation limits the conformations that this amino acid can assume. Proline is not found in α-helices or β-sheets. Proline often occurs at bends, and in collagen, it promotes the formation of a left-handed helix. *Biochemistry,* p. 49.
7. The answer is C: cysteine. Cysteine contains a thiol group on its β-carbon. The combination of two cysteine residues results in the formation of a disulfide bond; three such disulfide bonds occur in insulin (two interchain and one within the A chain). Disulfide bonds are more prevalent in proteins that function extracellularly than in those that function intracellularly. The circulating form of this amino acid is cystine, made up of two cysteine residues. The other standard amino acid (found in proteins) that contains sulfur is methionine. *Biochemistry,* p. 40.
8. The answer is D: glycine. In the formation of the collagen triple helix, every third amino acid is glycine. This amino acid, which lacks an R group, is the only one of the standard amino acids that is small enough to fit on the inside of this structure. Mutations that change these periodic glycines are the basis of most of the collagenopathies of Ehlers-Danlos syndrome. *Biochemistry,* p. 475.
9. The answer is A: serine. The three amino acids that contain a hydroxyl group and that occur in the phosphorylated state are serine, threonine, and tyrosine. The ratio of phosphoserine/phosphothreonine/phosphotyrosine in cells is about 1000/10/1. The enzymes that are responsible for attaching the phosphoryl group to these amino acids in proteins are called protein kinases. *Biochemistry,* p. 41.
10. The answer is D: methionine. The methio group (CH_3S–) of methionine participates in many reactions of one-

carbon metabolism. This amino acid initiates the synthesis of proteins in humans and in bacteria. This amino acid, along with tryptophan, occurs infrequently in proteins, but both are essential in humans. The amino-terminal methionine that is found in the nascent protein is often removed by a posttranslational hydrolysis reaction. The codon that corresponds to methionine is AUG. *Biochemistry,* p. 39.

11. The answer is B: threonine. Both the α- and β-carbons of threonine are attached to four different substituents. The other standard amino acid that bears two chiral carbon atoms is isoleucine. Glycine, in contrast, lacks a chiral carbon atom. *Biochemistry,* p. 41.
12. The answer is B: diabetes mellitus. Postprandial blood glucose levels higher than 170 mg/dL (9.4 mM) are indicative of diabetes mellitus. This is further confirmed by glucosuria. The highest attainable urinary specific gravity under physiological conditions is about 1.035. The higher specific gravity in this instance is due to the glucose in the urine. The history of polydipsia, polyphagia, and polyuria are also classical. Diabetes insipidus is due to a deficiency of antidiuretic hormone or nonresponsiveness to the hormone. In this instance, the urine is very dilute with a low specific gravity of 1.005 or less. In contrast to hypoglycemia, the patient has hyperglycemia. Starvation and malabsorption are possible causes of weight loss. Based upon the history of increased food intake, the patient is not starving. Malabsorption is usually associated with abnormal bowel function, not noted in the history. *Biochemistry,* p. 46; *Nelson,* p. 391.
13. The answer is A: metabolic acidosis. The acidosis is indicated by the pH. The basis of the acidosis is the excessive generation of acetoacetic and β-hydroxybutyric acids, which are buffered by reaction with $NaHCO_3$:

    $NaHCO_3$ + acetoacetic acid $\rightleftharpoons$ Na-acetoacetate $+ H_2CO_3$.

    The H_2CO_3 is lost as CO_2 from the lungs, and the net result is a decrease in pH due to the decrease in $[HCO_3^-]$, the numerator of the fraction in the log term of the Henderson-Hasselbalch equation ($pH = pK_a + \log [HCO_3^-]/[H_2CO_3]$). *Biochemistry,* p. 39.
14. The answer is E: increased respiratory rate. To compensate for the metabolic acidosis, the patient exhibited tachypnea (rapid breathing rate). The purpose of this is to lower the pCO_2 or the $[H_2CO_3]$, which occurs in the denominator of the Henderson-Hasselbalch equation, by expiring carbon dioxide. The labored respirations of diabetic ketoacidosis are characteristic and are given the name Kussmaul respirations. There is decreased urinary excretion of bicarbonate and increased urinary excretion of ammonium ion, hydrogen ions, and phosphate as $H_2PO_4^-$. *Nelson,* p. 391.
15. The answer is B: parenteral insulin. The primary defect in this disorder, type I diabetes mellitus, is insulin deficiency. Insulin is ordinarily given subcutaneously because it is ineffective by mouth owing to digestion of the protein hormone. Patients with acute diabetic ketoacidosis are often treated with intravenous insulin. Pig and beef insulin are effective in humans and were the mainstay of treatment for five decades until the advent of recombinant human insulin. Patients with diabetic ketoacidosis are hypovolemic, and they must be treated with intravenous fluids. Although these individuals have an elevated serum potassium initially, insulin drives the potassium into cells and hypokalemia results unless potassium supplements are given after the potassium is normalized (too much potassium can cause cardiac arrest). The sulfonylureas stimulate the release of insulin from pancreatic β-cells, and they are used in the treatment of some type II diabetics. These agents are not used for the treatment of diabetic ketoacidosis, and they are not used in people with type I diabetes owing to the paucity or deficiency of β-cell function. Antidiuretic hormone is used for the treatment of diabetes insipidus. Ammonium chloride produces acidosis and is contraindicated in this patient. Carbohydrate in food is used to counteract hypoglycemia in individuals receiving insulin. *Biochemistry,* p. 46; *Cecil,* p. 1291.

ANSWERS TO SUPPLEMENTARY QUESTIONS

16. See Figure 3–1.
17. (a) $pH = -\log [H^+] = -\log 4.6 \times 10^{-5} = -(-4.34) = 4.34$.
    (b) $pH = -\log [H^+] = -\log 7.9\ 10^{-9} = -(-8.10) = 8.1$.
18. $pH = -\log [H^+]$; $7.4 = -\log [H^+]$; $-7.4 = \log [H^+]$; $[H^+] = 3.98 \times 10^{-8}$.
19. $pH = pK_a + \log [HPO_4^{2-}]/[H_2PO_4^-]$; $7.4 = 6.8 + \log [HPO_4^{2-}]/[H_2PO_4^-]$; $0.6 = \log [HPO_4^{2-}]/[H_2PO_4^-]$; $3.98 = [HPO_4^{2-}]/[H_2PO_4^-]$.
20. $[HPO_4^{2-}] + [H_2PO_4^-]$ is 5.00 mM; $[HPO_4^{2-}] = 5.00\text{ mM} - [H_2PO_4^-]$; $3.98 = [HPO_4^{2-}]/[H_2PO_4^-]$; $3.98 = (5.00\text{ mM} - [H_2PO_4^-])/[H_2PO_4^-]$; by cross-multiplying, we obtain $3.98 [H_2PO_4^-] = 5.00\text{ mM} - [H_2PO_4^-]$; and $4.98 [H_2PO_4^-] = 5.00$ mM; $[H_2PO_4^-] = 5.00\text{ mM}/4.98 = 1.00$ mM; and $[HPO_4^{2-}] = 5.00\text{ mM} - [H_2PO_4^-] = 5.00\text{ mM} - 1.00\text{ mM} = 4.00$ mM and $[HPO_4^{2-}] = 4.00$ mM.
21. $pH = pK_a + \log [HPO_4^{2-}]/[H_2PO_4^-]$; $pH = 6.8 + \log 0.32$; $pH = 6.8 + (-0.49) = 6.31$.
22. $pH = pK_a + \log [HCO_3^-]/[CO_2 + H_2CO_3]$; $7.4 = 6.1 + \log [HCO_3^-]/[CO_2 + H_2CO_3]$; $1.3 = \log [HCO_3^-]/[CO_2 + H_2CO_3]$; $19.95 = [HCO_3^-]/[CO_2 + H_2CO_3]$; $[HCO_3^-]/[CO_2 + H_2CO_3] \approx 20$.
23. $([HCO_3^-] + [CO_2 + H_2CO_3]) = 24$ mM; $[CO_2 + H_2CO_3] = 24\text{ mM} - ([HCO_3^-]$; $[HCO_3^-]/(24\text{ mM} - [HCO_3^-]) \approx 20$; by cross-multiplying, $[HCO_3^-] = 480\text{ mM} - 20 [HCO_3^-]$; $21 [HCO_3^-] = 480$ mM; $[HCO_3^-] = 480\text{ mM}/21 = 22.9$ mM; and $[CO_2 + H_2CO_3] = 24\text{ mM} - [HCO_3^-] = 24\text{ mM} - 22.9\text{ mM} = 1.1$ mM.
24. $[HCO_3^-] + [CO_2 + H_2CO_3] = 16$ mM; $16\text{ mM} = 15\text{ mM} + [CO_2 + H_2CO_3]$; $1.0\text{ mM} = [CO_2 + H_2CO_3]$; $pH = 6.1 + \log 15\text{ mM}/1\text{ mM}$; $pH = 6.1 + \log 15 = 6.1 + 1.18 = 7.28$.

REFERENCES

Behrman, R. E. *Nelson Textbook of Pediatrics,* 14th ed. W. B. Saunders Company, Philadelphia, 1992.

Roskoski, R., Jr. *Biochemistry.* Philadelphia, W. B. Saunders Company, 1996.

Wyngaarden, J. B., L. H. Smith, Jr., and J. C. Bennett (eds.). *Cecil Textbook of Medicine,* 19th ed. Philadelphia, W. B. Saunders Company, 1992.

CHAPTER FOUR

ENZYMES

SYNOPSIS

OBJECTIVES

1. To define the distinguishing properties of enzymes.
2. To use the Michaelis-Menten and Lineweaver-Burk formulations of enzyme kinetics.
3. To distinguish among competitive, noncompetitive, and uncompetitive inhibition and to explain the action of certain therapeutic agents.
4. To enumerate the general mechanisms of enzyme action including that of serine proteases.
5. To compare and contrast the various mechanisms of enzyme regulation including the role of positive cooperativity.
6. To interpret serum enzyme and isozyme activities in the diagnosis of clinical conditions.

Objective 1: To define the distinguishing properties of enzymes.

I. General properties of enzymes
  A. An enzyme is a protein catalyst (PRINCIPLE 5 OF BIOCHEMISTRY)
    1. A protein is a polypeptide made up of amino acid residues
    2. A catalyst is a substance that alters the rate of a chemical reaction
  B. The rate of a catalyzed reaction ranges from 10^3- to 10^{11}-fold greater than that of an uncatalyzed reaction
  C. *A catalyst accelerates the rate of a reaction by decreasing the free energy of activation of a reaction ($\Delta G^{\ddagger}$)* (Fig. 4–1)
  D. A catalyst increases the rate at which a thermodynamically feasible reaction attains its equilibrium *without* altering the position of the equilibrium
  E. The structures and classes of enzymes are based upon common characteristics
    1. Some enzymes are simple proteins that contain only amino acid residues, such as the digestive enzymes trypsin, chymotrypsin, and elastase
    2. Other enzymes are complex proteins that contain amino acid residues and a nonamino acid cofactor
      a. The complete, active enzyme is called a **holoenzyme,** and it is made of a protein portion (**apoenzyme**) and **cofactor**
      b. **Prosthetic groups** are tightly bound cofactors
    3. The six major classes of enzymes are **oxidoreductases, transferases, hydrolases, isomerases, lyases,** and **ligases**

II. Unisubstrate and multisubstrate reactions catalyzed by enzymes
  A. Uni, bi, ter, and quad reactions involve one, two, three, and four substrates, respectively
  B. The order of addition of reactants and the release of products can be random or ordered
  C. If one product is released prior to the addition of some of the substrates, the reaction is described as a ping-pong reaction

Objective 2: To use the Michaelis-Menten and Lineweaver-Burk formulations of enzyme kinetics.

III. Enzyme kinetics
  A. The Michaelis-Menten equation expresses velocity as a function of substrate concentration
    1. A plot of velocity as a function of substrate concentration yields a rectangular hyperbola (Fig. 4–2)
    2. Such data show that enzymes exhibit saturation
    3. The **Michaelis-Menton equation** is given by the following expression:

$$v = \frac{V_{max}[S]}{K_m + [S]} \tag{4.1}$$

      a. The $\mathbf{V_{max}}$ is the maximal velocity exhibited when the enzyme is completely saturated with substrate
      b. The $\mathbf{K_m}$ (Michaelis constant) is the substrate concentration at half the maximal velocity ($V_{max}/2$)
  B. The **Lineweaver-Burk equation,** which yields a linear double-reciprocal plot, is given by the following expression:

$$\frac{1}{v} = \frac{K_m}{V_{max}}\left(\frac{1}{[S]}\right) + \frac{1}{V_{max}} \tag{4.2}$$

    1. This plot provides a convenient procedure for determining steady-state kinetic values
    2. The *y*-intercept equals $1/V_{max}$
    3. The *x*-intercept equals $-1/K_m$

Objective 3: To distinguish among competitive, noncompetitive, and uncompetitive inhibition and to explain the action of certain therapeutic agents.

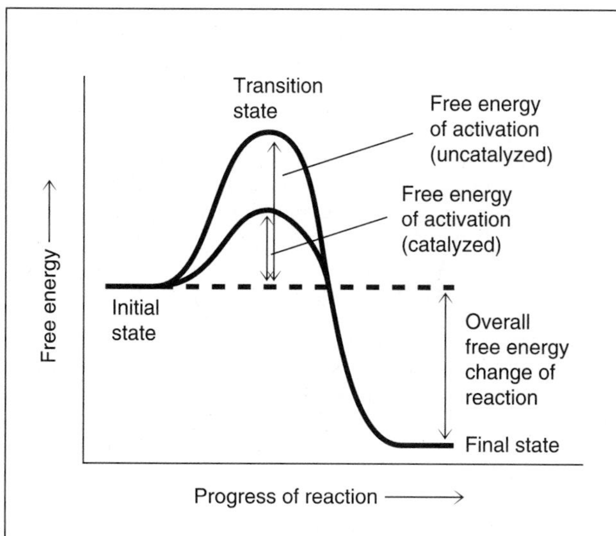

FIGURE 4-1. Free energies of activation of catalyzed and uncatalyzed reactions.

IV. Enzyme inhibition
  A. Irreversible inhibition
    1. Irreversible inhibition occurs when the inhibitor reacts with an enzyme to form a very stable complex, and the enzyme is permanently inactivated
    2. Usually an irreversible inhibitor forms a covalent bond with the enzyme
    3. The inhibition of cyclooxygenase by aspirin, which involves the acetylation of a serine residue, is an example of this type of inhibition
  B. Reversible inhibition
    1. Competitive inhibition
      a. Compounds that produce this type of inhibition are structural analogues of the varied substrate
      b. Inhibition is overcome at high substrate concentration

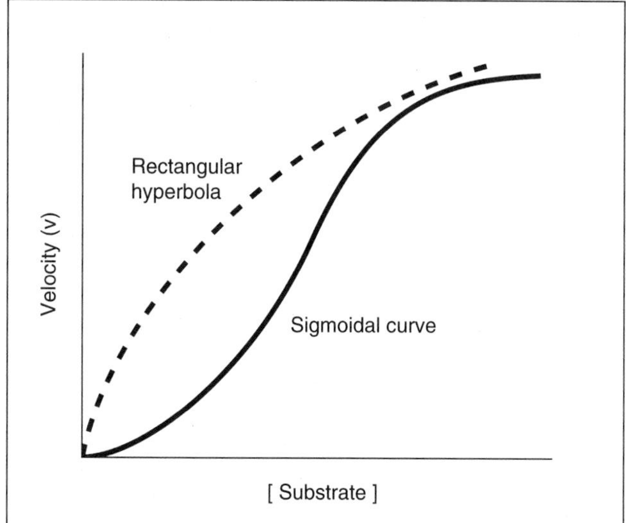

FIGURE 4-2. A rectangular hyperbola and a sigmoidal curve. The rectangular hyperbola illustrates saturation kinetics, and the sigmoidal curve is the *sine qua non* of positive cooperativity.

      c. The Lineweaver-Burk plots for the inhibited and noninhibited enzyme have the same *y*-intercept (Fig. 4–3*A*)
    2. Noncompetitive inhibition
      a. Compounds that produce this type of inhibition are not structural analogues of the varied substrate
      b. Inhibition is not overcome at high substrate concentration
      c. The Lineweaver-Burk plots for the inhibited and noninhibited enzyme have different *y*-intercepts (Fig. 4–3*B*)
      d. The *x*-intercepts, which reflect K_m values, are the same for the inhibited and noninhibited enzyme
    3. Uncompetitive inhibition
      a. Compounds that produce uncompetitive inhibition have no effect on the slope but increase the *y*-intercept of a Lineweaver-Burk plot (Fig. 4–3*C*)
      b. This pattern of inhibition is observed with some multisubstrate enzymes
    4. Drugs whose structures resemble substrates
      a. Captopril and enalapril, which are used in the treatment of hypertension and congestive heart failure, produce competitive inhibition of angiotensin converting enzyme (ACE)
      b. Lovastatin and mevinolin, which are used in the treatment of hypercholesterolemia, produce competitive inhibition of the rate-limiting enzyme for cholesterol synthesis (HMG-CoA reductase)

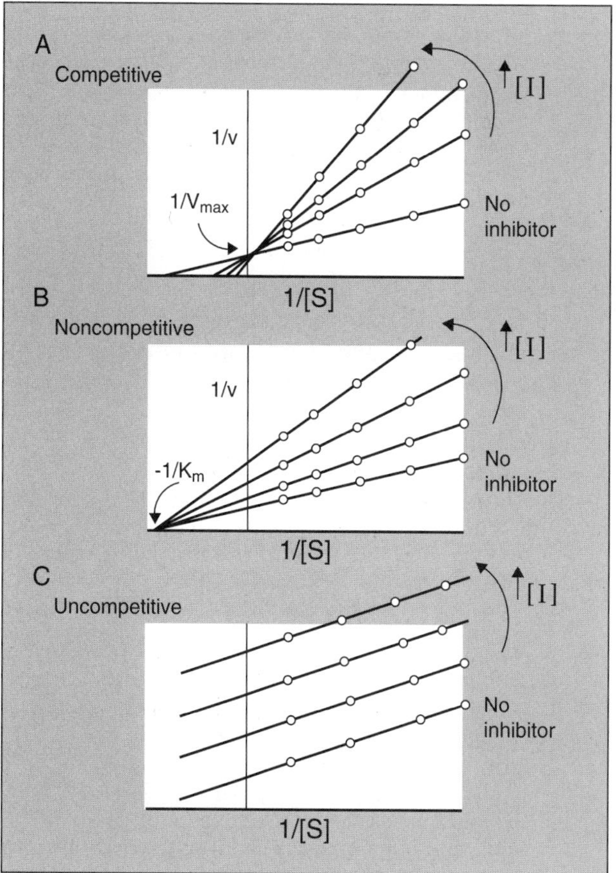

FIGURE 4-3. Reversible enzyme inhibition. *A.* Competitive inhibition. *B.* Noncompetitive inhibition. *C.* Uncompetitive inhibition.

Objective 4: To enumerate the general mechanisms of enzyme action including that of serine proteases.

V. Factors that contribute to rate enhancement by enzymes
  A. Enzymes can enhance the rate of a reaction by placing the reactive species close together (proximity and covalent catalysis) according to Fischer's lock and key hypothesis (PRINCIPLE 7 OF BIOCHEMISTRY)
  B. Enzymes can enhance the rate of a reaction by orienting the substrates in a reactive mode
  C. Enzymes whose conformation is altered by substrate binding are said to undergo induced fit
  D. Enzymes can act by producing strain and distortion in the substrates
  E. Enzymes can function as general acids and bases
  F. Enzymes can force the substrates to resemble the transition state

VI. Biochemical mechanism of serine proteases
  A. Serine proteases exhibit considerable substrate specificity
    1. *Trypsin, a serine protease, cleaves on the carboxyterminal side of lysine and arginine*
    2. Chymotrypsin cleaves on the carboxyterminal side of phenylalanine, tyrosine, tryptophan, and other hydrophobic residues
    3. Elastase cleaves on the carboxyterminal side of alanine
  B. The catalytic triad of amino acids consists of **serine, histidine,** and **aspartate**
    1. Histidine bridges serine and aspartate
    2. A covalent adduct is formed between the active site serine and the carbonyl group of a specific peptide bond, allowing displacement of the amino group from the peptide bond and release of the carboxyterminal portion of the original polypeptide
    3. The remainder of the original polypeptide is released from the active site by hydrolysis

Objective 5: To compare and contrast the various mechanisms of enzyme regulation including the role of positive cooperativity.

VII. Regulation of enzyme activity
  A. Enzymes can be controlled through their synthesis and degradation
    1. An increased rate of synthesis is called **enzyme induction**
    2. A decreased rate of synthesis is called **enzyme repression**
  B. Enzymes can be regulated by allosteric effectors (PRINCIPLE 8 OF BIOCHEMISTRY)
    1. Effectors bind noncovalently to a site distinct from the active site called the allosteric site
    2. Effectors can be stimulatory or inhibitory
  C. Enzymes can be regulated by phosphorylation
    1. Protein kinases catalyze the phosphorylation of proteins, and phosphatases catalyze the hydrolytic removal of the phosphoryl group
    2. Phosphorylation represents regulation by covalent modification
    3. Phosphorylation of some enzymes is stimulatory and of others is inhibitory
      a. The effects of phosphorylation make physiological sense and can be rationalized
      b. Protein-serine/threonine phosphorylation mediated by protein kinase A generally promotes catabolic processes and inhibits anabolic processes
  D. Positive cooperativity results in relatively large changes in effect over small changes in ligand concentration
    1. Positive cooperativity results when binding of the first ligand to a protein increases the binding of the second and subsequent ligands
    2. The distinguishing feature of positive cooperativity is the increase in slope at the lower concentrations of ligand that produces a sigmoidal concentration-dependence curve, the *sine qua non* for positive cooperativity (see Fig. 4–2)
    3. The binding of oxygen to hemoglobin exhibits a sigmoidal binding curve and is the prototypical example of positive cooperativity
  E. Principles of regulation provide guidelines for explaining metabolic control
    1. Regulation of the activity of a single enzyme may involve a variety of mechanisms
    2. Metabolic regulation makes physiological sense according to the molecular logic of the cell (PRINCIPLE 9 OF BIOCHEMISTRY)

Objective 6: To interpret serum enzyme and isozyme activities in the diagnosis of clinical conditions.

VIII. Clinical significance of enzymes
  A. Transaminases
    1. Aspartate aminotransferase (AST) and alanine aminotransferase (ALT) catalyze the reversible transfer of the α-amino group of the substrate amino acid to α-ketoglutarate
    2. Transaminases are released from damaged cells such as the myocardium following a myocardial infarction
    3. Transaminases are also elevated modestly (5×) with hepatic cirrhosis and obstructive liver disease and greatly (25×) with hepatitis
  B. Phosphatases
    1. Alkaline phosphatase
      a. Serum levels are elevated with obstructive liver disease and with bone disease
      b. Serum levels are elevated physiologically during adolescence, an indication of active bone growth; this increase can be used by dentists in deciding when to perform orthodontic procedures
    2. Acid phosphatase
      a. Serum levels are elevated with metastatic carcinoma of the prostate
      b. Serum levels can decrease when therapy for metastatic carcinoma of the prostate is efficacious
  C. Transferases
    1. γ-Glutamyl transpeptidase, which occurs in liver, is elevated in liver disease including subclinical alcoholism

2. Creatine phosphokinase (CPK) occurs in cardiac and skeletal muscle and brain
   a. CPK is elevated following a myocardial infarction
      (1) The MB isozyme (see below) of heart muscle is a sensitive and specific marker of myocardial necrosis
      (2) Elevation occurs within 6 hours in 50% and within 12 hours in >90% of patients
   b. CPK is elevated in males with muscular dystrophy and in carrier mothers

D. Amylase
   1. This enzyme, which is produced by the parotid and pancreas, catalyzes the hydrolysis of starch and glycogen
   2. Amylase is elevated in pancreatitis, and it can be elevated by mumps

E. Dehydrogenases
   1. Lactate dehydrogenase, which is found in all human cells, is elevated following a myocardial infarction, liver disease, and hemolytic anemia
      a. The LDH_1 isozyme (HHHH, see below) occurs principally in the heart
      b. When LDH_1 exceeds LDH_2 (HHHM), myocardial infarction is likely
   2. β-Hydroxybutyrate dehydrogenase is elevated following a myocardial infarction

F. Isozymes
   1. Isoenzymes are different but closely related protein molecules that catalyze the same reaction
   2. Creatine phosphokinase is a dimer made up of two kinds of subunits (M, for muscle, and B, for brain) that can be combined in three different ways: MM, MB, BB
   3. LDH is a tetrameric enzyme made up of two types of subunits (H, for heart, and M, for muscle) that can be combined in five different ways to form LDH_1 through LDH_5, respectively: HHHH, HHHM, HHMM, HMMM, MMMM

QUESTIONS

DIRECTIONS. (Items 1–18): Each of the numbered items or incomplete statements in this section is followed by answers or by completions of the statement. Select the ONE lettered answer or completion that is BEST in each case. Correct answers and explanations are given at the end of the chapter.

1. Trypsin catalyzes the hydrolysis of peptide bonds on the carboxyterminal side of which of the following amino acids?

   (A) Alanine
   (B) Arginine and lysine
   (C) Aspartate
   (D) Histidine
   (E) Phenylalanine, tyrosine, tryptophan, and hydrophobic amino acids

2. A mutation that results in an increase in the K_m (Michaelis constant) of an enzyme has the following effect on the rate of the reaction.

   (A) The V_{max} of the enzyme-catalyzed reaction is increased
   (B) The rate of the reaction at a given subsaturating substrate concentration is increased
   (C) The V_{max} of the enzyme-catalyzed reaction is decreased
   (D) The rate of the reaction at a given subsaturating substrate concentration is decreased
   (E) The rate of the reaction at saturating substrate concentration is decreased

3. The inhibition of cyclooxygenase by aspirin is based upon which of the following types of reaction?

   (A) A covalent chemical reaction at an active site serine
   (B) A covalent chemical reaction at an allosteric site
   (C) A noncovalent chemical reaction at an active site serine
   (D) A noncovalent chemical reaction at an allosteric site
   (E) A noncovalent chemical reaction with the enzyme's heme prosthetic group

4. All of the following are components of the catalytic triad found in trypsin and chymotrypsin EXCEPT

   (A) histidine
   (B) aspartate
   (C) serine
   (D) lysine

5. Hemoglobin Raleigh is the result of a mutation that converts valine 1 of the β-chain to an alanine (the alanine residue is then *N*-acetylated). The oxygen-binding curve is sigmoidal and is shifted toward the right. Hemoglobin Raleigh exhibits which of the following types of cooperativity?

   (A) Negative cooperativity with a decreased oxygen affinity
   (B) Negative cooperativity with an increased oxygen affinity
   (C) No cooperativity
   (D) Positive cooperativity with an increased oxygen affinity
   (E) Positive cooperativity with a decreased oxygen affinity

6. A protein consists of a dimer that can be made up of A and B subunits. What is the total number of possible isozymes?

   (A) One
   (B) Two
   (C) Three
   (D) Four
   (E) Five

7. The reaction shown below is catalyzed by which one of the following classes of enzymes?
   (A) Hydrolase
   (B) Isomerase
   (C) Ligase
   (D) Lyase
   (E) Oxidoreductase

$$\begin{array}{c} COO^- \\ | \\ C-H \\ \| \\ H-C \\ | \\ COO^- \\ + \\ H_2O \end{array} \rightleftharpoons \begin{array}{c} COO^- \\ | \\ HO-C-H \\ | \\ H-C-H \\ | \\ COO^- \end{array}$$

8. Note that $v = (V_{max} \times [S])/(K_m + [S])$. If the V_{max} of an enzyme-catalyzed reaction is 100 μmol/min, and the K_m is 1 mM, what is the velocity at a substrate concentration of 10 mM?
   (A) 9.1 μmol/min
   (B) 50 μmol/min
   (C) 91 μmol/min
   (D) 99 μmol/min
   (E) 100 μmol/min

9. The K_m of hexokinase for glucose is 30 μM, and the K_m of glucokinase for glucose is 10 mM. Which one of the following statements regarding hexokinase, glucokinase, or both enzymes is true when the blood glucose concentration is 10 mM (as found in the hepatic portal vein after a meal)?
   (A) Both hexokinase and glucokinase are operating near maximal velocity
   (B) Hexokinase is operating near maximal velocity
   (C) Glucokinase is operating near maximal velocity
   (D) Neither hexokinase nor glucokinase is operating near maximal velocity

10. A 65-year-old man complains of back pain and has difficulty urinating. Laboratory examination reveals an elevated acid phosphatase and alkaline phosphatase. What is the likely diagnosis?
   (A) Cancer of the kidney
   (B) Metastatic cancer of the prostate
   (C) Myopathy
   (D) Obstructive jaundice
   (E) Osteoporosis

11. Which one of the following serum enzymes is characteristically elevated within 12 hours of a myocardial infarction (heart attack)?
   (A) Alkaline phosphatase
   (B) Amylase
   (C) Aspartate aminotransferase
   (D) Creatine phosphokinase
   (E) β-Hydroxybutyrate dehydrogenase

12. Infants fed a diet deficient in pyridoxine (the precursor of pyridoxal phosphate) develop seizures owing to altered neurotransmitter biosynthesis. Which one of the following holoenzymes consists of an apoenzyme combined with pyridoxal phosphate?
   (A) Choline acetyltransferase
   (B) Dopamine β-hydroxylase
   (C) Glutamate decarboxylase
   (D) Tyrosine hydroxylase
   (E) Tryptophan hydroxylase

Items 13–18

History

A 51-year-old woman retailer with a long history of alcoholism sought evaluation because of a skin rash (dermatitis). The rash involved her arms, trunk, and legs. She also experienced nausea, vomiting, diarrhea, and abdominal pain during the previous 3 months. Her family noticed that the patient exhibited increasing forgetfulness. The patient was restless, irritable, and confused about the day and date. She recognized family members but was unable to focus attention, and her mental status waxed and waned.

Physical Examination

Her temperature was 36.1 °C (97 °F); pulse, 110/min; respiration, 14/min; and blood pressure, 90/60 mm Hg. Her skin showed angular cheilitis (inflammation in the corners of the mouth) and a generalized rash involving the hands, elbows, feet, and trunk. Her sclerae were jaundiced. Abdominal examination revealed hepatomegaly.

Laboratory

Hematocrit 28% (normal ♀, 35–45%)
White cell count, 3200/μL (normal, 4500–11,000/μL)
Red blood cell indices, normal
Alanine aminotransferase (ALT, SGPT), 42 U/L (normal, 8–20 U/L)
Amylase, 512 U/L (normal, 25–125 U/L)
Aspartate aminotransferase (AST, SGOT), 82 U/L (normal, 10–30 U/L)
Alkaline phosphatase, 331 U/L (normal ♀, 42–98 U/L)
Creatine phosphokinase (CPK), 56 U/L (normal ♀, 26–140 U/L)
γ-Glutamyl transpeptidase, 719 U/L (normal, 8–40 U/L)
Prothrombin time, normal
Total and direct bilirubin, 5.1 and 1.2 mg/dL (normal, 0.2–1.0 and 0.0–0.2 mg/dL)

13. Abnormalities in which of the following laboratory values are helpful in the diagnosis of liver disease?
   (A) Acid phosphatase and alkaline phosphatase
   (B) Aspartate aminotransferase, alanine aminotransferase, alkaline phosphatase, and total and direct bilirubin
   (C) Amylase
   (D) Blood urea nitrogen (BUN) and creatinine
   (E) Creatine phosphokinase, β-hydroxybutyrate dehydrogenase, and lactate dehydrogenase

14. Which one of the following laboratory values in this patient suggests a diagnosis of pancreatitis?
    (A) Alanine aminotransferase
    (B) Alkaline phosphatase
    (C) Amylase
    (D) Aspartate aminotransferase
    (E) γ-Glutamyl transpeptidase

15. Which one of the following laboratory values is the most sensitive indicator of mild alcoholic liver disease?
    (A) Alanine aminotransferase
    (B) Alkaline phosphatase
    (C) Bilirubin
    (D) γ-Glutamyl transpeptidase
    (E) Prothrombin time

16. Which one of the following laboratory values in this patient is suggestive of an obstructive component to liver disease?
    (A) Alanine aminotransferase
    (B) Alkaline phosphatase
    (C) Aspartate aminotransferase
    (D) Creatine phosphokinase
    (E) γ-Glutamyl transpeptidase

17. Liver disease may result in an elevation of any one of the following serum enzymes EXCEPT
    (A) alanine aminotransferase
    (B) alkaline phosphatase
    (C) aspartate aminotransferase
    (D) creatine phosphokinase
    (E) γ-glutamyl transpeptidase

18. The most efficacious treatment of this patient's dermatitis, diarrhea, and dementia is
    (A) niacin
    (B) ascorbate
    (C) riboflavin
    (D) thiamin
    (E) vitamin B_{12}

ANSWERS AND EXPLANATIONS

1. The answer is B: arginine and lysine. The portion of the binding site of trypsin that determines specificity is occupied by a negatively charged residue that attracts the positively charged peptidyl lysine or arginine. Hydrolysis at such sites is a familiar motif in metabolism because many proteases, such as the blood clotting factors, also catalyze hydrolysis reactions on the carboxyterminal side of basic residues. Chymotrypsin catalyzes hydrolysis on the carboxyterminal side of phenylalanine, tyrosine, tryptophan, and hydrophobic amino acids, and elastase catalyzes hydrolysis on the carboxyterminal side of alanine. Aspartate is found at the active site of pepsin, a stomach protease. *Biochemistry,* p. 59.
2. The answer is D: decreases the rate of the reaction at a given subsaturating substrate concentration. The K_m of an enzyme is the substrate concentration that results in a reaction velocity that is one-half of the V_{max}. By increasing the K_m, a higher substrate concentration is required to produce a half-maximal velocity. The K_m of an enzyme can vary independently of the V_{max}. *Biochemistry,* p. 56.
3. The answer is A: based upon a chemical reaction at an active site serine. Aspirin acetylates the active site serine of cyclooxygenase to inhibit the enzyme irreversibly by chemical modification. Aspirin does not modify the allosteric sites of the enzyme nor does it react with the enzyme's heme prosthetic group. Nonsteroidal antiinflammatory drugs such as ibuprofen inhibit cyclooxygenase through noncovalent interaction with the enzyme's active site, but the reaction with aspirin is covalent. *Biochemistry,* p. 57.
4. The answer is D: lysine. Lysine is NOT part of the catalytic triad. The catalytic triad involves the interaction of serine, histidine, and aspartate. Histidine interacts with the serine hydroxyl group by accepting and donating protons. Aspartate neutralizes charges that develop on histidine. Lysine does not form part of the catalytic triad. *Biochemistry,* p. 59.
5. The answer is E: exhibits positive cooperativity with a decreased oxygen affinity. The concentration dependence of a positively cooperative process is a sigmoidal curve. The increasing slope in the early part of the curve indicates that an increase in substrate (or ligand) concentration has a magnified effect. The shift to the right indicates that a higher oxygen concentration is required to produce a given degree of saturation and that the mutant hemoglobin has decreased oxygen affinity. The sigmoidal concentration-dependence curve is not exhibited by proteins that exhibit negative cooperativity or no cooperativity. *Biochemistry,* p. 485.
6. The answer is C: three. The three combinations of two different subunits taken two at a time are AA, AB, and BB. *Biochemistry,* p. 61.
7. The answer is D: lyase. Lyase reactions involve the splitting of one molecule into two with the formation of an additional double bond (or the reverse reaction). A hydrolase catalyzes the cleavage or lysis of a chemical bond by water. Isomerase reactions involve the conversion of one molecule into another with the same chemical formula. A ligase joins two molecules in an ATP-dependent process. Oxidation-reduction reactions generally involve an electron donor and acceptor. *Biochemistry,* p. 55.
8. The answer is C: 91 μmol/min. The Michaelis-Menton equation, the starting point for this calculation, is given as $v = (V_{max}[S])/(K_m + [S])$. Filling in the appropriate values, it becomes

$$v = (100\ \mu\text{mol/min} \times 10\ \text{mM})/(1\ \text{mM} + 10\ \text{mM})$$
$$v = (1000\ \mu\text{mol/min} \times \text{mM})/(11\ \text{mM})$$
$$v = 91\ \mu\text{mol/min}$$

This value shows that the enzyme is operating at 91% capacity with a substrate concentration that is 10 times the K_m. Similar calculations show that the enzyme is operating at 9% of its capacity when the substrate concentration is one-tenth the K_m, 50% at the K_m, and 99% at 100 times the K_m value. Note that increasing the substrate concentration from 0.1 mM to 1 mM increases the reaction rate from 9% to 50%, but increasing the substrate concentration from 10 mM to 100 mM increases the reaction rate from 91% to 99%, or just 8%. At lower substrate concentration, the enzyme follows first-order kinetics, and near saturation, the enzyme follows zero-order kinetics. *Biochemistry,* p. 56.

9. The answer is B: hexokinase is operating near maximal velocity. The substrate concentration is 333 times the K_m (the substrate concentration at one-half maximal velocity) of hexokinase, which is, therefore, operating near its maximal velocity. The substrate concentration is at the K_m value for glucokinase, which is, therefore, only operating at half-maximal velocity. The physiological advantage for having glucokinase in the liver is that it is not saturated at the physiological concentrations of glucose found in the portal vein. *Biochemistry,* p. 56.
10. The answer is B: metastatic cancer of the prostate. Difficulty in urination and back pain can be related to a large number of conditions. Cancer of the prostate, however, is uniquely associated with an elevated serum acid phosphatase. Because the tumor has metastasized to bone (the probable cause of back pain), there is also an increase in serum alkaline phosphatase. Elevated serum alkaline phosphatase can also result from obstructive liver disease. Acid phosphatase, however, is not elevated with obstructive jaundice. Elevated serum alkaline phosphatase is not characteristic of a primary tumor of the kidney, osteoporosis, or myopathy. Males with muscular dystrophy and their carrier mothers often exhibit elevated creatine phosphokinase levels. *Biochemistry*, p. 62.
11. The answer is D: creatine phosphokinase. This enzyme is localized to skeletal and cardiac muscle and brain, and it is commonly elevated when there is damage to muscle. Many other enzymes are elevated following a myocardial infarction including the transaminases and lactate dehydrogenase. Aspartate aminotransferase is elevated about 24 hours and β-hydroxybutyrate dehydrogenase is elevated about 36 hours post-myocardial infarction, whereas creatine phosphokinase is elevated about 12 hours following the insult. *Biochemistry,* p. 64.
12. The answer is C: glutamate decarboxylase. Glutamate decarboxylase, which catalyzes the biosynthesis of GABA, requires pyridoxal phosphate as a cofactor. In the 1950s, infants fed formulas deficient in pyridoxine (vitamin B_6) developed seizures. This response was postulated to be due to the deficiency of GABA, the chief inhibitory neurotransmitter in brain. All human transaminases also consist of an apoenzyme and pyridoxal phosphate. Choline acetyltransferase does not contain a cofactor. Tyrosine hydroxylase and probably tryptophan hydroxylase contain ferrous iron as a cofactor, and dopamine β-hydroxylase contains copper as a cofactor. *Biochemistry,* p. 410.
13. The answer is B: aspartate aminotransferase, alanine aminotransferase, alkaline phosphatase, and total and direct bilirubin. Transaminases are elevated in a variety of disorders including liver disease, heart disease, hemolytic anemia, and following a myocardial infarction. Alkaline phosphatase is elevated when there is obstruction of the bile ducts (either primary or secondary to inflammation) and bone disease. Bilirubin, a bile pigment, is elevated with hemolysis and with liver disease. Acid phosphatase is indicative of metastatic prostate cancer. Elevations of blood urea and creatinine are indicative of renal disease. *Biochemistry,* p. 61.
14. The answer is C: amylase. Amylase is a digestive enzyme that is produced by the pancreas and the parotid gland. Inflammation of either of these organs can produce elevated enzyme levels. *Biochemistry,* p. 63.
15. The answer is D: γ-glutamyl transpeptidase. A variety of enzyme and metabolite levels are altered in liver disease, and they show a progression depending upon the severity of the pathology. γ-Glutamyl transpeptidase is the most sensitive indicator of liver pathology, and it may be the only abnormality in a person with excess ethanol intake. Transaminases and alkaline phosphatase are elevated with more extensive pathology. Elevations of bilirubin that are due to liver pathology occur later in the disease. Alterations in prothrombin (measured by the prothrombin time) and serum albumin, plasma proteins synthesized by liver, occur only after severe liver dysfunction. *Biochemistry,* p. 63.
16. The answer is B: alkaline phosphatase. Elevation of this enzyme is characteristic of obstruction of the bile ducts that may be secondary to a gallstone or tumor. With inflammation such as hepatitis, alkaline phosphatase may be elevated because of biliary obstruction caused by the inflammation. Bilirubin and direct bilirubin are elevated because of inflammation or obstruction, and this produces jaundice. Patients with severe obstruction may experience itching because of increased levels of circulating bile acids. *Biochemistry,* p. 62.
17. The answer is D: creatine phosphokinase. This enzyme is present in cardiac and skeletal muscle and brain, and it plays a role in maintaining cellular ATP during active cellular metabolism. This enzyme is NOT present in liver, and elevation of creatine phosphokinase is NOT indicative of hepatic cirrhosis or other liver disease. *Biochemistry,* p. 63.
18. The answer is B: niacin. The classic triad of dermatitis, diarrhea, and dementia is a result of pellagra caused by a deficiency of niacin. Pellagra as a primary disorder is uncommon in the United States, but it is common in individuals with alcoholism. Another vitamin deficiency that is common in people with alcoholism is thiamine deficiency. The major symptoms of thiamine deficiency are related to the nervous system (dry beriberi) and cardiovascular system (wet beriberi). The nervous system manifestations include peripheral neuritis with sensory disturbances and diminished muscle strength. Thiamine deficiency leads to Wernicke's encephalopathy with ataxia, ophthalmoplegia, and nystagmus that respond to thiamine but to no other vitamin. This encephalopathy is also characterized by impaired learning and memory and confabulation (making conversation without regard for the truth). Although this patient had altered mental status, dermatitis and diarrhea are not characteristic of thiamine deficiency. Riboflavin deficiency is accompanied by dermatitis, glossitis, neuropathy, and anemia. This patient lacks the anemia of riboflavin deficiency and has dementia, not characteristic of riboflavin deficiency. Deficiency of vitamin B_{12} produces a megaloblastic anemia and neuropathy. Deficiency of ascorbate produces hemorrhages in the skin (ecchymosis and petechiae). *Biochemistry,* p. 26; *Cecil,* pp. 1170 and 2127.

REFERENCES

Roskoski, R., Jr. *Biochemistry.* Philadelphia, W. B. Saunders Company, 1996.

Wyngaarden, J. B., L. H. Smith, Jr., and J. C. Bennett (eds.). *Cecil Textbook of Medicine,* 19th ed. Philadelphia, W. B. Saunders Company, 1992.

CHAPTER FIVE

BIOENERGETICS AND OXIDATION-REDUCTION REACTIONS

SYNOPSIS

OBJECTIVES

1. To analyze biochemical processes by their free energy changes.
2. To delineate the four main types of biochemical oxidation-reduction reactions.
3. To describe the metabolism of superoxide, peroxide, and hydroxyl free radicals.
4. To describe the role of myeloperoxidase in the white blood cell.

Objective 1: To analyze biochemical processes by their free energy changes.

I. Free energy change as a criterion of feasibility
   A. The Gibbs **free energy change** (ΔG) is the most important thermodynamic function used in biochemistry because of its ability to predict whether a process or reaction is possible at constant temperature and pressure
   B. The criteria for the feasibility of a reaction are given as follows
      1. $\Delta G < 0$ (process is feasible and is **exergonic**); exergonic reactions proceed with the liberation of free energy
      2. $\Delta G = 0$ (equilibrium conditions prevail, and process is **isoergonic**); no free energy is liberated during isoergonic reactions
      3. $\Delta G > 0$ (process is not feasible and is **endergonic**); endergonic reactions require added energy in order to proceed

II. Standard free energy change and the equilibrium constant
   A. For the following reaction $A + B \rightleftharpoons C + D$, the equilibrium constant is expressed as $\mathbf{K_{eq} = [C][D]/[A][B]}$, where the concentrations of the reactants ([A] and [B]) and the products ([C] and [D]) correspond to concentrations at equilibrium
   B. The relationship between the standard free energy change and equilibrium constant is given by the following exponential relationship: $\mathbf{\Delta G° = -RT \ln K_{eq}}$
      1. $\Delta G°$ is the standard free energy change
      2. R is the temperature-energy coefficient (8.314 J K^{-1} mol^{-1})
      3. T is the absolute temperature in degrees Kelvin (273 + °C)
      4. The standard free energy change of the reaction is the energy change when one mole of A and one mole of B are converted to one mole each of C and D when they are present in aqueous solution at a concentration of 1.0 M
      5. The concentration of water at standard conditions is given a relative value of 1.00 (and not 55.5 M)
      6. Because most biochemical reactions occur near neutrality (pH 7.0), this pH value is used for the biochemical standard state and this convention is denoted by the prime (′) as in $\Delta G°'$ (standard free energy change at pH 7.0)
         a. Note that $[H^+] = 1 \times 10^{-7}$ M is given a relative value of 1.00
         b. Moreover, the expression for the free energy change (*not* standard free energy change) at pH = 7.0 is $\Delta G'$

III. Standard free energy change as a state function
   A. If we know the free energy change associated with each portion of a chemical process or pathway, we can calculate the free energy change for the entire process because free energy changes are state functions
   B. From the thermodynamic data of two reactions, we can calculate the standard free energy change at pH 7 ($\Delta G°'$) for a third reaction:

	$\Delta G°'$ (kJ/mol)
Glucose 1-phosphate → glucose 6-phosphate	−6.32
Glucose 6-phosphate + H_2O → glucose + P_i	−13.8
Glucose 1-phosphate + H_2O → glucose + P_i	−20.1

IV. The concentration-dependence of the free energy change

A. The free energy change at pH 7 ($\Delta G'$) is given by the following expression:

$$\Delta G' = \Delta G^{\circ\prime} - RT \ 1n \frac{[C][D]}{[A][B]}$$

B. The free energy change is a function of the standard free energy change and the actual concentrations of the reactants and products

1. Increasing the concentrations of the reactants makes the free energy change of a process more negative (more favorable)
2. Increasing the concentrations of the products makes the free energy change of a process more positive (less favorable)

Objective 2: To delineate the four main types of biochemical oxidation-reduction reactions.

V. Bioenergetics of oxidation-reduction reactions

A. There are four types of oxidation-reduction reactions in biochemistry

1. An electron can be transferred directly from donor to acceptor
2. An electron can be transferred from donor to acceptor with a proton by a process formally equivalent to the transfer of a hydrogen atom (H·)
3. Two electrons can be transferred with one proton as a hydride ion ($H:^-$)
4. There may be a direct reaction between a reductant (AH) and molecular oxygen: $2\ AH + O_2 \rightarrow 2\ AOH$

B. Oxidation-reduction reactions are considered as half-reactions

1. Half-reactions are written as reductions (the electron is a reactant): $A^+ + e^- \rightarrow A$
2. The reference standard for oxidation-reduction reactions is the hydrogen electrode; its half-reaction is written $2\ H^+ + 2\ e^- \rightarrow H_2$ and is given a value of 0.00 V, where V refers to volts
3. Electrons bear a negative charge, and compounds with a tendency to donate electrons have a negative reduction potential
4. Electrons flow to the more positive half cell
   a. By convention, the difference in the electrical potential ($\Delta\mathscr{E}$) of the acceptor (oxidant) minus the donor (reductant) is positive during electron transfer
   b. A difference in reduction potential that is positive corresponds to a negative free energy change, and both positive reduction potential and negative free energy change are associated with thermodynamically feasible reactions

VI. Standard reduction potentials

A. The greater the tendency to donate electrons and act as a reducing agent, the more negative is the reduction potential

B. *Electrons tend to go from the compound with the more negative reduction potential to that with the less negative reduction potential*

C. The compound with the more positive reduction potential accepts electrons and is reduced

D. The standard reduction potential for oxygen is highly positive (+0.818 V), and oxygen has little tendency to donate electrons and act as a reducing agent

E. The lactate dehydrogenase reaction serves as a useful prototype for an oxidation-reduction reaction

1. This reaction is given by the following chemical equation: $\text{pyruvate}^{-1} + NADH + H^+ \rightarrow \text{lactate}^{-1} + NAD^+$
2. This process consists of two half-reactions and standard reduction potentials ($\mathscr{E}^{\circ\prime}$), where the prime (′) indicates pH 7.0:
   a. $\text{Pyruvate}^- + 2\ H^+ + 2e^- \rightarrow \text{lactate}^-$ $\quad \mathscr{E}^{\circ\prime} = -0.19$ V
   b. $NAD^+ + 2\ H^+ + 2e^- \rightarrow NADH + H^+$ $\quad \mathscr{E}^{\circ\prime} = -0.32$ V
   c. Subtracting equation b from equation a yields $\text{Pyruvate}^- + NADH + H^+ \rightarrow \text{lactate}^- + NAD^+$ $\quad \Delta\mathscr{E}^{\circ\prime} = +0.13$ V
   d. Under standard conditions, electrons go to the more positive half-cell (in this case to pyruvate)
   e. By convention, a positive value for the difference in reduction potentials corresponds to actual electron flow
   f. Under standard biochemical conditions (1 M reactants and products and pH 7), the reaction will proceed from reactants to products as written
3. *The reduction of a ketone by NADH to produce an alcohol is a favorable reaction*

F. The reduction potential varies with the concentrations of the reactants and products as given by the following equation (called the Nernst equation):

$$\Delta\mathscr{E}' = \Delta\mathscr{E}^{\circ\prime} - \frac{RT}{n\mathfrak{F}} 1n \frac{[C][D]}{[A][B]}$$

1. $\Delta\mathscr{E}'$ is the actual difference in reduction potentials, and $\Delta\mathscr{E}^{\circ\prime}$ is the difference in the standard reduction potentials (1.00 M reactants and products)
2. R is the temperature-energy coefficient given above, T is the absolute temperature, and n is the number of electrons that are transferred per molecule (usually 1 or 2)
3. $\mathfrak{F}$ is the voltage-energy coefficient, or Faraday constant (96.485 kJ [V equivalent]$^{-1}$

G. Standard free energy changes

1. The following equation gives the relationship between the standard free energy change and the difference in the standard reduction potentials: $\Delta G^{\circ\prime} = -n\mathfrak{F}\,\Delta\mathscr{E}^{\circ\prime}$
2. For the lactate dehydrogenase reaction, $\Delta G^{\circ\prime} = -2 \times 96.485\ \text{kJ}\ V^{-1}\ \text{mol}^{-1} \times 0.13\ V$, or -25.1 kJ/mol, thereby indicating a great tendency to convert pyruvate to lactate

Objective 3: To describe the metabolism of superoxide, peroxide, and hydroxyl free radicals.

VII. Chemistry of oxygen, superoxide, peroxide, and hydroxyl free radicals

A. Chemical properties of oxygen

1. Oxygen is very electronegative (second only to fluoride) and attracts electrons

2. The valence shell of each oxygen atom in molecular oxygen lacks an electron, and atomic oxygen attracts electrons to form compounds in which the oxygen atom has eight electrons in its valence shell
3. The reduction of molecular oxygen by organic compounds to form water is very exergonic (PRINCIPLE 8 OF BIOENERGETICS)

B. Reactive oxygen intermediates
1. The reduction of molecular oxygen by one electron yields superoxide
   a. **Superoxide dismutase** catalyzes the dismutation of superoxide to oxygen and peroxide as follows: $2\ O_2^- + 2\ H^+ \rightarrow O_2 + H_2O_2$
   b. Cytosolic superoxide dismutase contains copper and zinc
   c. Mitochondrial (and bacterial) superoxide dismutase contains manganese
2. The reduction of molecular oxygen by two electrons yields peroxide
   a. **Catalase** catalyzes the breakdown of peroxide to oxygen and water
   b. **Glutathione peroxidase,** an enzyme that contains selenocysteine, catalyzes the reaction of glutathione with peroxide to form oxidized glutathione and water
3. The hydroxyl free radical ($OH^·$) can be formed from water by high-energy radiation (x-rays and γ-rays)
   a. The radical is more reactive than superoxide and peroxide
   b. The hydroxyl free radical, which reacts readily with nucleic acids, proteins, and lipids, can be scavenged nonenzymatically by vitamin C, vitamin E, glutathione, and β-carotene

Objective 4: To describe the role of myeloperoxidase in the white blood cell.

VIII. Bactericidal metabolism of leukocytes

A. Physiology: the generation of peroxide and hypochlorite, toxic oxygen metabolites
1. **NADPH oxidase** of leukocytes catalyzes the conversion of molecular oxygen to superoxide
2. Hydrogen peroxide and hypochlorite, formed from superoxide, are bactericidal
   a. **Superoxide dismutase** catalyzes the formation of hydrogen peroxide
   b. **Myeloperoxidase** catalyzes the formation of hypochlorite (OCl^-)

B. Pathology: the basis of chronic granulomatous disease
1. This rare disorder is due to a deficiency of NADPH oxidase
2. Neutrophils are unable to generate superoxide anion, and they are unable to kill catalase-positive microbes
   a. Nitroblue tetrazolium, a yellow, soluble compound, is a redox dye that reacts with and is reduced by superoxide produced by neutrophils to form blue precipitates
   b. Paradoxically, catalase-positive bacteria are overwhelmed by the peroxide that is produced by normal neutrophils, and catalase-negative bacteria are less sensitive to peroxide (catalase-negative bacteria adapt to endogenously generated peroxides)
   c. Catalase-positive bacteria that are cultured from infected sites in affected individuals include gram-positive and gram-negative bacteria such as *Staphylococcus aureus, Shigella, Salmonella,* and *Escherichia coli*
   d. Catalase-negative bacteria (not found in infected sites) include *Streptococcus* and *Haemophilus influenzae*

QUESTIONS

DIRECTIONS (Items 1–16): Each of the numbered items or incomplete statements in this section is followed by answers or by completions of the statement. Select the ONE lettered answer or completion that is BEST in each case. Correct answers and explanations are given at the end of the chapter.

1. The equilibrium constant for the reaction ATP + creatine $\rightleftharpoons$ ADP + creatine phosphate, which is catalyzed by creatine phosphokinase, is about 5.94×10^{-3}. What does the equilibrium constant indicate with regard to this reaction?

(A) Reaction will proceed from left to right under standard conditions
(B) Free energy of the products is less than the free energy of the reactants
(C) Standard free energy change ($\Delta G°'$) for this reaction is positive
(D) Enzyme alters the standard free energy change *in vivo*

2. The standard free energy changes ($\Delta G°'$) for reactions 5.1 and 5.2 are noted below. What is the standard free energy change for reaction 5.3?

	$\Delta G°'$ (kJ/mol)	
$ATP + H_2O \rightarrow ADP + P_i$	−30.4	(5.1)
ATP + formate + tetrahydrofolate → N^{10}–Formyltetrahydrofolate + ADP + P_i	−4.5	(5.2)
N^{10}–Formyltetrahydrofolate + H_2O → formate + tetrahydrofolate		(5.3)

(A) −25.9 kJ/mol
(B) −34.9 kJ/mol
(C) + 6.8 kJ/mol
(D) +25.9 kJ/mol
(E) +34.9 kJ/mol

3. The standard free energy changes ($\Delta G^{\circ\prime}$) of reactions 5.4 and 5.5 are noted below. What is the standard free energy change for reaction 5.6?

	$\Delta G^{\circ\prime}$ (kJ/mol)	
Asparagine + $H_2O \rightarrow$ Aspartate$^-$ + NH_4^+	−15.1	(5.4)
ATP + $H_2O \rightarrow$ AMP + PP_i	−37.4	(5.5)
ATP + aspartate$^-$ + $NH_4^+ \rightarrow$ AMP + PP_i + asparagine		(5.6)

(A) − 52.5 kJ/mol
(B) + 52.5 kJ/mol
(C) − 22.3 kJ/mol
(D) + 22.3 kJ/mol
(E) + 2.5 kJ/mol

4. McArdle disease, which results in the inability to perform anaerobic exercise, results from a deficiency of muscle phosphorylase. At 25 °C and pH 7.0, the standard free energy change ($\Delta G^{\circ\prime}$) for the phosphorylase reaction is 14.2 kJ/mol : Glycogen$_n$ + $P_i \rightleftharpoons$ glycogen$_{n-1}$ + glucose 1-phosphate. Which of the following describes the phosphorylase reaction?

(A) The equilibrium constant is greater than 1
(B) Under standard conditions (1 M reactant and product), the reaction proceeds from product to reactant
(C) The reactant possesses more free energy than the product
(D) The reaction proceeds readily in the absence of an enzyme
(E) The reaction proceeds to the right only if the equilibrium constant changes

5. When NAD^+ is reduced, what does it accept from the reductant molecule?

(A) One electron
(B) Two electrons and two protons
(C) Molecular oxygen
(D) Two electrons and one proton ($H:^-$, a hydride ion)
(E) A hydronium ion (H_3O^+)

6. Lactic acid is a normal metabolite of glucose metabolism. Lactic acidosis occurs when there is a deficiency of oxidative metabolism (myocardial infarction) and in a variety of metabolic abnormalities such as type I glycogen storage disease (von Gierke disease). The standard reduction potentials ($\mathscr{E}^{\circ\prime}$) for the reduction of pyruvate (to form lactate) and NAD^+ (to form NADH + H^+) are noted in the following diagram.

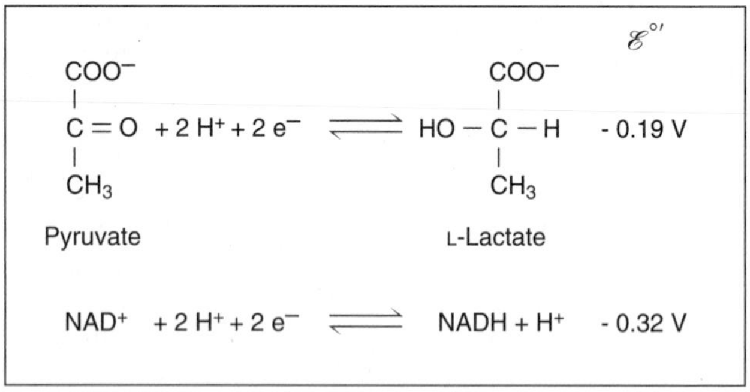

Pyruvate (COO^-–C=O–CH_3)		L-Lactate (COO^-–HO–C–H–CH_3)	$\mathscr{E}^{\circ\prime}$
C=O + 2 H^+ + 2 e^-	$\rightleftharpoons$	HO − C − H	- 0.19 V
NAD^+ + 2 H^+ + 2 e^-	$\rightleftharpoons$	NADH + H^+	- 0.32 V

What is the $\Delta\mathscr{E}^{\circ\prime}$ for the following reaction: pyruvate^{-1} + NADH + $H^+ \rightarrow$ lactate^{-1} + NAD^+?

(A) − 0.52 V
(B) + 0.52 V
(C) − 0.13 V
(D) + 0.13 V

7. Molecular oxygen is a good oxidant because

(A) each oxygen atom contains a complete octet of electrons in the outer shell
(B) it is very electronegative
(C) it has a low affinity for electrons
(D) it is inert
(E) it readily donates its electrons to many acceptors

8. Addition of one electron to molecular oxygen, which occurs following coronary thrombosis and cardiac reperfusion, yields which of the following molecules?

(A) Hydroxyl free radical
(B) Hydroperoxy free radical
(C) Peroxide
(D) Superoxide

9. Which of the following metals is found in cytosolic superoxide dismutase, which is an enzyme that may be defective in amyotrophic lateral sclerosis?

(A) Copper and zinc
(B) Iron
(C) Magnesium
(D) Manganese
(E) Molybdenum

10. Which one of the following substances, which is generated by ionizing radiation, is most reactive with biological molecules such as DNA, RNA, protein, and lipids?

(A) Hydroxyl free radical
(B) Molecular oxygen
(C) Peroxide
(D) Superoxide

11. A deficiency of which one of the following enzymes occurs in a peroxisomal disorder?

(A) Catalase
(B) Glutathione peroxidase
(C) Succinate dehydrogenase
(D) Superoxide dismutase
(E) Xanthine dehydrogenase

12. An individual is exposed to hypoxia at high altitudes (20,000 feet above sea level) during decompression in an airplane. What would be the first symptom to occur?

(A) Decreased bowel motility
(B) Decreased myocardial contraction
(C) Decreased urine output
(D) Easy fatigability
(E) Unconsciousness

Items 13–16

History

The patient is a 6-month-old male who was brought to the pediatrician by his mother because of fever of 38.9 °C (102 °F) and the recent onset of skin lesions. He had several previous bouts of upper respiratory infection. The parents are not in a high-risk group for AIDS. The patient has two sisters (aged 3 and 5 years), who are healthy, and two maternal male cousins who succumbed to pneumonia before 3 years of age.

Physical Examination

Temperature, 39.2 °C (102.6 °F); respiratory rate, 44/min (normal, 33/min); pulse, 176/min (normal, 150/min); weight, 13.5 lb (5th percentile). He has marked cervical lymphadenopathy, purulent circumoral skin lesions, and hepatosplenomegaly. Rales (abnormal sounds detected with a stethoscope) were heard on both the left and right sides of the posterior thorax.

Laboratory

Hematocrit and hemoglobin, normal
White blood count, 26,000/μL (normal, 5000–17,000/μL)
Neutrophils, 72% (normal, 54–62%)
Lymphocytes, 23% (normal, 25–33%)
Monocytes, 5% (normal, 3–7%)
IgG, 410 mg/dL (normal, 240–620 mg/dL)
IgM, 52 mg/dL (normal, 25–60 mg/dL)
IgA 35 mg/dL (normal, 25–75 mg/dL)
IgE, trace (normal, trace)
Adenosine deaminase, normal
Nucleoside phosphorylase, normal
Skin lesion, gram-positive bacteria, and no acid-fast bacilli
Stimulated neutrophil nitroblue tetrazolium (NBT) test, no reaction (normal, positive reaction)
Neutrophil phagocytosis, normal
Chest x-ray, diffuse interstitial infiltration

13. Nitroblue tetrazolium is reduced directly by which of the following compounds?
    (A) Oxygen (O_2)
    (B) Superoxide (O_2^-)
    (C) Peroxide (H_2O_2)
    (D) Water (H_2O)

14. Inability to react with nitroblue tetrazolium indicates that the patient's neutrophils lacked normal activity of which one of the following enzymes?
    (A) Cathepsin
    (B) Lysozyme
    (C) Myeloperoxidase
    (D) NADPH oxidase
    (E) Superoxide dismutase

15. Myeloperoxidase catalyzes the physiological reaction of hydrogen peroxide (H_2O_2) and
    (A) chloride ion
    (B) glutathione
    (C) hydroxyl free radical ($OH^·$)
    (D) NADPH
    (E) superoxide (O_2^-)

16. What is the most likely diagnosis for this patient?
    (A) Agammaglobulinemia
    (B) AIDS
    (C) Myeloperoxidase deficiency
    (D) Tuberculosis
    (E) Chronic granulomatous disease

ANSWERS AND EXPLANATIONS

1. The answer is C: the standard free energy change ($\Delta G^{\circ\prime}$) for this reaction is positive. An equilibrium constant less than 1 corresponds to a positive standard free energy change, and the reaction will proceed from products to reactants under standard conditions. Moreover, the free energy of the products is greater than that of the reactants ($G_{products} - G_{reactants}$ is positive), and the reaction will proceed from right to left under standard conditions. Enzymes do not alter the free energy change of a reaction; enzymes accelerate the rate of a reaction by decreasing the free energy of activation ($\Delta G^{\ddagger}$). Creatine phosphate is a storage form of energy-rich bonds in cardiac and skeletal muscle and brain. When the cellular concentration of ATP falls, creatine phosphate readily donates its phosphoryl group to ADP to regenerate ATP. Elevation of serum creatine phosphokinase occurs within 6 hours in half of the patients following a myocardial infarction and in almost all patients within 12 hours. After release into the circulation, the M isozyme form of the enzyme undergoes a hydrolysis of its carboxyterminal lysine residue catalyzed by plasma carboxypeptidase N. The recently released and unmodified isozyme can be differentiated from the previously released isozyme. Moreover, it is possible to detect increases in the proportion of the unmodified form following a myocardial infarction before changes in the total activity occur, and this is helpful in establishing the diagnosis within 6 hours in most cases. Serum creatine phosphokinase is also elevated in muscular dystrophy. *Biochemistry*, p. 67.
2. The answer is A: −25.9 kJ/mol. Equation 5.2 (ATP + formate + tetrahydrofolate → N^{10}–formyltetrahydrofolate + ADP + P_i) and the sign of the standard free energy change are reversed before addition to equation 5.1 to yield equation 5.3. The corresponding free energy change is now obtained by addition: −30.4 kJ/mol + (4.5 kJ/mol) = −25.9 kJ/mol. This calculation is valid because free energy changes are state functions, and free energy changes do not depend upon the pathway but on the initial and final states. N^{10}-Formyltetrahydrofolate functions as a formyl group donor; although this compound does not have the group transfer potential of a high-energy bond, the transfer potential is more than

adequate to allow its participation in purine nucleotide synthesis.

3. The answer is C: –22.3 kJ/mol. If equation 5.4 is subtracted from equation 5.5, equation 5.6 results. The standard free energy changes are –37.4 kJ/mol–(–15.1 kJ/mol) = –22.3 kJ/mol.
4. The answer is B: Under standard conditions (1 M reactant and product), the reaction proceeds from product to reactant. A positive standard free energy change indicates that the reaction is endergonic, the equilibrium constant is less than 1, and the reaction can proceed from products to reactants under standard conditions (1 M reactants and products). At physiological concentrations of phosphate and glucose 1-phosphate, however, the reaction proceeds from reactants to products. This reaction, which has a standard free energy change of +14.2 kJ/mol, has an equilibrium constant of 3.24×10^{-3} at 25 °C. If the reactant possessed more free energy than products, the difference ($G_{products}-G_{reactants}$) would be negative and not positive as noted. Almost all biochemical reactions are catalyzed by enzymes, and the enzyme that catalyzes this reaction is glycogen phosphorylase. This enzyme provides substrate for glycolysis and ATP production. A hereditary deficiency of muscle glycogen phosphorylase (McArdle disease) is accompanied by easy fatigability and a failure to generate lactate following exercise. Thermodynamic data provide information on whether a process or reaction can or cannot occur and no information on the rate of a process. The science of kinetics deals with reaction rates. The equilibrium constant does not vary at constant temperature, pressure, pH, and ionic strength. *Biochemistry*, p. 68.
5. The answer is D: two electrons and one proton ($H:^-$, a hydride ion). The transfer of a hydride ion yields NADH, the bona fide product. There are only a few biochemical reactions that involve one-electron transfers and free radicals. Redox substrates, such as FMN and FAD, transfer reductants as two electrons and two protons, although these transfers may involve two successive one electron–one proton transfers. Molecular oxygen is an oxidant and not a reductant. *Biochemistry*, p. 69.
6. The answer is D: +0.13 V. $\Delta\mathscr{E}^{\circ\prime} = \mathscr{E}^{\circ\prime}_{oxidant} - \mathscr{E}^{\circ\prime}_{reductant}$; $\Delta\mathscr{E}^{\circ\prime}$ = –0.19 V–(–0.32 V) = +0.13 V. A positive standard reduction potential is associated with a negative standard free energy change, and such reactions are exergonic and proceed from reactants to products under standard conditions. The reduction potential and free energy change vary with the concentrations of reactants and products. Increasing the concentrations of the reactants makes a process more favorable, and increasing the concentrations of the products makes a process less favorable. That the reduction of pyruvate is exergonic explains why the circulating lactate/pyruvate ratio favors lactate. Lactate dehydrogenase is a cytosolic enzyme, and the ratio of lactate to pyruvate reflects the cytosolic redox state. The ratio of β-hydroxybutyrate to acetoacetate reflects the mitochondrial redox state.
7. The answer is B: it is very electronegative. Oxygen is the second-ranking element in electronegativity (fluoride is the most electronegative). Oxygen has a strong propensity to attract electrons because of its high affinity for them. The valence shell of each oxygen atom in molecular oxygen lacks an electron, and oxygen has a strong tendency to form compounds, such as water, with a complete octet of electrons in its valence shell. *Biochemistry*, p. 72.
8. The answer is D: superoxide. The addition of one electron to molecular oxygen yields superoxide ($O_2^{\bar{}}$). The addition of two electrons results in peroxide (O_2^{2-}). The hydroxyl free radical is the compound made of oxygen and hydrogen atoms ($OH^{\cdot}$), a species that readily reacts with a variety of organic compounds including lipids, proteins, and nucleic acids. The hydroperoxy free radical is represented by $HOO^{\cdot}$, also a reactive substance. *Biochemistry*, p. 73.
9. The answer is A: copper and zinc. Molecular oxygen is a singlet molecule (it contains two unpaired electrons) and does not react readily with organic compounds or hydrogen in the absence of a transitional metal ion. Superoxide dismutase and other enzymes that catalyze reactions with oxygen contain transition metals to promote reaction of molecular oxygen. Cytosolic superoxide dismutase contains copper and zinc. Both mitochondrial and bacterial superoxide dismutase contain manganese. Several enzymes that react with oxygenated species contain heme (e.g., catalase); heme contains iron, also a transition metal. Molybdenum, a transition metal, is a component of xanthine oxidase of purine metabolism and aldehyde oxidase of catecholamine metabolism. Magnesium is not a transition metal, but it forms complexes with ATP and other nucleotides to form enzyme substrates. *Biochemistry*, p. 73.
10. The answer is A: hydroxyl free radical. The hydroxyl free radical reacts with most biological molecules. The hydroxyl free radical can result from the interaction of high-energy x-rays and γ-rays with water. This reactivity explains the mutagenicity of these high-energy rays in cells. Moreover, deletions, fragmentation, and mutations of DNA that result from ionizing radiation can cause cancer. Peroxide is also a reactive substance. Superoxide and molecular oxygen are less reactive. *Biochemistry*, p. 73.
11. The answer is A: catalase. A deficiency of catalase is called acatalasemia (acatalasia), and this disorder is often accompanied by lesions of the oral cavity that result from bacterial infections due to increased sensitivity to oral bacteria. Catalase mediates the transformation of hydrogen peroxide to water and molecular oxygen according to the following equation: $H_2O_2 \rightarrow \frac{1}{2}O_2 + H_2O$. Most catalase occurs in the peroxisomes of cells, but some occurs in the cytosol. Red blood cells, which lack peroxisomes, also contain catalase. Succinate dehydrogenase occurs in the inner mitochondrial membrane. Superoxide dismutase, different forms of which occur in mitochondria and in the cytosol, catalyzes the conversion of two molecules of superoxide (plus two protons) to form hydrogen peroxide (H_2O_2) and molecular oxygen (O_2). Glutathione peroxidase, a cytosolic enzyme, catalyzes the destruction of peroxide to water and oxidized glutathione according to the following equation: $H_2O_2 + 2\,GSH \rightarrow 2\,H_2O + GSSG$. Glutathione peroxidase contains selenium, an essential element. That selenium is essential suggests that glutathione peroxidase is vital for the life of the cell. *Xanthine dehydrogenase,* a cytosolic enzyme, catalyzes the oxidation of xanthine to uric acid according to the following equation: xanthine + H_2O + $NAD^+ \rightarrow$ uric acid + NADH + H^+. When thiol groups of xanthine dehydrogenase are oxidized, forming disulfide bonds, the activity changes from xanthine dehydrogenase to xanthine oxidase. *Xanthine oxidase* activity is represented by the following: xanthine + O_2 + $H_2O \rightarrow$ uric acid + H_2O_2. *Biochemistry,* p. 74.
12. The answer is E: unconsciousness. The central nervous system is the organ most sensitive to hypoxia and anoxia, and unconsciousness is the first symptom that results from these conditions. Brain cells survive only 3–5

minutes without oxygen; brain cells die when anoxic conditions are longer. Heart, liver, and kidney cells can survive from 30 minutes to 2 hours without oxygen. In contrast, skeletal muscle, fibroblasts, and skin cells can survive several hours without oxygen.

13. The answer is B: superoxide (O_2^-). Oxygen, peroxide, and water are not good reducing agents and do not react with nitroblue tetrazolium. In contrast, superoxide can undergo either oxidation (and reduce nitroblue tetrazolium) or reduction (to form peroxide). *Nelson,* p. 567.
14. The answer is D: NADPH oxidase. Neutrophils rely on anaerobic glycolysis for their energy. When activated by bacteria, oxygen consumption is activated 100-fold. This is catalyzed by a four-component system called NADPH oxidase (sometimes called the respiratory burst oxidase). The enzyme consists of a cytochrome *b* made of an α- and β-chain, integral plasma membrane and lysosomal membrane proteins, and two cytosolic proteins of unknown function. The gene corresponding to the ß-chain is X linked, and the other genes are autosomal. Superoxide *per se* is not highly bactericidal. It is the precursor of peroxide, hydroxyl free radicals, and hypochlorite, all of which are bactericidal. The nitroblue tetrazolium test can be easily performed on a drop of fresh whole blood on a glass slide followed by microscopic examination. The water-soluble, yellow precursor is converted to an insoluble blue pigment generated by the activated oxidase complex. Lysozyme is an enzyme that degrades specific carbohydrates in bacterial cell walls; cathepsins degrade proteins. *Nelson,* p. 567.
15. The answer is A: chloride ion. Myeloperoxidase catalyzes the formation of hypochlorous acid (HOCl) from hydrogen peroxide and chloride ion. Hypochlorous acid, which is present in commercial household disinfectants, is a bactericidal substance produced by neutrophils. Although NADPH oxidase deficiency is very rare (one per million live births), myeloperoxidase deficiency is very common (one in 2000). Individuals with myeloperoxidase deficiency, however, rarely exhibit symptoms, indicating that this reaction is redundant. *Nelson,* p. 567.
16. The answer is E: chronic granulomatous disease. In contrast to myeloperoxidase deficiency, NADPH oxidase deficiency is associated with chronic infections. Granulomas, which are walled-off collections of inflammatory debris, result from the inability to digest and kill all bacteria. The serum tests rule out agammaglobulinemia (an absence of gamma globulins). The absence of acid-fast bacilli rule unlikely the presence of tuberculosis, and the absence of lymphopenia (decreased number of white cells) rules unlikely the presence of AIDS. Individuals with myeloperoxidase deficiency suffer from unusual infections only when they also have diabetes mellitus. The bacteria that are troublesome in patients with chronic granulomatous disease are catalase positive. NADPH oxidase-deficient white cells cannot scavenge peroxide from catalase-positive bacteria, hence the failure to kill all such bacteria and the resulting granuloma formation. It is postulated that bacteria that lack catalase generate peroxide that can be scavenged by the white cell for killing bacteria. Individuals with chronic granulomatous disease are treated with antibiotics. *Biochemistry,* p. 74; *Nelson,* p. 567.

REFERENCES

Behrman, R. E. *Nelson Textbook of Pediatrics,* 14th ed. Philadelphia, W. B. Saunders Company, 1992.

Roskoski, R., Jr. *Biochemistry.* Philadelphia, W. B. Saunders Company, 1996.

CHAPTER SIX

PRINCIPLES OF METABOLISM

SYNOPSIS

OBJECTIVES

1. To define and identify high-energy bonds.
2. To use the fundamental principles of bioenergetics to analyze biochemical reactions.
3. To describe the reactions of ATP.
4. To explain the role of energy charge in metabolic regulation.
5. To state Lipmann's law and its relationship to metabolism.

Objective 1: To define and identify high-energy bonds.

I. Energy-rich and energy-poor bonds
   A. Classification of energy-rich and energy-poor compounds
      1. Definitions
         a. Compounds with a standard free energy of hydrolysis of –30 kJ/mol and more negative possess a high-energy bond and are energy rich
         b. Compounds with a standard free energy of hydrolysis less negative than –30 kJ/mol possess a low-energy bond and are energy poor
         c. The group transfer potential of a compound is the positive value corresponding to its free energy of hydrolysis
      2. Principles of biochemical usage
         a. The transfer of a group to water (hydrolysis) provides a standard for use in comparing reactions
         b. The more positive the standard group transfer potential (the more negative the standard free energy of hydrolysis), the greater is the tendency to transfer the group to an acceptor
   B. Examples of energy-rich compounds (Table 6–1)
      1. Special oxygen esters (aminoacyl-tRNAs and acylcarnitines) are oxygen monoesters that invariably possess high group transfer potential
      2. Special phosphodiesters involving nucleotide bonds in DNA and RNA are energy rich
      3. **ATP** is the historical prototype of a high-energy compound, and ATP's importance in the energy economy of the cell is emphasized throughout the study of biochemistry
         a. The hydrolysis reactions of ATP are illustrated in Figure 6–1
         b. *ATP possesses two high-energy bonds, and each is a simple acid anhydride of phosphoric acid*
         c. The hydrolysis of 5′-AMP is accompanied by a standard free energy change of only –9.6 kJ/mol
         d. 5′-AMP is a phosphomonoester and is a low-energy compound
   C. Examples of energy-poor compounds
      1. Ordinary oxygen esters with phosphate, sulfate, or carboxylate are energy-poor compounds with a low group transfer potential
      2. Ordinary phosphodiesters, for example, those occurring in complex lipids, are energy poor

Objective 2: To use the fundamental principles of bioenergetics to analyze biochemical reactions.

II. Principles of bioenergetics and the feasibility of biochemical reactions
   A. Counting high-energy bonds in transferase reactions, where ~ represents a high-energy bond
      1. PRINCIPLE 1 states that when an equal number of energy-rich bonds occur in the reactants and products, the transferase reaction is functionally isoergonic and can proceed in either direction
         a. The reaction catalyzed by creatine phosphokinase illustrates PRINCIPLE 1

$$\text{ATP } (2\sim) + \text{creatine } (0\sim) \rightleftharpoons \text{ADP } (1\sim) + \text{phosphocreatine } (1\sim) \quad (6.1)$$

         b. The only exception to PRINCIPLE 1 is the inability of ATP to phosphorylate pyruvate; the reverse reaction between ADP and phosphoenolpyruvate to form ATP and pyruvate is unidirectional
      2. PRINCIPLE 2 states that when the number of energy-rich bonds is greater in the reactants than in the products, the reaction is exergonic and the conversion of reactants to products is favored
         a. The reaction catalyzed by hexokinase illustrates PRINCIPLE 2

$$\text{ATP } (2\sim) + \text{glucose } (0\sim) \rightarrow \text{ADP } (1\sim) + \text{glucose 6-phosphate } (0\sim) \quad (6.2)$$

TABLE 6–1. Energy-Rich and Energy-Poor Compounds

General Class	Examples
Energy rich	
Cyclic phosphodiester	Cyclic 3′,5′-adenosine monophosphate (cyclic AMP)
Glycoside diphosphate	UDP-glucose
Mixed acid anhydride	1,3-Bisphosphoglycerate, carbamoyl phosphate
Nucleotide phosphodiester	RNA, DNA
Phosphoramidate (P–N)	Phosphocreatine
Phosphoenolpyruvate	Phosphoenolpyruvate
Simple acid anhydride	ATP, ADP
Special oxygen esters	Acylcarnitine, aminoacyl-tRNA
Sulfonium derivative	*S*-Adenosylmethionine
Thioester	Acetyl coenzyme A
Energy poor	
Amide	Glutamine
Glycoside	Glycogen, lactose
Ordinary oxygen ester	Glucose 6-phosphate
Peptide bond	Glutathione, insulin
Phosphodiester	Phosphatidylcholine

b. This reaction proceeds with the loss of one high-energy bond and, in this case, is unidirectional

3. PRINCIPLE 3 states that when the number of energy-rich bonds is greater in the products than in the reactants, the reaction is endergonic and the conversion of products to reactants is favored

   a. This is equivalent to PRINCIPLE 2 except that the products contain more high-energy bonds than do the reactants

   b. The synthesis of uridine diphosphate glucose provides an example of this situation

$$\text{UTP } (2\sim) + \text{glucose 1-phosphate } (0\sim) \rightleftharpoons \text{UDP-glucose } (2\sim) + PP_i\ (1\sim) \qquad (6.3)$$

   c. This reaction is bidirectional

4. PRINCIPLE 4 states that when the number of energy-poor bonds in the reactants and products of a transferase reaction is the same (no energy-rich bonds), the reaction is functionally isoergonic and can proceed in either direction

   a. The interconversion of glucose 6-phosphate (a low-energy compound) and glucose 1-phosphate (a low-energy compound) as catalyzed by phosphoglucomutase illustrates PRINCIPLE 4

$$\text{Glucose 6-phosphate } (0\sim) \rightleftharpoons \text{glucose 1-phosphate } (0\sim) \qquad (6.4)$$

   b. This reaction is bidirectional

5. PRINCIPLE 5 states that the hydrolysis of energy-rich or energy-poor compounds is exergonic and thermodynamically favored; such reactions, moreover, are unidirectional

B. Oxidation-reduction and decarboxylation reactions

1. PRINCIPLE 6 states that decarboxylation reactions are exergonic

2. PRINCIPLE 7 of bioenergetics states that simple oxidation-reduction reactions are bidirectional and functionally isoergonic

   a. Simple oxidation-reduction reactions do not involve molecular oxygen, a simultaneous decarboxylation, or the formation of a carboxylic acid

$$\underset{\text{ATP}}{RO-PO_2^-\!-O\sim PO_2^-\!-O\sim PO_3^{-}} + HO-H \longrightarrow \underset{\text{ADP}}{RO-PO_2^-\!-O\sim PO_2^-\!-OH} + \underset{P_i}{HO-PO_2^-} \qquad \Delta G^{\circ\prime} = -35.5\ \text{kJ mol}^{-1}$$

$$\underset{\text{ADP}}{RO-PO_2^-\!-O\sim PO_3^{-}} + HO-H \longrightarrow \underset{\text{AMP}}{RO-PO_2^-\!-OH} + \underset{P_i}{HO-PO_2^-} \qquad \Delta G^{\circ\prime} = -36.3\ \text{kJ mol}^{-1}$$

$$\text{AMP} + HO-H \longrightarrow \underset{\text{Adenosine}}{R-O-H} + \underset{P_i}{HO-PO_2^-} \qquad \Delta G^{\circ\prime} = -9.6\ \text{kJ mol}^{-1}$$

FIGURE 6-1. Hydrolysis of ATP.

b. The reaction catalyzed by lactate dehydrogenase is an example of a simple oxidation-reduction reaction

$$\text{Pyruvate} + \text{NADH} + \text{H}^+ \rightleftharpoons \text{lactate} + \text{NAD}^+ \quad (6.5)$$

3. PRINCIPLE 8 states that reactions of organic substances with oxygen are exergonic and unidirectional

C. Other reactions
1. Lyase reactions, except for decarboxylation reactions, are generally bidirectional
2. Generation and deprotonation of a carboxylic acid from an aldehyde is exergonic and unidirectional; these are simple oxidation-reduction reactions, but they result in the formation of a carboxylic acid that dissociates into a carboxylate and proton

Objective 3: To describe the reactions of ATP.

III. Four reactions of ATP (Fig. 6–2)
A. Type I reactions: transfer of the phosphoryl group
1. *The phosphoryl group, or phosphorylium ion (PO_3^-), is transferred and not the phosphate group ($-OPO_3^{2-}$)*
2. This distinction between phosphoryl and phosphate is often a source of confusion, and the term "phosphate transfer," although commonly used, is imprecise

B. Type II reactions: transfer of the adenylyl group
1. Transfer of the adenylyl group to an acceptor and the displacement of intact inorganic pyrophosphate is the second most common class of reaction undergone by ATP
2. Besides ATP, a variety of other nucleotides undergo a similar reaction

C. Type III reactions: transfer of the pyrophosphoryl group
1. The conversion of ribose 5-phosphate to phosphoribosylpyrophosphate (PRPP) is an example of this class of reaction
2. The attachment of pyrophosphate to a hemiacetal group results in a glycoside diphosphate, and each glycoside diphosphate possesses two high-energy bonds

D. Type IV reaction: displacement of triphosphate
1. *S*-Adenosylmethionine biosynthesis is the only example of this process
2. The displaced triphosphate is hydrolyzed to phosphate and pyrophosphate prior to its liberation from the enzyme

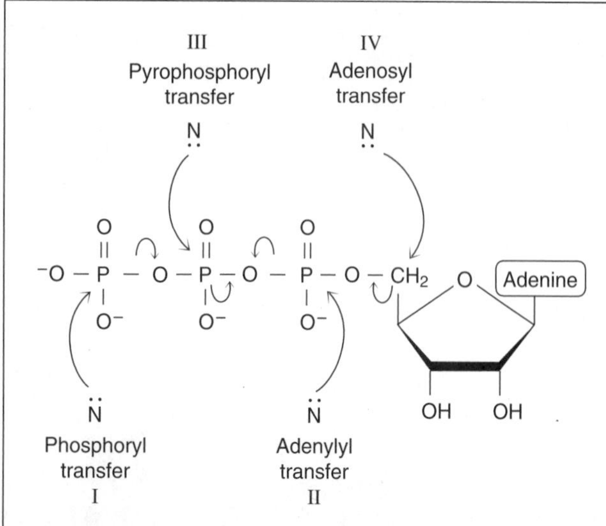

FIGURE 6-2. The four types of reactions of ATP.

IV. Phosphorylation of purine and pyrimidine nucleosides
A. The structures of the common purine and pyrimidine bases are shown in Figure 14–1
B. A family of enzymes catalyze the phosphorylation of (1) AMP and dAMP; (2) GMP and dGMP; (3) CMP, dCMP, and UMP; and (4) dTMP
C. **Nucleoside diphosphokinase** catalyzes the reaction of the nucleoside diphosphates (NDP) according to the following equation, where NTP represents any of the physiological nucleoside triphosphates

$$\text{ATP } (2\sim) + \text{NDP } (1\sim) \rightleftharpoons \text{ADP } (1\sim) + \text{NTP } (2\sim) \quad (6.6)$$

Objective 4: To explain the role of energy charge in metabolic regulation.

V. Maintenance of a nearly constant energy charge in cells by regulation of energy-producing and energy-consuming reactions
A. The energy charge is defined by the following equation:

$$\text{Energy charge} = \frac{[\text{ATP}] + 0.5\,[\text{ADP}]}{[\text{ATP}] + [\text{ADP}] + [\text{AMP}]} \quad (6.7)$$

1. The energy charge reflects the molar fraction of the total adenine nucleotide pool (ATP + ADP + AMP) that contains high-energy bonds
2. The factor of 0.5 before ADP reflects ADP's high-energy bond content as one-half that of ATP

B. Rates of energy-producing and energy-consuming reactions are often controlled by the relative concentration of ATP, ADP, and AMP
C. Under physiological conditions in all organisms and cells, the energy charge value hovers around 0.85

Objective 5: To state Lipmann's law and its relationship to metabolism.

VI. ATP and energy exchange: Lipmann's law (PRINCIPLE 10)
A. Lipmann's law states that all forms of life (plants, animals, and microorganisms) use ATP as the fundamental unit of biochemical energy
1. Besides transfer of the phosphoryl group, ATP is able to generate pyrophosphate, and the subsequent hydrolysis of pyrophosphate serves to pull many reactions forward
2. ADP cannot generate pyrophosphate by a comparable mechanism
3. This characteristic explains why ATP and not ADP is the common currency of energy exchange in biochemistry

B. There are no exceptions to PRINCIPLE 10, and this principle assumes the status of a law

C. It must be emphasized that *the source of energy for most metabolic transformations does not result directly from a simple hydrolysis of ATP*

D. ATP is able to function as the universal currency of exchange because it exists in cells at concentrations in the cell that are far removed from hydrolytic equilibrium

VII. The high-energy bond and group activation

A. The combination of a fatty acid with coenzyme A through a high-energy thioester bond confers a high group transfer potential on the acyl group

1. Acyl-CoA can then react with an acceptor to form an acyl derivative and the coenzyme A leaving group

2. Coenzyme A is said to "activate" the acyl group; acetyl-CoA, for example, is sometimes called "active" acetate

B. This same principle and terminology are applicable to the other groups that participate in the formation of the energy-rich bonds

1. Amino acyl-tRNAs, for example, represent activated amino acids that are used in protein synthesis (PRINCIPLE 17 OF BIOCHEMISTRY)

2. Uridine diphosphate sugars represent activated monosaccharides that are used in carbohydrate synthesis

QUESTIONS

DIRECTIONS Each of the numbered items or incomplete statements in this section is followed by answers or by completions of the statement. Select the ONE lettered answer or completion that is BEST in each case. Correct answers and explanations are given at the end of the chapter.

1. The standard free energy of hydrolysis of acetyl-CoA is about –35 kJ/mol:

$$\text{Acetyl-CoA} + H_2O \rightleftharpoons \text{acetate}^- + H^+ + \text{CoA}$$

Which of the following is a true statement regarding the biochemical properties of acetyl-CoA?

(A) It is an energy-poor compound
(B) It possesses a low group transfer potential
(C) It rapidly decomposes in water
(D) It represents an activated donor of the acetyl group
(E) It can be formed from acetate and coenzyme A in the absence of added energy

2. Type I glycogen storage disease is due to a deficiency of glucose-6-phosphatase. This enzyme catalyzes the following reaction:

$$\text{Glucose 6-phosphate} + H_2O \rightleftharpoons \text{glucose} + P_i$$

What are the bioenergetics and direction of this process?

(A) endergonic and unidirectional
(B) isoergonic and bidirectional
(C) isoergonic and unidirectional
(D) exergonic and bidirectional
(E) exergonic and unidirectional

3. A deficiency of pyruvate kinase in erythrocytes causes a hemolytic anemia. This enzyme catalyzes the following reaction:

$$\text{ATP} + \text{pyruvate} \rightleftharpoons \text{ADP} + \text{phosphoenolpyruvate}$$

Which one of the following is a true statement regarding this reaction?

(A) The reactants contain more high-energy bonds than the products
(B) The products contain more high-energy bonds than the reactants
(C) The reaction proceeds from right to left under standard conditions
(D) The reaction is bidirectional *in vivo*

4. The following reaction is catalyzed by uridine diphosphate glucose (UDP-glucose) pyrophosphorylase:

$$\text{UTP} + \text{glucose 1-phosphate} \rightleftharpoons \text{UDP-glucose} + PP_i$$

Which one of the following is a true statement regarding this reaction?

(A) The reactants contain two high-energy bonds
(B) The products contain two high-energy bonds
(C) The reaction is exergonic
(D) The conversion of reactants to products is favored under standard conditions

5. The following reaction is catalyzed by phosphoglucose isomerase:

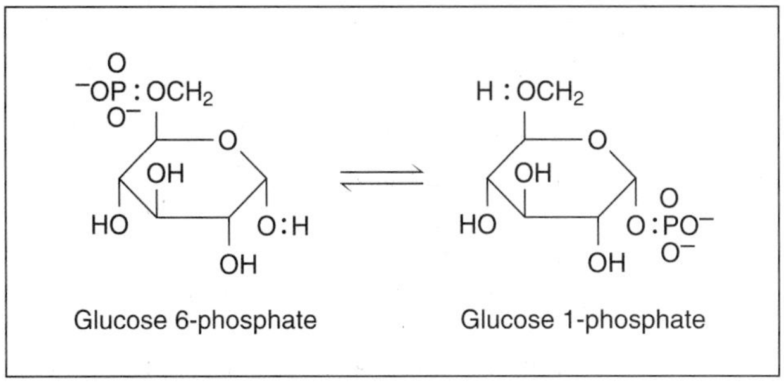

Glucose 6-phosphate ⇌ Glucose 1-phosphate

Which one of the following is a true statement regarding this reaction?

(A) There is one high-energy bond in the reactant
(B) There is no high-energy bond in the product
(C) The reaction is pulled forward by hydrolysis
(D) The reaction is unidirectional

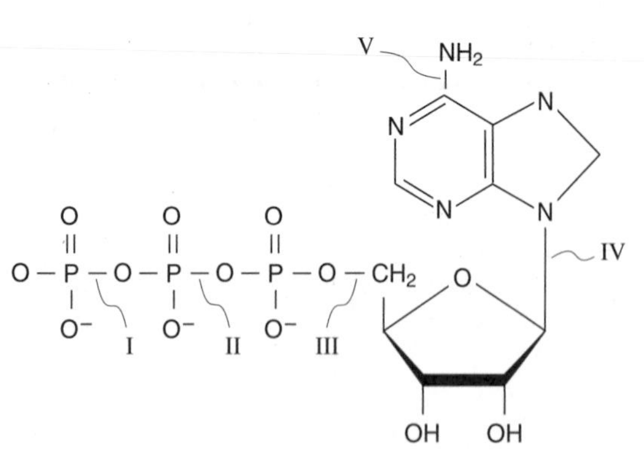

V NH2
N N N N
O O O
O – P – O – P – O – P – O – CH2 O IV
O⁻ O⁻ O⁻
I II III
OH OH

DIRECTIONS. (Items 6–7): Each set of matching questions in this section refers to the above illustration with several labeled options followed by numbered items. For each numbered item, select the ONE lettered option that is most closely associated with it.

6. The synthesis of glucose 6-phosphate from ATP and glucose involves cleavage of which one of the following bonds?
   (A) I
   (B) II
   (C) III
   (D) IV
   (E) V

7. Cleavage of which of the following bonds occurs during the synthesis of *S*-adenosylmethionine from methionine?
   (A) I only
   (B) II only
   (C) I and II
   (D) I and III
   (E) II and III

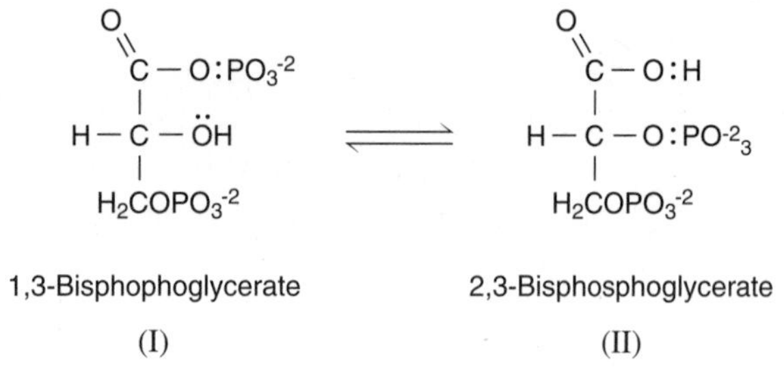

$$\underset{\text{1,3-Bisphophoglycerate (I)}}{O{=}C(-O{:}PO_3^{-2})-H-C-\ddot{O}H-H_2COPO_3^{-2}} \rightleftharpoons \underset{\text{2,3-Bisphosphoglycerate (II)}}{O{=}C(-O{:}H)-H-C-O{:}PO^{-2}_3-H_2COPO_3^{-2}}$$

1,3-Bisphophoglycerate (I)

2,3-Bisphosphoglycerate (II)

8. Based upon the fundamental principles of bioenergetics, which statement is true regarding the above reaction?
   (A) The equilibrium constant is about 1
   (B) There is one high-energy bond in the reactant
   (C) There is one high-energy bond in the product
   (D) The reaction is functionally isoergonic
   (E) The standard free energy change of this reaction is positive

9. Cytidine diphosphocholine is formed from CTP and choline phosphate according to the reaction shown in the diagram at the top of page 43. Based upon the fundamental principles of bioenergetics, which of the following is a true statement regarding this reaction?
   (A) the number of high-energy bonds in the reactants is one
   (B) the number of high-energy bonds in the products is two
   (C) the reaction is endergonic
   (D) the equilibrium constant is much greater than 1

Items 10–15

History

A 34-year-old male auto mechanic presents with malaise, fatigue, and an unintentional 4.5 kg (10 lb) weight loss over the past 2 months. The patient acknowledged that he is homosexual. Several of his close friends, who were taking daily medication, had been hospitalized with pneumonia and other infections. The patient was unaware of exposure to individuals with tuberculosis. The patient denied drug abuse. He had never received a blood transfusion. The patient stated that he had infectious mononucleosis 15 years previously.

Physical Examination

Temperature, 37°C (98.6°F), pulse 65/min, respirations, 14/min, blood pressure 124/76 mm Hg. Painless oral leukoplakia was observed on the lateral aspect of the tongue. There was no lymphadenopathy, thrush, petechiae, hepatosplenomegaly, skin lesions, or evidence of Kaposi sarcoma.

Laboratory

White blood cell count, 3500/μL (normal, 4500–11,000/μL)
Polymorphonuclear leukocytes, 52% (normal, 54–62%)
Lymphocytes, 24% (normal, 23–33%)
Monocytes, 4% (normal, 3–7%)
Red blood cell count, 3.7 million/μL (normal ♂, 4.3–5.7 million/μL)
Hematocrit, 36% (normal ♂, 39–49%)
Hemoglobin, 11.1 g/dL (normal ♂, 13.5–17.5 g/dL)
Mean cell volume, 97 fL (normal, 80–100 fL)
Mean corpuscular hemoglobin concentration (MCHC), 33% Hb/cell (normal, 31–37%)
Platelets, 100,000/μL (normal, 150,000–450,000/μL)
Corrected reticulocyte count, 1 (normal, 1)
CD4$^+$ lymphocyte count, 220/μL (normal, >500/μL)
Serum glucose, 88 mg/dL (normal, 70–105 mg/dL)
Total/direct bilirubin, 0.8/0.1 mg/dL (normal, 0.2–1.0/0.0–0.2 mg/dL)
Serum iron 78 μg/dL (normal, 65–175 μg/dL)
Total serum protein, 8.5 g/dL (normal, 6.4–8.3 g/dL)
Albumin, 4.2 g/dL (normal, 3.5–5.0 g/dL)
Globulin, 4.3 g/dL (normal, 2.2–4.0 g/dL)
Chest x-ray, normal
Blood was taken for HIV antibody determination

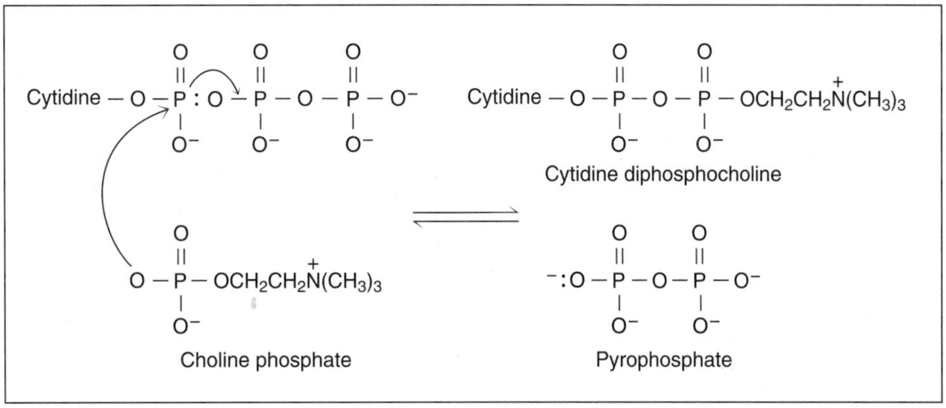

10. This patient has
   (A) a hemolytic anemia
   (B) a microcytic anemia
   (C) a megaloblastic anemia
   (D) polycythemia (excessive amount of red blood cells)
   (E) pancytopenia (deficiency of all types of blood cells)

The patient tested positive for HIV, and treatment with azidothymidine (AZT) was initiated. AZT is a nucleoside analogue of thymidine in which the 3′-hydroxyl group is replaced by the azido group. AZT is converted to the triphosphate in reactions catalyzed by thymidine kinase, thymidylate kinase, and nucleoside diphosphate kinase (shown below). AZT triphosphate is a more potent inhibitor of the reverse transcriptase of the AIDS virus than of the nuclear DNA polymerases of the host.

DIRECTIONS. (Items 11–15): Each set of matching questions in this section refers to the numbered reactions in the illustration below. For each numbered item, select the ONE lettered option that is most closely associated with it.

11. Which one of the following characteristics best describes the reaction catalyzed by thymidine kinase in reaction I?
   (A) There are three high-energy bonds in the reactants
   (B) There are two high-energy bonds in the products
   (C) The reaction proceeds with the loss of one high-energy bond
   (D) The reaction is endergonic
   (E) The equilibrium constant is near 1

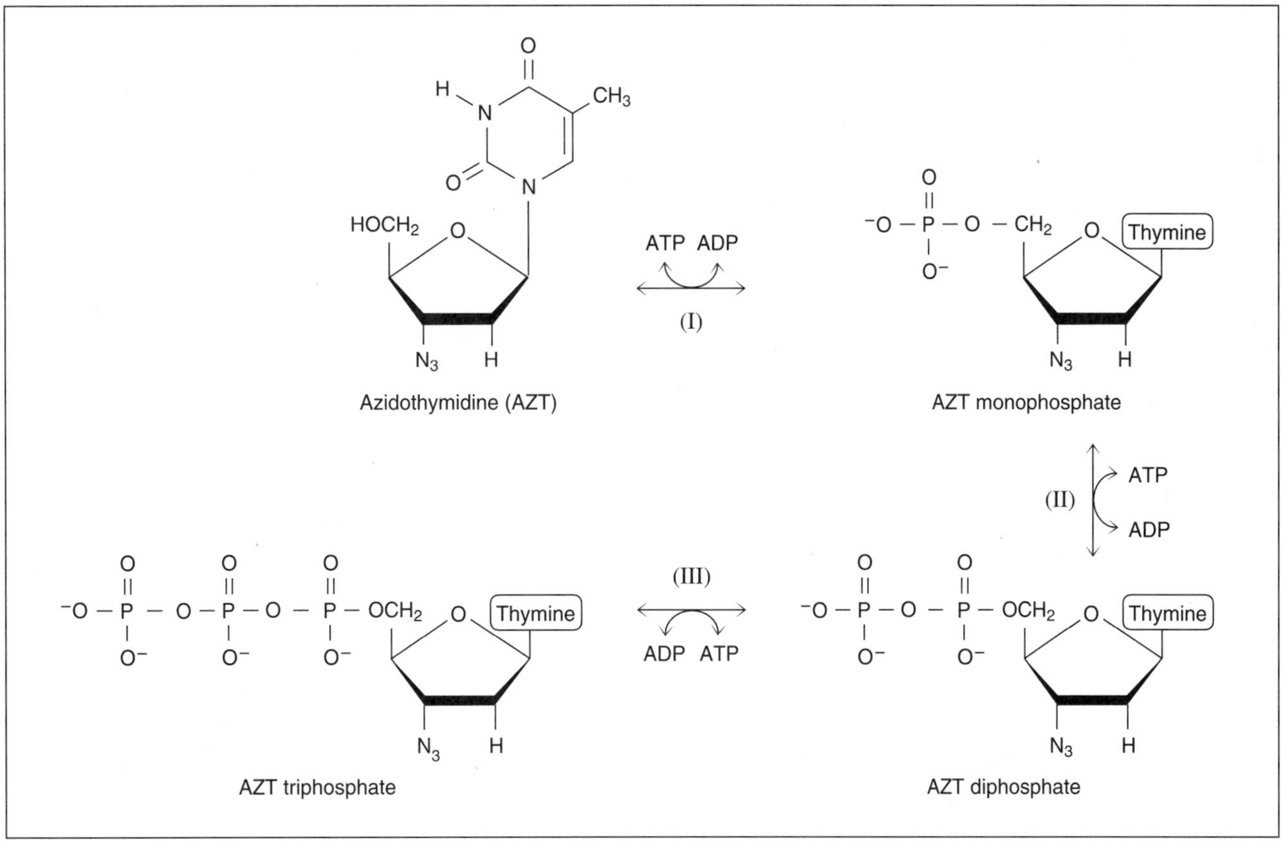

12. Which one of the following bioenergetic characteristics best describes the reaction catalyzed by thymidylate kinase (reaction II)?
    (A) The reaction is exergonic
    (B) The equilibrium constant is much less than 1
    (C) The reaction proceeds with the loss of one high-energy bond
    (D) There are two high-energy bonds in the reactants
    (E) There is one high-energy bond in the products

13. Which one of the following bioenergetic characteristics best describes the reaction catalyzed by nucleoside diphosphate kinase (reaction III)?
    (A) There are three high-energy bonds in the reactants
    (B) There are two high-energy bonds in the products
    (C) The reaction proceeds with the loss of one high-energy bond
    (D) The reaction is exergonic
    (E) The equilibrium constant is much less than 1

14. Reverse transcriptase requires dATP, dGTP, dTTP, and dCTP as substrates. What would be the pattern of inhibition if steady-state enzyme kinetic studies were performed by varying **dTTP** with and without AZT triphosphate?
    (A) Allosteric
    (B) Noncompetitive
    (C) Uncompetitive
    (D) Competitive
    (E) Irreversible

15. Reverse transcriptase requires dATP, dGTP, dTTP, and dCTP as substrates. What would be the pattern of inhibition if steady-state enzyme kinetic studies were performed by varying **dGTP** with and without AZT triphosphate?
    (A) Allosteric
    (B) Noncompetitive
    (C) Uncompetitive
    (D) Competitive
    (E) Irreversible

ANSWERS AND EXPLANATIONS

1. The answer is D: It represents an activated donor of the acetyl group. The arbitrary boundary for the standard free energy of hydrolysis of high-energy compounds is –30 kJ/mol or more negative; acetyl-CoA is thus an energy-rich compound. The group transfer potential is the negative of the free energy of hydrolysis, and acetyl-CoA possesses a high group-transfer potential. Acetyl-CoA is stable in water; the standard free energy of hydrolysis is a thermodynamic value and provides no information on the rate of a process such as the rate of breakdown or hydrolysis of a compound. The terms "high-energy compound" and "energy-rich compound" are synonymous, and the energy-rich acetyl-CoA is a suitable donor of the acetyl group for biochemical reactions. Acetyl-CoA participates in the synthesis of acetylcholine, platelet activating factor, and the acetylation of the amino-terminal amino acid of several proteins during posttranslational modification. Acetyl-CoA cannot be formed from acetate and coenzyme A without the input of additional energy. *Biochemistry,* p. 88.
2. The answer is E: the reaction is exergonic and unidirectional. The reactant contains a low-energy bond (a phosphate ester). The hydrolysis of both low-energy and high-energy compounds is exergonic. This corresponds to PRINCIPLE 5 OF BIOENERGETICS. Hydrolysis reactions, moreover, are unidirectional. *Biochemistry,* p. 82.
3. The answer is C: the reaction proceeds from right to left under standard conditions. Although the number of high-energy bonds is the same in the reactants and products, this reaction proceeds from products to reactants in a unidirectional fashion. This is the sole exception to PRINCIPLE 1 OF BIOENERGETICS, since other reactions with the same number of high-energy bonds in the reactants and products are functionally isoergonic and bidirectional. The inability of ATP to phosphorylate pyruvate is due, in part, to the high group transfer potential of phosphoenolpyruvate. The conversion of pyruvate to phosphoenolpyruvate during gluconeogenesis is mediated by a two-step process involving pyruvate carboxylase and phosphoenolpyruvate carboxykinase. *Biochemistry,* p. 82.
4. The answer is A: the reactants contain two high-energy bonds. UTP possesses two acid anhydride bonds, and glucose 1-phosphate possesses a low-energy phosphate ester. The products contain three high-energy bonds (two in UDP-glucose and one in pyrophosphate). Under standard conditions, the reaction proceeds from products to reactants according to PRINCIPLE 3 OF BIOENERGETICS. In the physiological situation, however, the hydrolysis of pyrophosphate pulls the reaction forward. UDP-glucose is the activated donor of glucose in human metabolism. *Biochemistry,* p. 82.
5. The answer is B: there is no high-energy bond in the product. Glucose 6-phosphate (the reactant) and glucose 1-phosphate (the product) are simple oxygen esters that lack a high-energy bond. Their interconversion is functionally isoergonic according to PRINCIPLE 4 OF BIOENERGETICS. Because there is no thermodynamic barrier for this interconversion, this process is bidirectional. *Biochemistry,* p. 82.
6. The answer is A: bond I at the γ-phosphoryl group. This is a type I reaction of ATP, which is its most common class of reaction, and the reaction involves the transfer of the terminal phosphoryl group to an acceptor (in this example, glucose). *Biochemistry,* p. 83.
7. The answer is E: II and III. *S*-Adenosylmethionine biosynthesis is a type IV reaction of ATP. Methionine is attached to the 5′-carbon of adenosine, and this requires the cleavage at the bond labeled III. During the course of this reaction, bond II is cleaved, resulting in pyrophosphate. *Biochemistry,* p. 86.
8. The answer is B: there is one high-energy bond in the reactant. The acylphosphate is a mixed acid anhydride and is energy rich. The resulting phosphate ester on C^2 in the product is energy poor. The phosphate ester on C^3 in both the reactant and product is energy poor. The reaction proceeds with the loss of a high-energy bond and is therefore exergonic according to PRINCIPLE 2 OF BIOENERGETICS. The standard free energy change is therefore negative, and the equilibrium constant is much larger than 1. This reaction toward product is unidirectional.

2,3-Bisphosphoglycerate is an allosteric regulator of hemoglobin that promotes oxygen dissociation. The concentration of this metabolite in red cells increases at high altitudes. *Biochemistry,* p. 77.

9. The answer is B: the number of high-energy bonds in the products is two. Each of the products, CDP-choline and pyrophosphate, contains one energy-rich acid anhydride for a total of two. CTP, a reactant, contains two energy-rich acid anhydride bonds. The number of high-energy bonds is the same in the reactants and products, and the reaction is functionally isoergonic. The hydrolysis of pyrophosphate, not included in this example, helps pull the reaction forward to produce CDP-choline, an important compound for biosynthetic reactions. *Biochemistry,* p. 178.
10. The answer is E: pancytopenia. The patient has a normochromic, normocytic anemia based upon the red blood cell indices, and the decreased red blood cell count, hematocrit, and hemoglobin. The total white blood cell count and platelet counts are also subnormal, and the total picture is that of pancytopenia. The normal values for bilirubin rule unlikely a hemolytic anemia. The hematocrit, hemoglobin, and white cell counts are increased in polycythemia, but not in this patient. The pancytopenia is most likely due to AIDS. The patient is in a high-risk group for this disease. The depressed $CD4^+$ favors the diagnosis. There is a past history of infectious mononucleosis, but this does not explain the pancytopenia. The elevation of gamma globulin levels in AIDS is paradoxical in an immunodeficiency disease. Many of these antibodies are produced autogenously and not in response to antigenic stimulation. *Cecil,* p. 831.
11. The answer is C: the reaction proceeds with the loss of one high-energy bond. ATP contains two high-energy bonds. AZT monophosphate is a low-energy phosphate ester, and ADP contains one high-energy bond. The products thus contain one high-energy bond. The reaction proceeds with the loss of a high-energy bond and is exergonic. The equilibrium constant is much greater than 1. *Biochemistry,* p. 87.
12. The answer is D: there are two high-energy bonds in the reactants. There are two high-energy bonds in the products (ADP and AZT diphosphate each contain an energy-rich simple acid anhydride). The reaction is functionally isoergonic according to PRINCIPLE 1 OF BIOENERGETICS, and the equilibrium constant is about 1. *Biochemistry,* p. 87.
13. The answer is A: there are three high-energy bonds in the reactants. ATP contains two high-energy bonds, and AZT diphosphate contains one high-energy bond for a total of three. The products also contain a total of three high-energy bonds (two in AZT triphosphate and one in ADP). The reaction is thus functionally isoergonic, and the equilibrium constant is about 1. *Biochemistry,* p. 87.
14. The answer is D: competitive. AZT triphosphate is an analogue of dTTP. Increasing the concentration of dTTP overcomes the inhibition caused by AZT triphosphate, and the pattern of inhibition is competitive. A Lineweaver-Burk plot would show no change in the *y*-intercept and a less negative *x*-intercept. Dideoxycytidine (ddC) and dideoxyinosine (ddI), which have been tested in AIDS patients, are metabolized by successive reactions that parallel reactions I–III. *Biochemistry,* p. 57.
15. The answer is B: noncompetitive. AZT triphosphate is not a structural analogue of dGTP, and increasing the concentration of dGTP will not overcome inhibition by AZT triphosphate. A Lineweaver-Burk plot would show an increase in the *y*-intercept and no change in the *x*-intercept. AZT triphosphate binds to the active site of reverse transcriptase noncovalently. Therefore, its pattern of inhibition is neither allosteric nor irreversible. Besides its inhibitory effect on reverse transcriptase, AZT triphosphate is incorporated into nascent DNA during elongation, causing premature chain termination; these actions of AZT triphosphate are responsible for both its therapeutic and toxic effects. *Biochemistry,* p. 57.

REFERENCES

Roskoski, R., Jr. *Biochemistry.* Philadelphia, W. B. Saunders Company, 1996.

Wyngaarden, J. B., L. H. Smith, Jr., and J. C. Bennett (eds.). *Cecil Textbook of Medicine,* 19th ed. Philadelphia, W. B. Saunders Company, 1992.

CHAPTER SEVEN

GLYCOLYSIS AND THE PENTOSE PHOSPHATE PATHWAY

SYNOPSIS

OBJECTIVES

1. To draw the Haworth structures of the common monosaccharides.
2. To describe the Embden-Myerhof glycolytic pathway and its regulation.
3. To cite the main functions of the pentose phosphate pathway.
4. To describe monosaccharide metabolism and the metabolic lesions of galactosemia.

Objective 1: To draw the Haworth structures of the common monosaccharides.

I. Carbohydrate chemistry
  A. Monosaccharides and disaccharides
    1. Carbohydrates are polyhydroxy aldehydes or ketones
    2. The Haworth structure of the β-anomer of D-glucose, in which the hydroxyl groups alternate above and below the plane of the ring, should be mastered (Fig. 7–1)
    3. Galactose is the isomer of glucose that differs by the hydroxyl configuration about C^4, and mannose differs at C^2
    4. The aldehyde groups of glucose, mannose, galactose (monosaccharides), lactose, maltose, and isomaltose (disaccharides) are easily oxidized by copper in alkaline solution, and these compounds are therefore designated as reducing sugars
    5. Sucrose, in contrast, is not a reducing sugar
      a. The hemiacetal group of glucose and hemiketal group of fructose form an acetal bond
      b. The absence of a hemiacetal group makes sucrose a nonreducing sugar in alkaline copper solution, and this is a noteworthy property
  B. Polysaccharides
    1. Starch is a polymer of D-glucose that is made in plants
      a. Amylose is a straight-chain polymer that consists of D-glucosyl units linked by α-1,4-glycosidic bonds
      b. Amylopectin has a tree-like structure with straight-chain portions linked by α-1,4-glycosidic bonds and branches, which occur every 24–30 residues, linked by α-1,6-glycosidic bonds
      c. Nutritionists regard starch and other polysaccharides as complex carbohydrates, whereas glucose and sucrose are simple carbohydrates
    2. Glycogen has a structure like that of amylopectin with straight-chain portions with branches
      a. Glycogen has a greater degree of branching (about every 12 residues) than does amylopectin
      b. Glycogen has a greater molecular mass (1 million Da) than does amylopectin (100,000 Da)
    3. Cellulose consists of long, straight chains of glucosyl residues that are linked by β-1,4-glycosidic bonds
      a. Since humans lack an enzyme that will hydrolyze the β-1,4-glycosidic bonds of cellulose, it cannot be digested and absorbed
      b. Cellulose is a component of fiber (nondigestible carbohydrate) in the diet, and fiber aids intestinal motility and acts as a stool softener
    4. Glycans are extracellular polymers of glucose produced by bacteria, and glycans are important in dental cariogenesis
      a. *Streptococcus mutans*, which is responsible for the initiation of dental caries, produces a polymer containing α-1,6 and α-1,3 linkages

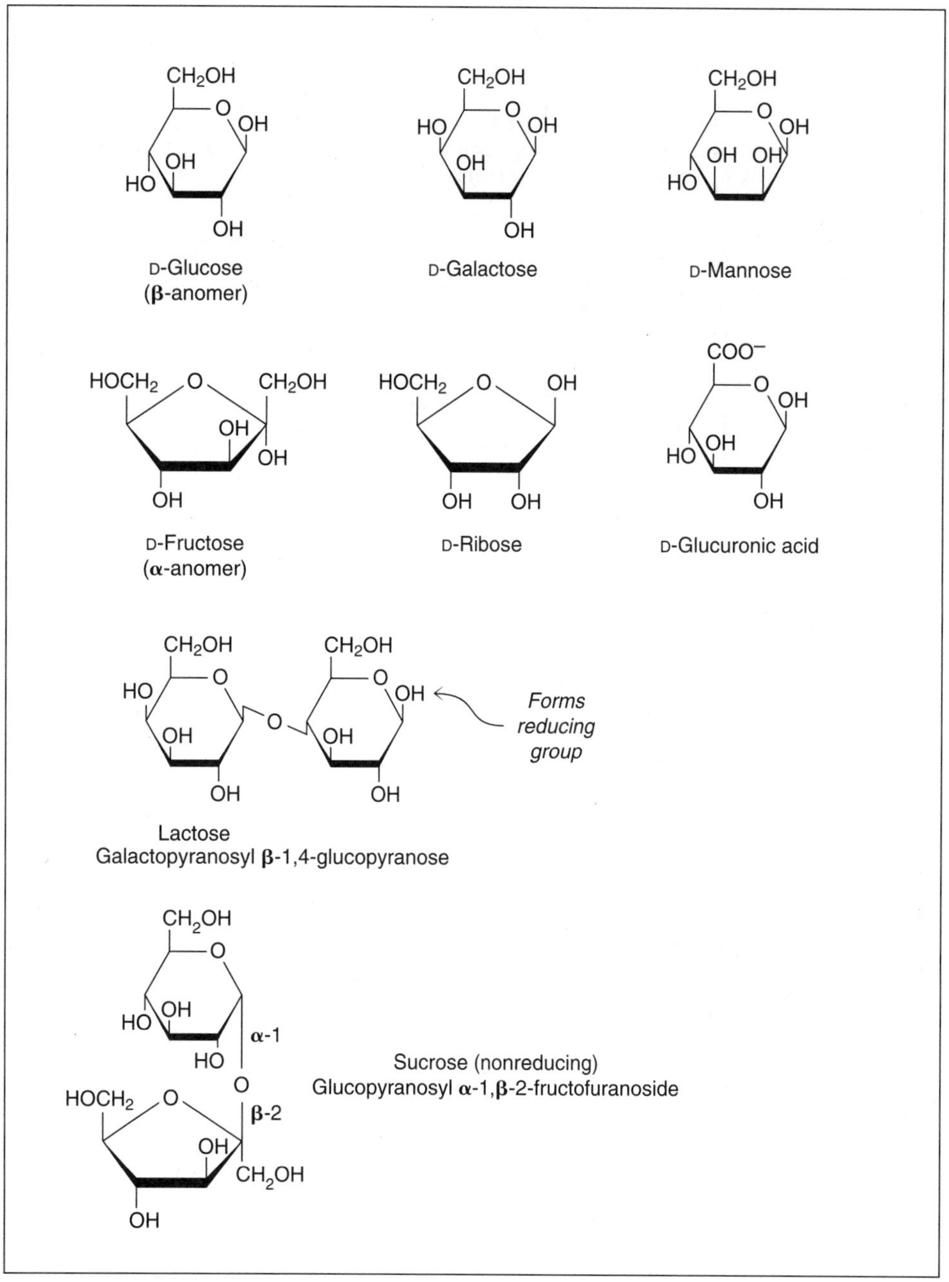

D-Glucose (β-anomer)

D-Galactose

D-Mannose

D-Fructose (α-anomer)

D-Ribose

D-Glucuronic acid

Forms reducing group

Lactose
Galactopyranosyl β-1,4-glucopyranose

α-1

β-2

Sucrose (nonreducing)
Glucopyranosyl α-1,β-2-fructofuranoside

FIGURE 7-1. Structures of several important monosaccharides and disaccharides (lactose and sucrose). The α-1,β-2–glycosidic bond in sucrose ties up the potential aldehyde of glucose and thereby makes it a nonreducing sugar.

b. Mutan is formed from sucrose in reactions catalyzed by extracellular glucosyl transferases:

$$\text{Sucrose} + \text{mutan}_n \rightarrow \text{mutan}_{n+1} + \text{fructose}$$

(1) The glycosidic bond of sucrose is a high-energy bond with a standard free energy of hydrolysis of −30 kJ/mol

(2) The product is a low-energy glycosidic bond, and the overall reaction is exergonic (PRINCIPLE 2 OF BIOENERGETICS)

(3) Sucrose is the most cariogenic sugar in the diet, and its role in mutan formation explains this phenomenon

c. The α-1,3 linkages of mutan are critically important in cariogenesis because they confer insolubility and promote bacterial colonization

Objective 2: To describe the Embden-Myerhof glycolytic pathway and its regulation.

II. Essentials of the Embden-Myerhof glycolytic pathway

A. Stoichiometry of the glycolytic pathway

1. The net process is expressed by the following equation:

$$\text{Glucose} + 2\ \text{ADP} + 2\ P_i + 2\ \text{NAD}^+ \rightarrow 2\ \text{pyruvate} + 2\ \text{ATP} + 2\ H_2O + 2\ \text{NADH} + 2\ H^+ \quad (7.1)$$

2. This pathway generates ATP anaerobically (in the absence of oxygen), and this is a distinctive attribute

B. First phase of glycolysis (Fig. 7–2)
1. The first phase involves the conversion of one mole of glucose to two moles of glyceraldehyde 3-phosphate
2. The reactions are catalyzed by hexokinase (or glucokinase in liver), phosphoglucose isomerase, phosphofructokinase, aldolase, and triose phosphate isomerase

C. Second phase of glycolysis
1. The reactions are catalyzed by glyceraldehyde-3-phosphate dehydrogenase, phosphoglycerate kinase, phosphoglycerate mutase, enolase, and pyruvate kinase
2. NAD^+ is regenerated anaerobically by the lactate dehydrogenase reaction or aerobically by oxidative phosphorylation
3. *The net yield of ATP by anaerobic glycolysis is two moles per mole of glucose,* and generation of ATP occurs during the second phase of glycolysis

D. Metabolism of 2,3-bisphosphoglycerate (2,3-BPG), an allosteric agent that promotes oxygen dissociation from hemoglobin
1. A mutase catalyzes the conversion of 1,3-bisphosphoglycerate to 2,3-BPG, and a hydrolase catalyzes the conversion of 2,3-BPG to 3-phosphoglycerate
2. The mutase and hydrolase form a bifunctional protein

E. Regulation of glycolysis
1. The three irreversible steps of glycolysis are catalyzed by hexokinase (glucokinase), phosphofructokinase, and pyruvate kinase; the only reversible kinase reaction in glycolysis is catalyzed by phosphoglycerate kinase
2. Phosphofructokinase is the main regulatory enzyme
   a. ATP and citrate inhibit this enzyme
   b. AMP and fructose 2,6-bisphosphate activate this enzyme
      (1) Fructose 2,6-bisphosphate is the main regulatory molecule

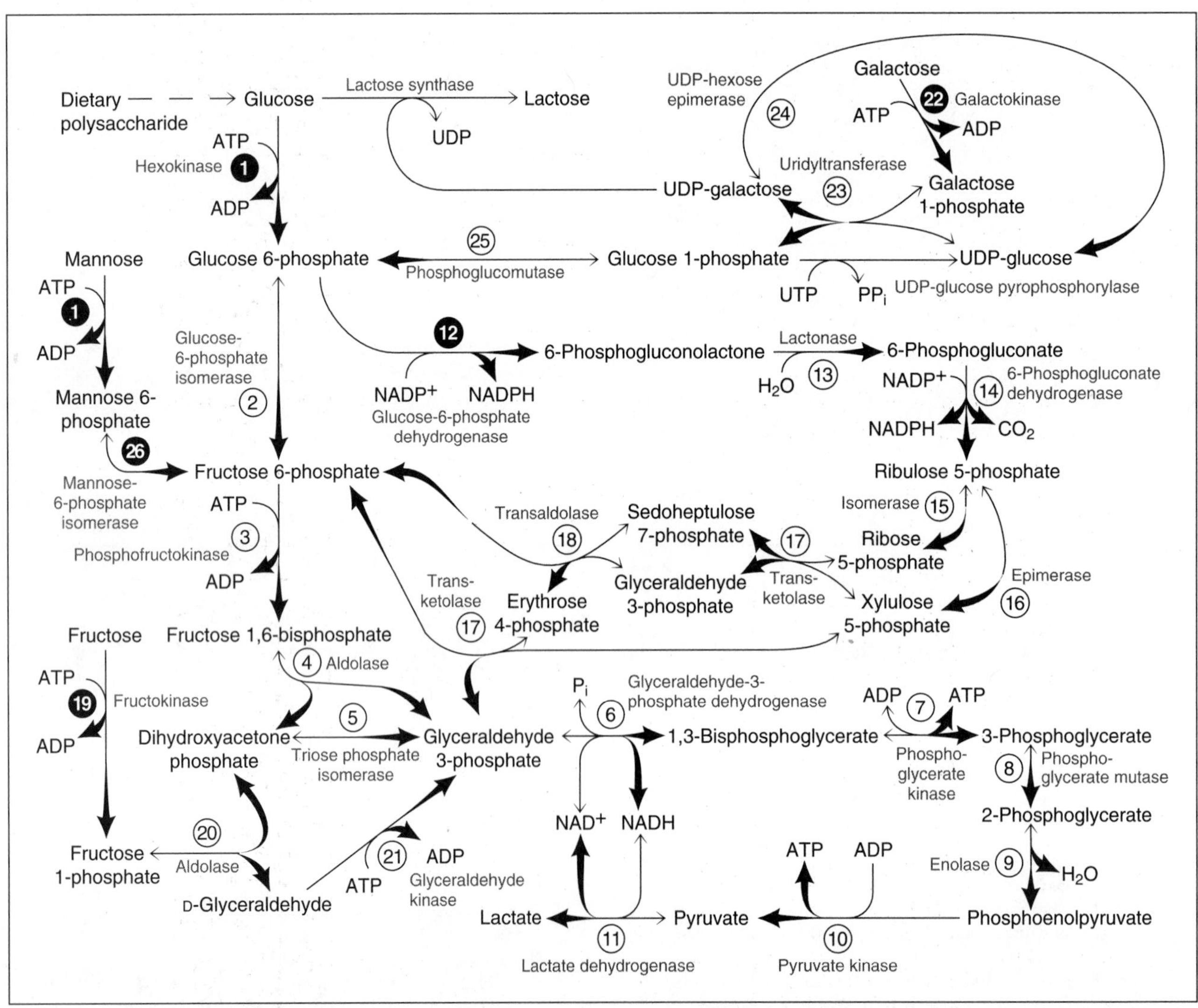

FIGURE 7–2. Overview of glycolysis, the pentose phosphate pathway, lactose, and monosaccharide metabolism.

(2) The cyclic AMP signal transduction pathway decreases the concentration of fructose 2,6-bisphosphate in liver (but not muscle), thereby decreasing the rate of glycolysis
(a) A bifunctional kinase/phosphatase mediates the formation and degradation of fructose 2,6-bisphosphate
(b) Phosphorylation by protein kinase A decreases the kinase activity and increases the phosphatase activity of the dual-function protein

F. Requirement for regenerating NAD^+, P_i, and ADP
1. These three components are required in stoichiometric amounts for the continued metabolism of glucose by the glycolytic pathway (Equation 7.1)
2. The lactate dehydrogenase reaction is responsible for the regeneration of NAD^+ under anaerobic conditions

$$\text{Pyruvate}^- + \text{NADH} + \text{H}^+ \rightleftharpoons \text{lactate}^- + \text{NAD}^+ \quad (7.2)$$

3. ADP is formed by the many reactions that use ATP as reactant

G. Clinical aspects of glycolysis
1. Acute and chronic lactic acidosis, caused by a variety of conditions, is important clinically
a. Inability to oxidize pyruvate or acetyl-CoA because of a metabolic lesion prompts anaerobic glycolysis and lactic acid generation
b. Ischemia, hypoxia or anoxia, and inability to extract oxygen from blood are common clinical conditions that promote lactic acid production
2. *S. mutans* is a gram-positive, anaerobic bacterium that inhabits dental plaque and derives its energy from glycolysis
a. *S. mutans* produces dental caries by converting any of the common sugars to lactic acid, the cariogenic agent
(1) As a result, plaque pH decreases from about 6.8 to 5 or less, and lactic acid dissolves enamel
(2) This microbe also produces formic acid and acetic acid by bacterial fermentation
(3) A carbohydrate-containing meal, especially that with simple sugars (monosaccharides and disaccharides), produces a prompt and brisk decrease in plaque pH
(4) Caries is common in conditions associated with decreased salivary flow (xerostomia) as a result of salivary gland irradiation, anticholinergic medication, or Sjögren syndrome, an autoimmune disorder
b. *S. mutans* is inhibited by fluoride
(1) Fluoride's anticariogenic and bacteriostatic properties are postulated to be due to inhibition of *S. mutans* enolase (enolase from most organisms is inhibited by fluoride)
(2) Bacterial phosphoglucomutase and proton-translocating (F_0F_1) ATPase may also be inhibited by low concentrations ($\approx$0.25 mM) of fluoride

Objective 3: To cite the main functions of the pentose phosphate pathway.

III. Essentials of the Warburg-Dickens pentose phosphate pathway
A. Functions of the pathway
1. The pentose phosphate pathway is responsible for the biosynthesis of the five-carbon ribose found in nucleotides (ATP, NAD^+, $NADP^+$, coenzyme A, FAD), RNA, and DNA
2. Another important characteristic of the pathway is that it generates NADPH + H^+ for reductive biosynthesis

B. Oxidative segment of the pentose phosphate pathway (Figure 7–2)
1. This segment mediates the formation of NADPH and pentose phosphates
2. The three reactions in this segment are catalyzed by glucose-6-phosphate dehydrogenase, lactonase, and 6-phosphogluconate dehydrogenase
a. The irreversible lactonase reaction makes this portion of the pathway unidirectional
b. The glucose-6-phosphate dehydrogenase and 6-phosphogluconate dehydrogenase reactions are important because they generate NADPH
(1) Glucose-6-phosphate dehydrogenase deficiency in the red blood cell is one of the commonest enzyme deficiencies in humans
(2) The administration of antimalarial drugs, sulfonamides, antipyretics, and a host of other drugs can produce a hemolytic anemia in people with inadequate glucose-6-phosphate dehydrogenase activity
(3) Without NADPH generation, the reduction of glutathione is impaired, and the glutathione-mediated reduction of hemoglobin is thereby diminished

C. Nonoxidative segment of the pentose phosphate pathway
1. This portion of the pathway is a network of reactions that interconverts 3-, 4-, 5-, 6-, and 7-carbon sugar phosphates
2. **Epimerase** catalyzes the interconversion of ribulose 5-phosphate and xylulose 5-phosphate
3. **Isomerase** catalyzes the interconversion of ribulose 5-phosphate and ribose 5-phosphate
4. **Transketolase** mediates the transfer of two-carbon fragments
a. This enzyme contains thiamine pyrophosphate as cofactor
b. Transketolase activity may be decreased in individuals who consume excessive ethanol
5. **Transaldolase** mediates the transfer of three-carbon fragments

Objective 4: To describe monosaccharide metabolism and the metabolic lesions of galactosemia.

IV. Metabolism of fructose and galactose (see Fig. 7–2)
A. Monosaccharide metabolism
1. Fructose can be converted to glycolytic intermediates in three steps
a. **Fructokinase,** a liver enzyme, catalyzes the formation of fructose 1-phosphate
b. Aldolase catalyzes the formation of glyceraldehyde and dihydroxyacetone phosphate
c. **Glyceraldehyde kinase** catalyzes the formation of glyceraldehyde 3-phosphate
d. This pathway of fructose metabolism bypasses the phosphofructokinase reaction, the chief regulatory step of glycolysis

2. Galactose metabolism involves three reactions
   a. **Galactokinase** is the only enzyme that will catalyze the phosphorylation of galactose, and phosphorylation involves the hydroxyl group attached to C^1
   b. Galactose 1-phosphate reacts with UDP-glucose to form glucose 1-phosphate and UDP-galactose as catalyzed by **uridyltransferase**
   c. An **epimerase** catalyzes the conversion of UDP-galactose to UDP-glucose, which can then react with another molecule of galactose 1-phosphate to form glucose 1-phosphate
3. Galactosemia results from the inability to metabolize galactose
   a. *Classic galactosemia, a severe malady, is due to a deficiency of galactose-1-phosphate uridyltransferase*
      (1) As a result of this deficiency, galactose 1-phosphate accumulates in red cells and in liver to produce disease
      (2) Treatment consists of a diet lacking milk and milk products (specifically lactose)
   b. A variant form of galactosemia, due to a deficiency of galactokinase, is less severe because phosphorylated galactose does not accumulate in cells

QUESTIONS

DIRECTIONS: Each of the numbered items or incomplete statements in this section is followed by answers or by completions of the statement. Select the ONE lettered answer or completion that is BEST in each case. Correct answers and explanations are given at the end of the chapter.

Items 1–3

Select the most appropriate compound(s) shown below that possess the specified features.

1. Which of the compounds shown below are anomers?

(A) I and II
(B) II and III
(C) I and III
(D) I and IV
(E) IV and V

2. This sugar, which gives a positive Clinitest result (oxidized by alkaline copper) but negative Clinistix result (oxidized by glucose oxidase), can occur in the urine of individuals with galactosemia who drink milk or eat milk products

(A) I
(B) II
(C) III
(D) IV
(E) V

3. This sugar, which gives a positive Clinitest (oxidized by alkaline copper) and Clinistix (oxidized by glucose oxidase) tests, can occur in the urine of individuals with diabetes mellitus

(A) I
(B) II
(C) III
(D) IV
(E) V

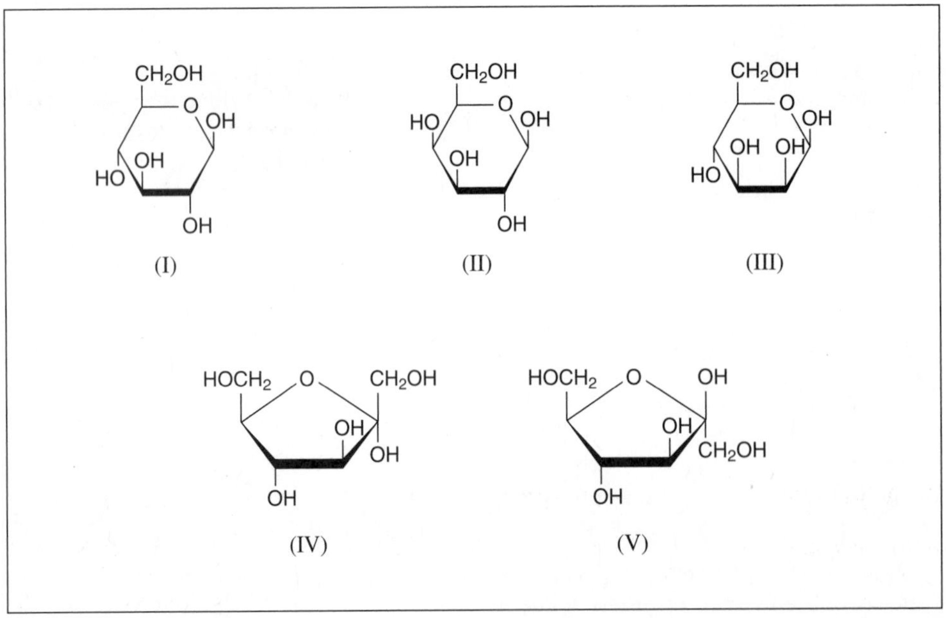

(I) (II) (III)

(IV) (V)

Items 4–6

Refer to the Roman numerals in the illustration below to answer Questions 4–6.

4. For reactions proceeding in the direction indicated by the arrows, which reactions involve expenditure of ATP (i.e., conversion of ATP to ADP)?
   (A) I and III
   (B) II and IX
   (C) IV and V
   (D) VI and XI
   (E) VII and X

5. Which reactions can be diminished in patients with pellagra?
   (A) I and III
   (B) II and IX
   (C) IV and V
   (D) VI and XI
   (E) VII and X

6. Which reactions are physiologically irreversible?
   (A) IV, VI, and XI
   (B) VI, VII, and IX
   (C) I, III, and X
   (D) V, VIII, and IX
   (E) VII only

7. Muscle phosphofructokinase deficiency (Tarui disease) is accompanied by muscle weakness, pain, exercise intolerance, and a mild hemolytic anemia. Biopsies show increased muscle glycogen, and exercise evokes little or no increase in venous lactate. Phosphofructokinase is characterized by all of the following properties EXCEPT
   (A) the enzyme is allosterically inhibited by citrate
   (B) the enzyme is allosterically activated by ATP
   (C) the enzyme is the principal regulatory enzyme of glycolysis
   (D) the decreased catabolism of glucose accounts for glycogen accumulation in the deficiency state
   (E) the decreased catabolism of glucose accounts for the decreased lactate production during exercise

8. 2,3-Bisphosphoglycerate in red cells binds preferentially to deoxyhemoglobin (the T state) and promotes the release of oxygen from oxyhemoglobin. 2,3-BPG concentrations increase in people with chronic hypoxia (e.g., at high altitudes or with pulmonary dysfunction). For glucose metabolized to lactate via 2,3-bisphosphoglycerate in erythrocytes, what is the net yield of ATP molecules per molecule of glucose?
   (A) 0
   (B) 1
   (C) 2
   (D) 30
   (E) 32

9. All of the following are true statements regarding phosphorylation of the dual-activity hepatic polypeptide, 6-phosphofructo-2-kinase/fructose-2,6-bisphosphate-2-phosphatase, EXCEPT
   (A) it decreases the kinase activity and increases the phosphatase activity
   (B) it is catalyzed by a cAMP-dependent protein kinase (protein kinase A)
   (C) it is triggered when glucagon binds to its plasma membrane receptor in liver
   (D) it results in a decrease in fructose 2,6-bisphosphate concentration
   (E) it leads to an increase in glycolytic activity in liver

10. A deficiency of each of the following enzymes of the Embden-Myerhof glycolytic pathway leads to nonspherocytic hemolytic anemia. A deficiency of which of the following enzymes leads to an increase in 2,3-bisphosphoglycerate levels in red cells?
   (A) Aldolase
   (B) Phosphoglucose isomerase
   (C) Hexokinase
   (D) Pyruvate kinase
   (E) Triose phosphate isomerase

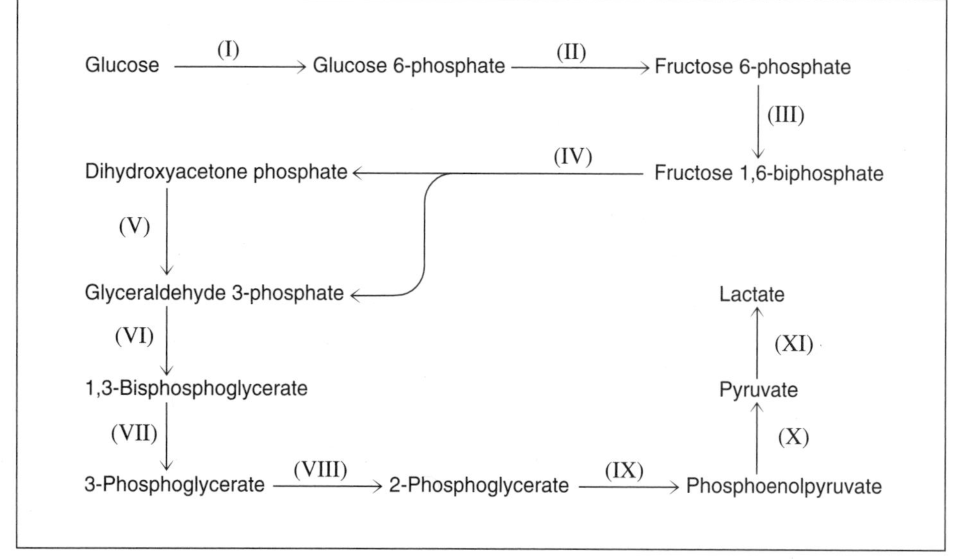

11. Deficiency of glucose-6-phosphate dehydrogenase and partial deficiency of 6-phosphogluconate dehydrogenase produce hemolytic anemia. Which one of the following is a true statement regarding the function of these enzymes?
    (A) They catalyze the interconversion of 3-, 4-, 5-, 6- and 7-carbon sugar phosphates
    (B) They provide NADH for the conversion of pyruvate to lactate
    (C) They provide NADPH for regeneration of glutathione in erythrocytes for protection against oxidative damage
    (D) They provide NADH for ATP production via oxidative phosphorylation
    (E) They catalyze two of the steps in the conversion of ribulose 5-phosphate to glucose 6-phosphate

12. All of the following monosaccharides are substrates for hexokinase EXCEPT
    (A) glucose
    (B) fructose
    (C) galactose
    (D) mannose

DIRECTIONS. This set consists of a list of several lettered options followed by two numbered items. For each numbered item, select the ONE lettered option that is most closely associated with it. Each lettered option may be selected once, more than once, or not at all.

(A) Amylose
(B) Cellulose
(C) Fructan
(D) Glycogen
(E) Mutan

13. A polymer with straight-chain portions (containing α-1,4-glycosidic bonds) linked to branches by α-1,6-glycosidic bonds; found in liver, muscle, and a variety of other human cells
14. A major component of dietary fiber

Items 15–18

History

The patient is a 47-year-old female cashier who came to the dental clinic because of dental caries. She noted that her mouth seemed dry, and she had difficulty swallowing dry foods. Moreover, she noted a sensation of burning of the eyes over the past year. The patient is not in a high-risk group for AIDS. The patient is not taking any anticholinergic or other medication nor has she ever received any irradiation treatments. She denies any weight loss.

Physical Examination

Physical examination revealed nine carious lesions. She had a fissured tongue, angular cheilitis (inflammation of the lips), and bilateral parotid gland swelling.

Laboratory

Red blood cell count, normal
Hemoglobin, normal
White blood cell count, normal
Serum glucose, 84 mg/dL (normal, 70–105 mg/dL)
HIV antibody, negative (normal, negative)
Nucleoprotein (La or SS–B) antibody, positive (normal, negative)
Salivary gland biopsy of lower lip showed lymphocytic infiltration of the minor salivary glands, an abnormal finding.

15. The caries in this patient are attributable to which one of the following disorders?
    (A) Antibodies to nucleoprotein antigen
    (B) Inability to mount an immune response against *S. mutans*
    (C) Niacin deficiency
    (D) Inadequate production of insulin
    (E) Inadequate production of saliva

16. *S. mutans* is a unique dental microbe because of its ability to synthesize extracellular
    (A) amylose
    (B) amylopectin
    (C) cellulose
    (D) glycan
    (E) glycogen

17. In dental caries, the demineralization is caused by acidification of the saliva, bathing the enamel, to pH values of less than 5.5 by which one of the following acids?
    (A) Propionic acid
    (B) Lactic acid
    (C) Formic acid
    (D) Butyric acid
    (E) Acetic acid

18. The most likely diagnosis for this patient is
    (A) Sjögren syndrome
    (B) pellagra
    (C) AIDS
    (D) mumps
    (E) diabetes mellitus

ANSWERS AND EXPLANATIONS

1. The answer is E: IV and V. IV is α-D-fructose, and V is β-D-fructose; these differ only at the anomeric carbon and are therefore anomers. The anomeric carbon of aldoses and ketoses refers to the carbonyl carbon that combines with an alcohol to form a hemiacetal or hemiketal, respectively. Compounds I, II, and III are all aldohexoses having the same (β) configuration at the anomeric carbon. I (β-D-glucose) and II (β-D-galactose) differ only at (the nonanomeric) C^4 and are epimers; II and III (β-D-mannose) differ at both C^2 and C^4 and are stereoisomers but neither anomers nor epimers; I and III differ only at C^2 and are therefore epimers. *Biochemistry,* p. 91.
2. The answer is B: II. D-Galactose is a reducing sugar that gives a positive Clinitest result but does not give a positive Clinistix result, which is based upon a specific reaction involving glucose oxidase. D-Galactose is bonded to D-glucose to produce lactose or milk sugar, a disaccharide. Lactose is digested by lactase; lactase and other disaccharidases are found in the brush-border of the small intestine. Galactose metabolism requires galactokinase, galactose-1-phosphate uridyltransferase, and UDP-galactose epimerase. A deficiency of uridyltransferase produces classical galactosemia, a severe disease involving the liver, kidney, and brain due to the excessive accumulation of galactose 1-phosphate. A deficiency of galactokinase is not as severe because galactose is not entrapped within cells as the anionic metabolite. In both conditions, galactose, a nonglucose reducing substance, is excreted in the urine in patients receiving human or cow's milk or another formula containing lactose. The use of the less specific Clinitest in pediatric patients is recommended by many authorities because it detects reducing substances in the urine that are Clinistix negative. Fructosuria is another example in which a urinary sugar gives a positive Clinitest but negative Clinistix result. The loss of lactase in adults leads to milk intolerance, and this is one of the most common enzyme deficiencies in the world. Such individuals decrease their intake of milk and milk products voluntarily, and this disorder is inconsequential. *Biochemistry,* p. 93.
3. The answer is A: I. Compound I is β-D-glucose. D-Glucose gives both a positive Clinitest result (as a reducing substance) and Clinistix result (based upon glucose oxidase). The hydroxyl groups in β-D-glucose alternate from top to bottom in the Haworth projection formula as shown, and the minimized interaction of these groups makes β-D-glucose the most stable and prevalent hexose in nature. The hyperglycemia results from increased production by gluconeogenesis and the decreased ability to transport glucose into muscle cells and adipocytes. When the transport maximum for glucose in kidney is exceeded (about 200 mg/dL), excessive glucose is excreted in the urine accounting for glucosuria. *Biochemistry,* p. 93.
4. The answer is A: reactions I and III. Reactions I (catalyzed by hexokinase or glucokinase) and III (catalyzed by phosphofructokinase) are the "priming" reactions that involve an initial expenditure of ATP, and both of these reactions are physiologically irreversible. Reactions VII (catalyzed by phosphoglycerate kinase) and X (catalyzed by pyruvate kinase) are reactions that use ADP as substrates and generate ATP as products in the direction of the arrows. *Biochemistry,* p. 98.
5. The answer is D: VI and XI. The three D's of pellagra (diarrhea, dermatitis, and dementia) are due to a deficiency of niacin, a component of $NAD(P)^+$. NAD^+ is a substrate in reaction VI (catalyzed by glyceraldehyde-3-phosphate dehydrogenase) and reaction XI (catalyzed by lactate dehydrogenase). Because $NAD(P)^+$ is involved in so many reactions, it is difficult to pinpoint the precise relationship between pellagra symptoms and specific reactions such as those occurring in glycolysis. *Biochemistry,* pp. 26 and 98.
6. The answer is C: reactions I, III, and X. The hexokinase (and glucokinase) reactions (I), the phosphofructokinase reaction (III), and the pyruvate kinase reaction (X) are physiologically irreversible. In the conversion of pyruvate to glucose during gluconeogenesis, alternative reactions exist to bypass these three steps. *Biochemistry,* p. 99.
7. The answer is B: the enzyme is NOT allosterically activated by ATP. It is allosterically inhibited by ATP. Phosphofructokinase is allosterically inhibited by citrate and is the principal regulatory enzyme of glycolysis. The decreased catabolism of glucose accounts for glycogen accumulation in the deficiency state, and the decreased catabolism of glucose accounts for the markedly decreased lactate production during exercise. One purpose of glycolysis is to generate ATP, and this is the only human metabolic pathway that can do this anaerobically. ATP serves as a signal to decrease glycolysis when ATP levels are ample. *Biochemistry,* p. 100.
8. The answer is A: 0 ATP. When 2,3-bisphosphoglycerate is formed from 1,3-bisphosphoglycerate, the high-energy mixed acid anhydride linkage at C^1 is lost. The conversion of 2,3-BPG to 3-phosphoglycerate by hydrolysis is catalyzed by a bifunctional mutase/phosphatase that mediates both synthesis and degradation of 2,3-BPG, and this overall process occurs without the concomitant formation of ATP. Thus, for each molecule of 2,3-BPG formed (two from each glucose), an ATP is lost. ATP is still formed at the pyruvate kinase reaction (2 per glucose unit) and since 2 ATP are required in the priming reactions, the net ATP yield is zero. Since erythrocytes contain no mitochondria, the NADH formed by the glyceraldehyde 3-phosphate dehydrogenase reaction cannot be used in oxidative phosphorylation reactions and must be used instead to form lactate from pyruvate. *Biochemistry,* p. 100.
9. The answer is E: phosphorylation of the kinase/phosphatase does NOT lead to an increase in glycolytic activity in liver. Glucagon, which interacts with its receptor in the liver plasma membrane, activates adenylyl cyclase. Following the phosphorylation of the kinase/phosphatase by activated cyclic AMP-dependent protein kinase, fructose-6-phosphate-2-kinase activity is decreased, and phosphatase activity is increased. The resulting decrease in fructose 2,6-bisphosphate concentration removes an allosteric activator of phosphofructo-1-kinase and thus decreases the flux through the glycolytic pathway. Muscle fructose-6-phosphate-2-kinase lacks a protein kinase A phosphorylation site, and glycolysis in muscle is not decreased in response to activation of the cyclic AMP signal transduction pathway. *Biochemistry,* p. 101.
10. The answer is D: pyruvate kinase. In pyruvate kinase

deficiency, there is an accumulation of all of the glycolytic intermediates up to phosphoenolpyruvate. There is increased conversion of 1,3-bisphosphoglycerate to 2,3-bisphosphoglycerate. In hexokinase, phosphoglucose isomerase, aldolase, and triose phosphate isomerase, intermediates prior to the formation of 1,3-bisphosphoglycerate accumulate, and there is a decreased, and not increased, production of 2,3-bisphosphoglycerate. Distinct enzyme deficiencies in the red blood cells that lead to nonspherocytic hemolytic anemias include hexokinase (reaction I), glucose phosphate isomerase (reaction II), aldolase (reaction IV), triose phosphate isomerase (reaction V), phosphoglycerate kinase (reaction VII), and pyruvate kinase (reaction X) and have been described. There are two genes but three types of pyruvate kinase. The M (muscle) type of pyruvate kinase is encoded by one gene. The L (liver) and R (red cell) enzymes are encoded by the same gene. Different L and R enzymes result from the use of two promoters and alternative splicing in the conversion of hnRNA to mRNA. A deficiency of phosphofructokinase (reaction III) leads to increased hemolysis (which is compensated by increased erythrocytosis) and a myopathy. *Biochemistry,* p. 98.

11. The answer is C: They provide NADPH for regeneration of glutathione in erythrocytes for protection against oxidative damage. The function of glucose-6-phosphate dehydrogenase and 6-phosphogluconate dehydrogenase is to generate NADPH in the oxidative branch of the pentose phosphate pathway. Transketolase and transaldolase catalyze the interconversion of 3-, 4-, 5-, 6-, and 7-carbon sugar phosphates. Glyceraldehyde-3-phosphate dehydrogenase and other reactions provide NADH for the lactate dehydrogenase reaction and for oxidative phosphorylation. The oxidative branch of the pentose phosphate pathway is not reversible, because the lactonase reaction is unidirectional (PRINCIPLE 5 OF BIOENERGETICS); thus, ribulose 5-phosphate is not converted to glucose 6-phosphate using these enzymes. *Biochemistry,* p. 103.
12. The answer is C: galactose. Galactose is NOT a substrate for hexokinase; glucose, fructose, and mannose are substrates for hexokinase. Liver also contains fructokinase, an enzyme that catalyzes the phosphorylation of the hydroxyl group at C^1. *Biochemistry,* p. 105.
13. The answer is D: glycogen is a polymer in which the straight-chain portions are glucosyl units in α-1,4 linkage, and the branch points also have α-1,6 linkages. Amylopectin, one form of energy storage carbohydrate (starch) in plants, is also made of glucosyl units in α-1,4 linkage, and the branch points also have α-1,6 linkages. Glycogen, the carbohydrate storage form in animals, is larger and more highly branched than amylopectin. *Biochemistry,* p. 95.
14. The answer is B: cellulose. Fiber is the dietary component of plants that is resistant to digestion by human enzymes. Fiber includes a variety of soluble and insoluble plant products. Cellulose is a large, indigestible, insoluble polymer of D-glucosyl units bound by β-1,4-glycosidic bonds and is a major component of dietary fiber. Diets high in fiber are postulated to have a protective effect against developing colorectal and breast cancers and atherosclerosis. *Biochemistry,* p. 95.
15. The answer is E: inadequate production of saliva. Caries are the result of demineralization of enamel caused by acid, and the ability of saliva to buffer and neutralize acid produced by oral microbes is one of saliva's anticariogenic actions. Buffers in saliva counteract the decrease in plaque pH. The pH of saliva at rest is normally between 6 and 7. The pH of saliva increases with increased flow, and this is protective. When salivary flow is stimulated by eating, the pH can increase to pH 7.6. This provides protection against the acid that is produced by anaerobic glycolysis in bacteria. As with blood plasma, the most important buffer is bicarbonate–carbonic acid. The next most important are phosphate and protein. Saliva also promotes remineralization of enamel. The antibodies to nucleoprotein antigen are a reflection of an aberrant autoimmune response. The absence of dermatitis, diarrhea, and dementia rule out niacin deficiency; niacin deficiency is not characterized by xerostomia as seen in this patient. Resistance to caries in nonsusceptible individuals does not appear to be related to the ability to mount an immune response against *S. mutans* or other oral bacteria. The blood glucose is not consistent with a diagnosis of insulin deficiency (diabetes mellitus). *Cecil,* p. 1535.
16. The answer is D: glycan. Glycans are polysaccharides that are synthesized extracellularly from sucrose. This unique bacterial pathway uses energy-rich sucrose as a glucosyl donor for the biosynthesis of glucan, a polymer. This reaction does not depend directly on ATP, an intracellular compound. *S. mutans* can also synthesize fructan by a related mechanism. Glucan, but not fructan, is implicated in promoting bacterial aggregation and colonization of the pellicle and plaque. Amylose and amylopectin occur in starch and are plant products. Cellulose is also a plant product. Glycogen occurs intracellularly in animals and in bacteria. *Biochemistry,* p. 148.
17. The answer is B: lactic acid. Although dental microbes can produce acetic, butyric, formic, and propionic acids, lactic acid is the most abundant of these fermentation products. *Biochemistry,* p. 148.
18. The answer is A: Sjögren syndrome. The combination of dry mouth with rampant caries and dry eyes in an adult is consistent with the diagnosis of Sjögren syndrome. There was no indication that these symptoms were the result of medication, AIDS, or irradiation effects. If there were signs and symptoms of joint disease and rheumatoid arthritis, a diagnosis of the secondary form of Sjögren syndrome would be in order. Mumps would explain the parotid swelling but not the other signs and symptoms given in the history. The antibody against nucleoprotein antigen is characteristic of several autoimmune diseases and is consistent with the diagnosis. *Cecil,* p. 1535.

REFERENCES

Roskoski, R., Jr. *Biochemistry.* Philadelphia, W. B. Saunders Company, 1996.

Wyngaarden, J. B., L. H. Smith, Jr., and J. C. Bennett (eds.). *Cecil Textbook of Medicine*, 19th ed. Philadelphia, W. B. Saunders Company, 1992.

CHAPTER EIGHT

THE KREBS CYCLE

SYNOPSIS

OBJECTIVES

1. To describe the role of the Krebs cycle in metabolism.
2. To describe the bioenergetics of decarboxylation reactions.
3. To outline the eight reactions of the Krebs cycle.
4. To describe the pathways for generating Krebs cycle intermediates.
5. To explain the regulation of pyruvate dehydrogenase and the Krebs cycle.
6. To identify possible metabolic defects that produce hepatic encephalopathy.

Objective 1: To describe the role of the Krebs cycle in metabolism.

I. Biochemical functions of the Krebs cycle
   A. The Krebs cycle is responsible for the oxidation of acetyl groups to carbon dioxide, the generation of reducing equivalents (three NADH and one $FADH_2$), and the formation of GTP by substrate level phosphorylation
   B. The Krebs cycle is the final common pathway of metabolism
   C. It is a prominent part of stage III of aerobic metabolism and provides reducing equivalents that sustain oxidative phosphorylation, the chief source of ATP in humans
   D. Krebs cycle reactions, which play an integral role in the conversion of carbohydrate to fat, also provide precursors for the synthesis of aspartate, glutamate, amino acids derived from them, and heme

Objective 2: To describe the bioenergetics of decarboxylation reactions.

II. Overview of decarboxylation reactions
   A. PRINCIPLE 6 OF BIOENERGETICS states that *decarboxylation reactions are exergonic*
   B. Most decarboxylation reactions are unidirectional
      1. Simple decarboxylation reactions, which are generally unidirectional, are not accompanied by a concomitant oxidation
      2. Oxidative decarboxylation reactions are accompanied by a concomitant reduction of NAD^+ or $NADP^+$
         a. Some oxidative decarboxylation reactions are unidirectional, and others are bidirectional
         b. The uni- or bidirectional nature of decarboxylation reactions must be considered on a case-by-case basis

III. Conversion of pyruvate to acetyl-CoA, a transition between the glycolysis and Krebs cycle pathways
   A. The oxidative decarboxylation of pyruvate yields acetyl-CoA, carbon dioxide, and NADH and H^+ in a *unidirectional* reaction catalyzed by **pyruvate dehydrogenase**
   B. The pyruvate dehydrogenase reaction requires the participation of three distinct enzyme activities (E1, E2, and E3) and five different cofactors including thiamine pyrophosphate, NAD^+, coenzyme A, FAD, and lipoate (the first four being vitamin derivatives); other reactions that involve three similar enzyme activities and these five cofactors are also exergonic and unidirectional
   C. The pyruvate dehydrogenase reaction, not part of the Krebs cycle *per se,* provides substrate for the Krebs cycle

Objective 3: To outline the eight reactions of the Krebs cycle.

IV. Overview of the Krebs cycle
   A. A reaction between acetyl-CoA (the stoichiometric substrate) and oxaloacetate (the regenerating substrate) to form the six-carbon citrate initiates the cyclic process (Fig. 8–1)
   B. The first phase of the Krebs cycle involves two decarboxylation reactions to form succinyl-CoA
   C. After the formation of GTP by substrate level phosphorylation, succinate is converted to oxaloacetate

V. Reactions of the Krebs cycle
   A. Initiation of the cycle
      1. The cycle is initiated by the **citrate synthase** reaction

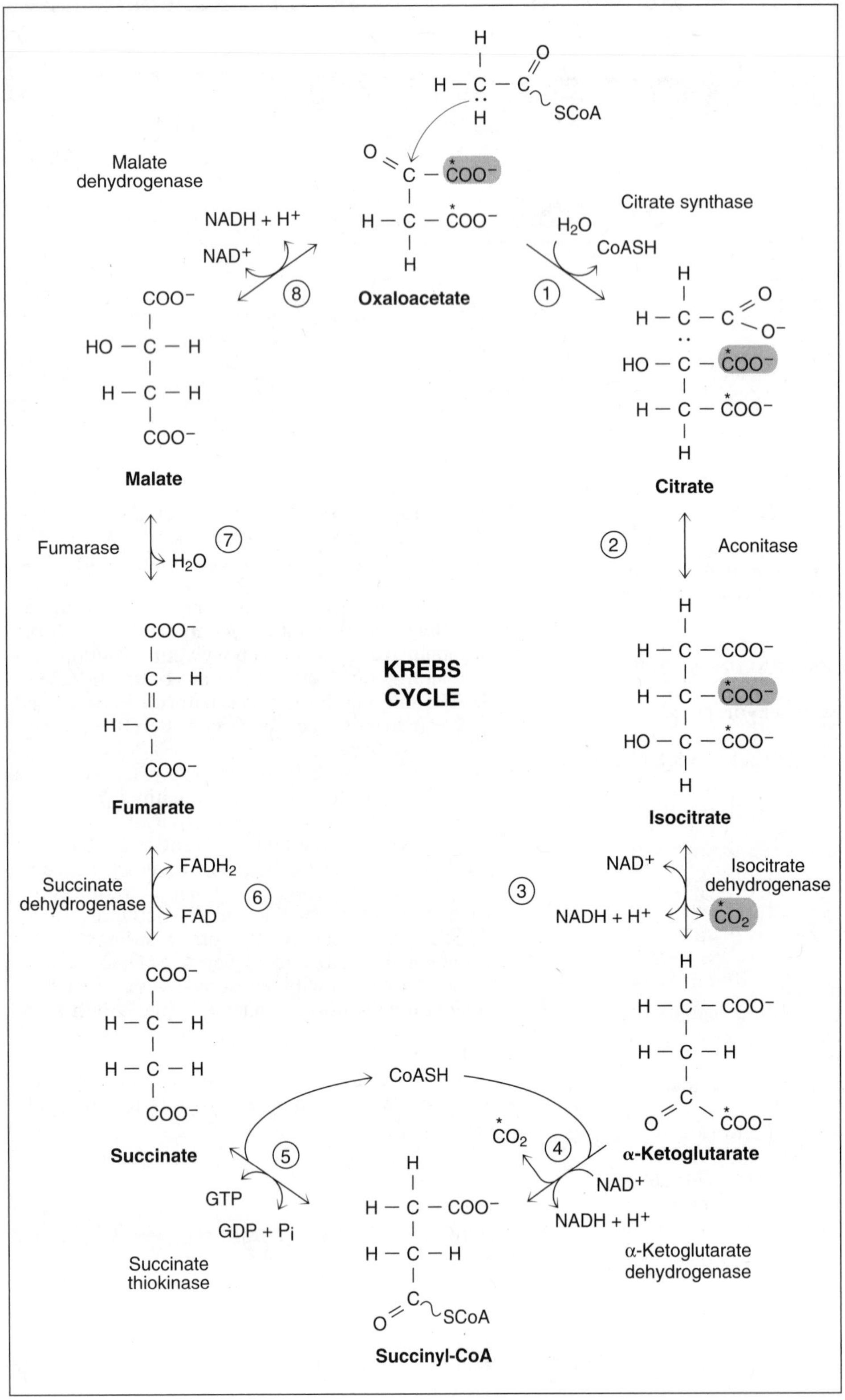

FIGURE 8-1. Reactions of the Krebs cycle.

2. This reaction is unidirectional and is driven by the hydrolysis of a high-energy thioester bond

B. Conversion of citrate to succinate
   1. **Aconitase** catalyzes the conversion of citrate to isocitrate
   2. **Isocitrate dehydrogenase** catalyzes an oxidative decarboxylation to form α-ketoglutarate in the main regulatory reaction of the pathway
   3. **α-Ketoglutarate dehydrogenase** catalyzes a unidirectional oxidative decarboxylation yielding succinyl-CoA
      a. This reaction makes the overall cycle unidirectional

b. This enzyme-catalyzed process is analogous to that of pyruvate dehydrogenase with three enzymes and five cofactors
4. **Succinate thiokinase** catalyzes the substrate level phosphorylation of GDP to form GTP at the expense of succinyl-CoA

C. Conversion of succinate to oxaloacetate
1. **Succinate dehydrogenase** catalyzes the oxidation of succinate to fumarate by FAD
2. **Fumarase** catalyzes the hydration of fumarate to malate, a lyase reaction
3. **Malate dehydrogenase** catalyzes the NAD^+-dependent oxidation of malate to oxaloacetate, the regenerating substrate, and the cycle is completed

VI. ATP yield for Krebs cycle and oxidative phosphorylation reactions
A. One turn of the cycle generates three molecules of NADH and one $FADH_2$
1. Oxidation of one mole of NADH yields 2.5 moles of ATP, or a total of 7.5 per mole of acetyl-CoA metabolized
2. Oxidation of one mole of $FADH_2$ yields 1.5 moles of ATP

B. One mole of GTP (= ATP) is generated by substrate level phosphorylation per mole of acetyl-CoA metabolized by the Krebs cycle
C. A total of 10 moles of ATP ($7.5 + 1.5 + 1$) result from the oxidation of one mole of acetyl-CoA by the combined activity of the Krebs cycle and oxidative phosphorylation

VII. Bioenergetics of dehydrogenase reactions
A. *Simple oxidation-reduction reactions are reversible* (PRINCIPLE 7 OF BIOENERGETICS)
1. Simple oxidation-reduction reactions do not involve molecular oxygen, a decarboxylation, or generation of a carboxylate
2. The lactate dehydrogenase reaction is a prototype of a simple oxidation-reduction reaction

B. Reduction of molecular oxygen to water, R—OH, or R=O is physiologically irreversible (PRINCIPLE 8 OF BIOENERGETICS)

Objective 4: To describe the pathways for generating Krebs cycle intermediates.

VIII. The amphibolic nature of the Krebs cycle
A. The Krebs cycle participates in catabolic and anabolic reactions and is thus amphibolic
B. When intermediates of the Krebs cycle are consumed in anabolic processes, they can be replenished by the following two anaplerotic reactions
1. The **pyruvate carboxylase** reaction is an important reaction in generating Krebs cycle intermediates
a. Pyruvate and carbon dioxide are converted to oxaloacetate
b. The endergonic carboxylation is sustained by the conversion of ATP to ADP and P_i
c. Biotin, covalently bonded to the enzyme, is a participant in this process
2. The reaction catalyzed by **malic enzyme** is a minor process with the potential to generate Krebs cycle intermediates
a. Pyruvate, carbon dioxide, and NAD(P)H are converted to malate and $NAD(P)^+$
b. Both cytosolic and mitochondrial enzymes can be involved in this process

Objective 5: To explain the regulation of pyruvate dehydrogenase and the Krebs cycle.

IX. Regulatory steps in the oxidation of pyruvate and acetyl-CoA
A. Pyruvate dehydrogenase catalyzes an important regulatory step in oxidative metabolism
1. This enzyme is phosphorylated by ATP in a reaction catalyzed by mitochondrial pyruvate dehydrogenase kinase, and phosphorylation is inhibitory
2. The phosphorylated enzyme is dephosphorylated by a phosphatase
3. The kinase is activated by acetyl-CoA, NADH, and ATP, and regulation thus follows the molecular logic of the cell (PRINCIPLE 9 OF BIOCHEMISTRY)

B. Isocitrate dehydrogenase is the main regulatory enzyme of the Krebs cycle
1. It is activated by **ADP,** and this step follows the metabolic logic of the cell
2. Because the Krebs cycle participates in the oxidation of fuel molecules and in fatty acid biosynthesis from carbohydrate, it is important to regulate Krebs cycle activity downstream from the citrate synthase reaction
3. The availability of substrates, e.g., acetyl-CoA and NAD^+, can also regulate Krebs cycle activity

Objective 6: To identify possible metabolic defects that produce hepatic encephalopathy.

X. Hepatic encephalopathy
A. Because of the pivotal nature of pyruvate dehydrogenase and the Krebs cycle in human metabolism, metabolic defects in these pathways are rare; hepatic encephalopathy, however, is common
B. There is a decrease in oxidative metabolism in brain in hepatic encephalopathy, which may be related to the following
1. Conversion of α-ketoglutarate and ammonium ion to glutamate in an NAD(P)H-dependent reduction catalyzed by **glutamate dehydrogenase** depletes Krebs cycle intermediates and thereby decreases energy production
2. Ammonium ion inhibits pyruvate and α-ketoglutarate dehydrogenase activity, decreasing the provision of substrate for the Krebs cycle and decreasing Krebs cycle activity
3. Ammonium ion inhibits the shuttle for transporting reducing equivalents into brain mitochondria (Chapter 9), thereby decreasing the rate of glycolysis and the provision of substrate for oxidative phosphorylation
4. An increase in the number of GABA receptors during hepatic encephalopathy (GABA is the chief inhibitory neurotransmitter in brain) decreases neuronal activity; decreased oxidative metabolism accompanies the quiescent state of nerve cells

QUESTIONS

DIRECTIONS (Items 1–18): Each of the numbered items or incomplete statements in this section is followed by answers or by completions of the statement. Select the ONE lettered answer or completion that is BEST in each case. Correct answers and explanations are given at the end of the chapter.

Items 1–2

(I) α-Ketoglutarate dehydrogenase
(II) Glyceraldehyde-3-phosphate dehydrogenase
(III) Isocitrate dehydrogenase
(IV) Lactate dehydrogenase
(V) 6-Phosphogluconate dehydrogenase
(VI) Pyruvate dehydrogenase

Use the list of enzymes above to answer Questions 1–2.

1. Which of the enzymes listed above catalyze(s) an oxidative decarboxylation?
   (A) I and VI only
   (B) II and IV only
   (C) I, III, V, and VI only
   (D) III and V only
   (E) VI only

2. A deficiency of E_3 (lipoamide dehydrogenase), which results in an inborn error of metabolism, leads to diminished activity of which of the enzymes listed above?
   (A) I and VI only
   (B) II and IV only
   (C) I, III, V, and VI only
   (D) III and V only
   (E) VI only

3. Which of the following metabolites is the stoichiometric substrate of the Krebs cycle?
   (A) Oxaloacetate
   (B) Acetyl-CoA
   (C) Citrate
   (D) Pyruvate
   (E) NADH

Items 4–10

Use the numbered enzyme-catalyzed reactions outlined below to answer Questions 4–10.

4. For reactions moving in the direction of the arrows, which reactions yield NADH as one product?
   (A) I, IV, V, and IX only
   (B) II, III, and VI only
   (C) I, IV, V, VII, and IX only
   (D) IV, V, and IX only
   (E) IV, V, and VII only

5. A deficiency of this activity in humans leads to fumaric aciduria
   (A) I
   (B) II
   (C) VII
   (D) VIII
   (E) IX

6. This reaction yields GTP via substrate level phosphorylation
   (A) I
   (B) II
   (C) V
   (D) VI
   (E) VII

7. This reaction yields $FADH_2$ but not NADH
   (A) I
   (B) IV
   (C) V
   (D) VI
   (E) VII

8. Which of the reactions is (are) physiologically irreversible?
   (A) I only
   (B) I, II, and V only
   (C) VI and VII only
   (D) III and IX only
   (E) IV only

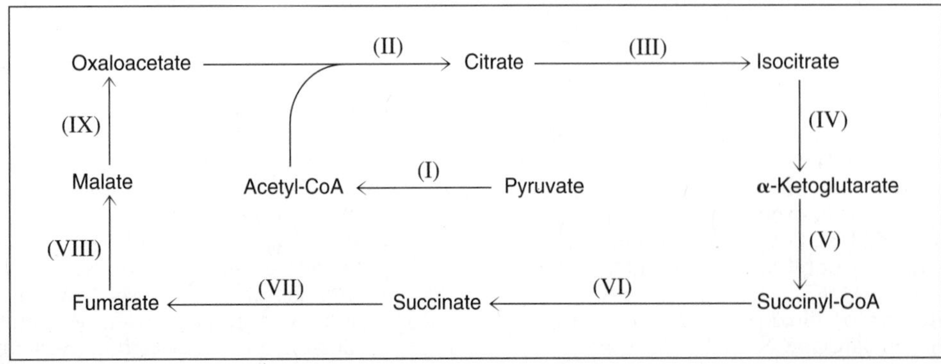

9. Which of the reactions is the primary site of Krebs cycle regulation?
   (A) I
   (B) II
   (C) IV
   (D) V
   (E) VII

10. This reaction is inhibited by the following compound: $^{-}OOC-CH_2-COO^{-}$
   (A) I
   (B) II
   (C) VII
   (D) VIII
   (E) IX

11. The deficiency of pyruvate carboxylase leads to a decrease in cellular
   (A) acetyl-CoA
   (B) Krebs cycle intermediates
   (C) lactate
   (D) biotin
   (E) alanine

12. Malic enzyme performs all of the following functions EXCEPT
   (A) catalyzing an oxidative decarboxylation
   (B) catalyzing the generation of malate from pyruvate
   (C) supplementing the pentose phosphate pathway in the production of NADPH
   (D) catalyzing the interconversion of malate and oxaloacetate

13. Pyruvate dehydrogenase phosphatase deficiency in humans has which one of the following effects?
   (A) It leads to lactic acidemia
   (B) It increases the rate of conversion of pyruvate to acetyl-CoA
   (C) It increases the flux of metabolites through the Krebs cycle
   (D) It causes a lysosomal disease
   (E) It increases protein-tyrosine phosphate levels

Items 14–18

History

The patient is a 62-year-old male (a retired dentist) who was brought to the emergency room in an ambulance accompanied by his spouse. She reported that her husband had become incoherent. The patient had contracted hepatitis 24 years previously. His wife reported that he has complained of fatigue during the past several months, and he recently became jaundiced. He purposely ate a low-protein diet with ample leafy vegetables and fruit, and he avoided alcohol.

Physical Examination

The patient did not answer questions and was nonresponsive. His sclera and skin were jaundiced, and he had numerous spider hemangiomas (named for the shape of skin lesions produced by proliferating vascular endothelium). He responded only mildly to deep pain, and exhibited asterixis (a type of tremor; sometimes called liver flap). Pupillary reflexes were intact; deep tendon reflexes were brisk and equal bilaterally. There was no pedal edema or ascites. The liver was palpated 12 cm below the right costal margin. His blood pressure was 90/60 mm Hg; heart rate, 88/min; respirations, 12/min; temperature, 36.2 °C (97.2 °F).

Laboratory

Blood urea nitrogen (BUN), 12 mg/dL (normal, 7–18 mg/dL)
Creatinine, 0.7 mg/dL (normal ♂, 0.7–1.3 mg/dL)
Serum glucose, 77 mg/dL (normal, 70–105 mg/dL)
Hematocrit, 42% (normal ♂, 39–49%)
Hemoglobin, 15.6 g/dL (normal ♂, 13.5–17.5 g/dL)
White blood count, 13,500/μL (normal, 4500–11,000/μL)
Platelets, 278,000/μL (normal, 150–450 × 10^3/μL)
Bilirubin, total/direct, 6.8/1.2 mg/dL (normal, 0.2–1.0/0–0.2 mg/dL)
Amylase, 118 U/L (normal, 25–125 U/L)
Alkaline phosphatase, 144 U/L (normal ♂, 53–128 U/L)
Aspartate aminotransferase (AST, SGOT), 86 U/L (normal, 10–30 U/L)
γ-Glutamyl transpeptidase, 420 U/L (normal ♂, 9–50 U/L)
Blood ammonia, 620 μM (normal, 11–32 μM)
Prothrombin time, 29 sec (control, 19 sec)
Albumin, 4.2 g/dL (normal, 3.5–5.0 g/dL)
Globulins, 2.6 g/dL (normal, 2.2–4.0 g/dL)

Serum electrolytes and blood pH were normal. A drug screen including an analysis for ethanol was negative. A computerized axial tomography (CT) scan of the head revealed no tumor, but was suggestive of cerebral edema. An electroencephalogram (EEG) revealed diminished generalized (not localized) cerebral activity. The following data were obtained from femoral arterial and jugular vein samples (femoral arterial blood is representative of all arterial blood, and the jugular vein provides the effluent from the brain).

Determination	Arterial Blood	Venous Blood
Oxygen	8.75 mM (normalized, 8.75 mM)	6.75 mM (normalized, 5.75 mM)
Carbon dioxide	21.5 mM (normalized, 21.5 mM)	22.5 mM (normalized, 24.5 mM)
Glucose	5.11 mM (normalized, 5.11 mM)	3.15 mM (normalized, 4.56 mM)
	92 mg/dL (normalized, 92 mg/dL)	57 mg/dL (normalized, 82 mg/dL)
Lactate	1.10 mM (normalized, 1.10 mM)	3.27 mM (normalized, 1.27 mM)
pH	7.42 (normalized, 7.42)	7.32 (normalized, 7.37)

14. Which one of the following analyses is the most sensitive indicator of abnormal liver function?
   (A) Prothrombin time
   (B) Hepatomegaly
   (C) Serum ammonia
   (D) Serum albumin
   (E) γ-Glutamyl transpeptidase

15. Without regard to possible mechanism, which one of the following laboratory values in this patient indicates that there is decreased activity of the Krebs cycle enzymes?
   (A) Oxygen supply
   (B) Carbon dioxide production
   (C) Glucose consumption
   (D) Acid production
   (E) Plasma pH

16. The most likely diagnosis in this patient is
    (A) hepatic encephalopathy
    (B) Wernicke-Korsakoff syndrome
    (C) marasmus
    (D) an astrocytoma of the brain
    (E) hemolytic anemia

17. Cerebral ATP levels, despite diminished oxygen consumption, were maintained by which one of the following compensatory actions?
    (A) Decreased urea production
    (B) Decreased glucose consumption
    (C) Increased glycolysis
    (D) Decreased lactate production
    (E) Decreased carbon dioxide production

18. All of the following are possible mechanisms for producing coma in this patient EXCEPT
    (A) The concentration of Krebs cycle intermediates is decreased in brain as ammonium ion combines with α-ketoglutarate to form glutamate
    (B) The transport of reducing equivalents into brain mitochondria is inhibited by high levels of ammonium ion
    (C) Both the number and sensitivity of GABA (γ-aminobutyric acid) receptors is increased leading to diminished neuronal and oxidative activity
    (D) Brain pyruvate and α-ketoglutarate dehydrogenase activities are increased as a result of hyperammonemia

ANSWERS AND EXPLANATIONS

1. The answer is C: I, III, V, and VI only. Glyceraldehyde-3-phosphate dehydrogenase and lactate dehydrogenase catalyze oxidation-reduction reactions, but these reactions do not involve a decarboxylation reaction. Isocitrate dehydrogenase, 6-phosphogluconate dehydrogenase, pyruvate dehydrogenase, and α-ketoglutarate dehydrogenase catalyze decarboxylation reactions that are accompanied by the reduction of $NAD(P)^+$. *Biochemistry,* p. 110.
2. The answer is A: I and VI only. Even though four of the enzymes catalyze oxidative decarboxylations, only pyruvate dehydrogenase and α-ketoglutarate dehydrogenase utilize three enzyme activities (E_1, E_2, and E_3) and five cofactors (thiamine pyrophosphate, lipoamide, coenzyme A, FAD, and NAD^+). E_3 is lipoamide dehydrogenase and mutations of this subunit decrease the activity of both pyruvate and α-ketoglutarate dehydrogenase. Diminished activity of both enzymes can result in lactic acidosis and excretion of α-ketoglutarate in the urine. *Biochemistry,* p. 111.
3. The answer is B: acetyl-CoA. Since two molecules of CO_2 are released with each turn of the cycle, the equivalent of an acetate (or acetyl) unit is completely oxidized, so acetyl-CoA is the stoichiometric substrate. Oxaloacetate, which is regenerated with each turn of the cycle, is called the regenerating substrate. Catalytic amounts of Krebs cycle intermediates can promote the catabolism of large (stoichiometric) amounts of the acetyl group. Pyruvate is not a Krebs cycle intermediate, and NADH is produced, not consumed, when the cycle is oxidizing acetyl units. *Biochemistry,* p. 111.
4. The answer is A: I, IV, V, and IX only. Pyruvate dehydrogenase (I), isocitrate dehydrogenase (IV), α-ketoglutarate dehydrogenase (V), and malate dehydrogenase (IX) all yield NADH when the reactions proceed in the direction shown. *Biochemistry,* p. 112.
5. The answer is D: VIII. Inborn errors of metabolism involving the Krebs cycle are extremely rare because this pathway is of pivotal importance in intermediary metabolism. A deficiency of fumarase has been described that results in fumaric aciduria. Synthesis of fumarate occurs, but the subsequent conversion of fumarate to malate is defective. This disease is characterized by mental retardation. A second metabolic defect in the Krebs cycle is due to a deficiency of α-ketoglutarate dehydrogenase activity. This disease is accompanied by excretion of α-ketoglutarate in the urine; affected individuals exhibit delayed development. The partial enzyme activities in these disorders account for the nonlethal nature, but affected individuals do not survive childhood. *Biochemistry,* p. 114.
6. The answer is D: VI. Reaction VI, catalyzed by succinate thiokinase, conserves the energy-rich thioester bond of coenzyme A as the energy-rich acid anhydride bond of GTP. Since formation of this high-energy phosphate bond does not involve the electron transport chain, it is termed substrate level phosphorylation. *Biochemistry,* p. 114.
7. The answer is E: VII. The enzyme catalyzing this reaction, succinate dehydrogenase, contains FAD as cosubstrate and feeds electrons into the electron transport chain at site 2. Succinate dehydrogenase is the only enzyme of the Krebs cycle that is an integral inner mitochondrial membrane protein. The other enzymes of the Krebs cycle are hydrophilic and occur within the mitochondrial matrix. *Biochemistry,* p. 113.
8. The answer is B: I, II, and V only. Reactions I (pyruvate dehydrogenase), II (citrate synthase), and V (α-ketoglutarate dehydrogenase) are physiologically irreversible. All the other reactions are reversible. Two of the dehydrogenase reactions (I and V), those involving an α-keto acid that undergoes a decarboxylation and the formation of a thioester, are very exergonic and unidirectional. The isocitrate dehydrogenase reaction, which involves an α-hydroxy acid, undergoes a decarboxylation and conversion of the alcohol to a keto acid. This reaction is exergonic, but it is bidirectional. The citrate synthase reaction is accompanied by a hydrolysis reaction, and hydrolysis of high-energy bonds (as occurs here) and low-energy bonds is exergonic (PRINCIPLE 5 OF BIOENERGETICS). *Biochemistry,* p. 112.
9. The answer is C: IV. The isocitrate dehydrogenase reaction is the first oxidative step in the Krebs cycle, is the primary site of metabolic control, and is stimulated allo-

sterically by ADP, a compound whose concentration rises when ATP is being used, i.e., when the energy charge is low. Secondary regulatory steps including the α-ketoglutarate dehydrogenase and citrate synthase reactions have been proposed. The regulation of metabolic pathways at several steps is called the dispersive control of metabolism. Substrate availability (acetyl-CoA, NAD^+) may also play a regulatory role. *Biochemistry,* p. 117.

10. The answer is C: VII. The compound shown is malonate, a homologue of succinate and a competitive inhibitor of succinate dehydrogenase. This compound was important historically in the elucidation of the pathway by Krebs, who showed that, in the presence of malonate, precursors of acetyl-CoA were converted quantitatively to succinate; in the absence of malonate, these compounds were oxidized to carbon dioxide. *Biochemistry,* p. 113.
11. The answer is B: Krebs cycle intermediates. The pyruvate carboxylase reaction, which is an ATP-dependent process involving a carboxy-biotinyl intermediate, generates oxaloacetate in the mitochondrial matrix. This anaplerotic reaction produces the regenerating substrate of the Krebs cycle (oxaloacetate) that reacts with acetyl-CoA and mediates its complete oxidation. A deficiency of oxaloacetate leads to a buildup and not a decrease in acetyl-CoA. A deficiency of pyruvate carboxylase results in a decrease in Krebs cycle intermediates, and pyruvate oxidation is diminished. Inability to oxidize pyruvate and demand for ATP lead to substantial increases in glycolysis and lactic acid and pyruvic acid production. One alternative route for disposal of pyruvate is formation of alanine by transamination, and patients with carboxylase deficiency exhibit elevated alanine levels in the blood. Pyruvate carboxylase, which requires acetyl-CoA for expression of its activity, contains covalently linked biotin; inability to synthesize the enzyme results in increased cellular biotin levels. Besides mutations of pyruvate carboxylase, mutations that decrease the covalent coupling of biotin to pyruvate carboxylase exist that produce a similar clinical picture. Other anaplerotic reactions that replenish Krebs cycle intermediates yield α-ketoglutarate, succinyl-CoA, fumarate, or oxaloacetate from the catabolism of amino acids, and malate, derived from pyruvate via the malic enzyme reaction. A deficiency of pyruvate carboxylase also decreases gluconeogenesis and can lead to fasting hypoglycemia. *Biochemistry,* p. 116.
12. The answer is D: malic enzyme does NOT catalyze the interconversion of malate and oxaloacetate, a reaction not involving decarboxylation (or carbon dioxide fixation). Although production of NADPH may be the primary purpose for the oxidative decarboxylation of malate by a cytosolic form of malic enzyme, the reverse reaction may also occur under certain conditions, thus serving an anaplerotic function. Thus, malate can be formed from pyruvate either by the one-step reaction catalyzed by malic enzyme or via the two-step mitochondrial sequence involving pyruvate carboxylase and malate dehydrogenase. Cytosolic malic enzyme plays an important role in generating NADPH for fatty acid biosynthesis and may account for about half of the required NADPH in adipose cells. *Biochemistry,* p. 116.
13. The answer is A: it leads to lactic acidemia. Enzyme phosphorylation by pyruvate dehydrogenase kinase decreases the activity of pyruvate dehydrogenase (and thus conversion of pyruvate to acetyl-CoA). In the absence of pyruvate dehydrogenase phosphatase, the inhibited enzyme form accumulates, and there is decreased conversion of pyruvate to acetyl-CoA and a decreased flux of metabolites through the Krebs cycle due to decreased availability of the stoichiometric substrate (i.e., acetyl-CoA). As a result of diminished pyruvate oxidation, lactic acid accumulates. Diminished pyruvate oxidation, moreover, decreases aerobic ATP production. This increases the requirement for anaerobic ATP production by glycolysis with augmented lactic acid production. Pyruvate dehydrogenase, its kinase, and its phosphatase occur within the mitochondrion and not lysosome. Pyruvate dehydrogenase kinase is activated by acetyl-CoA and NADH. As a result of this activation, generation of acetyl-CoA and NADH is inhibited, following the metabolic logic of the cell (PRINCIPLE 9 OF BIOCHEMISTRY). Pyruvate dehydrogenase phosphatase catalyzes the removal of phosphate from protein-serine residues and not protein-tyrosine residues. *Biochemistry,* p. 117.
14. The answer is E: γ-glutamyl transpeptidase. This enzyme is a sensitive indicator and may be the only abnormality in a person who has excessive ethanol intake (and who may also deny excessive alcohol intake). In contrast, serum ammonia, prothrombin time, and serum albumin levels require extensive liver damage before abnormal values occur. Increased liver size is an indication of liver dysfunction, and it can occur early or late in the disease, depending upon the nature of the primary disorder. *Biochemistry,* p. 63; *Cecil,* p. 761.
15. The answer is B: carbon dioxide production. The Krebs cycle generates carbon dioxide and reducing equivalents, and diminished carbon dioxide production (indicated by the less than expected venous carbon dioxide) demonstrates this. The oxygen supply, as indicated by normal arterial oxygen levels, is not limiting. Altered glucose consumption, increased acid production, and decreased venous plasma pH can result from many causes that are not directly related to aberrant Krebs cycle activity. *Biochemistry,* p. 112.
16. The answer is A: hepatic encephalopathy. Jaundice, abnormal liver function tests (bilirubin, alkaline phosphatase, aspartate aminotransferase, γ-glutamyl transpeptidase, prothrombin time, and blood ammonia), hepatomegaly, and a history of hepatitis all point to liver disease. The encephalopathy is evidenced by his inability to respond to various sensory stimuli. Wernicke-Korsakoff syndrome due to diminished thiamine availability is not characterized by coma but by confabulation (providing a fluent answer without regard to facts). Marasmus is a disease of children with inadequate protein and calorie intake. Comas can be due to brain tumors (either primary such as an astrocytoma, or secondary from metastasis). The normal CT scan makes this an unlikely cause of coma. Jaundice and elevated bilirubin occur in hemolytic anemia. This person, however, lacks an anemia. A recommended therapy for those with chronic liver disease and the potential to develop encephalopathy is a low-protein diet. Such diets produce less ammonium ion and require less urea production (a function of the liver). *Biochemistry,* p. 118; *Cecil,* p. 796.
17. The answer is C: increased glycolysis. The brain derives its energy from the oxidative metabolism of glucose. Unlike heart, liver, and muscle, the brain does not oxidize fatty acids. After a few days of starvation, brain is able to use ketone bodies derived from the liver as an energy source. When the oxidative capacity of the brain decreases, increased anaerobic glycolysis to maintain ATP results. A variety of mechanisms increase the rate of glycolysis. Increased AMP levels that result from less

oxidative phosphorylation activate phosphofructokinase. Although brain contains creatine phosphate, oxidative metabolism is required to generate and maintain this storage form of high-energy phosphate bond energy. *Biochemistry,* p. 102.

18. The answer is D: brain pyruvate and α-ketoglutarate dehydrogenase activities are NOT increased as a result of hyperammonemia. The activity of these two enzymes is decreased by elevated ammonium ion concentrations. In hepatic encephalopathy, the liver fails to dispose of nitrogen via urea formation, the blood levels of ammonium ion are increased, and the oxidative capacity of the brain is decreased, leading to central nervous system dysfunction. Decreasing the concentrations of Krebs cycle intermediates or inhibiting the translocation of reducing equivalents into brain mitochondria would lower oxidative capacity in response to high ammonium ion levels. The number of γ-aminobutyric acid (GABA) receptors is increased in hepatic encephalopathy, and sensitivity to inhibitory neurotransmitters is increased. The action of GABA is to inhibit neuronal activity, and this is accompanied by decreased oxidative metabolism. *Biochemistry,* p. 119.

REFERENCES

Roskoski, R., Jr. *Biochemistry.* Philadelphia, W. B. Saunders Company, 1996.

Wyngaarden, J. B., L. H. Smith, Jr., and J. C. Bennett (eds.). *Cecil Textbook of Medicine,* 19th ed. Philadelphia, W. B. Saunders Company, 1992.

CHAPTER NINE

OXIDATIVE PHOSPHORYLATION

SYNOPSIS

OBJECTIVES

1. To provide an overview of mitochondrial metabolism.
2. To describe electron transport from NADH and succinate to oxygen.
3. To identify inhibitors and uncouplers of oxidative phosphorylation.
4. To describe the F_oF_1 ATP synthase and ATP synthesis.
5. To calculate the ATP yield from the complete oxidation of glucose.
6. To explain the control of glycolysis, the Krebs cycle, and oxidative phosphorylation.
7. To describe aberrant oxidative reactions in mitochondria.

Objective 1: To provide an overview of mitochondrial metabolism.

I. Oxidative phosphorylation, oxygen consumption, and ATP generation
   A. The purpose of oxidative phosphorylation is to generate ATP, the common currency of energy exchange (PRINCIPLE 10 OF BIOCHEMISTRY)
   B. Oxidative phosphorylation, but not substrate level phosphorylation, requires an electron transport chain, oxygen, and ATP synthase
   C. More than 90% of ATP generated and oxygen consumed in humans involves oxidative phosphorylation
   D. Inadequate oxygen and inability to perform oxidative phosphorylation is a major cause of death due to coronary occlusion and stroke
II. Mitochondria, the powerhouses of the cell
   A. Membranes and matrix
      1. The inner mitochondrial membrane, in contrast to the outer membrane, exhibits restricted permeability; except for oxygen, carbon dioxide, and a few other compounds, only substances with translocases are able to cross the inner membrane
      2. Oxaloacetate, $NAD(P)^+$l/NAD(P)H, and coenzyme A are unable to traverse the inner membrane because they lack translocases
      3. The inner membrane contains succinate dehydrogenase, but the other Krebs cycle enzymes are hydrophilic and occur in the matrix
   B. Malate-aspartate shuttle
      1. This is an intricate shuttle that moves reducing equivalents across the membrane, especially in liver and heart
      2. It consists of two carrier proteins in the inner membrane: the glutamate-aspartate translocase and the malate–α-ketoglutarate translocase
      3. The shuttle also consists of cytosolic and mitochondrial aspartate aminotransferase and malate dehydrogenase
      4. *The yield of ATP is 2.5 moles per mole of cytosolic NADH that is translocated by this shuttle*
   C. Glycerol phosphate shuttle
      1. This is a simpler shuttle that moves cytosolic reducing equivalents into the electron transport chain of the inner mitochondrial membrane, especially in brain and muscle
      2. It consists of a cytosolic and integral inner mitochondrial membrane glycerol phosphate dehydrogenase
      3. *The yield of ATP is 1.5 moles per mole of cytosolic NADH that is translocated by this shuttle*

Objective 2: To describe electron transport from NADH and succinate to oxygen.

III. Components of the electron transport chain
   A. Flavoproteins that contain flavin mononucleotide (FMN) or flavin adenine dinucleotide (FAD) are two-electron and two-proton carriers
   B. Coenzyme Q is a diffusible carrier of two electrons and two protons
   C. Iron-sulfur proteins—which consist of iron, sulfur (as sulfide, or S^{2-}), and cysteine sulfur atoms—are one-electron carriers
   D. Cytochromes, which contain heme, are one-electron carriers
IV. Pathway of mitochondrial electron transport (Fig. 9–1)
   A. Complexes I, II, III, and IV
      1. **NADH** donates its electrons to complex I
      2. Electrons from succinate are transported as **$FADH_2$** via complex II
      3. **Coenzyme QH_2** carries electrons from complexes I and II to complex III
         a. Coenzyme Q accepts electrons from the $FADH_2$

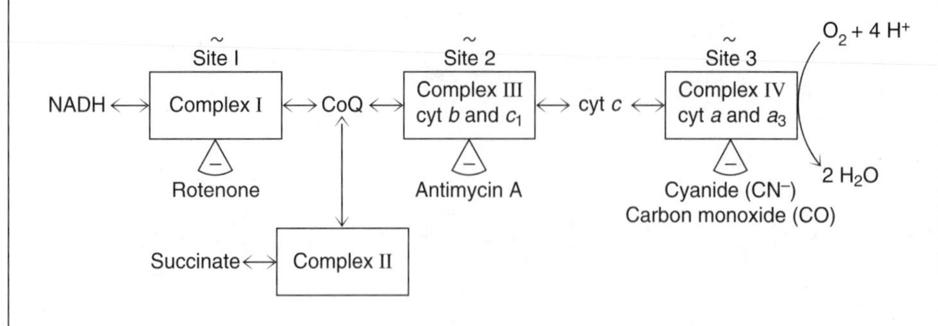

FIGURE 9-1. Components of the mitochondrial electron transport chain.

b. Mitochondrial acyl-CoA dehydrogenase (fatty acid oxidation) is an important source of reducing equivalents for coenzyme Q
4. Complex III contains cytochromes *b* and c_1
5. **Cytochrome *c*,** the only hydrophilic cytochrome, carries electrons from complex III to complex IV
6. *Complex IV, or cytochrome oxidase, which contains iron and copper, reacts physiologically with molecular oxygen*

V. Reactions of molecular oxygen
A. The reactions of electron transport from reductant to molecular oxygen are exergonic
B. An entire molecule of oxygen (and not a half-molecule) is the reactant
1. The cytochrome oxidase reaction involves molecular oxygen, 4 e^-, and 4 H^+
2. The cytochrome oxidase reaction is intricate because of the requirement for multiple components
C. The reduction of molecular oxygen to water, as catalyzed by cytochrome oxidase, is exergonic and unidirectional in accordance with PRINCIPLE 8 OF BIOENERGETICS

Objective 3: To identify inhibitors and uncouplers of oxidative phosphorylation.

VI. Characteristics of oxidative phosphorylation
A. Site-specific inhibitors and 2,4-dinitrophenol
1. Site-specific inhibitors block electron transport and proton translocation
a. **Rotenone,** a site 1–specific inhibitor, blocks electron transport in complex I
b. **Antimycin A,** a site 2–specific inhibitor, blocks electron transport in complex III
c. **Cyanide** and **carbon monoxide** are site 3–specific inhibitors that block electron transport in complex IV
2. **2,4-Dinitrophenol** uncouples electron transport and ATP synthesis by dissipating the proton gradient
a. Electron transport (oxygen consumption) is able to proceed in the absence of a proton gradient
b. ATP generation is not able to proceed in the absence of a proton gradient across the inner mitochondrial membrane
B. P/O ratios
1. The P/O ratio is the number of molecules of ATP formed per oxygen atom reduced to water
2. With NADH as reductant, the P/O ratio is 2.5
3. With $FADH_2$ as reductant, the P/O ratio is 1.5
C. Role of proton translocation
1. *The exergonic reactions of electron transport sustain proton translocation from the inside to the outside of the mitochondrion*
2. Proton translocation is sustained by a proton pump (sites 1 and 3) and by a redox loop mechanism (site 2)

Objective 4: To describe the F_oF_1 ATP synthase and ATP synthesis.

VII. F_0F_1 ATP synthase
A. Structure
1. The $\mathbf{F_0}$ portion spans the inner mitochondrial membrane
2. The $\mathbf{F_1}$ portion, which converts ADP and P_i to ATP and water, occurs within the matrix and is attached to F_o by a stalk
B. Mechanism of action
1. Three protons moving down their electrochemical gradient (from the outside to the inside of the mitochondrion) sustain the synthesis of one ATP
2. The F_1 component of each ATP synthase contains three ATP binding sites with tight, loose, and open configurations

VIII. Chemiosmotic theory
A. The three components of this theory include a proton-impermeable membrane, proton translocation coupled to electron transport, and an ATP synthase
B. This theory combines vectorial reactions across a membrane and chemical reactions on the ATP synthase
C. The number of protons translocated at site 1 (4), site 2 (2), and site 3 (4) is given in parentheses
D. *The synthesis of each ATP is sustained by the translocation of four protons*
1. Three protons are required for the synthesis of ATP
2. One proton is required for the translocation of phosphate from the exterior to the interior of the mitochondrion

Objective 5: To calculate the ATP yield from the complete oxidation of glucose.

IX. The ATP yield from the complete oxidation of one mole of glucose involves the following:
A. Conversion of one mole of cytosolic glucose to two moles of pyruvate occurs with the concomitant generation of two moles of ATP (net) and two moles of NADH

TABLE 9–1. ATP Yield from the Complete Oxidation of Glucose*

	ATP Produced
Glycolysis *per se*	2
2 NADH from glycolysis	3 or 5 (glycerol phosphate or malate-aspartate shuttles, respectively)
Pyruvate dehydrogenase (2 NADH)	5
Isocitrate dehydrogenase (2 NADH)	5
α-Ketoglutarate dehydrogenase (2 NADH)	5
Succinate thiokinase (2 GTP or 2 ATP)	2
Succinate dehydrogenase (2 $FADH_2$)	3
Malate dehydrogenase (2 NADH)	5
	30 or 32

1 Glucose → 30 ATP (glycerol phosphate shuttle) or 32 ATP (malate-aspartate shuttle)
1 Acetyl-CoA → 10 ATP
1 Pyruvate → 12.5 ATP

* Based on the values of Hinkle and coworkers. *In* P. C. Hinkle, A. Kumar, A. Resetar, and D. L. Harris. Mechanistic stoichiometry of mitochondrial oxidative phosphorylation. Biochemistry 30:3576–3582, 1991.

(which leads to the formation of 3 moles of ATP via the glycerol phosphate shuttle or 5 moles of ATP via the malate-aspartate shuttle)

B. Two moles of intramitochondrial pyruvate are converted into two moles of acetyl-CoA with the concomitant generation of two moles of NADH (5 moles of ATP)

C. Two moles of intramitochondrial acetyl-CoA are oxidized via the Krebs cycle and the electron transport chain with the concomitant formation of 2×10, or 20, moles of ATP including two moles of GTP (via substrate level phosphorylation)

D. The total yield of ATP is $2 + 3 + 5 + 20$, or 30, moles of ATP using the glycerol phosphate shuttle or $2 + 5 + 5 + 20$, or 32, moles of ATP using the malate-aspartate shuttle (Table 9–1)

Objective 6: To explain the control of glycolysis, the Krebs cycle, and oxidative phosphorylation.

X. Regulation of glycolysis, the citric acid cycle, and oxidative phosphorylation
- A. The metabolic logic of the cell (PRINCIPLE 9 OF BIOCHEMISTRY) and regulation
  1. The main function of glycolysis, the Krebs cycle, and oxidative phosphorylation is to mediate ATP formation
  2. Low energy charge, directly and indirectly, activates these processes
- B. Glycolysis
  1. ATP and citrate inhibit **phosphofructokinase,** the controlling enzyme of glycolysis
  2. Fructose 2,6-bisphosphate and AMP activate phosphofructokinase
  3. *Fructose 2,6-bisphosphate levels in liver (but not muscle) are decreased by the cyclic AMP second messenger system*
- C. Pyruvate dehydrogenase
  1. Enzyme activity is controlled by its phosphorylation and dephosphorylation
  2. ATP, NADH, and acetyl-CoA activate pyruvate dehydrogenase kinase
  3. *Phosphorylated pyruvate dehydrogenase is inhibited*
- D. Krebs cycle
  1. **Isocitrate dehydrogenase** is the pace-setting enzyme of the Krebs cycle
  2. ADP activates isocitrate dehydrogenase allosterically

Objective 7: To describe aberrant oxidative reactions in mitochondria.

XI. Mitochondrial dysfunction
- A. Cyanide is one of the most toxic and rapidly acting poisons known, and death can occur within a few minutes of exposure because of its inhibition of oxidative phosphorylation as a site 3 inhibitor
- B. Under anoxic conditions secondary to vascular occlusion, oxidative phosphorylation is impaired because of the absence of substrate (oxygen) and secondarily because of a paucity of oxidizable fuel molecules
  1. Cellular glycogen provides a substrate for anaerobic glycolysis, which can provide energy for a short time
  2. After glycogen is depleted, cells lack substrate for continued anaerobic energy production
- C. Oxygen and free radicals
  1. The major sources of aberrant oxygen radical generation occur between complex I and CoQ and CoQ and complex III
  2. Reduced flavins and quinones react with oxygen to yield oxygen radicals at these sites
  3. Even under physiological conditions, from 1% to 3% of oxygen produces reactive oxygen intermediates

QUESTIONS

DIRECTIONS (Items 1–18): Each of the numbered items or incomplete statements in this section is followed by answers or by completions of the statement. Select the ONE lettered answer or completion that is BEST in each case. Correct answers and explanations are given at the end of the chapter.

1. Leber's hereditary optic neuropathy (LHON) is a maternally inherited disorder causing blindness due to death of the optic nerve at a mean age of 27 years. Affected individuals may also have cardiac conduction aberrations and behavioral abnormalities. One group of mutations that produces LHON involves one of the mitochondrially encoded proteins of complex I. Which one of the following mobile electron carriers normally accepts electrons from complex I (NADH-Q reductase) but does not do so efficiently in patients with LHON?

   (A) Coenzyme Q (ubiquinone)
   (B) Cytochrome c_1
   (C) NAD^+
   (D) Retinol
   (E) α-Tocopherol

2. Which one of the following cytochromes is a hydrophilic, mobile protein that ferries electrons from complex III (cytochrome reductase) to complex IV (cytochrome oxidase)?

   (A) Cytochrome a,a_3
   (B) Cytochrome b_{566}
   (C) Cytochrome *c*
   (D) Cytochrome c_1
   (E) Cytochrome P-450

3. Menkes disease, which is a pleiotropic disorder characterized by arterial and neuronal degeneration, is due to defective intestinal absorption of copper and a decrease in intracellular copper. Copper deficiency results in a secondary deficit of

   (A) complex I (NADH-Q reductase)
   (B) complex II (succinate-Q reductase)
   (C) complex III (cytochrome reductase)
   (D) complex IV (cytochrome oxidase)
   (E) cytochrome *c*

4. Mitochondria from a group of patients with lactic acidosis and muscle weakness were unable to (i) oxidize QH_2, (ii) translocate protons across the mitochondrial membrane against a concentration gradient with succinate as substrate, and (iii) reduce cytochrome *c*. The biochemical defect resides in

   (A) complex I (NADH-Q reductase)
   (B) complex II (succinate-Q reductase)
   (C) complex III (cytochrome reductase)
   (D) complex IV (cytochrome oxidase)
   (E) ATP synthase

5. Which of the following systems provides for a maximum yield of 1.5 ATP from oxidation of a cytosolic NADH?

   (A) The glycerol phosphate shuttle
   (B) The malate-aspartate shuttle
   (C) The intermembrane space shuttle
   (D) NADH-Q reductase (complex I)

6. The salient features of the chemiosmotic theory include all of the following EXCEPT

   (A) a membrane impermeable to hydrogen ions
   (B) formation of energy-rich phosphorylated intermediates at sites 1, 2, and 3 during electron transport
   (C) oxidation-reduction–driven proton translocation
   (D) a proton-driven ATP synthase
   (E) exergonic electron transport reactions

7. Oligomycin binds to and inhibits which of the following enzymes?

   (A) NAD^+-dependent dehydrogenases
   (B) Succinate-Q reductase
   (C) Cytochrome reductase
   (D) Cytochrome oxidase
   (E) F_0F_1 ATP synthase

8. When the F_1 portion of ATP synthase is experimentally separated from the membrane-bound F_o fragment, which of the following metabolic effects is observed?

   (A) F_1 forms ATP at an accelerated rate
   (B) Protons pass through F_0, but they do not sustain ATP formation
   (C) The inner membrane remains impermeable to protons
   (D) Electron transport and phosphorylation of ADP remain tightly coupled
   (E) Electron transport is inhibited

9. How many protons must pass down the transmembrane electrochemical gradient in the synthesis of one ATP from ADP and P_i and the transport of one P_i into the mitochondrion?

   (A) 3
   (B) 4
   (C) 6
   (D) 8
   (E) 10

10. Peroxidative damage to the inner mitochondrial membrane can affect directly all of the following processes EXCEPT

    (A) synthesis of ATP from ADP and P_i
    (B) transport of electrons from NADH to O_2
    (C) generation of $FADH_2$ by oxidation of succinate
    (D) translocation of protons from one side of the membrane to the other
    (E) oxidation of fuel substrates by NAD^+

11. Atractyloside inhibits which of the following transport systems?

    (A) The ATP-ADP antiport system
    (B) The malate-aspartate shuttle
    (C) The P_i-OH^- antiport system
    (D) The malate-oxaloacetate antiport system
    (E) The glycerol phosphate shuttle

Items 12–18

History

A 49-year-old unemployed male is brought to the emergency room by ambulance within 30 minutes after collapsing on the street. He reports that he experienced chest discomfort, which he attributed to heat. The discomfort intensified to a crushing sensation in the sternal area that radiated to his neck and left arm. He has smoked two packs of cigarettes per day for 30 years. His father died of a heart attack at 52 years of age.

Physical Examination

During the interview, the patient lapsed into unconsciousness. He did not respond to deep pain, and his skin became cool, clammy, and pale. The pulse was weak, thready, and irregular at a rate of 90/min; his respiratory rate was 14/min. His blood pressure was unobtainable with an arm cuff. The cardiac monitor displayed a sinus rhythm with frequent premature ventricular complexes. Oxygen was administered by mask at 10 L/min. A dopamine drip was started intravenously. A 12-lead electrocardiogram (ECG or EKG) showed evidence of an acute injury of the anterior myocardium. Blood was drawn to check cardiac enzyme and electrolyte levels. His peripheral pulses were all present and equal but faint. There was no pedal edema. The chest x-ray showed no cardiomegaly (enlarged heart). The patient was admitted to the critical care unit. Initial arterial pressures (in mm Hg) were as follows: direct arterial systolic pressure, 85; diastolic pressure, 40; mean arterial pressure, 55. The patient was treated with intravenous recombinant tissue plasminogen activator.

Laboratory

Initial serum electrolytes, normal
Creatine phosphokinase (CPK), 44 U/L (normal ♂, 40–175 U/L)
Aspartate aminotransferase (AST, SGOT), 14 U/L (normal, 10–30 U/L)
Lactate dehydrogenase (LDH), 276 U/L (normal, 208–378 U/L)
Total cholesterol, 280 mg/dL (recommended, <200 mg/dL)
LDL cholesterol, 166 mg/dL (recommended, <130 mg/dL)

The following analyses were obtained from arterial and central venous sampling.

	Arterial Blood	Venous Blood
Oxygen	7.75 mM (normalized, 8.75 mM)	5.15 mM (normalized, 5.25 mM)
Carbon dioxide	23.5 mM (normalized, 21.5 mM)	26.5 mM (normalized, 24.5 mM)
Glucose	5.10 mM (normalized, 5.10 mM)	4.05 mM (normalized, 4.90 mM)
	92 mg/dL(normalized, 92 mg/dL)	73 mg/dL (normalized, 88 mg/dL)
Lactate	1.10 mM (normalized, 1.10 mM)	4.65 mM (normalized, 1.27 mM)
Free Fatty acid	0.60 mM (normalized, 0.60 mM)	0.52 mM (normalized, 0.45 mM)
β-Hydroxybutyrate	240 nM (normalized, 240 nM)	210 nM (normalized, 180 nM
pH	7.32 (normalized, 7.42)	7.02 (normalized, 7.37)

Six hours after the onset of pain, the creatine phosphokinase value was 140 U/L with a preponderance of the MB form; aspartate aminotransferase, 16 U/L; lactate dehydrogenase, 318 U/L.

12. The diagnosis of a myocardial infarction is based upon
    (A) arterial pressure
    (B) chest x-ray
    (C) history and electrocardiography
    (D) initial serum enzyme levels
    (E) serum cholesterol

13. The primary cause of cellular death following vascular occlusion is lack of
    (A) ADP
    (B) NADH and lactate
    (C) P_i
    (D) thiamine
    (E) oxygen and ATP

14. Activation of glycolysis in anoxic cells is due to
    (A) increased AMP
    (B) increased NAD^+
    (C) increased P_i
    (D) decreased acetyl-CoA
    (E) increased pH

15. Myoglobin is released from dysfunctional cardiac cells. Which of the following is a true statement regarding myoglobin?
    (A) It is a tetrameric protein
    (B) It binds oxygen cooperatively
    (C) It is an oxygen-storage protein
    (D) It transfers electrons from complex III to complex IV of the electron transport chain
    (E) It releases oxygen to hemoglobin when the hemoglobin is half-saturated with oxygen

16. The first measurable change in metabolites in myocardial cells following ischemia is
    (A) an increased level of ADP
    (B) a decreased level of creatine phosphate
    (C) a decreased level of NAD^+
    (D) a decreased level of P_i
    (E) a decreased level of AMP

17. The source of lactate in the venous blood is
    (A) free fatty acids
    (B) acetoacetate/β-hydroxybutyrate
    (C) lactose
    (D) glucose and/or myocardial glycogen
    (E) sucrose

18. The number of moles of ATP that can be obtained anaerobically from one mole of β-hydroxybutyrate is
    (A) 0
    (B) 2.5
    (C) 6
    (D) 22.5
    (E) 130

ANSWERS AND EXPLANATIONS

1. The answer is A: coenzyme Q (ubiquinone). Coenzyme Q is a small, lipid-soluble compound that accepts electrons from complex I (NADH-Q reductase). After adding protons from the matrix, reduced coenzyme Q transfers electrons to complex III and protons are released into the intermembrane space. This combination of electron transfer and proton translocation occurs in what is called a redox loop. Coenzyme Q also accepts electrons from complex II (succinate-Q reductase), from the mitochondrial glycerol phosphate dehydrogenase, or from the acyl-CoA dehydrogenase used in β-oxidation of fatty acids in the mitochondrial matrix. Cytochrome c_1 (a component of complex III) is a relatively immobile integral membrane protein. NAD^+ is a hydrophilic carrier that does not occur in the membrane as such. Retinol and α-tocopherol are lipid-soluble vitamins that do not play a role in mitochondrial electron transport. Some patients with LHON have been treated with ubiquinone and have experienced beneficial effects. *Biochemistry,* p. 124.
2. The answer is C: cytochrome *c*. Cytochrome *c* is the small, very basic hydrophilic protein used to carry electrons from complex III to complex IV. Cytochromes b_{566} and c_1 are components of the immobile complex III, cytochromes a,a_3 are part of the immobile complex IV, and cytochrome P-450, which occurs in the endoplasmic reticulum and in mitochondria, does not form part of the respiratory electron transport chain. *Biochemistry,* p. 124.
3. The answer is D: complex IV (cytochrome oxidase). Of the four major complexes used in electron transport, only complex IV (cytochrome oxidase) contains copper. Complex IV and the other complexes contain iron as cytochrome or as an iron-sulfur complex. Complex IV is at the end of the electron transport chain and is involved in a physiological reaction with molecular oxygen. This cytochrome oxidase reaction is a four-electron, four-proton reduction of O_2, yielding 2 H_2O, and is physiologically irreversible. Cytochrome *c* contains heme iron but not copper. *Biochemistry,* p. 124.
4. The answer is C: complex III (cytochrome reductase). Only cytochrome reductase (complex III) oxidizes QH_2 and reduces cytochrome *c*. With succinate as substrate, protons cannot be translocated across the inner membrane. With NADH as substrate, however, protons can be translocated at site 1 by NADH-Q reductase. NADH-Q reductase and cytochrome oxidase translocate protons across the membrane but do not oxidize QH_2 or reduce cytochrome *c*. Succinate-Q reductase reduces Q, does not translocate protons, and does not directly reduce cytochrome *c* (only complex III does that). Metabolic defects in each of the four complexes have been described in humans. The downhill flow of protons through ATP synthase sustains ATP formation, but ATP synthase performs no redox functions. Defects in human ATP synthase have not been described. *Biochemistry,* p. 126.
5. The answer is A: the glycerol phosphate shuttle. The glycerol phosphate shuttle transports electrons from NADH to membranous FAD to form $FADH_2$, and electrons enter the transport chain at complex III (via QH_2). Oxidation of QH_2 yields only 1.5 ATP per electron pair, while oxidation of a mitochondrial NADH (the product of the aspartate-malate shuttle) yields 2.5 ATP. Oxidation of NADH by NADH-Q reductase usually provides for a maximum yield of 2.5 ATP per electron pair, since the proton translocation occurring at this site allows production of one additional ATP when compared to the ATP yield from oxidation of QH_2. An intermembrane space shuttle has not been described. *Biochemistry,* p. 122.
6. The answer is B: formation of energy-rich phosphorylated intermediates at sites 1, 2, and 3 during electron transport does NOT occur. Although early theories posited the formation of energy-rich phosphorylated intermediates at each site of electron transport where free energy changes were sufficient to support ATP synthesis, no such intermediates were ever found. The occurrence of such intermediates in the familiar reactions of substrate-level phosphorylation had made such expectations seem eminently reasonable. The Mitchell chemiosmotic theory, which requires a proton-impermeable membrane, redox-driven proton translocation, and a proton-driven ATP synthase, was a radical departure that helped to explain a wide variety of biological phenomena including oxidative phosphorylation and photosynthetic phosphorylation. *Biochemistry,* p. 126.
7. The answer is E: F_0F_1 ATP synthase. Oligomycin binds specifically to an oligomycin sensitivity conferring protein, a subunit of the F_0 portion of the F_0F_1 ATP synthase, and thereby inhibits synthase activity. Oligomycin does not inhibit any of the components of the electron transport chain. *Biochemistry,* p. 126.
8. The answer is B: protons pass through F_0 but they do not sustain ATP formation. Free F_1 is unable to mediate the formation of any ATP. Membrane-bound F_0 becomes freely permeable to protons and thus dissipates any proton gradient. Since there is no proton gradient impeding further proton translocation, electron transport can continue, even in the absence of ATP formation, and oxidative phosphorylation is uncoupled. *Biochemistry,* p. 129.
9. The answer is B: 4. Synthesis of one ATP from ADP and P_i requires the downhill passage of three protons through ATP synthase. ATP synthesis reduces the intramitochondrial phosphate level by one, which must be replenished by passage of a cytosolic phosphate into the mitochondrion. The latter process uses a P_i-OH^- antiport system, which is formally equivalent to symport, or concurrent passage of one P_i and one H^+ from cytosol to matrix. *Biochemistry,* p. 130.
10. The answer is E: peroxidative damage to the inner mitochondrial membrane does NOT directly affect oxidation of fuel substrates by NAD^+. NADH is formed from NAD^+ by dehydrogenase reactions occurring in the mitochondrial matrix. For example, pyruvate dehydrogenase, isocitrate dehydrogenase, α-ketoglutarate dehydrogenase, and malate dehydrogenase are hydrophilic enzymes that occur in the mitochondrial matrix. In contrast, synthesis of ATP from ADP and P_i, transport of electrons from NADH to O_2, and translocation of protons from one side of the membrane to the other are performed by components of the inner mitochondrial membrane. Moreover, succinate dehydrogenase, which mediates the generation of $FADH_2$ by oxidation of succinate, is an integral inner mitochondrial membrane. (It is likely, however, that oxidation of fuel substrates by NAD^+ would be indirectly affected as NADH accumulates). Oxygen radicals are adventitious by-products of oxidative phosphorylation, and they account for about 1–3% of total oxygen

uptake. The most likely cause of mitochondrial damage is oxidation by peroxides. These substances react with lipids, proteins, and nucleic acids. The major sources of radical generation are between complex I and CoQ and between CoQ and complex III. Reduced flavins and quinones react with oxygen to yield oxygen radicals at these sites. *Biochemistry,* p. 124.

11. The answer is A: the ATP-ADP antiport system. The ATP-ADP antiport system translocates ADP from the cytosol into the mitochondrion in exchange for mitochondrial ATP, and this antiport process is inhibited by atractyloside. The malate-aspartate shuttle and P_i-OH^- antiport system, along with transporters for such compounds as pyruvate, acylcarnitine, ornithine, and citrulline, all utilize integral membrane translocases that are not affected by atractyloside. A translocase for oxaloacetate in human mitochondria does not exist, and it is for this reason that oxaloacetate must be converted to malate or to aspartate prior to translocation of four-carbon compounds through the inner mitochondrial membrane. Mitochondrial glycerol phosphate dehydrogenase is located on the outer surface of the inner mitochondrial membrane. Its FAD accepts electrons from glycerol phosphate and forms $FADH_2$, which is oxidized by the electron transport chain within the membrane. There is no metabolite translocation from cytosol to matrix or from matrix to cytosol with this shuttle. *Biochemistry,* p. 121.

12. The answer is C: history and electrocardiography. A crushing left sternal chest pain with radiation into the neck or arm is a classical description of the pain suffered during a myocardial infarction (heart attack). The electrocardiogram (ECG) as described is consistent with such an episode. The ECG contains P, Q, R, S, and T waves, and several leads exhibit ST segment depression following damage to the anterior myocardium as a result of occlusion of the left anterior descending branch of the left coronary artery. The initial serum enzyme levels are normal and are therefore not diagnostic. It often requires 6 or more hours before creatine phosphokinase levels are elevated after the insult. New tests that can distinguish between newly released and existing creatine phosphokinase are more sensitive. The chest x-ray is reported as normal. Other causes of chest pain such as pulmonary embolus or pneumothorax can be diagnosed on the basis of the chest x-ray. The serum cholesterol is elevated, but this is elevated in asymptomatic people. The arterial pressure is subnormal, and the patient is in shock. Only a minority of people suffering from a myocardial infarction develop cardiogenic shock. Other causes of shock include trauma with blood loss and shock secondary to bacterial infection (septic shock). Septic shock occurs in the elderly who become comatose. Without the history of chest pain, septic shock would have been a valid provisional diagnosis in this patient. The heart normally derives most of its ATP by oxidative metabolism that involves the Krebs cycle and oxidative phosphorylation. The most likely cause of the infarction is atherosclerosis. The importance of this process in heart is underscored by the morbidity and mortality resulting from localized anoxia that is due to coronary artery disease. *Cecil,* p. 304.

13. The answer is E: oxygen and ATP. An infarction is ischemic necrosis or cell death that results from inadequate blood supply. The limiting component in blood is oxygen, and a deficiency of oxygen leads to decreased oxidative phosphorylation and decreased ATP formation. Anaerobic glycolysis using endogenous cellular glycogen is effective in maintaining cellular ATP for only a short time. Cells without adequate ATP die, a corollary of Lipmann's law. ATP is converted to P_i and ADP by cardiac myosin ATPase, and P_i and ADP are not limiting. Some NADH is oxidized by pyruvate in a reaction catalyzed by lactate dehydrogenase; in the absence of oxygen and oxidative phosphorylation, NADH and lactate accumulate. Thiamine deficiency decreases the activity of oxidative metabolism at the pyruvate dehydrogenase and α-ketoglutarate dehydrogenase steps, but there is no indication of thiamine deficiency in this person. Wet beriberi, which results from thiamine deficiency, is accompanied by heart failure (inability of the heart to maintain the circulation; this differs from a heart attack) and edema (which prompted the term "wet"). *Biochemistry,* p. 132.

14. The answer is A: increased AMP. Myocardial myosin ATPase results in the formation of ADP. To provide additional ATP, myokinase (adenylate kinase) catalyzes the following reaction: 2 ADP $\rightleftharpoons$ ATP + AMP. This provides another ATP for muscle contraction and generates an allosteric activator of phosphofructokinase, the rate-limiting reaction of glycolysis. Acetyl-CoA accumulates (not diminishes) because of decreased aerobic metabolism; P_i is generally present in excess and is not limiting in metabolism. Cellular pH is decreased, not increased, inanoxic cells, owing to generation of excess lactic acid. NADH and not NAD^+ accumulates during periods of inadequate oxidative metabolism. AMP is further metabolized to adenosine, which is released from myocardial cells and functions at an adenosine receptor linked to a G-protein to produce vasodilatation. *Biochemistry,* p. 100.

15. The answer is C: myoglobin is an oxygen-storage protein. Myoglobin is a monomer (not a tetramer) that exhibits a rectangular hyperbolic oxygen-binding curve (and not a sigmoidal curve that reflects positive cooperativity). Myoglobin has a much higher affinity for oxygen than does hemoglobin and does not release oxygen to the carrier in the erythrocyte. Cytochrome *c* is the protein that transfers electrons from complex III to complex IV. New tests for myocardial infarction are being developed based on the measurement of myoglobin in serum. Normal levels of myoglobin in serum range from 20 to 90 μg/L, and elevations occur following cardiac muscle damage. These changes may occur earlier than changes in creatine phosphokinase. *Biochemistry,* p. 48.

16. The answer is B: a decreased level of creatine phosphate. Although ATP is metabolized by myocardial myosin ATPase, it is regenerated by the creatine phosphokinase reaction. The levels of creatine phosphate are about five times those of ATP in the cell. Creatine phosphate also has a higher group transfer potential than ATP, and formation of ATP is favored. It is not until creatine phosphate is depleted that ATP levels fall. Because the levels of creatine phosphate fall before those of ATP, it was initially thought that creatine phosphate and not ATP was the substrate that provided energy for muscle contraction before the discovery of myosin ATPase. The levels of inorganic phosphate, AMP, and NADH increase in ischemic tissue. *Biochemistry,* p. 81.

17. The answer is D: glucose and/or myocardial glycogen. Glucose and glucosyl units derived from glycogen are converted to lactate during anaerobic glycolysis. Fatty acids and β-hydroxybutyrate cannot be converted to lactate in net amounts. Lactose and sucrose also would not yield lactate because lactose and sucrose *per se* do not occur in blood or myocardial tissues. Lactose is digested to form galactose and glucose, and sucrose to glucose

and fructose, prior to absorption from the gut. *Biochemistry,* p. 102.

18. The answer is A: 0. Glycolysis is the only multistep process that results in anaerobic ATP production. Fatty acids, ketone bodies (acetoacetate and β-hydroxybutyrate), and amino acids must be metabolized aerobically to provide ATP. This accounts for the levels of metabolites in the arterial and venous blood. Under normal conditions, the heart and most other cells of the body (except red blood cells and neural cells) use fatty acids and (during an overnight fast) ketone bodies in preference to glucose. Under anaerobic conditions, glucose and endogenous glycogen provide fuel molecules for ATP formation.

REFERENCES

Roskoski, R., Jr. *Biochemistry.* Philadelphia, W. B. Saunders Company, 1996.

Wyngaarden, J. B., L. H. Smith, Jr., and J. C. Bennett (eds.). *Cecil Textbook of Medicine,* 19th ed. Philadelphia, W. B. Saunders Company, 1992.

CHAPTER TEN

CARBOHYDRATE METABOLISM

SYNOPSIS

OBJECTIVES

1. To enumerate the principles of metabolite biosynthesis.
2. To describe the glycolytic bypass reactions of gluconeogenesis.
3. To describe the regulation of gluconeogenesis.
4. To outline the pathway and bioenergetics of glycogen biosynthesis.
5. To identify enzyme defects that produce glycogen storage diseases.

Objective 1: To enumerate the principles of metabolite biosynthesis.

I. Principles of biosynthesis
  A. Pathways for synthesis and degradation are exergonic (PRINCIPLE 18 OF BIOCHEMISTRY)
    1. The pathways for synthesis and degradation must therefore differ
    2. Some pathways (e.g., glycolysis and gluconeogenesis) vary by only a few steps, and others (e.g., protein synthesis and degradation) are completely independent
  B. The reaction of a high-energy donor and acceptor to produce a low-energy metabolite is a common strategy used in biosynthetic reactions (PRINCIPLE 17 OF BIOCHEMISTRY)

Objective 2: To describe the glycolytic bypass reactions of gluconeogenesis.

II. Gluconeogenesis
  A. Gluconeogenesis is the process whereby lactate, pyruvate derived from amino acids, Krebs cycle intermediates derived from amino acids, and glycerol are converted to glucose (Fig. 10–1)
  B. Gluconeogenesis is localized to the liver and kidney
  C. Erythrocytes and brain require a constant supply of glucose for energy production by glycolysis and oxidative phosphorylation (brain)
  D. Glycolysis and gluconeogenesis can occur simultaneously but in different cells of the body
  E. The pyruvate kinase bypass reactions require cooperation of the mitochondrion and cytosol
    1. **Pyruvate carboxylase** catalyzes the conversion of pyruvate to oxaloacetate in an ATP- and biotin-dependent process
      a. This enzyme requires acetyl-CoA as an allosteric activator for expression of its activity
      b. This enzyme occurs in the mitochondrion
    2. **Phosphoenolpyruvate (PEP) carboxykinase,** which occurs in the mitochondrion and cytosol, catalyzes the conversion of oxaloacetate to phosphoenolpyruvate in a GTP-requiring process
  F. **Fructose-1,6-bisphosphatase,** a cytosolic enzyme, catalyzes the phosphofructokinase bypass reaction
  G. **Glucose-6-phosphatase,** an enzyme of the endoplasmic reticulum, catalyzes the hexokinase bypass reaction

Objective 3: To describe the regulation of gluconeogenesis.

III. Regulation of glycolysis and gluconeogenesis
  A. Glycolysis and gluconeogenesis are reciprocally regulated
  B. High plasma glucagon activates the cyclic AMP second messenger system and activates gluconeogenesis
    1. *Fructose 2,6-bisphosphate, which declines in liver as a result of the action of cyclic AMP and protein kinase A, activates phosphofructokinase and inhibits fructose-1,6-bisphosphatase activity*
    2. As a result of the decline in fructose 2,6-bisphosphate, fructose-1,6-bisphosphatase activity increases

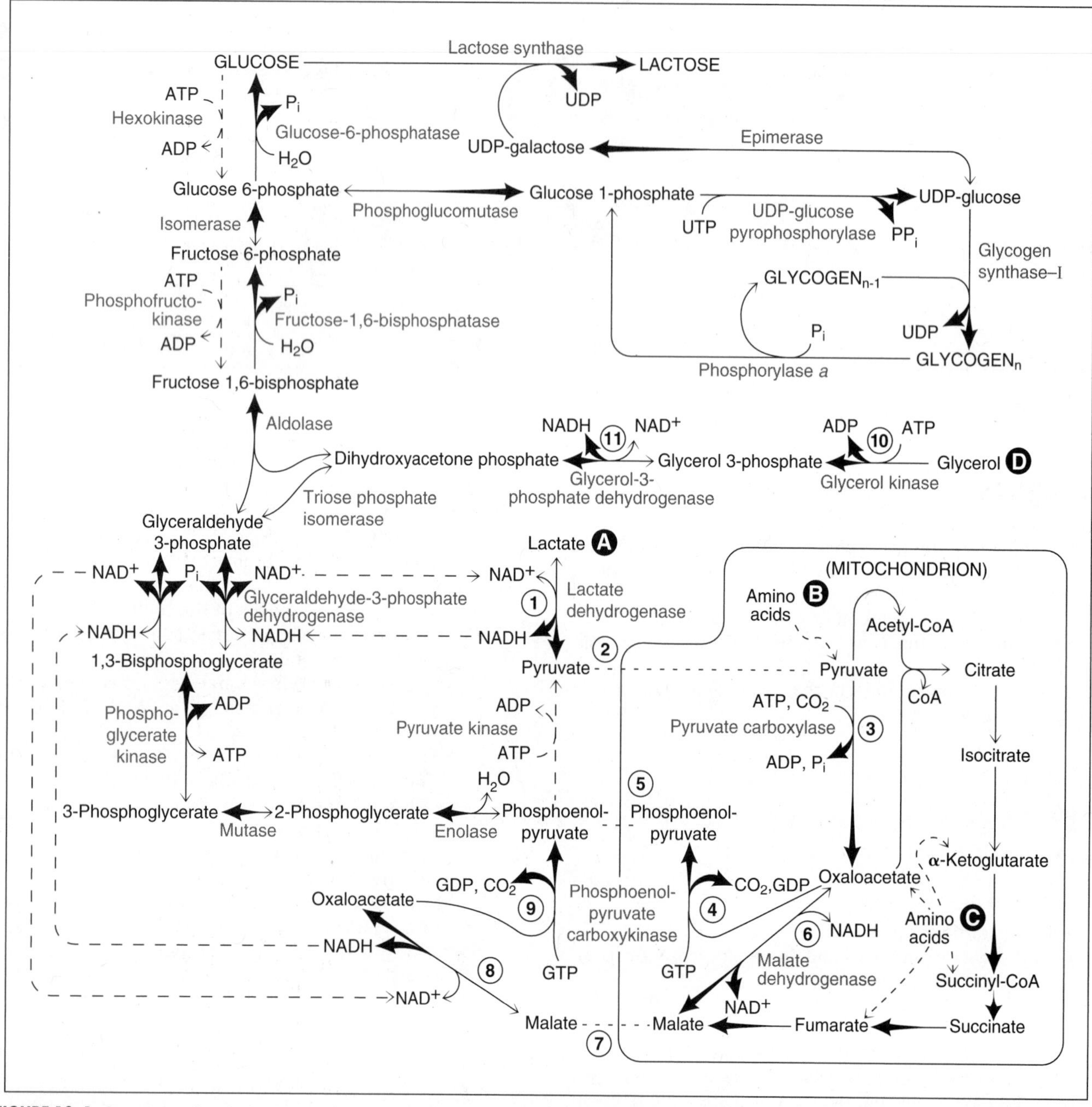

FIGURE 10–1. Overview of carbohydrate metabolism. The diagram illustrates the reactions of gluconeogenesis from (*A*) lactate, (*B*) and (*C*) amino acids, and (*D*) glycerol. The pathways from glucose to lactose and from glucose to glycogen and back are also indicated. *A.* The conversion of lactate to phosphoenolpyruvate involves steps 1–5 including the mitochondrial PEP carboxykinase. *B.* The conversion of mitochondrial pyruvate, derived from amino acids, to cytosolic phosphoenolpyruvate involves steps 3 and 6–9. *C.* The conversion of mitochondrial Krebs cycle intermediates to cytosolic phosphoenolpyruvate involves steps 7–9 plus step 6 for mitochondrial oxaloacetate. *D.* The conversion of glycerol to a glycolytic intermediate involves steps 10 and 11.

IV. Bioenergetics

A. The overall reaction for gluconeogenesis is as follows:

$$2\ \text{Pyruvate}^{-1} + 6\ \text{NTP}^{-4} + 2\ \text{NADH} + 6\ H_2O \rightarrow \text{Glucose} + 6\ \text{NDP}^{-3} + 6\ P_i^{-2} + 2\ \text{NAD}^+ + 2\ H^+ \quad (10.1)$$

B. Six high-energy bonds are expended per molecule of glucose synthesized from two molecules of pyruvate, and the process is energetically expensive

V. Diabetes mellitus

A. The metabolic derangements in diabetes mellitus are due to an increase in the ratio of glucagon to insulin action (Table 10–1)

TABLE 10–1. Hormonal Abnormalities and Metabolic Derangements of Diabetes Mellitus

Derangement	Insulin Deficiency	Glucagon Excess
Underutilization of glucose	++++	0
Overproduction of glucose	+	++++
Increased glycogenolysis	+	++++
Increased gluconeogenesis	+	++++
Increased release of amino acids	++++	0
Increased lipolysis	++++	+
Increased hepatic ketogenesis	+	++++

B. A hallmark of diabetes is hyperglycemia, which is aggravated by increased gluconeogenesis

Objective 4: To outline the pathway and bioenergetics of glycogen biosynthesis.

VI. Bioenergetics and metabolism of glycosidic diphosphates
   A. UDP-glucose is the prototype of glycosidic diphosphates
   B. The synthesis of UDP-glucose by pyrophosphorylase is illustrated in equation 10.2
      1. The reactants have two high-energy bonds, both in UTP
      2. The products have three high-energy bonds (UDP-glucose contains the energy-rich phosphoric acid anhydride and the energy-rich glycosidic-diphosphate bond; PP_i contains the energy-rich simple acid anhydride linkage):

$$\text{UTP} + \text{glucose 1-phosphate} \rightleftharpoons \text{UDP-glucose} + PP_i \qquad (10.2)$$

      3. Under standard conditions, the reaction proceeds from products to reactants (PRINCIPLE 3 OF BIOENERGETICS)
         a. The standard free energy change for the reaction is +6.9 kJ/mol, and the reaction is bidirectional
         b. This is an unusual example in a biosynthetic pathway because the products have more high-energy bonds than the reactants
         c. The enzyme-catalyzed hydrolysis of pyrophosphate pulls the reaction in the direction of UDP-glucose formation (PRINCIPLE 14 OF BIOCHEMISTRY)
VII. Glycogen metabolism (Figure 10–1)
   A. Glycogenesis
      1. **Glycogen synthase** catalyzes the reaction between glycogen containing n-1 glucosyl residues (glycogen_{n-1}) and UDP-glucose to form a new α-1,4-glycosidic linkage (glycogen_n) and UDP
         a. This transferase reaction proceeds with a loss of one high-energy bond and is exergonic (PRINCIPLE 2 OF BIOENERGETICS)
         b. This process is repeated until a chain extending 12–16 glucosyl groups from a branch point is formed
      2. **Branching enzyme** (amylo-1,4-1,6-transglycosylase) catalyzes the formation of an α-1,6 branch on the proximal portion of the donor chain
      3. The formation of a glycogen primer requires special enzymatic machinery
         a. A **glycogenin** protein-tyrosine reacts with UDP-glucose to form a glycosylated protein in an autocatalytic process
         b. After the addition of about eight glucosyl residues, the oligosaccharide-protein complex functions as a primer to which additional glucosyl residues can be added to form the glycogen macromolecule as catalyzed by glycogen synthase
   B. Glycogenolysis
      1. **Glycogen phosphorylase** (usually called phosphorylase) catalyzes a reaction between phosphate and glycogen_n to yield glucose 1-phosphate and glycogen_{n-1} by a phosphorolysis (*not* a hydrolysis) reaction
         a. This phosphorolysis (lysis by phosphate) reaction occurs at α-1,4-glycosidic bonds
         b. Phosphorylase contains pyridoxal phosphate as a covalently bound prosthetic group
      2. A single protein with two enzymatic activities, called **debranching enzyme,** eliminates the branch by a two-step process
         a. Transglycosylase activity of debranching enzyme transfers a triglucosyl unit from a tetraglucosyl branch to the end of a chain
         b. Hydrolysis of the remaining α-1,6 glucosidic bond is exergonic, and the reaction is unidirectional (PRINCIPLE 5 OF BIOENERGETICS)
VIII. Regulation of glycogenesis and glycogenolysis
   A. Activation of phosphorylase by the glucagon signal transduction system
      1. Following stimulation of G_s by the glucagon-receptor complex and activation of adenylyl cyclase, cyclic AMP is generated
      2. Cyclic AMP activates **protein kinase A** by binding to the regulatory subunits and dissociating them from the catalytic subunits, which are thereby activated according to the following equation:

$$R_2C_2 + 4\ \text{cAMP} \rightleftharpoons 2\ C + R_2(\text{cAMP})_4 \qquad (10.3)$$

      3. Protein kinase A catalyzes the phosphorylation of **phosphorylase kinase** on its α- and β-subunits and activates the enzyme (Fig. 10–2*A*)
      4. Phosphorylase kinase catalyzes the phosphorylation and activation of phosphorylase, converting phosphorylase *b* to phosphorylase *a* (Fig. 10–2*B*)
      5. Phosphorylase catalyzes the degradation of glycogen, producing glucose 1-phosphate
   B. Inhibition of glycogen synthase
      1. Protein kinase A also catalyzes the phosphorylation and inhibition of **glycogen synthase,** converting the I-form to the D-form (Fig. 10–2*C*)
      2. Other protein kinases also catalyze the phosphorylation and inhibition of glycogen synthase
   C. Inhibition of phosphoprotein phosphatase–1
      1. Protein kinase A also catalyzes the phosphorylation of protein phosphatase inhibitor–1 (Fig. 10–2*D*)
      2. This phosphorylated protein inhibits phosphoprotein phosphatase–1
      3. The action of protein kinase A results in the activation of phosphorylase, the inhibition of glycogen synthase, and the generation of an inhibitor of the dephosphorylation reactions
   D. Allosteric regulation of glycogen metabolism
      1. Glucose inhibits and AMP activates phosphorylase
      2. ATP and glucose 6-phosphate are allosteric inhibitors of phosphorylase
      3. Phosphorylase kinase is activated by calcium, and the δ-subunit of phosphorylase kinase is the calcium-binding protein called **calmodulin**

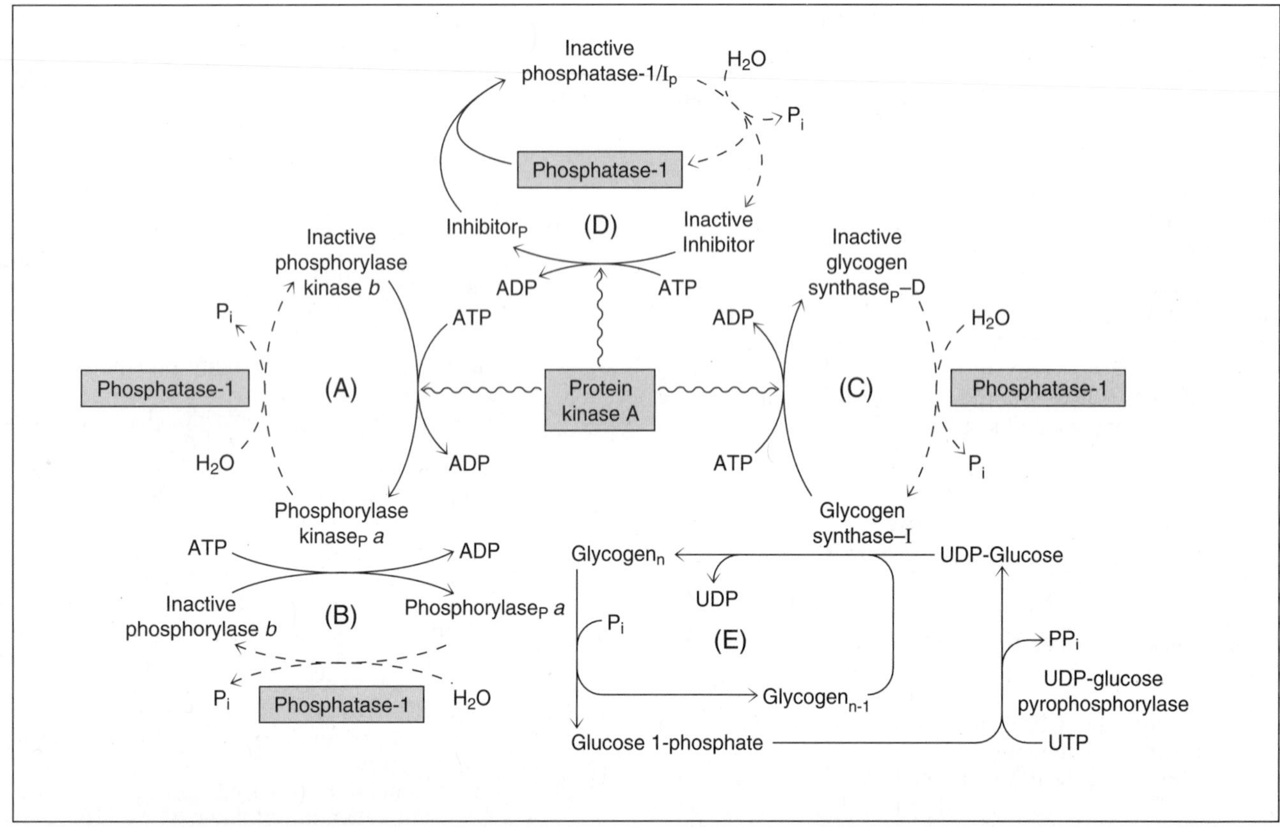

FIGURE 10-2. Regulation of glycogen metabolism. Phosphorylated proteins are denoted by a P subscript.

Objective 5: To identify enzyme defects that produce glycogen storage diseases.

IX. Glycogen storage diseases
  A. It is noteworthy that the type I glycogen storage disease (von Gierke disease) is due to a deficiency of glucose-6-phosphatase
    1. Affected individuals have hepatomegaly, and the kidneys are usually twice the normal size
    2. Hypoglycemia, lactic acidemia, and elevated blood triglycerides are hallmarks of the disorder
  B. Type II glycogen storage disease (Pompe disease) is due to a deficiency of acid α-glucosidase
    1. This disorder involves the heart, skeletal muscle, and nervous system
    2. This disorder is a lysosomal disease
  C. Type V glycogen storage disease (McArdle disease) is due to a deficiency of muscle phosphorylase
    1. Liver glycogen metabolism is normal, and there is no hypoglycemia
    2. Fatigue with exercise and muscle cramps appear in the second or third decade of life
    3. Patients fail to exhibit increased lactic acid production during exercise

QUESTIONS

DIRECTIONS. (Items 1–4): The set of matching questions in this section consists of a list of lettered options followed by several numbered items. For each numbered item, select the ONE lettered option that is most closely associated with it. Each lettered option may be selected once, more than once, or not at all. Correct answers and explanations are given at the end of the chapter.

Items 1–4

(A) Pyruvate → oxaloacetate
(B) Oxaloacetate → phosphoenolpyruvate
(C) Fructose 1,6-bisphosphate → fructose 6-phosphate
(D) Glucose 6-phosphate → glucose
(E) ATP + 3-phosphoglycerate → 1,3-bisphosphoglycerate + ADP

For each description of a chemical process, select the most appropriate item from the above list.

1. This process occurs in both the mitochondria and cytosol in human liver cells
2. A defect in this process, which requires biotin as cofactor and acetyl-CoA as an allosteric activator, causes lactic acidosis in children

3. A defect in this process is characterized by normal hyperglycemia following intravenous galactose, but not intravenous fructose, administration
4. All of the reactions are required for gluconeogenesis from amino acids degraded to succinyl-CoA EXCEPT

DIRECTIONS. (Items 5–18): Each of the numbered items or incomplete statements in this section is followed by answers or by completions of the statement. Select the ONE lettered answer or completion that is BEST in each case. Correct answers and explanations are given at the end of the chapter.

5. Ketogenic diets are under evaluation for the treatment of intractable forms of epilepsy. Such diets are designed to produce minimal substrates for gluconeogenesis. Which of the following compounds is (are) the most ketogenic?

(A) Glycerol
(B) Lactate
(C) Amino acids that are degraded to Krebs cycle intermediates
(D) Amino acids that are degraded to pyruvate
(E) Amino acids that are degraded to acetyl-CoA

6. Which of the following enzymes is used in both gluconeogenesis from amino acids and in glycolysis?

(A) Hexokinase
(B) Phosphofructokinase
(C) Phosphoglycerate kinase
(D) Pyruvate kinase
(E) Phosphoenolpyruvate carboxykinase

7. In liver, the increased glucagon/insulin ratio that occurs in diabetes mellitus leads to

(A) a decrease in glycogenolysis
(B) an increase in glycolysis
(C) an increase in glycogenesis
(D) a decrease in fructose 2,6-bisphosphate concentration
(E) an increase in pyruvate kinase activity

8. In liver, how many moles of nucleoside triphosphate (e.g., ATP or GTP) are required for the conversion of two moles of lactate to one mole of glucose?

(A) 2
(B) 4
(C) 6
(D) 8
(E) 32

9. Which of the following is a true statement regarding the formation of UDP-glucose from glucose 1-phosphate and UTP?

(A) It is catalyzed by phosphorylase
(B) It results in the formation of one less high-energy bond in products than in reactants
(C) It is pulled forward by the subsequent hydrolysis of pyrophosphate
(D) It is the primary regulatory step in glycogen synthesis
(E) It is an irreversible reaction

10. McArdle disease is a myopathy that results in an inability to perform anaerobic exercise. The disease is due to a deficiency of the enzyme that catalyzes the predominant reaction of glycogenolysis, and this enzyme involves which one of the following processes?

(A) Trisaccharide transfer
(B) Hydrolysis reaction
(C) Phosphorolysis reaction
(D) Lyase reaction
(E) Dephosphorylation reaction

11. All of the following types of phosphorylation are directly affected in rare individuals with deficient protein kinase A in liver EXCEPT

(A) phosphorylation of phosphorylase kinase
(B) phosphorylation of phosphorylase *b*
(C) phosphorylation of glycogen synthase
(D) phosphorylation of phosphoprotein phosphatase–1 inhibitor
(E) phosphorylation of fructose-6-phosphate-2-kinase/phosphatase

12. In muscle, the substance that triggers muscle contraction *and* allosterically activates phosphorylase kinase is

(A) cyclic AMP
(B) 5′-AMP
(C) calcium
(D) glucose 6-phosphate
(E) ATP

13. The extracellular "first messenger" that initiates the cyclic AMP-dependent glycogenolytic cascade in muscle is

(A) glucagon
(B) acetylcholine
(C) calcium
(D) epinephrine
(E) sodium

14. Hypoglycemia is characteristic of glycogen storage disease that results from a deficiency of any of the following enzymes EXCEPT

(A) glucose-6-phosphatase
(B) amylo-1,6-glucosidase (debranching enzyme)
(C) liver phosphorylase
(D) liver phosphorylase kinase
(E) branching enzyme

Items 15–18

History

A 56-year-old male accountant presents in the outpatient clinic with a chief complaint of bilateral cramping leg muscle pain brought on and aggravated by walking. The patient noted that he became tired with modest exertion. He denied joint pain, signs of inflammation (swelling or redness), dyspnea, palpitations, and dark amber colored urine (myoglobinuria). He has smoked about one pack of cigarettes per day for nearly 40 years. Family history was noncontributory.

Physical Examination

Funduscopic examination revealed dilated irregular retinal veins and white exudates. Examination of the chest revealed no abnormalities. There were no murmurs, or abnormal heart sounds, nor were there bruits (pronounced "brew eez"; abnormal auscultatory sounds) in the abdomen. Pulses in the upper extremity were normal. The femoral artery pulse was normal, but the dorsal pedal pulses and popliteal artery pulses were not palpable. The patient's muscle strength in the arms and legs was normal. He exhibited decreased deep tendon reflexes in the lower extremity and decreased vibratory sensation. His response to pinprick was normal. The patient was 180 cm tall (5 ft 11 in.) and weighed 96 kg (212 lb). Blood pressure was 116/80.

Laboratory

Glucose 320 mg/dL (normal, 70–105 mg/dL)
Creatine phosphokinase, 54 U/L (normal, 40–175 U/L)
Hemoglobin $A_{1,}$ 12% (normal, 5.6–7.5%)
Triglyceride, 240 mg/dL (normal, 40–160 mg/dL)
Cholesterol, 264 mg/dL (recommended, <200 mg/dL)
LDL cholesterol, 150 mg/dL (recommended, <130 mg/dL)
Creatinine, 2.4 mg/dL (normal, 0.7–1.3 mg/dL)
Blood urea nitrogen (BUN), 36 mg/dL (normal, 7–18 mg/dL)
Uric acid, 4 mg/dL (normal, 3.5–7.2 mg/dL)
Lactate, 14.2 mg/dL (normal, 4.5–19.8 mg/dL)
Lactate following exercise, 35 mg/dL (normal, >19.8 mg/dL)
Electrolytes, pH, hematocrit, hemoglobin, and white blood count, normal
Urinalysis
  Specific gravity, 1.030 (normal, 1.003–1.035)
  Glucosuria, 2+ (normal, 0)
  Proteinuria, 1+ (normal, 0)
  Ketonuria, 0 (normal, 0)
Chest x-ray, normal
Electrocardiogram, normal.

15. The primary diagnosis in this patient is
    (A) muscle phosphoglycerate mutase deficiency
    (B) muscle glycogen phosphorylase deficiency (McArdle disease)
    (C) hypertension
    (D) gout
    (E) diabetes mellitus

16. The pathogenesis for producing the hyperglycemia in this patient can be related to each of the following mechanisms EXCEPT
    (A) There is decreased transport of glucose into muscle and adipose cells
    (B) There is decreased transport of glucose into liver cells
    (C) There is increased gluconeogenesis due to induction of phosphoenolpyruvate carboxykinase by glucagon
    (D) There is increased glycogenolysis
    (E) There are decreased levels of hepatic fructose 2,6-bisphosphate owing to the action of glucagon

17. The muscle pain that results from walking (intermittent claudication) is the result of
    (A) atherosclerosis and peripheral vascular disease
    (B) McArdle disease
    (C) muscle phosphoglycerate mutase deficiency
    (D) peripheral neuropathy
    (E) renal disease and azotemia (elevated blood urea nitrogen and creatinine)

18. The patient's average blood glucose concentration during the previous few weeks was
    (A) decreased
    (B) normal
    (C) elevated
    (D) unpredictable

ANSWERS AND EXPLANATIONS

1. The answer is B: oxaloacetate → phosphoenolpyruvate. This reaction is catalyzed by phosphoenolpyruvate carboxykinase, which occurs in both a cytosolic and a mitochondrial form. When lactate is the primary precursor of glucose, the conversion of lactate to pyruvate provides the cytosolic NADH needed for the reversal of the glyceraldehyde-3-phosphate dehydrogenase step, and the mitochondrial form of phosphoenolpyruvate carboxykinase is used. Mitochondrial phosphoenolpyruvate is then transported to the cytosol for conversion to glucose. On the other hand, if alanine is the primary precursor, cytosolic NADH must be generated another way; after the mitochondrial conversion of pyruvate to oxaloacetate, oxaloacetate is reduced to mitochondrial malate, which is transported to the cytosol for subsequent oxidation to cytosolic oxaloacetate, generating NADH, and the cytosolic oxaloacetate is converted to phosphoenolpyruvate by the cytosolic form of phosphoenolpyruvate carboxykinase. Reaction A, catalyzed by pyruvate carboxylase, occurs only in the mitochondrion. Reaction C, catalyzed by fructose-1,6-bisphosphatase, occurs only in the cytosol. Reaction D, catalyzed by glucose-6-phosphatase, occurs in the endoplasmic reticulum, and reaction E, catalyzed by phosphoglycerate kinase, occurs in the cytosol. *Biochemistry,* p. 136.
2. The answer is A: pyruvate → oxaloacetate. A deficiency

of pyruvate carboxylase produces a fasting hypoglycemia and lactic acidosis. Pyruvate carboxylase utilizes a biotinyl cofactor to carry an "activated" CO_2, which condenses with pyruvate to form oxaloacetate, a substrate for gluconeogenesis and a Krebs cycle intermediate. A deficiency of pyruvate carboxylase explains the fasting hypoglycemia because of the failure to convert lactate and pyruvate (obtained via the degradation of selected amino acids) to oxaloacetate for gluconeogenesis. This reaction, which also requires ATP, does not occur to any appreciable extent in the absence of acetyl-CoA. Besides its role in gluconeogenesis, pyruvate carboxylase is responsible for the anaplerotic reactions that maintain the levels of Krebs cycle intermediates. With inadequate levels of Krebs cycle intermediates, pyruvate and acetyl-CoA cannot be metabolized to meet energy needs, and this increases anaerobic glycolysis. Failure to metabolize pyruvate aerobically increases lactic acid production, which also occurs in patients with pyruvate carboxylase deficiency. *Biochemistry,* p. 116; *Nelson,* p. 363.

3. The answer is C: fructose 1,6-bisphosphate $\rightarrow$ fructose 6-phosphate. Galactose is metabolized to galactose 1-phosphate, UDP-galactose, UDP-glucose, glucose 1-phosphate, and glucose 6-phosphate and is released as free glucose as catalyzed by glucose-6-phosphatase. This means that the glucose 6-phosphate $\rightarrow$ glucose reaction is functional. Fructose is converted to fructose 1-phosphate, dihydroxyacetone phosphate, and glyceraldehyde. Following conversion of glyceraldehyde to glyceraldehyde 3-phosphate, the dihydroxyacetone phosphate and glyceraldehyde 3-phosphate combine to form fructose 1,6-bisphosphate. The inability to convert this compound to fructose 6-phosphate prevents the release of glucose into the blood. These tests are used in infants in the diagnosis of fructose-1,6-bisphosphatase deficiency. These infants are free from symptoms as long as their diet is limited to human milk. If they receive formulas or food containing fructose or sucrose, they develop intermittent episodes of hypoglycemia and lactic acidosis. Treatment involves fructose and sucrose restriction. The metabolism of pyruvate and oxaloacetate is not required for the conversion of fructose to glucose. *Biochemistry,* p. 105; *Nelson,* p. 363.
4. The answer is A: pyruvate $\rightarrow$ oxaloacetate. The relevant pathway of gluconeogenesis is succinyl-CoA $\rightarrow$ succinate $\rightarrow$ fumarate $\rightarrow$ mitochondrial malate $\rightarrow$ cytosolic malate $\rightarrow$ cytosolic oxaloacetate (plus cytosolic NADH) $\rightarrow$ phosphoenolpyruvate (using the cytosolic phosphoenolpyruvate carboxykinase), etc. The pyruvate carboxylase reaction is NOT required for gluconeogenesis from any Krebs cycle intermediate (or from any amino acid degraded to a Krebs cycle intermediate). *Biochemistry,* p. 135.
5. The answer is E: amino acids that are degraded to acetyl-CoA. Acetyl-CoA, derived from ketogenic amino acids and exogenous fatty acids, is converted to fatty acids and to ketone bodies (acetoacetate and β-hydroxybutyrate). Leucine is the only amino acid that is entirely ketogenic; several amino acids are both glycogenic and ketogenic, and these amino acids in a ketogenic diet provide the minimum substrates for gluconeogenesis that are required for red blood cell and neuronal metabolism. Humans have no enzymatic mechanisms for the net conversion of acetyl-CoA (or acetate) to either pyruvate or Krebs cycle intermediates such as α-ketoglutarate, succinyl-CoA, fumarate, malate, or oxaloacetate. Acetyl-CoA enters the Krebs cycle as a two-carbon fragment attached to oxaloacetate. In one turn of the cycle, two carbon dioxide molecules are released, effectively removing the equivalent of the two-carbon acetate, so there is nothing remaining to provide net synthesis of glucose. It is unclear how the ketogenic diet decreases the severity of seizures, but carbohydrate in the diet or gluconeogenic substrates decrease ketogenesis and eliminate the beneficial effect of the ketogenic diet. Glycerol is converted to glycerol 3-phosphate, which is oxidized to dihydroxyacetone phosphate, an intermediate in gluconeogenesis. Lactate and some amino acids are converted to pyruvate, which then forms glucose after conversion to phosphoenolpyruvate (PEP) via oxaloacetate. Carbon chains from amino acids converted to α-ketoglutarate, succinyl-CoA, fumarate, or oxaloacetate all appear as malate, which is transported to the cytosol for conversion first to cytosolic oxaloacetate and then to cytosolic phosphoenolpyruvate. *Biochemistry,* p. 120.
6. The answer is C: phosphoglycerate kinase. In this reaction, reactants and products have the same number of high-energy bonds, so the enzyme catalyzes a functionally isoergonic reaction that is freely reversible and thus available for use in both glycolysis and gluconeogenesis. Hexokinase, phosphofructokinase, and pyruvate kinase catalyze physiologically irreversible reactions used only in glycolysis. Phosphoenolpyruvate carboxykinase is used only in gluconeogenesis. *Biochemistry,* p. 137.
7. The answer is D: a decrease in fructose 2,6-bisphosphate concentration. Glucagon binding to its receptor leads to a decrease in the concentration of fructose 2,6-bisphosphate because activation of protein kinase A results in phosphorylation of the dual-activity protein, fructose-6-phosphate-2-kinase/phosphatase, and this phosphorylation inhibits the kinase activity and activates the phosphatase activity. Fructose 2,6-bisphosphate is hydrolyzed to form fructose 6-phosphate, and the decrease in fructose 2,6-bisphosphate concentration removes an activator of phosphofructokinase (thus decreasing the rate of glycolysis) and an inhibitor of fructose-1,6-bisphosphatase (thus allowing more glucose formation from noncarbohydrate precursors). The activation of protein kinase A also leads to a decrease in glycogen synthesis and an increase in glycogenolysis (also resulting in more glucose production) and to a decrease in pyruvate kinase activity (thus decreasing glucose catabolism by glycolysis). The net result of all these actions is the liberation of glucose from the liver into the blood, thereby contributing to the hyperglycemia of diabetes mellitus. Under fasting conditions in nondiabetics, the physiological elevation of the glucagon/insulin ratio provides fuel for brain, red blood cells, and other tissues with a primary dependence on glucose for energy. It is low blood glucose that triggers the release of glucagon from the α-cells of the pancreatic islets of Langerhans, so these responses conform to the molecular logic of the organism (not just the cell). *Biochemistry,* p. 138.
8. The answer is C: 6. The conversion of two moles of lactate to two moles of pyruvate provides the two moles of cytosolic NADH that are required at the glyceraldehyde-3-phosphate dehydrogenase step. The conversion of each pyruvate to oxaloacetate requires ATP (for a total of two) and each oxaloacetate to phosphoenolpyruvate requires GTP (another two), and the phosphoglycerate kinase reaction requires an ATP for conversion of each 3-phosphoglycerate to 1,3-bisphosphoglycerate (another two). The fructose-2,6-bisphosphatase and glucose-6-phosphatase reactions do not generate ATP, so the total is $2 + 2 + 2 = 6$ moles of ATP (or equivalent, such as

GTP) required for conversion of two moles of lactate to one mole of glucose. *Biochemistry,* p. 138.

9. The answer is C: The formation of UDP-glucose from glucose 1-phosphate is pulled forward by the subsequent hydrolysis of pyrophosphate. UDP-glucose pyrophosphorylase (not phosphorylase) catalyzes the following reaction, glucose 1-phosphate + UTP $\rightleftharpoons$ UDP-glucose + PP_i. The reactants contain two high-energy bonds, both acid anhydride bonds in UTP, while the products contain a total of three, one in PP_i and two in UDP-glucose. This is an unusual situation in biochemistry, and the reaction would probably not proceed to the right if the high-energy acid anhydride bond in pyrophosphate were not subsequently hydrolyzed by a pyrophosphatase. The primary regulatory step in glycogenesis is catalyzed by glycogen synthase. *Biochemistry,* p. 139.
10. The answer is C: phosphorolysis reaction. Most (90%) of the linkages in glycogen are α-1,4-glycosidic bonds, and these are cleaved with inorganic phosphate in a reaction catalyzed by phosphorylase, yielding glucose 1-phosphate. Muscle glycogen phosphorylase is the enzyme whose activity is decreased in McArdle disease. As a result of this deficiency, muscle glycogen cannot serve as a substrate for glycolysis and anaerobic ATP production. The levels of muscle glycogen in McArdle disease (4 g/100 g wet weight) are about four times normal (1 g/100 g wet weight). A trisaccharide transfer occurs as part of the debranching reaction sequence, but this occurs less commonly than phosphorolysis. The α-1,6 bond at the branch point is cleaved by hydrolysis by one of the activities of the debrancher enzyme, yielding free glucose, but this reaction accounts for only about 10% of the glucosyl units released. Neither lyase nor dephosphorylation reactions occur during glycogenolysis. *Biochemistry,* p. 142.
11. The answer is B: phosphorylation of phosphorylase *b*. Inactive phosphorylase *b* is phosphorylated, forming the active phosphorylase *a,* by phosphorylase kinase, NOT by protein kinase A, so this step is a downstream stage of the glycogen cleavage cascade. All the other reactions are performed in liver by protein kinase A activated in response to glucagon binding. As a result of defective activation of phosphorylase *b* (owing to decreased phosphorylase kinase activity) in protein kinase A deficiency, both liver and muscle glycogen are elevated. Glucagon injection in such patients fails to elicit a hyperglycemic response. *Biochemistry,* p. 144; *Nelson,* p. 370.
12. The answer is C: calcium. In muscle, depolarization at the motor endplate results in release of calcium ions from the sarcoplasmic reticulum into the cytosol, where it binds to troponin C, one of the components of the contractile machinery in the muscle, to trigger muscle contraction. Calcium ion also binds to, and allosterically activates, phosphorylase kinase, which can then activate phosphorylase, allowing glycogen cleavage and subsequent ATP production to supply energy for the contraction. Note that, in this situation, phosphorylase kinase need not be phosphorylated by protein kinase A in order to be converted to an active conformation. None of the other compounds trigger muscle contraction, although ATP does supply the power for contraction. Cyclic AMP does not allosterically activate phosphorylase kinase (though it does lead to activation of phosphorylase kinase via protein kinase A action). 5′-AMP is an allosteric activator of phosphorylase, converting phosphorylase *b* to an active, glycogen-cleaving conformation, even without phosphorylation of serine 14. Glucose 6-phosphate and ATP are allosteric inhibitors of phosphorylase, and this makes sense (PRINCIPLE 9 OF BIOCHEMISTRY), since a high energy charge indicates that there is no need to break down any energy storage compounds. Glucose 6-phosphate in high enough concentration can allosterically activate the phosphorylated (inactive) form of glycogen synthase, but this may not be important physiologically. *Biochemistry,* p. 146.
13. The answer is D: epinephrine. The plasma membrane of muscle cells contains receptors for epinephrine, but not for glucagon, and these epinephrine receptors serve to activate adenylyl cyclase via the same type of G-protein intermediates used in liver after glucagon binding. Acetylcholine is the neurotransmitter used at the motor endplate upon nerve stimulation, but it does not directly initiate the activation of adenylyl cyclase. Calcium is an intracellular messenger, and sodium, though involved in depolarization of the cell membrane, is not considered to be a "first messenger." *Biochemistry,* p. 147.
14. The answer is E: branching enzyme. Branching enzyme deficiency results in normal amounts of liver glycogen but with very long outer branches. Although progressive cirrhosis and liver failure can lead to early death, hypoglycemia is NOT part of the clinical picture because the enzymes that catalyze glycogenolysis are functional. In glucose-6-phosphatase deficiency (von Gierke disease), the liver cannot release free glucose to maintain blood levels and hypoglycemia results. Liver glycogen with a normal branched structure accumulates, leading to hepatomegaly. A deficiency in the debranching enzyme (amylo-1,6-glucosidase) means that only the outer chains containing α-1,4 linkages can be cleaved during glycogenolysis, and significant hypoglycemia can result. In times of glucose abundance (e.g., after meals) the glycogen particles continue to grow, however, leading to increased accumulation of abnormally large glycogen molecules in the liver and resultant hepatomegaly. In liver phosphorylase deficiency, liver glycogen cannot be degraded, and hepatomegaly and hypoglycemia occur. In liver phosphorylase kinase deficiency, the capacity to degrade glycogen is compromised (because of the inability to convert phosphorylase *b* to phosphorylase *a*) and hypoglycemia results. Glycogen has a normal structure in this disorder. *Nelson,* p. 365.
15. The answer is E: diabetes mellitus. The diagnosis is based upon the hyperglycemia and an elevated level of hemoglobin A_1. Hemoglobin A_1 represents total glycohemoglobin, and it consists of hemoglobins A_{1a}, A_{1b}, and A_{1c}. Some clinical laboratories measure hemoglobin A_1, and others measure hemoglobin A_{1c} (which constitutes about two-thirds of total hemoglobin A_1). The hyperlipidemia seen in this patient is also a common complication of diabetes mellitus. The blood pressure is normal, indicating the lack of hypertension, and the normal uric acid levels rule out gout. In McArdle disease (muscle phosphorylase deficiency), which involves all the skeletal muscles of the body and not just those of the lower extremity, fatigue results from the inability to break down stored glycogen. There is deficient production of lactic acid from muscle glycogen in response to exercise, but this patient's response was normal. For reasons that are unclear, symptoms of McArdle disease develop during the second and third decades of life and are not present before. This patient is older than one would expect for a person presenting with McArdle disease (type V glycogen storage disease). Patients with deficient muscle phosphoglycerate mutase activity also have exercise intolerance and are unable to increase blood lactic acid following exercise. Myoglobinuria in response to

muscle breakdown occurs in McArdle disease and muscle phosphoglycerate mutase deficiency, but not in this patient. *Biochemistry,* p. 92; *Nelson,* p. 365.

16. The answer is B: there is decreased transport of glucose into liver cells. Hyperglycemia does NOT result from decreased glucose transport into liver because the transport of glucose into liver is not affected by insulin; liver contains GLUT1 glucose transporters, which are not regulated by insulin. Insulin, however, has many other effects on liver metabolism such as inducing glycogen synthase and acetyl-CoA carboxylase, leading to increased glycogen and fatty acid synthesis, respectively. Insulin also stimulates hepatic protein synthesis. In contrast to the lack of an effect in liver, insulin stimulates glucose transport into skeletal muscle and adipocytes that contain insulin-responsive GLUT4 glucose transporters. Glucagon induces phosphoenolpyruvate carboxykinase in liver cells, thereby promoting gluconeogenesis. Moreover, glucagon stimulates glycogenolysis and decreases glycolysis via the cyclic AMP second messenger system. Stimulation of glycogenolysis involves the phosphorylase cascade, and inhibition of glycolysis results from decreased fructose 2,6-bisphosphate levels. *Biochemistry,* pp. 508, 512.
17. The answer is A: atherosclerosis and peripheral vascular disease. This patient has elevated total cholesterol, LDL ("bad") cholesterol, smokes cigarettes, is overweight, and has diabetes mellitus, all of which are risk factors for atherosclerosis. Sometimes bruits, which are sounds produced by turbulent blood flow past an arterial lesion, indicate the general location of such lesions, but bruits were not heard in this patient. Peripheral neuropathies generally involve decreased sensation to vibration and decreased deep tendon reflexes, which were observed in this patient and are common in patients with diabetes. Exertional muscle pain, however, is not a result of peripheral neuropathy. The rise in blood lactate following exercise rules out the deficiencies of muscle phosphorylase (McArdle disease) and phosphoglycerate mutase, diseases that can lead to muscle cramps and pain. Azotemia (elevated nitrogen as indicated by blood urea and creatinine) is evident in this patient but does not usually lead to muscle pain. *Cecil,* p. 1308.
18. The answer is C: elevated. The amount of glycosylated hemoglobin, hemoglobin A_1, was 12%, while the normal levels range between 5.5% and 7.5%. The increase indicates that the patient experienced hyperglycemia during the previous few weeks. Hemoglobin glycosylation results from the nonenzymatic reaction of glucose with hemoglobin, and the extent of modification is proportional to the average blood glucose levels. Red cells and hemoglobin have a lifetime of about 120 days, and the extent of glycosylation reflects the blood glucose levels that were present over the previous few weeks. Abnormal protein glycosylation may also be responsible for diabetic retinopathy, nephropathy, and neuropathy, all observed in this patient. Abnormal protein glycosylation has also been suggested as one mechanism for elevating serum cholesterol by altering LDL transport into cells. Besides cessation of smoking (nicotine is a vasoconstrictor), recommended therapy for this person is weight reduction, and this treatment requires a trial lasting several months. Weight reduction alone increases insulin sensitivity (decreases insulin resistance). Treatment of the intermittent claudication and peripheral artery disease would be considered later. A worsening in symptoms might prompt surgery. *Biochemistry,* p. 92.

REFERENCES

Behrman, R. E. *Nelson Textbook of Pediatrics,* 14th ed. Philadelphia, W. B. Saunders Company, 1992.

Roskoski, R., Jr. *Biochemistry.* Philadelphia, W. B. Saunders Company, 1996.

Wyngaarden, J. B., L. H. Smith, Jr., and J. C. Bennett (eds.). *Cecil Textbook of Medicine,* 19th ed. Philadelphia, W. B. Saunders Company, 1992.

CHAPTER ELEVEN

FATTY ACID AND TRIGLYCERIDE METABOLISM

SYNOPSIS

OBJECTIVES

1. To describe the structures of fatty acids and lipid digestion.
2. To depict fatty acid activation and β-oxidation.
3. To present the pathway for the metabolism of propionyl-CoA.
4. To describe fatty acid biosynthesis by the fatty acid synthase multienzyme complex.
5. To describe the pathways for triglyceride biosynthesis.
6. To outline ketone body metabolism.

Objective 1: To describe the structures of fatty acids and lipid digestion.

I. Types of fatty acids
   A. Saturated and unsaturated fatty acids
      1. Myristate (C_{14}), palmitate (C_{16}), and stearate (C_{18}) are important saturated fatty acids
      2. Monounsaturated fatty acids have one double bond, and polyunsaturated fatty acids have two or more double bonds
      3. Physiological fatty acids have double bonds with the *cis* configuration, but hydrogenated fatty acids in processed foods have some *trans* double bonds
   B. Essential fatty acids
      1. Those fatty acids that are required for optimal health and cannot be synthesized are called essential fatty acids, and they must be obtained from the diet
      2. The parent fatty acids of the **ω-6 class (linoleate)** and the **ω-3 class (linolenate)** are two C_{18} essential fatty acids
      3. Linoleate is 18:2Δ9,12, and linolenate is 18:3Δ9,12,15
II. Digestion and absorption of lipids
   A. Role of the digestive enzymes
      1. **Gastric lipase** and **pancreatic lipase** (which requires **colipase** for activity) are broad-specificity lipases
      2. The pancreas secretes **esterase** and **phospholipase,** also required for lipid digestion
   B. Role of bile salts
      1. **Bile salts,** which are derived from cholesterol, aid in the emulsification and absorption of fats and fat-soluble vitamins (A, D, E, and K) and of β-carotene (a precursor of vitamin A)
      2. Cholesterol and bile salts are released from the liver and gallbladder into the gut
      3. Bile salts are taken up in the terminal ileum and recycled to the liver by a process called **enterohepatic circulation**
         a. Failure to reabsorb adequate bile acids in the terminal ileum can result in bile that is deficient in bile salts
         b. Bile lacking bile salts can lead to lipid malabsorption and steatorrhea (fat in the stool)

Objective 2: To depict fatty acid activation and β-oxidation.

III. Steps in β-oxidation of fatty acids
   A. Fatty acid activation as acyl-CoA and fatty acylcarnitine
      1. Fatty acid + ATP + coenzyme A ⇌ fatty acyl–CoA + AMP + PP_i
      2. Fatty acyl–CoA + carnitine ⇌ fatty acylcarnitine + CoA (catalyzed by carnitine acyltransferase I)
      3. Fatty acylcarnitine is translocated into the mitochondrion and fatty acyl–CoA is regenerated in a reaction catalyzed by carnitine acyltransferase II
   B. The first and repeating spirals of β-oxidation (Fig. 11–1)
      1. The reactions include an FAD-dependent oxidation by acyl–CoA dehydrogenase, a hydration, an NAD^+-dependent oxidation, and cleavage of the β-keto acid as catalyzed by thiolase to yield acetyl-CoA and fatty acyl–CoA

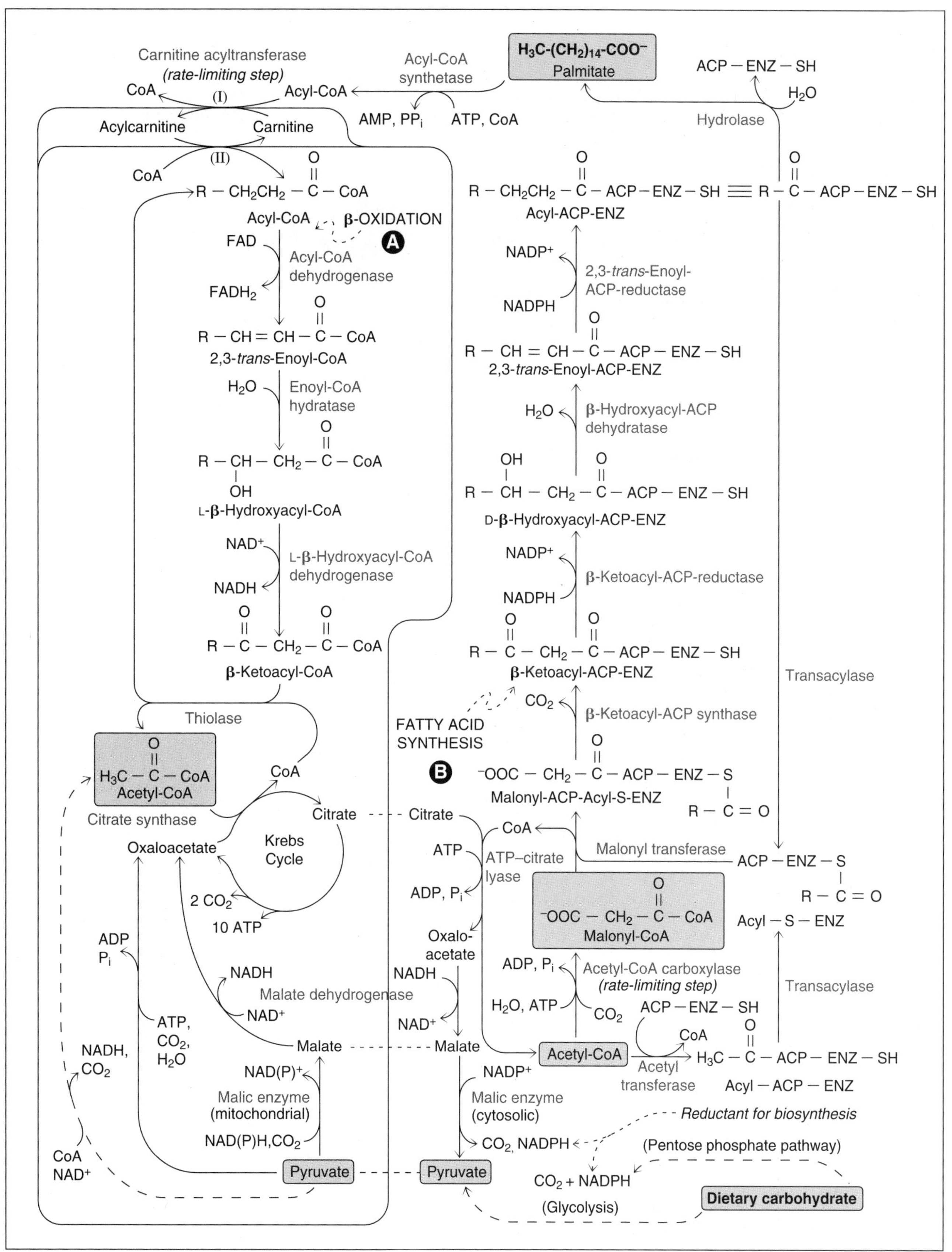

FIGURE 11-1. Pathways for β-oxidation (A) and fatty acid biosynthesis (B).

2. The process of oxidation, hydration, oxidation, and thiolysis is repeated sequentially until the carbon chain is too short (two or three carbon atoms) for subsequent β-oxidation

C. Carnitine acyltransferase I, the rate-limiting step of β-oxidation
1. Carnitine acyltransferase I is inhibited by malonyl-CoA, a reactant in fatty acid biosynthesis
2. β-Oxidation is inhibited when fatty acid synthesis is active, thereby following the molecular logic of the cell

D. ATP yield during the β-oxidation of fatty acids
1. Each spiral of β-oxidation generates $FADH_2$ (leading to 1.5 moles of ATP per mole of $FADH_2$) and NADH (leading to 2.5 moles of ATP per mole of NADH)
2. A 16-carbon fatty acid undergoes seven spirals of β-oxidation to produce eight molecules of acetyl-CoA
   a. During the seventh spiral, acetoacetyl-CoA is cleaved by coenzyme A to yield two molecules of acetyl coenzyme A
   b. The yield of ATP from seven moles of $FADH_2$, seven moles of NADH, and eight moles of acetyl-CoA is 108 moles of ATP
   c. Palmitate must first be converted into palmitoyl-CoA before β-oxidation
      (1) This reaction requires one molecule of ATP and the expenditure of two high-energy bonds
      (2) By convention, we denote the loss of an ATP to AMP as two ATP equivalents
   d. The net ATP yield is 106 moles of ATP (108 − 2 = 106) per mole of palmitate

E. Oxidation of unsaturated fatty acids
1. When an unsaturated fatty acid undergoes β-oxidation, an NADPH-dependent reduction is required for each double bond in the fatty acid
2. *Each double bond reduces the ATP yield by 2.5 when compared with the corresponding saturated fatty acid*
3. Three additional enzymes are required for the oxidation of unsaturated fatty acids: **enoyl-CoA isomerase,** NADPH-dependent **2,4-dienoyl-CoA reductase,** and for double bonds that begin at odd-numbered carbon atoms, **3,5-dienoyl-CoA isomerase**

Objective 3: To present the pathway for the metabolism of propionyl-CoA.

IV. Metabolism of propionyl coenzyme A

A. Vitamin B_{12} in the conversion of propionate to succinyl-CoA
1. Propionyl-CoA undergoes an ATP- and biotin-dependent carboxylation to form D-methylmalonyl-CoA
2. After an isomerization, L-methylmalonyl-CoA is converted to succinyl-CoA in a vitamin B_{12}-dependent reaction catalyzed by methylmalonyl-CoA mutase
3. *Adenosylcobalamin is the coenzyme in the methylmalonyl-CoA mutase reaction,* one of two reactions in human metabolism that requires B_{12}

B. Oxidation of succinyl-CoA
1. Krebs cycle intermediates must be converted to pyruvate and then acetyl-CoA prior to complete oxidation (the Krebs cycle catalyzes the oxidation of acetyl-CoA)
2. Malate, a Krebs cycle intermediate, undergoes an oxidative decarboxylation to form pyruvate, carbon dioxide, and NAD(P)H
   a. Enzymes that catalyze this process occur in the mitochondrion (and cytosol)
   b. Metabolism in the mitochondrion obviates any need for metabolite translocation

Objective 4: To describe fatty acid biosynthesis by the fatty acid synthase multienzyme complex.

V. Fatty acid and lipid biosynthesis

A. **Fatty acid synthase** as a multienzyme complex
1. The equation for palmitate biosynthesis is given as follows:

$$\begin{array}{lcl} \text{Acetyl-CoA} & & \text{palmitate}^- + H^+ \\ + & & + \\ 7\ \text{malonyl-CoA}^- + 7\ H^+ & \rightarrow & 7\ CO_2 + 8\ \text{CoA} \\ + & & + \\ 14\ \text{NADPH} + 14\ H^+ & & 14\ \text{NADP}^+ + 6\ H_2O \end{array} \quad (11.1)$$

2. Malonyl-CoA is formed by the ATP-and biotin-dependent carboxylation of acetyl-CoA in a reaction catalyzed by **acetyl-CoA carboxylase,** *the rate-limiting enzyme of fatty acid synthesis,* as illustrated below

$$\text{Acetyl-CoA} + \text{ATP} + HCO_3^- \rightarrow \text{malonyl-CoA}^- + \text{ADP} + P_i \quad (11.2)$$

3. Acetyl-CoA is a precursor for fatty acids
   a. Glucose and other substances are converted to pyruvate, which is converted to acetyl-CoA in the mitochondrion
   b. Acetyl-CoA reacts with oxaloacetate to form citrate, which is exported from the mitochondrion
   c. ATP-citrate lyase catalyzes the conversion of cytosolic citrate to acetyl-CoA (the precursor of fatty acids) and oxaloacetate

B. Pathway for fatty acid biosynthesis (Figure 11–1)
1. The stoichiometry for palmitate synthesis is given as follows:

$$\begin{array}{lcl} 8\ \text{Acetyl-CoA} & & \text{palmitate} + H^+ \\ + & & + \\ 7\ \text{ATP} & & 7\ \text{ADP} + 7\ P_i \\ + & \rightarrow & + \\ 7\ CO_2 + 7\ H_2O & & 7\ CO_2 + 6\ H_2O \\ + & & + \\ 14\ \text{NADPH} + 14\ H^+ & & 14\ \text{NADP}^+ + 8\ \text{CoA} \end{array} \quad (11.3)$$

2. Acetyl-CoA reacts with the central thiol of **acyl carrier protein** (ACP) and is translocated to the peripheral thiol (a protein-cysteine on *β-ketoacyl-ACP synthase* [KSase])
3. Malonyl-CoA combines with ACP
4. The following condensation reaction is a crucial step in fatty acid synthesis: malonyl-ACP reacts with acetyl–S-protein to form acetoacetyl-ACP with the liberation of carbon dioxide
5. β-Ketoacyl–ACP is reduced by NADPH, dehydrated, reduced again with NADPH, and parked on the peripheral thiol

6. Malonyl-CoA combines with ACP and undergoes a second spiral of chain elongation
7. The process occurs until palmitoyl-ACP is formed
   a. Palmitoyl-ACP is hydrolyzed from the fatty acid synthase complex to regenerate the enzyme and produce palmitate
   b. Note that synthesis stops at C_{16}

VI. Regulation of fatty acid oxidation and biosynthesis
   A. The reaction catalyzed by **acetyl-CoA carboxylase** is the chief regulatory step in fatty acid biosynthesis in eukaryotes (Table 25–1)
      1. This enzyme is activated by citrate (the precursor of the acetyl-CoA building blocks for biosynthesis) and is inhibited by palmitoyl-CoA (one of the products)
      2. **Citrate** promotes the conversion of less active monomeric enzymes to more active polymeric aggregates that take the shape of filaments
      3. Increased cytosolic citrate serves as a signal that fuel molecules are abundant, and this signal promotes the formation of fatty acid
   B. The regulation of fatty acid oxidation is coordinated with the regulation of fatty acid synthesis
      1. **Malonyl-CoA** inhibits carnitine acyltransferase I
         a. This is the rate-limiting process in β-oxidation
         b. As a result, fatty acid translocation into the mitochondrion is diminished
      2. Conditions that favor fatty acid biosynthesis thereby produce an inhibitor of a step required prior to fatty acid oxidation

VII. Source of reducing equivalents
   A. In *liver,* the most important human tissue for fatty acid biosynthesis, NADPH is generated mainly from the two $NADP^+$-requiring reactions of the *pentose phosphate pathway*
   B. In *adipose tissue,* NADPH is generated by *malic enzyme* and the *pentose phosphate pathway*
   C. NADPH is the donor for fatty acid biosynthesis in accordance with PRINCIPLE 16 OF BIOCHEMISTRY

Objective 5: To describe the pathways for triglyceride biosynthesis.

VIII. Triglyceride biosynthesis
   A. General pathway
      1. Glycerol phosphate, derived from glycerol or from dihydroxyacetone phosphate by reduction, undergoes two acylation reactions with acyl ~ CoA as the energy-rich donor
      2. Phosphatidate undergoes a dephosphorylation reaction yielding 1,2-diglyceride, which reacts with acyl ~ CoA to produce triglyceride
         a. The dephosphorylation is an exergonic hydrolysis reaction in accordance with PRINCIPLE 5 OF BIOENERGETICS
         b. The acyltransferase reactions proceed with a decrease in the number of high-energy bonds and are exergonic in accordance with PRINCIPLE 2 OF BIOENERGETICS
   B. Intestinal pathway for triglyceride biosynthesis
      1. 2-Monoglyceride and free fatty acids are taken up by intestinal mucosal cells
      2. The fatty acids are activated in ATP-dependent reactions (ATP → AMP + PP_i) as acyl-CoA thioesters
      3. 2-Monoglyceride is converted to triglyceride after two acyl transfer reactions from acyl ~ CoA

Objective 6: To outline ketone body metabolism.

IX. Steps in ketone body (acetoacetate and β-hydroxybutyrate) metabolism
   A. *Ketone body synthesis occurs in hepatocytes and degradation in extrahepatic cells*
      1. β-Oxidation yields acetoacetyl-CoA, which reacts with acetyl-CoA to form hydroxymethylglutaryl-CoA (HMG-CoA); this reaction is driven forward by the hydrolytic removal of coenzyme A
      2. HMG-CoA undergoes a lyase reaction to produce acetoacetate and acetyl-CoA
      3. **Acetoacetate** can be reduced to form **β-hydroxybutyrate,** a second ketone body
      4. Acetoacetate can undergo nonenzymatic decarboxylation to form **acetone,** the third ketone body but a metabolic dead end
   B. Ketone body oxidation
      1. In extrahepatic cells, acetoacetate reacts with succinyl-CoA to form acetoacetyl-CoA and succinate, an isoergonic process in accordance with PRINCIPLE 1 OF BIOENERGETICS
      2. Acetoacetyl-CoA is cleaved by coenzyme A in a reaction catalyzed by thiolase to form two molecules of acetyl-CoA, the stoichiometric substrate of the Krebs cycle
   C. Diabetic ketoacidosis
      1. Excess β-oxidation yields substrates for ketone body synthesis
      2. Excess production of ketone bodies produces a metabolic acidosis of modest severity in starvation and of potentially life-threatening severity in diabetes mellitus

QUESTIONS

DIRECTIONS. (Items 1–6): Each set of matching questions in this section consists of a list of lettered options followed by several numbered items. For each numbered item, select the ONE lettered option that is most closely associated with it. Each lettered option may be selected once, more than once, or not at all. Correct answers and explanations are given at the end of the chapter.

Items 1–4

For each of the enzyme-catalyzed reactions outlined in the illustration below (A–G), select those that correspond most closely to the following properties.

1. Which reaction yields AMP and PP_i as additional products?
2. Which oxidation-reduction reaction can be impaired in pellagra?
3. Which reaction is rate-limiting in this metabolic pathway?
4. A deficiency of the enzyme catalyzing this reaction, the product of which is translocated across the mitochondrial membrane in exchange for carnitine, results in a metabolic myopathy characterized by lipid accumulation and myoglobinuria.

Items 5–6

(A) Adenosylcobalamin
(B) Biotin
(C) Carnitine
(D) Citrate
(E) Cytochrome P-450

Select the biological compound that corresponds to the designated property.

5. Which compound leads to polymerization (and thus activation) of acetyl-CoA carboxylase monomers?
6. A deficiency of the enzyme that leads to the covalent attachment of this compound to pyruvate carboxylase, propionyl-CoA carboxylase, β-methylcrotonoyl-CoA carboxylase, and acetyl-CoA carboxylase leads to organic aciduria.

DIRECTIONS. (Items 7–18): Each of the numbered items or incomplete statements in this section is followed by answers or by completions of the statement. Select the ONE lettered answer or completion that is BEST in each case.

7. All of the following represent the fatty acid shown below EXCEPT

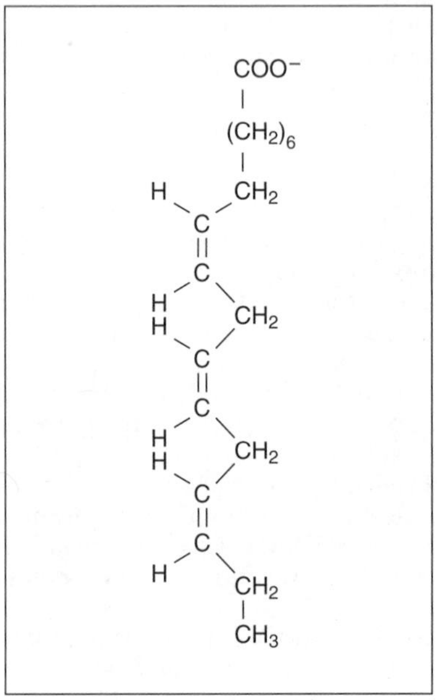

COO^-
$|$
$(CH_2)_6$
$|$
CH_2
$H\text{–}C{=}C\text{–}H$
CH_2
$H\text{–}C{=}C\text{–}H$
CH_2
$H\text{–}C{=}C\text{–}H$
CH_2
$|$
CH_3

(A) 18:3Δ9,12,15
(B) 18:3ω-3
(C) *cis,cis,cis*-9,12,15-octadecatrienoate
(D) 18:3n-3
(E) linoleate

8. Each of the following substances accumulates in one of the sphingolipidoses EXCEPT

(A) cerebroside
(B) ganglioside G_{M1}
(C) ceramide
(D) platelet activating factor
(E) sphingomyelin

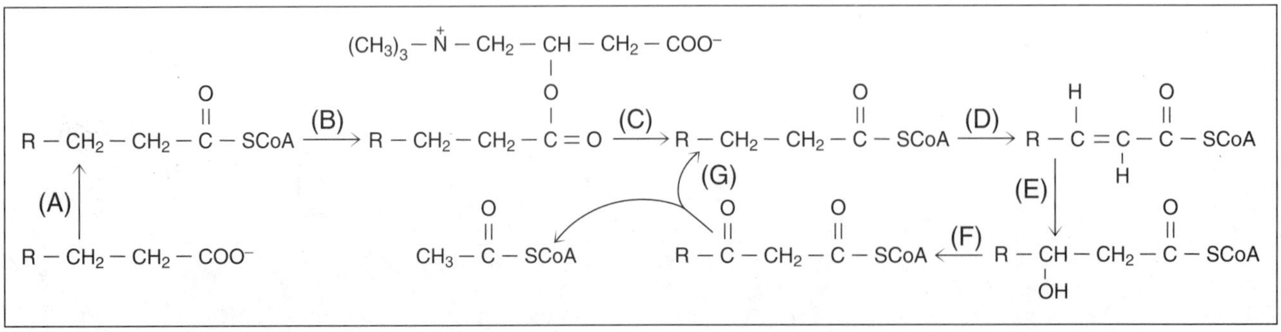

$$R-CH_2-CH_2-COO^- \xrightarrow{(A)} R-CH_2-CH_2-\overset{O}{\overset{\|}{C}}-SCoA \xrightarrow{(B)} R-CH_2-CH_2-\underset{|}{C}{=}O \text{ (O-linked to } (CH_3)_3-\overset{+}{N}-CH_2-CH-CH_2-COO^-) \xrightarrow{(C)} R-CH_2-CH_2-\overset{O}{\overset{\|}{C}}-SCoA \xrightarrow{(D)} R-\overset{H}{C}{=}\underset{H}{C}-\overset{O}{\overset{\|}{C}}-SCoA$$

$$\xrightarrow{(E)} R-\underset{OH}{CH}-CH_2-\overset{O}{\overset{\|}{C}}-SCoA \xrightarrow{(F)} R-\overset{O}{\overset{\|}{C}}-CH_2-\overset{O}{\overset{\|}{C}}-SCoA \xrightarrow{(G)} CH_3-\overset{O}{\overset{\|}{C}}-SCoA + R-CH_2-CH_2-\overset{O}{\overset{\|}{C}}-SCoA$$

9. The fasting hypoglycemia of patients with medium-chain fatty acyl–CoA dehydrogenase deficiency is due to
   (A) impaired acetyl-CoA production and subsequent inability to activate pyruvate carboxylase
   (B) decreased ability to convert acetyl-CoA to glucose
   (C) increased ratio of mitochondrial CoA/acyl-CoA
   (D) increased ratio of mitochondrial carnitine/acylcarnitine
   (E) increased conversion of acetyl-CoA to ketone bodies

10. What is the molar yield of ATP from the complete oxidation of one mole of myristic acid (14:0), using β-oxidation, the Krebs cycle, and oxidative phosphorylation?
   (A) 24
   (B) 70
   (C) 92
   (D) 94
   (E) 112

11. Which of the following enzymes is uniquely required for the oxidation of fatty acids containing a double bond at an odd carbon number?
   (A) Acyl-CoA dehydrogenase
   (B) 2,4-Dienoyl-CoA reductase
   (C) 3,5-Dienoyl-CoA isomerase
   (D) Enoyl-CoA isomerase
   (E) Thiolase

12. What is the molar yield of ATP from complete oxidation of one mole of propionyl-CoA, using Krebs cycle and other appropriate mitochondrial reactions, plus oxidative phosphorylation?
   (A) 10
   (B) 15
   (C) 16.5
   (D) 17.5
   (E) 32

13. All of the following are correct statements regarding fatty acid synthesis EXCEPT
   (A) *De novo* synthesis of fatty acids occurs outside the mitochondrion
   (B) Fatty acid elongation in the endoplasmic reticulum requires malonyl-CoA as a carbon donor
   (C) In *de novo* fatty acid synthesis, all the reductive steps take place while the acyl group is bound to acyl carrier protein (ACP)
   (D) The reductant used by the fatty acid synthase complex is NADPH
   (E) If the carboxyl group added to acetyl-CoA in the acetyl-CoA carboxylase reaction were radiolabeled, every third carbon of palmitate would be labeled

14. All of the following statements regarding the general pathway and the intestinal pathway for triglyceride synthesis are correct EXCEPT
   (A) Both pathways require formation of phosphatidate as an intermediate
   (B) Both pathways involve the formation of 1,2-diglyceride as an intermediate
   (C) Both pathways proceed with a loss in free energy
   (D) Both pathways require acyl-CoA as the activated acyl group donor
   (E) Both pathways involve conversion of ATP to AMP + PP_i

Items 15–18

History

A 32-year-old woman of Northern European ancestry experienced intermittent diarrhea (6–8 stools daily) and a 24-pound weight loss over a 6-week period despite normal food intake. The stools are described as loose, bulky, and foul-smelling. They are brown and not white or chalky. She experiences abdominal discomfort during the episodes of diarrhea as well as at other times. The patient denies jaundice, but she experiences fever, malaise, and night sweats. She denies cough, chest pain, and hemoptysis (blood in the sputum). Her family history is not contributory. She denies excess alcohol intake, HIV risk factors, recent travel abroad, and the use of any medications, but she says that she smoked one pack of cigarettes daily for 14 years.

Physical Examination

The patient is thin and pale and appears chronically ill. Her blood pressure, heart rate, and respiratory rates are normal. Her temperature is 38°C (100.4°F). There is tenderness in the right lower quadrant and hyperactive bowel sounds. There is no hepatosplenomegaly. The stool is negative for occult blood and parasites. Vibratory perception in the lower extremities is diminished. Peripheral pulses and muscular strength are good.

Laboratory

Hematocrit of 24% (normal ♀, 36–46%)
Red blood cell count, $2.0 \times 10^6/\mu L$ (normal ♀, $3.8–5.1 \times 10^6/\mu L$)
Hemoglobin, 6.1 g/dL (normal ♀, 12–16 g/dL)
Mean cell volume, 118 fl (normal, 80–100 fl)
Corrected reticulocyte count, 1 (normal, 1)
White blood count, $8{,}500/\mu L$ (normal, $4500–11{,}000/\mu L$)
Platelets, $150{,}000/\mu L$ (normal, $150–450 \times 10^3/\mu L$)
Peripheral blood smear, macrocytosis and hypersegmented neutrophils
Serum iron, 68 $\mu g/dL$ (normal, 50–170 $\mu g/dL$)
Bilirubin (total/direct), 1.6/0.3 mg/dL (normal, 0.2–1.0/0.0–0.2 mg/dL)
Serum albumin, 2.2 g/dL (normal, 3.5–5.0 g/dL)
Lactate dehydrogenase, 1800 U/L (normal, 210–380 U/L)
Globulin, 3.8 g/dL (normal, 2.2–4.0 g/dL)
Alkaline phosphatase, 55 U/L (normal ♀, 40–100 U/L)
Serum methylmalonate, 2400 nM (normal, 70–270 nM)
Thiamin, 2 $\mu g/dL$ (normal, 0–2 $\mu g/dL$)
Vitamin B_{12}, 44 ng/L (normal, 100–700 ng/L)
Folate, 1.2 $\mu g/dL$ (normal, 0.3–1.6 $\mu g/dL$)
Vitamin D_3, 1.2 ng/dL (normal, 2.5–4.5 ng/dL)
β-Carotene, 4 $\mu g/dL$ (normal, 10–85 $\mu g/dL$)
72-hour fecal fat (on 100-g fat/d diet) was 18 g/d (normal, <6 g/d).
D-Xylose absorption test, normal.

Schilling test for vitamin B_{12} absorption with (a) free cobalamin, (b) cobalamin with intrinsic factor, (c) cobalamin and pancreatic extract, and (d) cobalamin and antibiotics were abnormally low. An upper gastrointestinal radiologic examination with small bowel follow-through revealed inflammation of the distal portion of the small bowel consistent with Crohn disease.

15. The results of the differential Schilling test indicate that the patient had
    (A) classical pernicious anemia due to absence of intrinsic factor
    (B) bacterial overgrowth in the small bowel
    (C) chronic pancreatitis
    (D) ileal disease
    (E) dietary deficiency of cobalamin (vitamin B_{12})

16. What was the most likely cause of the moderate fat malabsorption (10–30 g of fat in the stool with 100-g daily intake), as observed in this patient?
    (A) Defective intestinal mucosal fat uptake
    (B) Deficient intrinsic factor production
    (C) Inadequate intestinal bile-salt concentrations
    (D) Iron deficiency anemia
    (E) Pancreatic disease

17. The anemia in this patient is due to a deficiency of
    (A) vitamin A
    (B) vitamin B_{12}
    (C) vitamin D
    (D) vitamin K
    (E) folate

18. The methylmalonate levels in this patient are due to a deficiency in the activity of which of the following enzymes?
    (A) Propionyl-CoA carboxylase
    (B) Ribonucleotide reductase
    (C) Methyltetrahydrofolate homocysteine transferase
    (D) Methylmalonyl-CoA epimerase
    (E) Methylmalonyl-CoA mutase

ANSWERS AND EXPLANATIONS

1. The answer is A: the formation of acyl-CoA from free fatty acid. This reaction involves cleavage of ATP between the α-and β-phosphoryl groups, yielding AMP and PP_i. The reactants contain two high-energy bonds, both in ATP, and the products also contain two—one the acid anhydride in PP_i, and the other the thioester bond in acyl-CoA. This functionally isoergonic reaction (PRINCIPLE 1 OF BIOENERGETICS) occurs in the cytosolic compartment, is pulled forward by the subsequent hydrolysis of PP_i (PRINCIPLE 14 OF BIOCHEMISTRY), and was the first example noted of this type of cleavage of nucleoside triphosphates. *Biochemistry,* p. 84.
2. The answer is F: the conversion of 3-hydroxyacyl-CoA to 3-ketoacyl-CoA. Pellagra is due to a deficiency of niacin, a component of NAD^+ and $NAD(P)^+$. The oxidation of an alcohol to a keto group typically involves formation of NADH, as seen earlier for the cytosolic reaction catalyzed by lactate dehydrogenase and for the Krebs cycle (and cytosolic) reaction catalyzed by malate dehydrogenase. Donation of reducing equivalents to the respiratory chain from mitochondrial NADH leads to the formation of 2.5 moles of ATP per mole of NADH. Reaction D, which is the other oxidation-reduction reaction of this pathway, mediates the conversion of acyl-CoA to 2,3-*trans*-enoyl-CoA. This mitochondrial reaction is catalyzed by acyl-CoA dehydrogenase, which transfers reducing equivalents as $FADH_2$ to intermediate carriers that will donate them to the electron transport chain at the level of coenzyme Q. The formation of a *trans* double bond in a saturated acyl carbon chain is almost always mediated by a flavin-dependent dehydrogenase. Conversion of succinate to fumarate in the Krebs cycle is an example encountered earlier (Chapter 8), and similar reactions occur in the degradation of the branched-chain amino acid carbon chains. *Biochemistry,* p. 24.
3. The answer is B: formation of acylcarnitine. The rates of the β-oxidation reactions within the mitochondrial matrix are largely dependent on substrate availability, and this is controlled by the rate of transport of fatty acids into the mitochondrion. Since transport is a function of acylcarnitine formation rate, this reaction is a logical place for regulatory control. Reaction A cannot serve as a regulatory step, since acyl-CoA is used anabolically to form glycerolipids, sphingolipids, and cholesterol esters and catabolically as a substrate for oxidation. *Biochemistry,* p. 158.
4. The answer is B: formation of acylcarnitine from acyl-CoA (and carnitine). This reaction, catalyzed by carnitine acyltransferase I at the outer surface of the inner mitochondrial membrane, is necessary because coenzyme A and its acylated derivatives cannot traverse the membrane. The acylcarnitine thus formed is translocated, in exchange for free carnitine, to the matrix side of the membrane, where it is converted to intramitochondrial acyl-CoA and carnitine by carnitine acyltransferase II. Reaction B (in the catabolic pathway) is inhibited by malonyl-CoA, an intermediate in the *anabolic* fatty acid synthesis pathway. *Biochemistry,* p. 157; *Nelson,* p. 338.
5. The answer is D: citrate. The relatively inactive monomers of acetyl-CoA carboxylase form active filamentous aggregates in the presence of citrate, which accumulates in the cytosol when energy supplies are abundant. *Biochemistry,* p. 172.
6. The answer is B: biotin. Acetyl-CoA carboxylase utilizes biotin as cofactor in the ATP-dependent carboxylation of acetyl-CoA to form malonyl-CoA. The carboxyl group is donated from an activated carboxy-biotinyl intermediate whose formation requires ATP cleavage. Similar reactions are required for the conversion of pyruvate to oxaloacetate by pyruvate carboxylase, propionyl-CoA to methylmalonyl-CoA by propionyl-CoA carboxylase, and β-methylcrotonoyl-CoA to β-methylglutaconyl-CoA. Biotin is a key factor in gluconeogenesis, lipogenesis, and amino acid (leucine, methionine, isoleucine, and valine) catabolism. Besides a deficiency of holoenzyme synthetase that attaches biotin to its apoenzymes, an inborn error of biotinidase exists in which there is a failure to cleave biotin from lysine, resulting in biotin deficiency.

The clinical pictures of the two defects are similar, but the holoenzyme synthetase deficiency becomes manifest soon after birth, and the biotinidase deficiency occurs at about 6 weeks of age. *Biochemistry,* p. 165; *Nelson,* p. 319.

7. The answer is E: linoleate. The common name for this essential 18-carbon fatty acid is linolenate. It contains three *cis* double bonds whose positions are denoted by the delta system as Δ9,12,15, meaning that the double bonds occur between carbons 9 and 10, 12 and 13, and 15 and 16, designating the carboxylate carbon as carbon 1. The ω-system (or n-system) is often used to describe families of polyunsaturated fatty acids, the two most common being the ω-6 (n-6) family, which includes linoleate and arachidonate, and the ω-3 (n-3) family, which includes linolenate (*cis,cis,cis*-octadecatetrieneoate). *Biochemistry,* p. 151.
8. The answer is D: platelet activating factor. Platelet activating factor is a glycerolipid containing an alkyl ether linkage at *sn*-1, an acetyl group at *sn*-2, and phosphocholine at *sn*-3. Sphingolipids contain the long-chain amino alcohol, sphingosine, to which a fatty acid is bound in amide linkage, and a variety of sphingolipids accumulate in the sphingolipidoses, which are lysosomal storage diseases. The combination of sphingosine and fatty acid is called a ceramide, and this accumulates in patients with ceramidase deficiency. The terminal alcohol group of sphingosine may be bound to phosphocholine, forming sphingomyelin, which accumulates in patients with sphingomyelinase deficiency. The terminal alcohol group of sphingosine may be bound to hexose such as glucose, forming glucosyl ceramide, or cerebroside, which accumulates in patients with Gaucher disease. The terminal alcohol group of sphingosine may be bound to a chain of sugars and amino sugars, forming a ganglioside. Gangliosides accumulate in patients with Tay-Sachs disease and several other disorders. *Biochemistry,* p. 155.
9. The answer is A: impaired acetyl-CoA production and subsequent inability to activate pyruvate carboxylase. The lack of medium-chain acyl-CoA dehydrogenase results in the accumulation of medium-chain acyl thioesters that cannot be metabolized at the normal rate. As a result, acetyl-CoA production by β-oxidation is diminished. This decreases the concentration of the activator of pyruvate carboxylase, an enzyme important in gluconeogenesis and in providing Krebs cycle intermediates. There is an increased ratio of mitochondrial acyl-CoA to CoA and an increased ratio of acylcarnitine to carnitine. Moreover, several medium-chain acylcarnitines such as octanoyl carnitine appear in the urine, and a secondary carnitine deficiency results. Decreased availability of acetoacetyl-CoA and acetyl-CoA as a result of the deficiency of β-oxidation decreases ketone body production. These patients are acidotic, but they are not ketotic. Human cells lack the ability to convert acetyl-CoA into net amounts of glucose (humans cannot convert fat into carbohydrate). Besides medium-chain acyl-CoA dehydrogenase, deficiencies in long-chain and short-chain acyl-CoA dehydrogenases have been reported. *Biochemistry,* p. 116; *Nelson,* p. 336.
10. The answer is C: 92. Formation of the activated myristyl-CoA requires two ATP equivalents (ATP → AMP + PP_i and PP_i → 2 P_i). Conversion of the 14-carbon myristyl group to seven acetyl-CoA requires six rounds of β-oxidation, each yielding one $FADH_2$ (1.5 ATP) and one NADH (2.5 ATP), for a total of four ATP per round. Oxidation of each acetyl-CoA yields 10 ATP, and the yield is calculated as follows: $(7 \times 10) + (6 \times 4) - 2 = 70 + 24 - 2 = 92$. *Biochemistry,* p. 159.
11. The answer is C: 3,5-dienoyl-CoA isomerase. 3,5-Dienoyl-CoA isomerase is required to convert a Δ3-*trans,* Δ5-*cis*-dienoyl-CoA, a reactant uniquely associated with the metabolism of fatty acids with a double bond beginning at an odd numbered carbon atom, to a Δ2-*trans,* Δ4-*trans*-dienoyl-CoA derivative. Enoyl-CoA isomerase and 2,4-dienoyl-CoA reductase are required for the metabolism of fatty acids that contain double bonds at both odd and even numbered carbon atoms. Thiolase and acyl-CoA dehydrogenase are required for the metabolism of saturated and unsaturated fatty acids. *Biochemistry,* p. 159.
12. The answer is C: 16.5 moles of ATP from oxidation of one mole of propionyl-CoA. Conversion of propionyl-CoA to succinyl-CoA requires one ATP in the propionyl-CoA carboxylase step. This is replenished when succinyl-CoA is converted to succinate, yielding the ATP equivalent, GTP. Additional ATP molecules are produced as follows: succinate → fumarate (1.5 from $FADH_2$), fumarate → malate (0), malate → pyruvate (2.5 ATP from the NADH produced by mitochondrial malic enzyme), pyruvate → CO_2 + H_2O (12.5 ATP). To summarize: $1.5 + 2.5 + 12.5 = 16.5$. *Biochemistry,* p. 162.
13. The answer is E: labeling the carboxyl carbon of malonyl-CoA would NOT result in the labeling of every third carbon in the finished fatty acid. The carboxyl added in the acetyl-CoA carboxylase reaction is released in the condensation step when two of the carbons of malonyl-CoA are added to the carboxyl end of the growing fatty acid chain. It is the exergonic decarboxylation that helps drive the reaction forward. Elongation of fatty acids beyond 16 carbons occurs in the endoplasmic reticulum and requires malonyl-CoA as carbon donor, as does *de novo* synthesis. Fatty acid elongation reactions within the mitochondrion use acetyl-CoA as reactant. Synthesis of fatty acids from acetyl-CoA (*de novo* synthesis) occurs in the cytosol, and, during reduction by NADPH, the fatty acid is attached to the acyl carrier protein portion of the polyprotein called fatty acid synthase. *Biochemistry*, p. 166.
14. The answer is A: both pathways do NOT require formation of phosphatidate as an intermediate. Phosphatidate is an intermediate in the general pathway of triglyceride synthesis but NOT in the intestinal pathway. Both pathways require acyl-CoA as an activated acyl group donor, involve formation of 1,2-diglyceride as an intermediate, and proceed with a net loss of free energy (as do all metabolic pathways in accordance with PRINCIPLE 18 OF BIOCHEMISTRY). The formation of the high-energy thioester bond in acyl-CoA is accompanied by cleavage of ATP to AMP + PP_i. *Biochemistry,* p. 169.
15. The answer is D: ileal disease. If the B_{12} deficit is due to a dietary deficiency, provision of free cobalamin restores the body reserves. If there is diminished B_{12} absorption because of a deficiency of intrinsic factor, administration of exogenous intrinsic factor leads to normal B_{12} uptake in people with classical pernicious anemia (not observed in this patient). If the inability to absorb B_{12} is due to the inability to liberate the vitamin from foods because of pancreatic enzyme deficiency, this is corrected by the concomitant administration of pancreatic extract (not observed in this patient). If bacteria occur abnormally in the distal ileum, the administration of antibiotics can eliminate these bacteria and normal absorption can occur (not observed in this patient). If the inability to absorb B_{12} is due to an abnormality of the ileal mucosa, none of these interventions will improve B_{12} absorption. Based upon the x-ray findings and clinical description,

this patient is suffering from Crohn disease, an inflammatory disease usually involving the small bowel. The pathogenesis of this disorder is unknown, and treatment is symptomatic. A female patient, slight fever, Northern European ancestry, and history of cigarette smoking are all positively correlated with Crohn disease. The diarrhea, weight loss, and steatorrhea are characteristic of Crohn disease. Besides these, the patient is suffering from an anemia due to vitamin B_{12} deficiency that is due to malabsorption and not to a deficiency of intrinsic factor. Pernicious anemia is B_{12} deficiency that is related to lack of intrinsic factor production by the stomach. Another cause of chronic diarrhea is parasitic infection. This prompted the question about foreign travel to places where parasitic infections can be more common; laboratory examination of the stool showed no evidence of parasitic infection. The patient suffered from fever and night sweats. Tuberculosis is characteristically associated with night sweats, which prompted the physician to ask about cough and blood in the sputum (hemoptysis), but these were lacking in the patient. *Biochemistry,* p. 27; *Cecil,* p. 692.

16. The answer is C: inadequate intestinal bile-salt concentrations. Bile salts are required for the emulsification, digestion, and absorption of dietary lipids. This patient's defect resides in the distal ileum, the site for bile salt reuptake in the process of enterohepatic circulation and vitamin B_{12} absorption. The terminal ileum reabsorbs about 95% of intestinal bile salts and returns them to the liver in a process called enterohepatic circulation. Because of diminished intestinal reuptake and supply of bile salts to the liver, inadequate bile salts are secreted, thus diminishing fat digestion and absorption. The defect was not great enough to produce a frank steatorrhea where the stool is white with fat. Absorption of fats occurs in the proximal portion of the small intestine, and the distal ileum is the site of the defect in this patient (and most patients with Crohn disease). Pancreatic deficiency usually leads to a much greater degree of lipid excretion (>40 g/d on a diet of 100 g of fat). Intrinsic factor is required for B_{12} but not lipid absorption. Iron deficiency anemia is not related to fat absorption. *Biochemistry,* p. 190; *Cecil,* p. 687.
17. The answer is B: vitamin B_{12}. A deficiency of B_{12} leads to a macrocytic anemia with hypersegmented white blood cells. As a result of increased cellular turnover, there is an elevation of lactate dehydrogenase and a modest elevation of serum bilirubin. B_{12} deficiency also leads to a peripheral neuropathy with diminished vibratory sensation. This patient has all of these characteristics. The other common cause of a macrocytic anemia is folate deficiency, but the patient's serum folate levels were normal. Iron deficiency anemia is a common nutritional problem but is characterized by a microcytic anemia (which this patient lacks); the serum iron in this person is normal. This patient suffers from a deficiency of the fat-soluble vitamins based upon serum analysis, but there are no signs and symptoms such as night blindness (vitamin A), rickets (vitamin D), or bleeding (vitamin K) that are readily attributable to their deficiency. Although the blood levels of these vitamins are decreased, adequate cell and tissue levels prevented the occurrence of these deficiency symptoms. *Cecil,* p. 846.
18. The answer is E: methylmalonyl-CoA mutase activity. The cofactor for this enzyme, which catalyzes the conversion of methylmalonyl-CoA to succinyl-CoA, is adenosylcobalamin. The cofactor for the conversion of homocysteine to methionine, catalyzed by methyltetrahydrofolate homocysteine transferase, is methylcobalamin. Methylmalonyl-CoA epimerase lacks a cofactor, and that for propionyl-CoA carboxylase is biotin. Human ribonucleotide reductase lacks vitamin B_{12} (but that from *Lactobacillus leishmanii* is unusual, even among microbes, because it uses B_{12} as cofactor). *Biochemistry,* p. 161.

REFERENCES

Roskoski, R., Jr. *Biochemistry.* Philadelphia, W. B. Saunders Company, 1996.

Wyngaarden, J. B., L. H. Smith, Jr., and J. C. Bennett (eds.). *Cecil Textbook of Medicine,* 19th ed. Philadelphia, W. B. Saunders Company, 1992.

CHAPTER TWELVE

COMPLEX LIPID METABOLISM

SYNOPSIS

OBJECTIVES

1. To outline the pathways for glycerolipid synthesis.
2. To describe sphingolipid synthesis and sphingolipidoses.
3. To outline the pathway for cholesterol and bile salt synthesis.
4. To describe the three major functions of lipoproteins.
5. To depict the pathways for chylomicron, VLDL, LDL, and HDL metabolism.
6. To enumerate the five classes of steroid hormones.

Objective 1: To outline the pathways for glycerolipid synthesis.

I. Principles of complex lipid biosynthesis
  A. Compounds with a high group-transfer potential donate their activated chemical fragments to substrates, yielding products with a low group-transfer potential (PRINCIPLE 17 OF BIOCHEMISTRY)
  B. Energy-rich donors in lipid metabolism include acyl-CoA and CDP-derivatives
  C. The following two equations illustrate the principle of group activation

$$\text{Acyl}{\sim}\text{SCoA} + \text{ROH} \rightarrow \text{Acyl-OR} + \text{CoASH} \quad (12.1)$$

$$\text{CMP}{\sim}\text{phosphocholine} + \text{ROH} \rightarrow \text{RO-phosphocholine} + \text{CMP} \quad (12.2)$$

    1. The reactants are energy-rich thioesters or acid anhydrides
    2. The products are low-energy oxygen esters (or amides) and phosphodiesters
    3. The reactions proceed with the loss of a high-energy bond and are exergonic (PRINCIPLE 2 OF BIOENERGETICS)

II. Glycerolipid metabolism
  A. Biosynthesis of glycerolipids
    1. Metabolism of **phosphatidate**
      a. Glycerol 3-phosphate is derived from glycerol or dihydroxyacetone phosphate (Fig. 12–1)
      b. Phosphatidate, a key intermediate in glycerolipid metabolism, is derived from glycerol 3-phosphate following two acyl transferase reactions
    2. Metabolism of **ethanolamine, choline,** and **serine**
      a. Ethanolamine reacts with ATP to form ethanolamine phosphate, which then reacts with CTP to form CDP-ethanolamine
      b. CDP-ethanolamine reacts with diglyceride to form phosphatidylethanolamine
      c. Phosphatidylethanolamine reacts with three molecules of *S*-adenosylmethionine to form phosphatidylcholine (Fig. 12–1)
      d. Phosphatidylethanolamine can also react with serine to form phosphatidylserine and ethanolamine by an exchange reaction
      e. Phosphatidylserine can undergo an exergonic decarboxylation reaction to form phosphatidylethanolamine in accordance with PRINCIPLE 6 OF BIOENERGETICS
  B. Metabolism of **phosphatidylinositol 4,5-bisphosphate** (PIP_2)
    1. CDP-diglyceride reacts with inositol to form phosphatidylinositol, which undergoes two successive phosphorylation reactions with ATP to form PIP_2
    2. PIP_2 undergoes a hydrolysis reaction catalyzed by phospholipase C to form diglyceride and inositol trisphosphate, two second messenger signaling molecules
    3. Inositol trisphosphate undergoes three successive dephosphorylation reactions
      a. The reactions are catalyzed by phosphatases to form inositol
      b. The final hydrolysis reaction is inhibited by **lithium ion**
    4. Diglyceride reacts with ATP to form phosphatidate
    5. Phosphatidate then reacts with CTP to form CDP-diglyceride, which can react with inositol and reinitiate the cycle
  C. Physiological actions of **diglyceride** and **inositol 1,4,5-trisphosphate** (second messenger molecules)
    1. Diglyceride activates protein kinase C, a broad-specificity enzyme
    2. Inositol trisphosphate interacts with a receptor in the endoplasmic reticulum membrane that stimulates the release of calcium into the cytosol

Objective 2: To describe sphingolipid synthesis and sphingolipidoses.

III. Biosynthesis of sphingolipids
  A. **Palmitoyl-CoA** and **serine** are the precursors of sphingosine (Fig. 12–2)

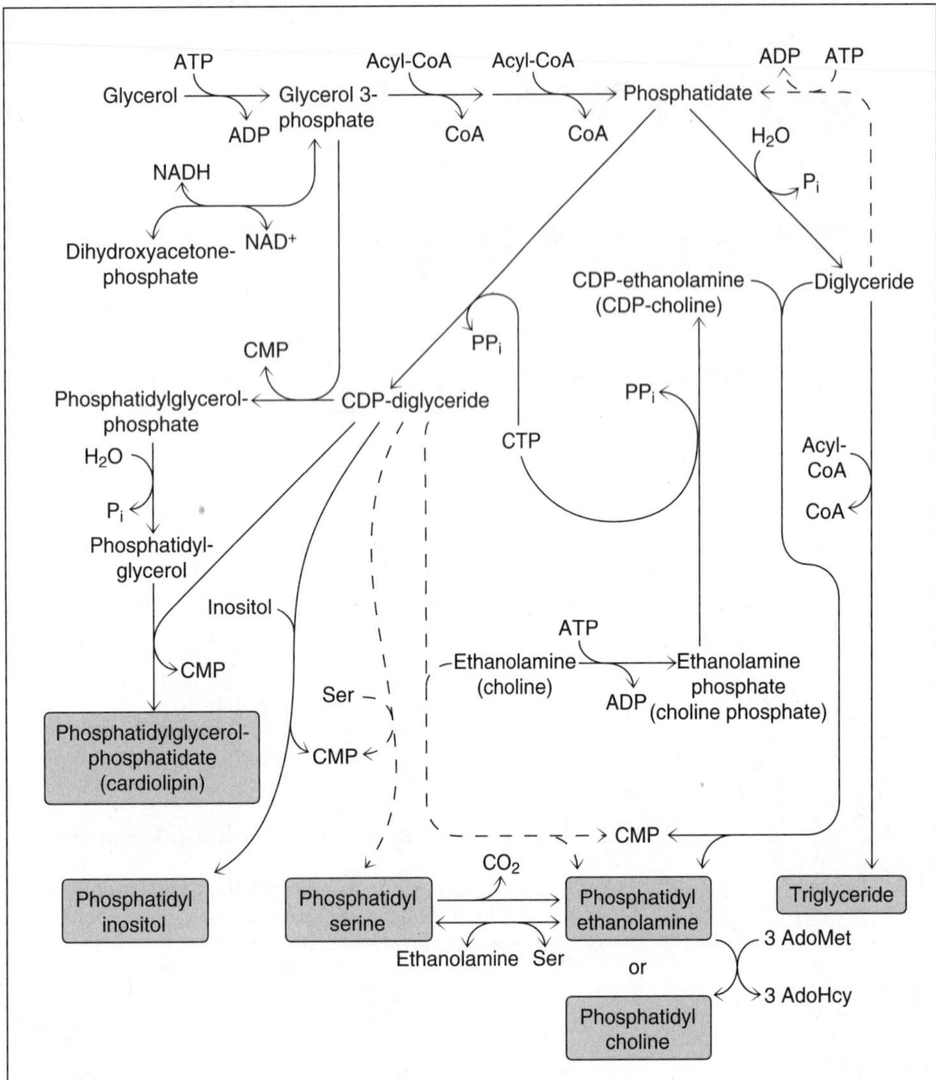

FIGURE 12-1. Overview of glycerolipid metabolism. AdoMet, *S*-adenosylmethionine; AdoHcy, *S*-adenosylhomocysteine.

B. Ceramide reacts with UDP-sugars to form **cerebrosides** (containing glucose or galactose) and **gangliosides** (containing a combination of two to six sugars and amino sugars, sulfate esters, and *N*-acetylneuraminate)
C. Ceramide reacts with phosphatidylcholine in an exchange reaction to form **sphingomyelin,** an unusual synthetic reaction since it lacks an activated donor

IV. Sphingolipid catabolism and sphingolipidoses
A. Sphingolipids are catabolized by sequential exergonic hydrolysis reactions that occur within lysosomes
B. Gaucher disease, the most common sphingolipidosis, is due to a deficiency of **β-glucosidase**
C. Tay-Sachs disease is due to a deficiency of **hexosaminidase A**

Objective 3: To outline the pathway for cholesterol and bile salt synthesis.

V. Cholesterol metabolism
A. Cholesterol biosynthesis
1. Three molecules of acetyl-CoA combine to form HMG-CoA
2. ***HMG-CoA reductase*** *is the rate-limiting and committed step in cholesterol biosynthesis;* the product is the six-carbon mevalonate
3. Mevalonate undergoes two successive phosphorylation reactions forming mevalonate pyrophosphate

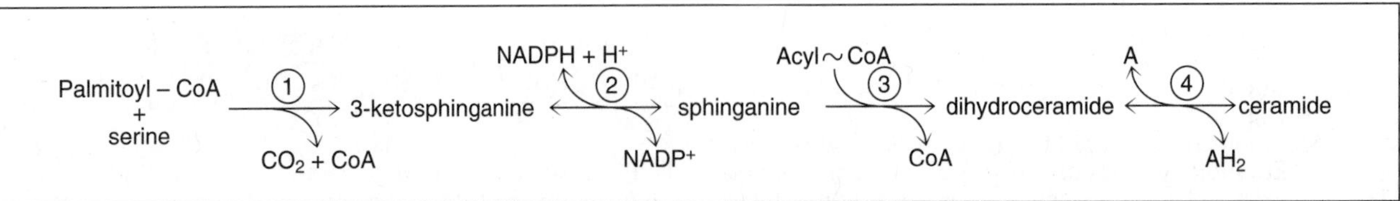

FIGURE 12-2. Pathway for ceramide biosynthesis.

4. Mevalonate pyrophosphate undergoes an exergonic decarboxylation reaction forming isopentenyl pyrophosphate
5. Isopentenyl pyrophosphate is converted in part to dimethylallyl pyrophosphate by isomerization
6. **Dimethylallyl pyrophosphate** and isopentenyl pyrophosphate combine to form **geranyl pyrophosphate**
7. Dimethylallyl pyrophosphate combines with geranyl pyrophosphate to form the 15-carbon **farnesyl pyrophosphate**
8. Two molecules of farnesyl pyrophosphate combine head-to-head to form **squalene,** a 30-carbon compound (Fig. 12–3)
9. Squalene reacts with molecular oxygen and undergoes an epoxidation and subsequent ring closures, yielding **lanosterol,** the first steroid in the pathway
10. The conversion of lanosterol to **cholesterol** requires about 20 reactions

B. Conversion of cholesterol to bile salts
   1. Hydroxyl groups are introduced in positions 7 and 12 in reactions involving oxygen, NADPH, and the cytochrome P-450 electron transport system
   2. A thioester is introduced at C^{24} by oxidation and thiolysis by coenzyme A
      a. The thioester, a high-energy bond, reacts with taurine or glycine to form conjugates

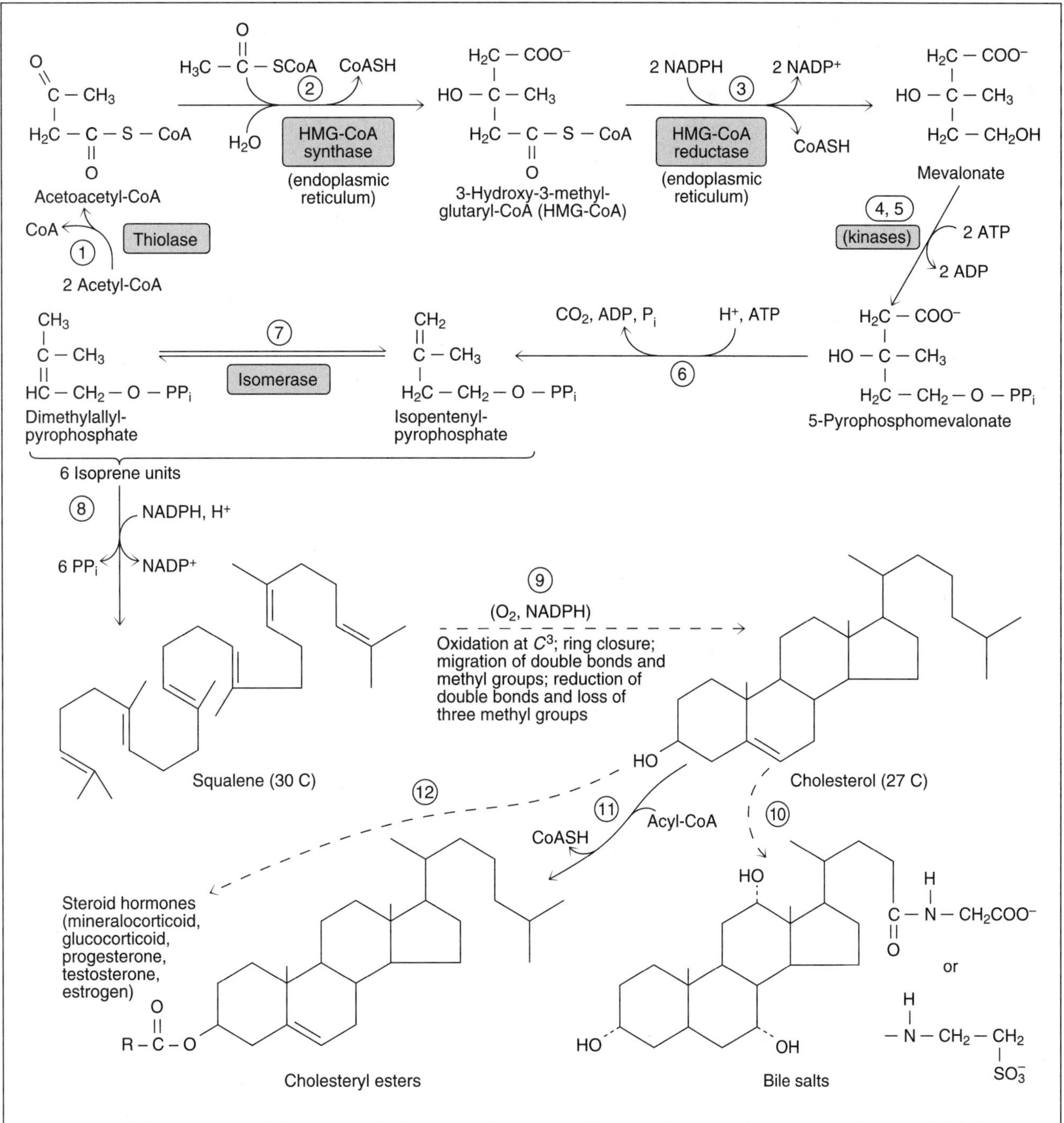

FIGURE 12–3. Overview of cholesterol biosynthesis and metabolism.

b. The reaction proceeds with the loss of a high-energy bond and is exergonic in accordance with PRINCIPLE 2 OF BIOENERGETICS

C. Enterohepatic circulation of bile salts
1. Bile salts, phospholipids, and cholesterol are released by the liver and enter the duodenum from the gallbladder and bile ducts; these compounds aid in the emulsification, digestion, and absorption of lipids
2. Bile salts are taken up in the terminal ileum and recirculated to the liver where they can again participate in lipid digestion and absorption (recall that vitamin B_{12} is also absorbed in the terminal ileum by a process that requires intrinsic factor)
3. The recirculation of bile salts is called enterohepatic (gut-liver) circulation

Objective 4: To describe the three major functions of lipoproteins.

VI. Lipoproteins and apolipoproteins (Table 12–1)
A. Three major functions of lipoproteins
1. Lipoproteins transport dietary fat from the intestinal mucosa, where it is absorbed, to other tissues by exogenous lipid transport involving chylomicrons
2. Lipoproteins transport triglyceride and cholesterol from liver to other tissues by endogenous lipid transport involving VLDL, IDL, and LDL
3. Lipoproteins transfer cholesterol from extrahepatic tissues to the liver by reverse cholesterol transport involving HDL

B. Enzymology of lipoprotein metabolism
1. **Lecithin-cholesterol acyltransferase** (LCAT) catalyzes the transfer of the *sn*-2 fatty acyl group of phosphatidylcholine to cholesterol; the products include cholesteryl ester and lysolecithin
2. **Lipoprotein lipase** catalyzes the hydrolysis of triglyceride in very low-density lipoprotein (VLDL) and chylomicrons to provide fatty acids to target cells; **apo-C-II** is an activator of this process
3. **Hepatic lipase** catalyzes the hydrolysis of triglyceride and phospholipids in high-density lipoprotein (HDL) and intermediate-density lipoprotein (IDL)
4. **Acid lipase,** present in most cells, catalyzes the hydrolysis of triglyceride and cholesteryl ester in lysosomes

Objective 5: To depict the pathways for chylomicron, VLDL, LDL, and HDL metabolism.

VII. Lipoprotein metabolism
A. Chylomicrons
1. Chylomicrons carry dietary lipid (triglyceride and cholesterol) from the small intestine to other tissues of the body
2. Capillary lipoprotein lipase (heparin-sensitive lipase) plays a key role in the delivery of fatty acids to extrahepatic cells

B. Endogenous lipid transport by VLDL, IDL, and LDL
1. VLDL synthesis occurs in the liver
2. The main function of VLDL is to transport triglyceride from the liver to other tissues
3. Triglyceride within VLDL is digested by lipoprotein lipase, and fatty acids and glycerol are discharged
4. VLDL is converted to IDL
5. Some IDL is taken up by the liver in a process that involves recognition by an apo-B-100/apo-E receptor, and the remaining IDL is converted to LDL
6. About half the LDL is taken up by the liver, and the remainder is taken up by extrahepatic tissues in a process that depends upon recognition by an apo-B-100/apo-E receptor

C. HDL and reverse cholesterol transport
1. HDL is synthesized in both liver and intestine and is released in discoidal form
2. Discoidal HDL interacts with cells and HDL_2 and is converted to HDL_3
3. *HDL_3 receives free cholesterol that is released from cells and is converted to cholesteryl ester in a reaction catalyzed by LCAT;* this is a pivotal reaction of reverse cholesterol transport
4. HDL_2 may also be taken up and degraded by the liver

VIII. Lipoprotein receptors
A. The LDL receptor
1. The LDL receptor, which is the best characterized of the lipoprotein receptors, recognizes both apo-B-100 and apo-E
2. The LDL receptor, which occurs in many cell types, participates in the removal of LDL from the plasma based upon the recognition of apo-B-100 by a process called receptor-mediated endocytosis

B. The chylomicron remnant receptor
1. The chylomicron remnant receptor, which is confined to the liver, recognizes apo-E

TABLE 12–1. Apoproteins of the Plasma Lipoproteins

Apoprotein	Plasma Lipoprotein Containing an Appreciable Amount	Major Site of Synthesis	Function
A-I	HDL, chylomicrons	Intestine, liver	LCAT activation
A-II	HDL	Intestine, liver	Structural
A-IV	Chylomicrons	Intestine	Structural
B-100	LDL, VLDL, IDL	Liver	Recognition by LDL receptor
B-48	Chylomicrons, chylomicron remnants	Intestine	Chylomicron formation
C-I	VLDL, HDL	Intestine	Structural
C-II	VLDL, HDL	Liver	Lipoprotein lipase activation
C-III	VLDL, HDL	Liver	Inhibition of VLDL uptake by liver
D	HDL	?	Structural
E	VLDL, chylomicron remnants, IDL	Liver, macrophages	Recognition by LDL and chylomicron remnant receptors

2. Although the LDL receptor also recognizes apo-E, these two receptors differ
3. The chylomicron remnant pathway accounts for the transport of dietary cholesterol and triglyceride to the liver from the intestine

IX. Disorders of lipoprotein metabolism
A. Hypercholesterolemia (>240 mg/dL) and hypertriglyceridemia (>160 mg/dL) occur commonly in the general population
B. Primary disorders of lipoprotein metabolism are those in which the primary abnormality is in lipoprotein metabolism *per se* (Table 12–2)
1. **Familial hypercholesterolemia,** which results from decreased cellular LDL uptake, is an autosomal dominant disorder that produces a type II hyperlipoproteinemia
2. **Lipoprotein lipase** deficiency is an autosomal recessive disease that results in type I (hyperchylomicronemia) or type V (hyperchylomicronemia and increased VLDL) hyperlipoproteinemias
3. **Apo-C-II** deficiency, a rare autosomal recessive disease, results in type I or type V hyperlipoproteinemia; apo-C-II activates lipoprotein lipase
4. **Hepatic lipase** deficiency, **LCAT** deficiency, and **lipid transfer protein deficiency** are rare disorders that do not produce distinctive changes in plasma lipoproteins
5. Other primary disorders are multigenetic and exhibit complex inheritance patterns, and their pathogenesis and mechanisms have not been worked out

C. Secondary disorders of lipoprotein metabolism are those occurring secondary to other abnormalities such as diabetes, hypothyroidism, or liver obstruction
1. Plasma samples are evaluated with sophisticated quantitative laboratory studies
a. Normal plasma is clear, and plasma electrophoresis reveals only HDL and LDL (no chylomicrons, VLDL, or IDL)
(1) HDL exhibits α-migration
(2) LDL exhibits β-migration
(3) VLDL, which is not present normally in a fasting sample, migrates in the pre-β region
(4) IDL, which is not present normally in a fasting sample, migrates in the β-region
b. Chylomicrons, which are not present physiologically after a 12- to 14-hour fast, do not migrate and remain at the origin
2. Plasma samples taken after a 12- to 14-hour fast and stored at 4°C for 18–24 hours also can provide valuable information
a. Persistent chylomicrons will cause the plasma to form a creamy layer that floats to the top
b. Persistent VLDL with a hypertriglyceridemia >400 mg/dL will cause plasma turbidity
c. Increased HDL will not increase plasma turbidity
d. A turbid plasma sample indicates hypertriglyceridemia due to elevated VLDL levels, and a creamy top layer indicates hyperchylomicronemia

Objective 6: To enumerate the five classes of steroid hormones.

X. Steroid hormones
A. Steroid hormone biosynthesis
1. The conversion of cholesterol to pregnenolone, a C_{21} compound, is the first step in biosynthesis (Fig. 12–4)
a. The C_{21} compound results from the action of the side-chain cleavage enzyme complex on 20,22-dihydroxycholesterol
b. Hydroxylation requires NADPH, oxygen, and the mitochondrial cytochrome P-450 system or adrenodoxin
2. The conversion of pregnenolone to **progesterone** (a progestin) occurs in two steps, and the conversion of progesterone to **aldosterone** (a mineralocorticoid) and **cortisol** (a glucocorticoid) requires a 21-hydroxylation reaction not required for testosterone and estradiol synthesis
3. Progesterone is converted to **testosterone** (a male sex hormone) and **estradiol** (a female sex hormone) in several steps

B. Structures of the steroid hormones
1. Progesterone, aldosterone, and cortisol are C_{21} compounds
a. Aldosterone is unique because of the aldehyde group on C^{18}, which is the basis of its name
b. Glucocorticoids and aldosterone contain a hydroxyl group on C^{11}, which progesterone lacks; glucocorticoids lack an aldehyde group
2. Testosterone is a C_{19} compound

TABLE 12–2. Classification of Hyperlipidemic Disorders

Type	Elevated Lipoprotein	Elevated Lipid	Possible Primary Cause	Cardiovascular Risk	Plasma Appearance
I	Chylomicrons	Triglyceride	Diabetes, hypothyroidism	→	Clear with creamy layer
IIa	LDL	Cholesterol	Hypothyroidism, biliary obstruction, nephrosis, pregnancy	↑ ↑	Clear
IIb	LDL and VLDL	Cholesterol and triglyceride	Same as IIa	↑ ↑	Clear to turbid
III	IDL	Cholesterol and triglyceride	Hypothyroidism, ethanol, diabetes	↑ ↑	Clear to turbid
IV	VLDL	Triglyceride	Diabetes, ethanol use, glucocorticoids, renal disease, pregnancy, glycogen storage diseases	?	Turbid
V	VLDL and chylomicrons	Triglyceride and cholesterol	Ethanol use, pancreatitis, diabetes	→	Turbid with creamy layer

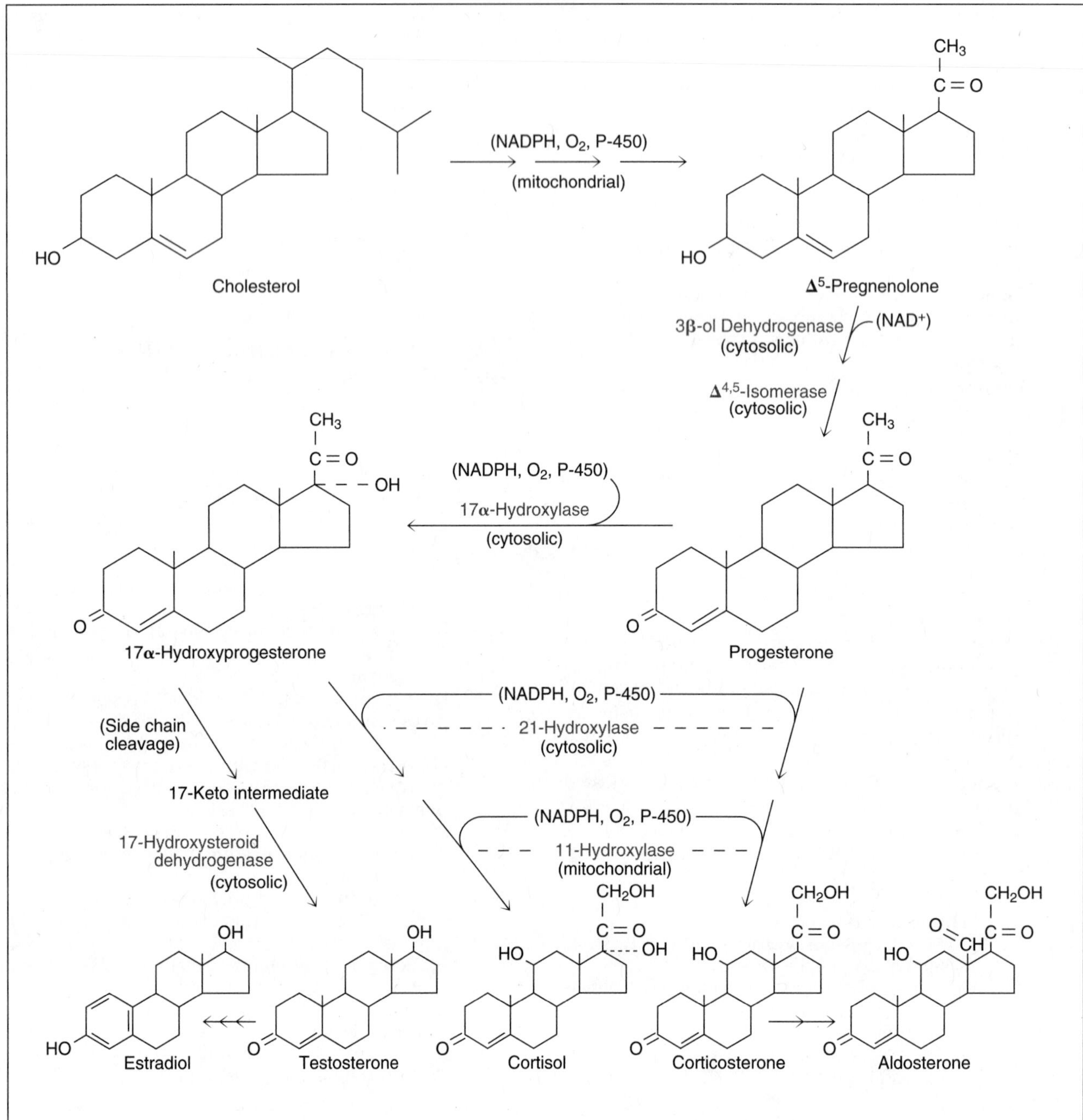

FIGURE 12-4. Overview of steroid hormone biosynthesis.

3. Estradiol is a C_{18} compound containing an aromatic A ring

C. Aberrant steroid hormone biosynthesis
   1. Congenital adrenal hyperplasia results most commonly from a deficiency of **progesterone 21-hydroxylase,** which is required for glucocorticoid and mineralocorticoid synthesis (Figure 12–4)
   2. As a result of 21-hydroxylase deficiency, there is increased production of dehydroepiandrosterone and masculinization

QUESTIONS

DIRECTIONS. (Items 1–8): Each set of matching questions in this section consists of a list of lettered options followed by several numbered items. For each numbered item, select the ONE lettered option that is most closely associated with it. Each lettered option may be selected once, more than once, or not at all.

Items 1–2

(A) Acylation
(B) Decarboxylation
(C) Hydroxylation
(D) Methylation
(E) Phosphorylation

For each biochemical process, select the most appropriate reaction.

1. The conversion of phosphatidylethanolamine to phosphatidylcholine involves three reactions of this type
2. Conversion of glycerol 3-phosphate to phosphatidate requires two reactions of this type

Items 3–4

(A) Chylomicrons
(B) Very low-density lipoprotein (VLDL)
(C) Intermediate-density lipoprotein (IDL)
(D) Low-density lipoprotein (LDL)
(E) High-density lipoprotein (HDL)

Match each characteristic with the correct lipoprotein.

3. Which lipoprotein is increased in familial hypercholesterolemia?
4. Tangier disease is characterized by low plasma cholesterol and normal or elevated triglyceride levels. Which lipoprotein is decreased in Tangier disease?

Items 5–6

(A) Apoprotein A-I gene
(B) Apoprotein B-100/B-48 gene
(C) Apoprotein C-II gene
(D) Apoprotein E gene
(E) LDL receptor gene

For each plasma lipid abnormality described, match the correct apoprotein gene.

5. A point mutation in this gene can lead to increased serum cholesterol and triglyceride due to the inability of chylomicron remnants and VLDL to be taken up by their liver receptor; LDL levels are low, and HDL levels are normal
6. A point mutation in this gene leads to a large elevation of plasma triglycerides due to decreased catabolism of chylomicrons because of decreased activity of lipoprotein lipase.

Items 7–8

(A) Aldosterone
(B) Cortisol
(C) Estradiol
(D) Progesterone
(E) Testosterone

For each structural characteristic described, select the corresponding steroid hormone.

7. A glucocorticoid containing 21 carbon atoms
8. A steroid containing an aromatic ring

DIRECTIONS. (Items 9–18): Each of the numbered items or incomplete statements in this section is followed by answers or by completions of the statement. Select the ONE lettered answer or completion that is BEST in each case. Correct answers and explanations are given at the end of the chapter.

9. The clinical effectiveness of ionic lithium in the treatment of bipolar disorders is related to its action as an inhibitor of
   (A) diglyceride kinase
   (B) inositol phosphate phosphatase
   (C) phosphatidate phosphatase
   (D) phosphatidylinositol kinase
   (E) phospholipase A_2

10. An intermediate in the synthesis of all three major classes of sphingolipid is
    (A) ceramide
    (B) UDP-galactose
    (C) phosphocholine
    (D) sphingosine
    (E) CMP-*N*-acetylneuraminate

11. *N*-Acetylglucosamine synthesis begins with a reaction between
    (A) fructose 6-phosphate and glutamine
    (B) glucose 6-phosphate and acetamide
    (C) glucose 6-phosphate, ammonium ion, and acetyl CoA
    (D) glucose 6-phosphate, glutamate, and NAD^+
    (E) galactose 6-phosphate, glutamine, and phosphoenolpyruvate

12. Most sphingolipidoses result from genetic deficiencies of which one of the following lysosomal enzymes?
    (A) DNAses
    (B) Glycosidases
    (C) Phosphatases
    (D) Proteases
    (E) RNAses

13. Females with adrenogenital syndrome generally show some degree of masculinization at birth, and males show premature sexual development. The most common cause of this disorder is a deficiency of 21-hydroxylase, an enzyme in the endoplasmic reticulum. As a result of this inborn error of metabolism, there is decreased synthesis of aldosterone and

(A) progesterone
(B) testosterone
(C) estradiol
(D) cortisol

14. All of the following metabolites play a role in the synthesis of steroid hormones from cholesterol EXCEPT

(A) NADPH
(B) O_2
(C) acetyl-CoA
(D) cytochrome P-450
(E) NAD^+

Items 15–18

History

The patient is a 24-year-old male freshman dental student being seen for a preschool physical examination. A dietary history indicates that the patient eats bacon and eggs nearly every day for breakfast. He has cheeseburgers, french fries, fried chicken, fried fish, and pizza at least seven times weekly. He also eats ample red meats, pork, and whole-milk dairy products. His father died of a myocardial infarction at age 48. The patient denies allergies or asthma and is not taking antihistamines, corticosteroids, β-adrenergic agonists, or antagonists. He denies polydipsia and polyuria and weight loss. The patient does not smoke, has an occasional beer (two per week), and jogs 4 miles five or six times weekly. He denies fatigue or difficulty sleeping.

Physical Examination

The patient is 181 cm (5 ft, 11 in.) and weighs 83 kg (182 lb). The heart rate is 52/min; blood pressure, 116/76 mm Hg; respiratory rate, 14/min; temperature, 37.6 °C (99.7 °F). Funduscopic examination is normal. Cardiac examination is normal. There is no lymphadenopathy or goiter. Peripheral pulses are good, and deep tendon reflexes are brisk but normal.

Laboratory

Blood urea nitrogen (BUN), 15 mg/dL (normal, 7–18 mg/dL)
Creatinine, 1.0 mg/dL (normal, 0.7–1.3 mg/dL)
Glucose, 86 mg/dL (normal, 70–105 mg/dL)
T_4, 8 μg/dL (normal, 5–12 μg/dL)
Thyroid-stimulating hormone, 4 μU/mL (normal, 2–10 μU/mL)
Cholesterol, 300 mg/dL (recommended, <200 mg/dL; moderate risk, 200–239 mg/dL; high risk, >240 mg/dL)
LDL cholesterol, 162 mg/dL (recommended, <130 mg/dL; moderate risk, 130–159 mg/dL; high risk, >160 mg/dL)
HDL cholesterol, 38 mg/dL (desirable, >50 mg/dL)
Triglyceride, 140 mg/dL (recommended ♂, 40–160 mg/dL)

Urinalysis, chest x-ray, red and white blood counts and differential, electrolytes, lactate dehydrogenase, γ-glutamyl transpeptidase, and creatine phosphokinase were normal. A second fasting blood specimen showed that glucose, cholesterol, HDL cholesterol, LDL cholesterol, and triglyceride values were within 5% of the initial values.

15. The lipid profile most closely matches that of which of the following types of hyperlipoproteinemia?

(A) I
(B) IIa
(C) IIb or III
(D) IV
(E) V

16. The cause of the hyperlipoproteinemia in this patient is due to

(A) diabetes mellitus
(B) glucocorticoid excess
(C) hypothyroidism
(D) nephrotic syndrome or uremia
(E) unknown causes

17. The first step in this patient's treatment is to decrease cholesterol intake. If this is ineffective after a suitable trial, administration of nonabsorbable anion exchange resins can be prescribed. The oral administration of ion exchange resins decreases body cholesterol by binding

(A) bile salts
(B) cholesterol
(C) cholesterol ester
(D) neutral sterols
(E) sterol 7α-hydroxylase

18. An additional therapeutic modality is to prescribe drugs that inhibit cholesterol synthesis. The rate-limiting enzyme of cholesterol biosynthesis that is inhibited by lovastatin is

(A) β-ketothiolase
(B) hydroxymethylglutaryl-CoA synthase
(C) hydroxymethylglutaryl-CoA reductase
(D) mevalonate kinase
(E) squalene synthase

ANSWERS AND EXPLANATIONS

1. The answer is D: methylation. In this conversion, three successive reactions occur in which a methyl group is transferred from the activated precursor, *S*-adenosylmethionine, to the amino group of the ethanolamine moiety, thereby forming phosphatidylcholine. Since a new choline group is formed, this is called the *de novo* pathway for choline synthesis. *Biochemistry,* pp. 177, 179.
2. The answer is A: acylation. Addition of acyl groups from acyl-CoA precursors to the *sn*-1 and *sn*-2 positions of glycerol 3-phosphate yields phosphatidate. Conversion

of phosphatidylserine to phosphatidylethanolamine involves a decarboxylation. The salvage pathways for choline and ethanolamine reutilization involve phosphorylation reactions. *Biochemistry,* pp. 175, 176.

3. The answer is D: low-density lipoprotein (LDL). This lipoprotein is the principal transporter of cholesterol in the plasma, and it transports cholesterol from liver to peripheral tissues. This is the "bad cholesterol" whose elevation in plasma is correlated with increased cardiovascular disease. Familial hypercholesterolemia is characterized by cutaneous xanthomas, juvenile atherosclerosis, and plasma cholesterol values of 650 mg/dL or greater in a nonjaundiced person. This autosomal dominant disease is due to mutations that reduce LDL-receptor mediated LDL uptake into the cell. *Biochemistry,* p. 201; *Nelson,* p. 355.
4. The answer is E: high-density lipoprotein (HDL). The major cholesterol-containing lipoproteins in the plasma are LDL and HDL, the major lipoproteins in normal plasma after an overnight fast. LDL contains cholesterol and triglyceride, and HDL contains mostly cholesterol. The deficiency that can produce low cholesterol with normal triglyceride is HDL. Tangier disease is due to the increased catabolism and decreased function of HDL. Consequently, cholesteryl esters accumulate in spleen, lymph nodes, intestinal mucosa, skin, and also liver. Because of a decrease in "good cholesterol," affected individuals are at increased risk for atherosclerosis and coronary artery disease, but only after the age of 40 years. *Biochemistry,* p. 197; *Nelson,* p. 358.
5. The answer is D: apoprotein E gene. Synthesized by the liver, apoprotein E and apoprotein B-100 are recognized and bound by the chylomicron remnant and VLDL receptor; binding leads to their endocytosis and disposal. Aberrant metabolism of VLDL leads to the accumulation of IDL, a type III hyperlipoproteinemia, and there is decreased conversion of VLDL to LDL. This type of hyperlipoproteinemia responds to decreased fat intake in the diet. Mutations in the Apo-B-100/B-48 gene lead to decreased catabolism and a consequent accumulation of chylomicrons and VLDL, which are not observed with Apo-E gene mutations. *Biochemistry,* p. 198; *Nelson,* p. 356.
6. The answer is C: apoprotein C-II gene. Apoprotein C-II is an activator of lipoprotein lipase (the enzyme that catalyzes the hydrolysis and release of triglyceride from lipoproteins), and mutations of apo-C-II or lipoprotein lipase lead to similar clinical syndromes. Because of decreased activity of lipoprotein lipase, fewer fatty acids are released from chylomicrons and VLDL in the capillary bed. Although there is a hyperchylomicronemia, VLDL levels are not significantly changed. The hyperchylomicronemia is due to diminished hydrolysis of chylomicron triglyceride. These rare patients are not at increased risk for atherosclerosis, but they have recurrent bouts of pancreatitis, which can be life-threatening. These people are treated with medium-chain triglyceride, the fatty acids of which are absorbed directly into the portal blood and are transported to the liver without the participation of chylomicrons and the systemic circulation. *Biochemistry,* p. 195; *Nelson,* p. 357.
7. The answer is B: cortisol. Progesterone, cortisol, and aldosterone all contain 21 carbons, but cortisol is the only glucocorticoid listed. Cortisol contains a C^{17} hydroxyl group, which progesterone and aldosterone lack. Aldosterone is characterized by an aldehyde group at C^{18}. *Biochemistry,* pp. 201, 202.
8. The answer is C: estradiol. The estrogens are the only steroid hormones containing an aromatic ring, which is formed when testosterone loses the methyl group at C^{19}, and the A ring is oxidized. *Biochemistry,* pp. 201, 202.
9. The answer is B: lithium inhibits inositol phosphate phosphatase. Phosphatidylinositol kinase and diglyceride kinase both participate in the "inositol cycle," in which phosphatidylinositol 4,5-bisphosphate is made and degraded within the cell. Phosphatidate phosphatase converts phosphatidate to diglyceride, and phospholipase A_2 hydrolyzes the ester bond at *sn*-2 of glycerophospholipids, but neither of these enzymes is directly involved in the inositol cycle. *Biochemistry,* p. 177.
10. The answer is A: ceramide. Sphingosine looks like an attractive option, since it is a component of all sphingolipids, but free sphingosine is not an intermediate in the pathway. The Δ^4 double bond of sphingosine is formed only after the addition of the fatty acyl group to the amino group. Phosphocholine is part of sphingomyelin but not of cerebrosides or gangliosides, and free phosphocholine is not added to ceramide in any case but is derived from phosphatidylcholine in an exchange reaction. UDP-galactose is an intermediate in the synthesis of gangliosides and some cerebrosides but not in the synthesis of sphingomyelin. CMP-*N*-acetylneuraminate donates *N*-acetylneuraminate groups in the synthesis of gangliosides, but this group is not found in cerebrosides or sphingomyelins. *Biochemistry,* p. 180.
11. The answer is A: fructose 6-phosphate and glutamine. In this reaction, the amide group of glutamine is transferred to C^2 of fructose 6-phosphate, yielding glucosamine 6-phosphate and glutamate. In the subsequent reaction, an acetyl group is transferred from acetyl-CoA to the amino group to form *N*-acetylglucosamine 6-phosphate. Following activation to the UDP derivative, other *N*-acetyl hexosamines may be formed via epimerase reactions. Note that the initial reaction in this sequence converts a ketose to an aldose. The product of the second reaction, *N*-acetylglucosamine 6-phosphate, would appear to represent a combination of glucose 6-phosphate and acetamide, or of glucose 6-phosphate, ammonium ion, and acetyl-CoA, but these reactions do not occur physiologically. *Biochemistry,* p. 184.
12. The answer is B: glycosidases. Most sphingolipidoses result from a failure to hydrolyze glycosidic bonds between the various monosaccharide or amino sugar units in gangliosides. Sphingomyelinase deficiency, which results in Niemann-Pick disease, is an exception because this enzyme is a phospholipase. Tay-Sachs disease is due to a deficiency of hexosaminidase A, and Gaucher disease, the most prevalent of the sphingolipidoses, is due to the deficiency of β-glucosidase. Neither DNAse, protease, phosphatase, nor RNAse is involved in the degradation of gangliosides. *Biochemistry,* pp. 187–189.
13. The answer is D: cortisol. As a result of the 21-hydroxylase deficiency, there is decreased conversion of progesterone to 11-deoxycorticosterone (the precursor of aldosterone) and of 17α-hydroxyprogesterone to 11-deoxycortisol (the precursor of cortisol). As a result of decreased feedback inhibition, adrenocorticotropic hormone from the anterior pituitary gland increases and stimulates the conversion of cholesterol to Δ^5-pregnenolone, the rate limiting reaction in steroid hormone synthesis. This multistep side-chain cleavage reaction is catalyzed by a mitochondrial complex that utilizes NADPH, O_2, and a cytochrome P-450 system in a series of hydroxylations and reduction of O_2 to water. Side-chain cleavage is an exergonic process in accordance with PRINCIPLE 8

OF BIOENERGETICS. There is a shunting of pregnenolone to dehydroepiandrosterone to account for the development of male sex characteristics in affected infants. Treatment with glucocorticoids such as hydrocortisone inhibits excessive production of androgen and stems virilization. Patients with dysregulation of electrolytes require maintenance therapy with synthetic mineralocorticoids such as 9α-fluorocortisol. The majority of mutations causing 21-hydroxylase deficiency are due to recombinations between the active gene and an adjacent pseudogene. *Biochemistry,* pp. 201–203; *Nelson,* p. 1444.

14. The answer is C: acetyl-CoA. Even a cursory examination of the pathways of steroid hormone synthesis will reveal the prevalence of NADPH, O_2, and cytochrome P-450 in the biosynthetic processes. NAD^+ is the oxidant used in conversion of the 3-hydroxyl group of pregnenolone to the 3-keto group in progesterone. Although acetyl-CoA is the source of all carbons in cholesterol, the precursor of steroid hormones, the reactions specific to steroid hormone synthesis from cholesterol do NOT involve acetyl-CoA. *Biochemistry,* p. 202.
15. The answer is B: IIa. There is an elevation of low-density lipoprotein (LDL) only, and this is, by definition, type IIa hypercholesterolemia. An elevation of LDL alone leads to an increase in cholesterol without an increase in triglyceride (Table 12–2). In type I hyperlipoproteinemia, there is an elevation of chylomicrons and triglyceride. In type IIb hyperlipoproteinemia, there is an elevation of VLDL, triglyceride, and cholesterol. In type III hyperlipoproteinemia, there is an elevation of IDL, triglyceride, and cholesterol. In type IV hyperlipoproteinemia, there is an increase in VLDL and triglyceride. Type V hyperlipoproteinemia is a combination of type I and type IV hyperlipoproteinemia with elevations of both chylomicrons and VLDL; this is accompanied by both elevated triglyceride and cholesterol. This classification provides a way to think about hyperlipidemia, but it is not precise. A single individual can change from one pattern to another during the course of a disease, and each can be due to simple or complex genetic disorders (primary hyperlipoproteinemia) or can be secondary to other diseases (secondary hyperlipoproteinemia). Elevations of LDL or IDL observed in type IIa, IIb, or III hypercholesterolemia are associated with increased risk of cardiovascular disease. *Cecil,* p. 1082.
16. The answer is E: unknown causes. His activity level, lack of fatigue, and normal thyroid hormone concentration (T_4) rule hypothyroidism unlikely. His fasting blood sugar levels on two occasions were normal, making diabetes unlikely. He denied taking glucocorticoids, and his physical description does not resemble that of Cushing disease. Normal electrolytes and plasma glucose also argue against excess glucocorticoid action. Normal serum electrolytes, urea nitrogen, creatinine, lack of hypertension, lack of edema, and a normal urinalysis do not support uremia or the nephrotic syndrome as a cause of the hyperlipidemia. That the father died at a young age from a myocardial infarction suggests that there may be a genetic component to the patient's hyperlipidemia. In the absence of other information, the cause is unknown. That this patient has ideal weight and exercises vigorously increases insulin sensitivity and may increase HDL. *Biochemistry,* p. 201.
17. The answer is A: bile salts. Neutral sterols, cholesterol, and cholesterol esters lack ionic charges and do not bind to ion exchange resins. Sterol 7α-hydroxylase catalyzes the rate-limiting reaction in bile acid synthesis in the liver, and it is not bound by the ion exchange resins in the gut lumen. Bile salts, in contrast, are ionic and bind to anion exchange resins with subsequent elimination in the stool. Bile salts normally are released into the gut, and about 94% of the total is taken up in the terminal ileum and transported back to the liver in the process called enterohepatic circulation. By depleting the body of bile salts, serum cholesterol can be lowered, at least to some degree. When the enteric circulation is disrupted, feedback inhibition of the 7α-hydroxylase is decreased and more cholesterol is converted into bile acid, thus decreasing cholesterol levels. Large amounts of resin (25-g portions) are taken, and constipation and bloating are common side effects. *Biochemistry,* p. 190; *Cecil,* p. 1082.
18. The answer is C: hydroxymethylglutaryl-CoA reductase. Among the enzymes of the cholesterol biosynthetic pathway listed, HMG-CoA reductase is the rate-limiting enzyme of the entire pathway. Administration of lovastatin and related drugs decreases circulating cholesterol levels by an indirect mechanism. The enzyme activity is acutely depressed, and this is followed by a compensatory increase in HMG-CoA reductase synthesis. There is a parallel and coordinate increase in LDL receptor synthesis, and the cholesterol-lowering effect is due to an increase in LDL receptor function. Prescription of lovastatin would not be initiated in this patient until the results of dietary therapy have been thoroughly evaluated. The identification and occurrence of a rate-limiting step of a metabolic pathway are not straightforward. There are suggestions that HMG-CoA synthase is regulatory, fitting the suggestion that metabolic pathways can be controlled at multiple steps (the dispersive control of metabolism). *Biochemistry,* p. 188; *Cecil,* p. 1082.

REFERENCES

Roskoski, R., Jr. *Biochemistry.* Philadelphia, W. B. Saunders Company, 1996.

Wyngaarden, J. B., L H. Smith, Jr., and J. C. Bennett (eds.). *Cecil Textbook of Medicine,* 19th ed. Philadelphia, W. B. Saunders Company, 1992.

CHAPTER THIRTEEN

AMINO ACID METABOLISM

SYNOPSIS

OBJECTIVES

1. To describe protein digestion.
2. To describe transamination and ammonium ion production.
3. To outline the reactions of the urea cycle.
4. To list the ten essential amino acids.
5. To outline the metabolism of the 20 amino acids.
6. To describe folate metabolism.
7. To provide an overview of inborn errors of amino acid metabolism.

Objective 1: To describe protein digestion.

I. Protein digestion and protease specificity
  A. Proteolytic digestive enzymes are synthesized and stored intracellularly as inactive precursors called zymogens
  B. Pepsin, which contains an active-site aspartate, is derived from pepsinogen produced by the stomach
  C. Trypsin, chymotrypsin, and elastase are pancreatic serine proteases
    1. *Trypsin, a serine protease, cleaves on the carboxyterminal side of lysine and arginine*
    2. Chymotrypsin cleaves on the carboxyterminal side of phenylalanine, tyrosine, tryptophan, and other hydrophobic residues
    3. Elastase cleaves on the carboxyterminal side of alanine
  D. Carboxypeptidases A and B are exopeptidases produced by the pancreas

Objective 2: To describe transamination and ammonium ion production.

II. Transamination reactions
  A. Transaminases, which contain pyridoxal phosphate as cofactor, catalyze isoergonic reactions
  B. The involvement of glutamate and α-ketoglutarate as one of the substrate-product pairs for most transaminases helps explain the predominant role attributed to glutamate in amino acid and nitrogen metabolism

III. Ammonium ion production
  A. Oxidation-reduction reactions
    1. Glutamate dehydrogenase catalyzes a reaction between glutamate, $NAD(P)^+$, and water to produce α-ketoglutarate, NAD(P)H, and ammonium ion, a reversible process
    2. D- And L-amino acid oxidase, found in the peroxisome, catalyze the reaction of their stereospecific amino acids with molecular oxygen to produce the corresponding α-keto acid and hydrogen peroxide
    3. Catalase catalyzes the breakdown of hydrogen peroxide to oxygen and water
  B. Glutaminase and asparaginase catalyze the hydrolysis of the amide group of their substrates to produce glutamate and aspartate, respectively, and ammonium ion
  C. Serine/threonine dehydratase catalyzes the production of ammonium ion from its corresponding substrates
  D. The glycine cleavage complex catalyzes the conversion of glycine, tetrahydrofolate, and NAD^+ to ammonia, carbon dioxide, N^{5-10} methylenetetrahydrofolate, and NADH.

Objective 3: To outline the reactions of the urea cycle.

IV. Urea cycle
  A. Overview
    1. Urea, which is synthesized in liver, accounts for 80–90% of excreted nitrogen
    2. Urate, ammonium ion, and creatinine are other end products of nitrogen metabolism
  B. Reactions
    1. The stoichiometry of urea synthesis is expressed as follows:

$$\begin{array}{ccc} NH_3 + HCO_3^- & & \text{Urea} \\ + & & + \\ \text{aspartate}^- & & \text{fumarate} \\ + & \rightarrow & + \\ 3\ \text{ATP} & & 2\ \text{ADP} + 2\ P_i \\ + & & + \\ H_2O & & \text{AMP} \end{array} \qquad (13.1)$$

a. **Carbamoyl-phosphate synthetase I** catalyzes the formation of products from bicarbonate, ammonia, and two moles of ATP (Fig. 13–1)
b. This enzyme is activated allosterically by *N*-acetylglutamate, formed from acetyl-CoA and glutamate, in a reaction catalyzed by an acetyltransferase
c. Carbamoyl-phosphate synthetase I provides one of the stoichiometric substrates for the urea cycle pathway
d. Carbamoyl phosphate provides one of the nitrogen atoms and the carbon atom of urea; the other stoichiometric substrate, aspartate, provides the second nitrogen atom of urea

2. Carbamoyl phosphate reacts with ornithine, the regenerating substrate, to produce citrulline in a reaction catalyzed by **ornithine transcarbamoylase**
   a. The reaction proceeds with the loss of one high-energy bond
   b. The reaction is exergonic in accordance with PRINCIPLE 2 OF BIOENERGETICS
3. Citrulline reacts with aspartate in an ATP-dependent process (with the formation of AMP and PP_i) to form argininosuccinate in a reaction catalyzed by **argininosuccinate synthetase**
   a. The generation of pyrophosphate and its hydrolysis pulls the reaction forward (PRINCIPLE 14 OF BIOCHEMISTRY)
   b. Hydrolysis of pyrophosphate (an energy-rich compound) is exergonic in accordance with PRINCIPLE 5 OF BIOENERGETICS
4. Argininosuccinate undergoes a lyase reaction to form arginine and fumarate in a reaction catalyzed by **argininosuccinate lyase**
5. Arginine reacts with water to form urea, the end product, and ornithine, the regenerating substrate (Fig. 13–1)
   a. **Arginase** catalyzes this hydrolysis reaction
   b. The hydrolysis of arginine (a low-energy compound) is exergonic in accordance with PRINCIPLE 5 OF BIOENERGETICS
6. Disorders of the urea cycle can involve any enzyme of the pathway
   a. The most common cause of hyperammonemia in infants is due to a defect either in one of the urea cycle enzymes or in carbamoyl-phosphate synthetase I
   b. Inborn errors of the urea cycle occur without acidosis, and this feature distinguishes these disorders from many other inborn errors of metabolism

V. Glycogenic and ketogenic amino acids (Table 13–1)
   A. Amino acids are designated as glycogenic if they can be converted to glucose
   B. Amino acids are designated as ketogenic if they can be converted to ketone bodies
   C. Amino acids are designated as both glycogenic and ketogenic if they can be converted to both types of compound
   D. *It is noteworthy that leucine is the only amino acid that is ketogenic only*

TABLE 13–1. Metabolic Classification of Amino Acids

Glycogenic	Both Glycogenic and Ketogenic	Ketogenic
Glycine	Isoleucine	Leucine
Alanine, serine, cysteine	Phenylalanine, tyrosine	
Aspartate, asparagine	Tryptophan, lysine	
Glutamate, glutamine		
Proline, histidine, arginine		
Methionine		
Threonine		
Valine		

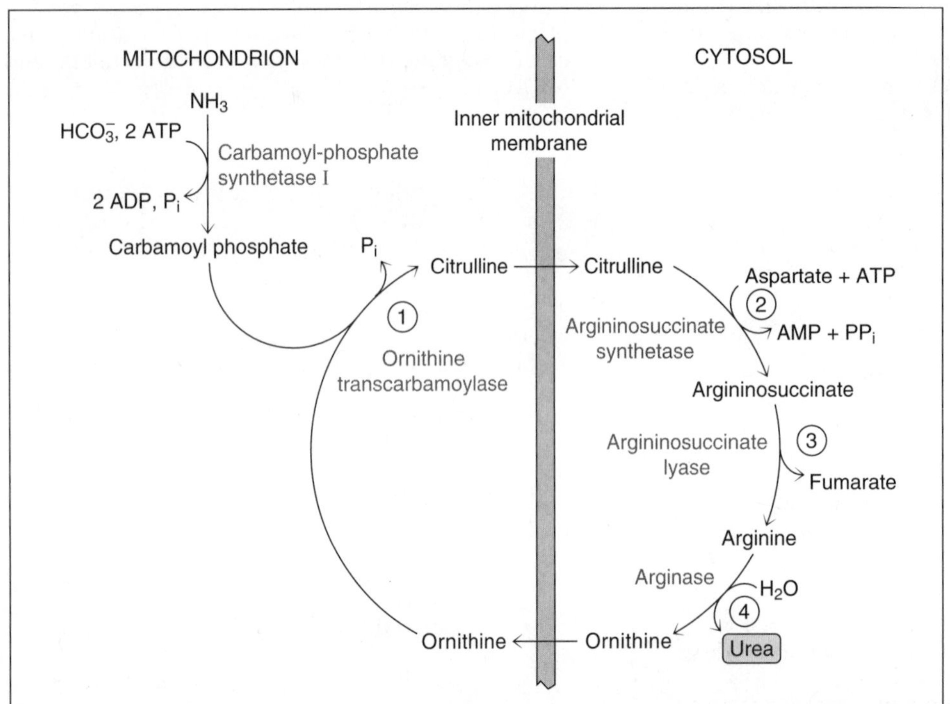

FIGURE 13-1. Urea cycle pathway.

Objective 4: To list the ten essential amino acids.

VI. Essential amino acids and nitrogen balance
- A. A mnemonic for the essential amino acids is the acronym PVT TIM *HA*LL ("private Tim Hall")
  1. This mnemonic corresponds to phenylalanine, valine, threonine, tryptophan, isoleucine, methionine, histidine, arginine, leucine, and lysine
  2. If one remembers that tyrosine is nonessential, since it is derived from phenylalanine (essential), then the mnemonic is less ambiguous
  3. HA is italicized to signify that these two additional amino acids are special cases
     - a. Arginine is required by infants and children
     - b. The essential nature of histidine is masked by the appreciable amount of carnosine (β-alanylhistidine) in muscle
- B. A deficiency in a single essential amino acid leads to negative nitrogen balance
  1. This is a condition in which nitrogen excretion exceeds nitrogen intake
  2. A deficiency of a single amino acid impairs protein synthesis and allows increased catabolism of the remaining amino acids

Objective 5: To outline the metabolism of the 20 amino acids.

VII. Amino acid metabolism based on families
- A. The C_2 and C_3 families of amino acids: alanine, serine, glycine, and cysteine
  1. Alanine is converted to pyruvate by transamination
  2. Glycine has at least two metabolic fates
     - a. A glycine cleavage complex catalyzes the formation of carbon dioxide, ammonia, and N^{5-10} methylenetetrahydrofolate in a reaction accompanied by the reduction of NAD^+
     - b. Glycine also reacts with N^{5-10} methylenetetrahydrofolate, formed in the previous reaction, and water to produce serine
  3. Serine undergoes a dehydration followed by hydrolysis as catalyzed by **serine dehydratase,** a pyridoxal phosphate-requiring enzyme, to produce pyruvate and ammonium ion
  4. Cysteine is converted into pyruvate in a series of reactions
- B. The nonessential C_4 family of amino acids: aspartate and asparagine
  1. Asparagine is hydrolyzed to form aspartate and ammonium ion
  2. Aspartate undergoes a transamination with α-ketoglutarate to form oxaloacetate
     - a. Oxaloacetate must be converted to pyruvate (via a malic enzyme pathway or a phosphoenolpyruvate carboxykinase pathway) prior to its oxidation by the Krebs cycle
     - b. In liver, aspartate can donate its amino group in the urea cycle while forming fumarate
- C. The C_5 family of amino acids: glutamine, glutamate, arginine, proline, and histidine
  1. Glutamine is hydrolyzed to form ammonium ion and glutamate, which is oxidized to form ammonium ion and α-ketoglutarate
  2. Arginine undergoes an exergonic hydrolysis reaction as catalyzed by arginase to form urea and ornithine, which is converted to α-ketoglutarate
  3. Proline catabolism begins with NAD^+-dependent oxidation to form Δ1-pyrroline 5-carboxylate, which is converted to α-ketoglutarate
  4. Histidine undergoes a lyase reaction with the elimination of ammonia and the formation of urocanate (originally isolated from canine urine); further catabolism yields *N*-formiminoglutamate (figlu) and then glutamate
- D. The essential C_4 family of amino acids: threonine and methionine
  1. Threonine undergoes a dehydration catalyzed by serine/threonine dehydratase to yield ammonium ion and α-ketobutyrate, which is converted to propionyl-CoA by oxidative decarboxylation
  2. Methionine is converted to *S*-adenosylmethionine, which donates its methyl group, forming *S*-adenosylhomocysteine (AdoHcy)
     - a. AdoHcy is cleaved to form homocysteine and adenosine
     - b. Homocysteine has at least two metabolic fates
       - (1) Most homocysteine is reconverted back to methionine in reactions involving methyltetrahydrofolate (in a B_{12}-dependent process) or betaine (*N*-trimethylglycine)
       - (2) Homocysteine combines with serine to form cystathionine and water as catalyzed by cystathionine synthase, a pyridoxal phosphate-dependent enzyme
     - c. Cystathionine lyase, also a pyridoxal phosphate-dependent enzyme, catalyzes the conversion of substrate to produce α-ketobutyrate, cysteine, and ammonia
     - d. α-Ketobutyrate can be converted to propionyl-CoA by oxidative decarboxylation
- E. The branched-chain amino acids: valine, isoleucine, and leucine
  1. Valine is converted sequentially to α-keto isovaleric acid (by transamination), isobutyryl-CoA (via branched-chain keto acid dehydrogenase), and propionyl-CoA
  2. Isoleucine is converted sequentially to α-keto-β-methylvalerate (by transamination), α-methylbutyryl-CoA (via branched-chain keto acid dehydrogenase), 2-methylcrotonyl-CoA, and acetyl-CoA plus propionyl-CoA
  3. Leucine undergoes a transamination, oxidative decarboxylation, and several more reactions to form HMG-CoA; thus, *leucine is entirely ketogenic*
  4. **Maple syrup urine disease** is caused by a deficiency of branched-chain keto acid dehydrogenase, which operates on metabolites of valine, leucine, and isoleucine
- F. Two aromatic amino acids: phenylalanine and tyrosine
  1. Phenylalanine is converted to tyrosine in liver by a reaction catalyzed by phenylalanine hydroxylase
  2. Tyrosine is converted in several steps to fumarate (glycogenic) and acetoacetate (ketogenic)
  3. Several inborn metabolic errors involve these aromatic amino acids
     - a. **Phenylketonuria** is caused by a deficiency in phenylalanine hydroxylase
     - b. **Alkaptonuria** is caused by a deficiency of homogentisate dioxygenase
     - c. Type I tyrosinemia is caused by a deficiency of fumarylacetoacetate hydrolase, which catalyzes

the last step of tyrosine degradation to mainstream metabolites

d. Type II tyrosinemia is caused by a defect in tyrosine aminotransferase, the first enzyme in the pathway for tyrosine catabolism

G. The ketoadipate family of amino acids: tryptophan and lysine

1. Tryptophan (another aromatic amino acid) is converted to alanine (glycogenic) and to acetyl-CoA via α-ketoadipate
2. Aminocarboxymuconate semialdehyde (ACS), a tryptophan metabolite, can also be converted to NAD^+, a vitamin derivative
3. Lysine forms saccharopine, an adduct of lysine and α-ketoglutarate, prior to conversion to α-ketoadipate

H. An overview of amino acid metabolism is shown in Figure 13–2

1. Amino acids that give rise to Krebs cycle intermediates or pyruvate are glycogenic
2. Amino acids that give rise to acetyl-CoA or acetoacetyl-CoA are ketogenic

Objective 6: To describe folate metabolism.

VIII. Tetrahydrofolate (THF) metabolism

A. Interconversion of tetrahydrofolate derivatives

1. One-carbon groups are attached to N^5, N^{10}, or both nitrogen atoms
2. Serine is the major source of one-carbon groups, and these are derived in a reaction catalyzed by serine hydroxymethyltransferase
3. N^5-Formyl-THF is used as a drug called leucovorin, and an ATP-dependent reaction is required for transfer of the one-carbon group from leucovorin
4. Methylene-THF can be reduced by NADH to yield N^5-methyl-THF and NAD^+
5. *N^5-Methyl-THF can transfer its methyl group to homocysteine in a vitamin B_{12}–dependent unidirectional reaction catalyzed by methyl-THF homocysteine methyltransferase to form methionine*

B. Folate and B_{12} interactions: the methyl trap hypothesis of vitamin B_{12} deficiency

1. The methyltransferase reaction is the only significant crossroad in human metabolism involving both folate and vitamin B_{12}
   a. This is the only reaction in humans that requires methyl-THF as methyl donor
   b. Methyl-THF cannot be retroconverted to methylene-THF because the reductase reaction is unidirectional; this represents an unusual situation for a "simple" oxidation-reduction reaction
2. In vitamin B_{12} deficiency, the cell cannot metabolize methyl-THF
   a. Consequently, methyl-THF accumulates
   b. Tetrahydrofolate cannot be made available for other reactions

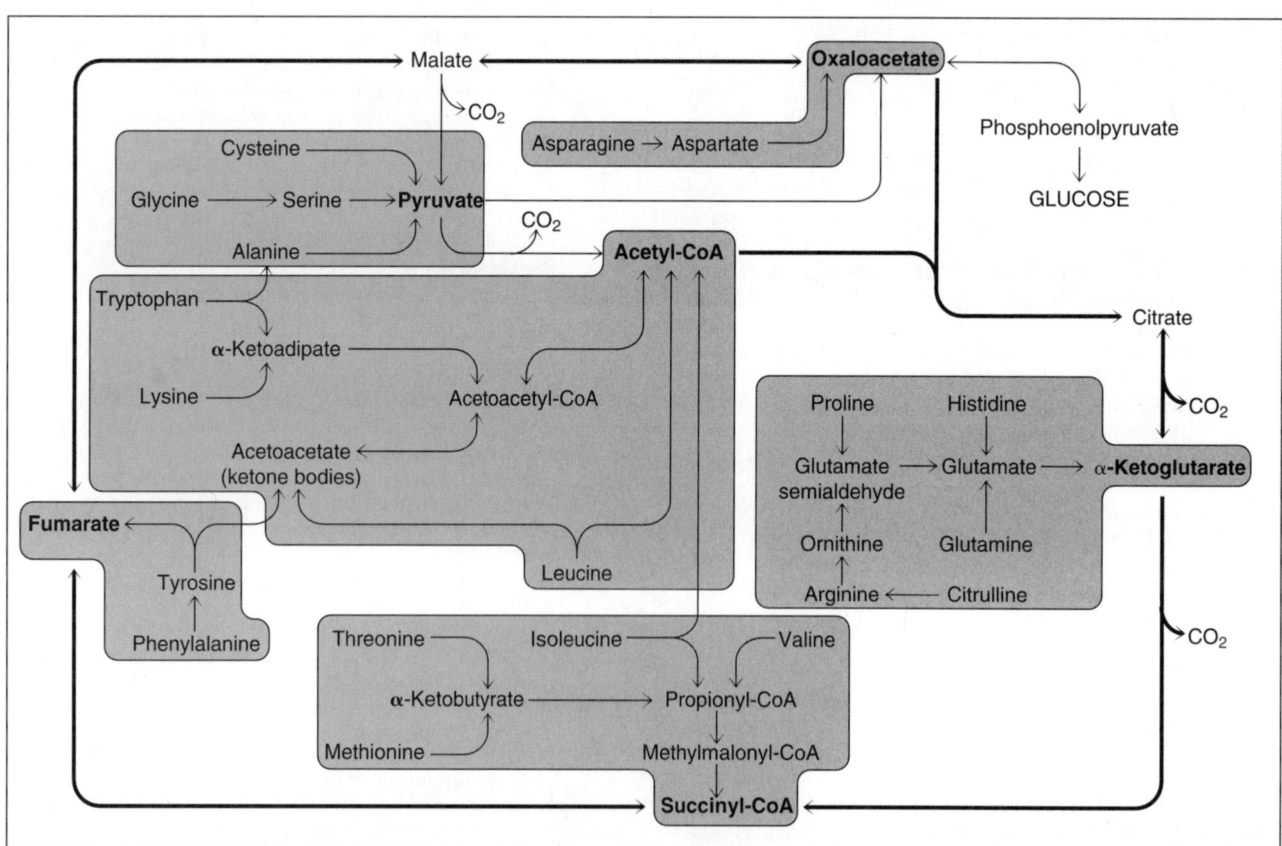

FIGURE 13-2. Overview of amino acid metabolism. Ketogenic amino acids yield acetyl-CoA or acetoacetyl–CoA. Glycogenic amino acids yield Krebs cycle intermediates or pyruvate.

Objective 7: To provide an overview of inborn errors of amino acid metabolism.

IX. Inborn errors of metabolism
  A. An overview of inborn errors of metabolism is provided in Table 13–2
    1. A clinical approach to newborn infants whose initial findings include poor feeding, vomiting, lethargy, convulsion or seizure, and coma is to determine whether these are related to infection
    2. If infection can be ruled unlikely, then metabolic diseases should be evaluated
    3. Plasma electrolytes, glucose, pH, carbon dioxide, and ammonia, along with a careful family history for hereditary disease, should be determined to aid in establishing a diagnosis
  B. Phenylketonuria (PKU) is probably the most prevalent of the inborn errors of amino acid metabolism
    1. The cause in 98% of cases is a deficiency of phenylalanine hydroxylase activity, a reaction that occurs in the liver
      a. Phenylalanine is converted to phenylpyruvate by a transamination reaction that is inconsequential in unaffected individuals
      b. Phenylpyruvate is excreted in the urine and accounts for the name "phenylketonuria"
    2. Variants are due to an inability to synthesize or metabolize tetrahydrobiopterin, the reductant of the phenylalanine hydroxylase reaction
    3. Because of widespread screening, undiagnosed PKU is uncommon in the United States and many other countries
      a. Amino acid analysis of blood reveals elevated phenylalanine (>1.2 mM) and normal tyrosine (40–100 μM)
      b. It is important to make the diagnosis and institute therapy early to minimize adverse neurological deficits
    4. Phenylketonuria is treated with a synthetic diet that contains minimal phenylalanine
  C. Selected inborn errors of metabolism with metabolic acidosis
    1. Maple syrup urine disease, which is due to a deficiency of branched-chain keto acid dehydrogenase, is characterized by urine with a maple syrup odor
    2. Propionic acidemia is due to a deficiency of propionyl-CoA carboxylase
      a. Propionyl-CoA is a metabolite of threonine, methionine, valine, isoleucine, and fatty acids that contain an odd number of carbon atoms
      b. Moderate to severe hyperammonemia and hypoglycemia commonly occur
      c. Carnitine deficiency occurs secondary to a loss of propionyl carnitine in the urine
      d. Treatment consists of a low-protein diet (with lowered levels of isoleucine, valine, methionine, and threonine) and supplemental carnitine
    3. Methylmalonic acidemia can be caused by a deficiency of methylmalonate mutase and defects in vitamin B_{12} metabolism
      a. Laboratory findings include acidosis, anemia, hyperammonemia, and hypoglycemia
      b. Hyperammonemia is due to inhibition of carbamoyl-phosphate synthetase I by organic acid metabolites
      c. Treatment is similar to that of propionic acidemia with a low-protein diet and carnitine
  D. Urea cycle defects are inborn errors of metabolism without metabolic acidosis
    1. These disorders occur with hyperammonemia and nonspecific elevations of plasma glutamine, aspartate, and alanine
    2. Defects of each of the enzymes of the urea synthesis have been described
      a. These include carbamoyl-phosphate synthetase I, ornithine transcarbamoylase, argininosuccinate synthetase, argininosuccinate lyase, and arginase
      b. There is one reported case of *N*-acetylglutamate synthase deficiency
    3. The clinical picture for all of these enzyme defects is similar, and the diagnosis is determined by laboratory analysis
      a. A deficiency of carbamoyl-phosphate synthetase I results in hyperammonemia without specific increases in any amino acids
      b. A deficiency of ornithine transcarbamoylase, like that of carbamoyl-phosphate synthetase I, results in hyperammonemia without specific increases in any amino acids
        (1) Translocation of carbamoyl phosphate from the mitochondrion to the cytosol results in increased orotic acid production and orotic aciduria
        (2) Some patients have orotic acid crystal formation and renal stones
      c. A deficiency of argininosuccinate synthetase results in increased plasma ornithine and citrulline levels
      d. A deficiency of argininosuccinate lyase results in increased plasma argininosuccinate
      e. A deficiency of arginase results in increased plasma arginine
    4. Metabolic treatment of urea cycle defects
      a. The goal of treatment is to provide enough amino acids for growth but not enough to produce toxicity
      b. The administration of benzoate results in the excretion of benzoylglycine (hippurate)
        (1) This results in the excretion of one atom of nitrogen (Fig. 13–3)
        (2) Benzoyl-CoA, a thioester, is the activated intermediate in hippurate synthesis
      c. The administration of phenylacetate results in the excretion of phenylacetylglutamine and the

TABLE 13–2. Selected Clinical Findings Associated with Inborn Errors of Metabolism

Sign or Symptom	Example
Abnormal urine odor	Maple syrup urine disease (maple syrup odor), phenylketonuria (mousy or musty odor)
Liver disease	Galactosemia, glycogen storage disease, lipidoses
Metabolic acidosis	All organic acidemias
Neurological abnormalities	Almost all categories
Poor feeding, persistent vomiting, and failure to thrive	Adrenal insufficiency, galactosemia, organic acidemias, urea cycle defects, phenylketonuria
Self-mutilation	Lesch-Nyhan syndrome

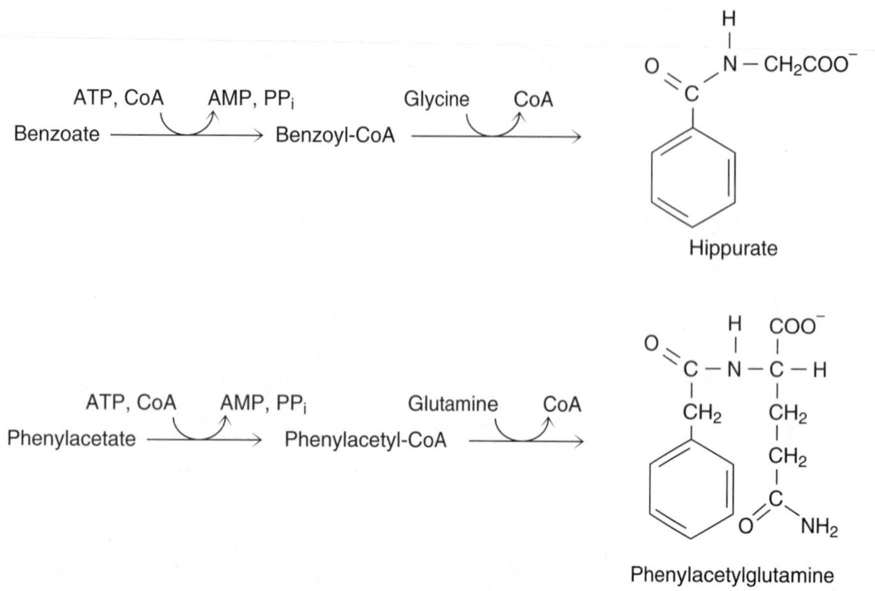

Benzoate —(ATP, CoA → AMP, PP_i)→ Benzoyl-CoA —(Glycine → CoA)→ Hippurate

Phenylacetate —(ATP, CoA → AMP, PP_i)→ Phenylacetyl-CoA —(Glutamine → CoA)→ Phenylacetylglutamine

FIGURE 13-3. Hippurate and phenylacetylglutamine biosynthesis.

excretion of two atoms of nitrogen per molecule (Fig. 13–3)

d. Arginine is administered in argininosuccinate synthetase and lyase deficiencies
   (1) Arginine is an essential amino acid in children
   (2) Arginine is hydrolyzed to produce urea (nontoxic) and ornithine
   (3) Ornithine can be metabolized to citrulline in synthetase deficiency, and citrulline can be excreted in the urine
   (4) Administration of arginine (four nitrogen atoms) results in excretion of five nitrogen atoms (two as urea and three as citrulline), so one additional nitrogen atom is eliminated
   (5) In argininosuccinate lyase deficiency, ornithine is converted to argininosuccinate, which is then excreted
      (a) In this case, six nitrogen atoms are excreted after administration of arginine (two as urea and four as argininosuccinate)
      (b) As a result, two additional nitrogen atoms are eliminated

e. Citrulline is administered in ornithine transcarbamoylase deficiency and is converted to arginine, an essential amino acid

QUESTIONS

DIRECTIONS. (Items 1–6): Each set of matching questions in this section consists of a list of several lettered options followed by several numbered items. For each numbered item, select the ONE lettered option that is most closely associated with it. Each lettered option may be selected once, more than once, or not at all. Correct answers and explanations are given at the end of the chapter.

Items 1–2

(A) Cystathionine lyase
(B) Cystathionine β-synthase
(C) Fumarylacetoacetate hydrolase
(D) Glutamate dehydrogenase
(E) Glutaminase

For each biochemical property described, select the correct enzyme.

1. A deficiency of this enzyme, which results in a disease characterized by liver, kidney, and central nervous system signs and symptoms, produces one form of tyrosinemia and tyrosinuria.
2. This enzyme is responsible for generating most of the ammonium ion in humans.

Items 3–4

(A) Glutamate
(B) Isoleucine
(C) Leucine
(D) Ornithine
(E) Tyrosine

For each metabolic property described, select the correct amino acid.

3. This amino acid is classified as a purely ketogenic and essential amino acid

4. Although this amino acid is not classified as essential in the normal population, it is required in patients with phenylketonuria

Items 5–6

(A) Alkaptonuria
(B) Homocystinuria and hypermethioninemia
(C) Hyperprolinemia
(D) Maple syrup urine disease
(E) Phenylketonuria

For each enzyme defect, select the correct metabolic disorder.

5. Results from a deficiency of branched-chain keto acid dehydrogenase activity
6. Results from a deficiency of homogentisate oxidase

DIRECTIONS. (Items 7–14): Each of the numbered items or incomplete statements in this section is followed by answers or by completions of the statement. Select the ONE lettered answer or completion that is BEST in each case.

7. The predominant nitrogen metabolite excreted in urine in humans is

   (A) ammonium ion
   (B) creatinine
   (C) urea
   (D) uric acid
   (E) xanthine

Items 8–11

For each description of a biochemical characteristic, select the correct enzyme-catalyzed reaction outlined below.

8. Which of the reactions require(s) an expenditure of two high-energy bonds?

   (A) I
   (B) II
   (C) III
   (D) I and III
   (E) II and IV

9. An inherited inability to transport the product of this reaction into the mitochondrion leads to the hyperammonemia, hyperornithinemia, and homocitrullinemia (HHH) syndrome.

   (A) I
   (B) II
   (C) III
   (D) IV
   (E) V

10. Which reaction is rate-limiting in this pathway?

    (A) I
    (B) II
    (C) III
    (D) IV
    (E) V

11. This reaction yields fumarate as one product.

    (A) I
    (B) II
    (C) III
    (D) IV
    (E) V

12. All of the following enzymes catalyze a reaction similar in mechanism to that catalyzed by pyruvate dehydrogenase EXCEPT

    (A) branched-chain keto acid dehydrogenase
    (B) glutamate dehydrogenase
    (C) α-ketoadipate dehydrogenase
    (D) α-ketobutyrate dehydrogenase
    (E) α-ketoglutarate dehydrogenase

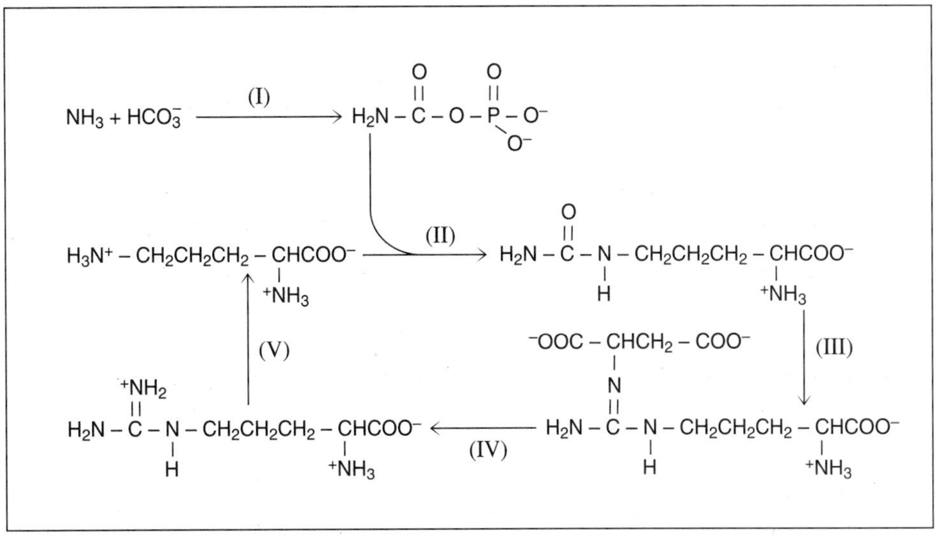

$$NH_3 + HCO_3^- \xrightarrow{(I)} H_2N-\overset{O}{\overset{\|}{C}}-O-\overset{O}{\overset{\|}{P}}(-O^-)-O^-$$

$$H_3N^+-CH_2CH_2CH_2-\underset{+NH_3}{\underset{|}{C}}HCOO^- \xrightarrow{(II)} H_2N-\overset{O}{\overset{\|}{C}}-\underset{H}{\underset{|}{N}}-CH_2CH_2CH_2-\underset{+NH_3}{\underset{|}{C}}HCOO^-$$

$$\xrightarrow{(III)} H_2N-\overset{N-CHCOO^-(CH_2-COO^-)}{\overset{\|}{C}}-\underset{H}{\underset{|}{N}}-CH_2CH_2CH_2-\underset{+NH_3}{\underset{|}{C}}HCOO^-$$

$$\xrightarrow{(IV)} H_2N-\overset{+NH_2}{\overset{\|}{C}}-\underset{H}{\underset{|}{N}}-CH_2CH_2CH_2-\underset{+NH_3}{\underset{|}{C}}HCOO^- \xrightarrow{(V)} H_3N^+-CH_2CH_2CH_2-\underset{+NH_3}{\underset{|}{C}}HCOO^-$$

13. An inborn inability to synthesize adequate methylcobalamin and adenosylcobalamin results in all of the following EXCEPT
(A) decreased methyltetrahydrofolate levels
(B) homocystinuria
(C) hypomethioninemia
(D) megaloblastic anemia
(E) methylmalonic acidemia

14. Combined lactic aciduria, propionic aciduria, and 3-methylcrotonic aciduria occur as a result of the deficiency of
(A) acetyl-CoA carboxylase
(B) holocarboxylase synthetase deficiency
(C) 3-methylcrotonyl-CoA carboxylase
(D) propionyl-CoA carboxylase
(E) pyruvate carboxylase

Items 15–18

History

The patient is a 4-day-old boy brought to the emergency room by his parents. The infant was the product of a normal pregnancy, labor, and delivery; his birth weight was 3240 g (7 lb, 2 oz) and height, 51 cm (20 in.), both normal. Between 2 and 3 days of age, he did not seek milk and had to be coaxed to feed. On the fourth day, he vomited several times and seemed to lack energy. The patient had a seizure, which prompted an immediate trip to the emergency room. The patient has two sisters (age 3 and 7 years) who are in good health. No family member has an upper respiratory infection. The patient had two maternal male cousins who died shortly after birth of unknown causes.

Physical Examination

Physical examination revealed a newborn in acute distress with a tense fontanelle and weighing 3000 g (6 lb, 10 oz). The respiratory rate was rapid and his temperature was 36.8°C (98.2°F).

Laboratory

Venous pH, 7.40 (normal, 7.35–7.45)
Blood urea nitrogen (BUN), 0.5 mg/dL (normal, 3–12 mg/dL)
The depressed BUN prompted the following studies:
Serum ammonia 320 μM (normal, <35 μM)
Alanine, 720 μM (normal, 240–410 μM)
Arginine, 44 μM (normal, 20–90 μM)
Argininosuccinate, 0 (normal, 0)
Aspartate, 44 μM (normal, 1–20 μM)
Citrulline, 14 μM (normal, 10–20 μM)
Glutamine, 1540 μM (normal, 540–960 μM)
Ornithine, 82 μM (normal, 50–150 μM)
The other amino acid levels were unremarkable
Urinalysis, abnormally high levels of orotic acid
The chest x-ray, hematocrit, white blood count and differential, serum electrolytes, and glucose were normal

15. Decreased blood urea nitrogen suggests that this disorder is
(A) a defect in urea synthesis
(B) ketothiolase deficiency
(C) maple syrup urine disease
(D) methylmalonic acidemia
(E) propionic acidemia

16. Elevated plasma ammonium levels occur in infants with a deficiency in any of the following enzymes EXCEPT
(A) argininosuccinate lyase
(B) argininosuccinate synthetase
(C) carbamoyl-phosphate synthetase I
(D) glycine cleavage complex
(E) ornithine transcarbamoylase

17. The plasma levels of amino acids in this patient could be explained by a deficiency of which one of the following enzymes?
(A) Arginase
(B) Argininosuccinate lyase
(C) Argininosuccinate synthetase
(D) Carbamoyl-phosphate synthetase I

18. The elevated urinary orotic acid in this patient can be explained by a deficiency of which one of the following enzymes?
(A) *N*-Acetylglutamate synthase
(B) Arginase
(C) Ornithine transcarbamoylase
(D) Argininosuccinate synthetase
(E) Argininosuccinate lyase

ANSWERS AND EXPLANATIONS

1. The answer is C: fumarylacetoacetate hydrolase. Type I tyrosinemia is due to a deficiency of fumarylacetoacetate hydrolase, the enzyme catalyzing the last step in the normal catabolism of phenylalanine and tyrosine. Affected infants exhibit liver, kidney, and central nervous system signs and symptoms. Type I tyrosinemia is accompanied by hypertyrosinemia. Because the phenylalanine hydroxylase reaction is unidirectional, hyperphenylalaninemia is absent. There is an accumulation of fumarylacetoacetate and nonenzymatic conversion to succinylacetoacetate and succinylacetone. The demonstration of these substances in the urine is diagnostic. There is an unexplained hypermethioninemia. Treatment with diets low in phenylalanine, tyrosine, and methionine is unsatisfactory, and most patients die within 2 years. Type II tyrosinemia is due to a deficiency of hepatic tyrosine aminotransferase. Infants with this inborn error of metabolism exhibit mental retardation, skin lesions, and corneal ul-

cers. They respond well to diets low in phenylalanine and tyrosine. *Biochemistry,* p. 232; *Nelson,* p. 310.

2. The answer is D: glutamate dehydrogenase. This enzyme catalyzes a reversible reaction that can be described as either the oxidative deamination of glutamate or the reductive amination of α-ketoglutarate. α-Ketoglutarate can receive amino groups from many other amino acids by transamination. The combination of transamination to form glutamate and the oxidative deamination of glutamate to yield ammonia and α-ketoglutarate provides a mechanism for funneling a large proportion of the α-amino groups to ammonia via glutamate and the glutamate dehydrogenase reaction. Of somewhat lesser importance is glutaminase, present in kidney and other tissues, which catalyzes a unidirectional hydrolysis of the amide bond of glutamine to yield ammonia (and glutamate). The activity of renal glutaminase is increased in long-term acidosis. The excretion of renal ammonia allows the kidney to excrete more acid than it otherwise could, since basic ammonia adds a proton and appears in the urine as the ammonium ion, NH_4^+. *Biochemistry,* p. 214.
3. The answer is C: leucine. Humans are incapable of synthesizing the carbon chain of this amino acid, so it must be acquired from the diet. In experimental conditions, humans may convert the appropriate α-keto acids to leucine and most other essential amino acids by transamination. This strategy has been used to advantage in some cases of uremia, in which a mixture of α-keto acids of essential amino acids has been provided in lieu of protein in an attempt to decrease the production of nitrogenous end products. Leucine is converted to hydroxymethylglutaryl-CoA, which is degraded to acetoacetate and acetyl-CoA; thus, this amino acid is entirely ketogenic. Isoleucine is essential, but it is both glycogenic and ketogenic. Lysine, also essential, is both ketogenic and glycogenic when given *in vivo;* the glycogenic nature is not discernible in the textbook reactions, indicating that its metabolism is incompletely understood. Ornithine and glutamate may be synthesized from other metabolic intermediates, and tyrosine (nonessential) is synthesized from phenylalanine (essential). *Biochemistry,* p. 220.
4. The answer is E: tyrosine. This amino acid is formed from the essential amino acid, phenylalanine, as catalyzed by hepatic phenylalanine hydroxylase, an enzyme utilizing tetrahydrobiopterin as reductant. This enzyme acts as a mixed function oxidase, adding one atom from O_2 to the benzene ring of phenylalanine and reducing the other atom to water. This reaction is exergonic in accordance with PRINCIPLE 8 OF BIOENERGETICS. A defect in this enzyme results in phenylketonuria. Because of a deficiency of this reaction, tyrosine becomes essential in patients with phenylketonuria, and tyrosine must be added in the diet. Infants on a normal diet (milk) with phenylketonuria have hyperphenylalaninemia ($>$ 1.2 mM) but normal plasma tyrosine concentrations (40–100 μM). *Biochemistry,* p. 230.
5. The answer is D: maple syrup urine disease. In branched-chain keto acid dehydrogenase deficiency, branched-chain keto acids occur in the urine and in the sweat, giving these fluids the odor of maple syrup. Patients with maple syrup urine disease have hyperleucinemia, hyperisoleucinemia, and hypervalinemia. This very rare but famous genetic disease results in failure to thrive, severe mental retardation, metabolic acidosis, and seizures. Keto acid dehydrogenase is made up of three components (E_1, E_2, and E_3, with the E_1 component consisting of $E_{1\alpha}$ and $E_{1\beta}$). Mutations of $E_{1\alpha}$, $E_{1\beta}$, or E_2 result in maple syrup urine disease, and some of these patients respond to thiamine treatment, a cofactor of E_1. A mutation of E_3 causes a deficiency of keto acid dehydrogenase and pyruvate dehydrogenase because these two multienzyme complexes share this subunit in common. Pyruvate dehydrogenase deficiency produces lactic acidosis. *Biochemistry,* pp. 229, 230; *Nelson,* p. 316.
6. The answer is A: alkaptonuria. One of the later steps in tyrosine catabolism is catalyzed by homogentisate dioxygenase, which converts homogentisate to maleylacetoacetate. A deficiency of homogentisate dioxygenase results in the accumulation of large amounts of homogentisate in the body and excretion in the urine. Arthritis resulting from this defect does not become apparent until midlife. The urine darkens owing to oxidation and polymerization of homogentisate at alkaline pH. Ochronosis, darkening tissue, is due to the slow accumulation of the polymeric derivative in sclera, conjunctiva, cornea, and ear cartilage. Affected patients may excrete up to 8 g of homogentisate daily, and this material can reduce alkaline copper solution (Fehling solution) to give a positive Clinitest test. This disease was among the first to be described as an "inborn error of metabolism" around the turn of the century by Archibald Garrod and thus is often mentioned on examinations because of its historical significance. *Biochemistry,* p. 230; *Nelson,* p. 310.
7. The answer is C: urea. Most (80–90%) of the nitrogen in the urine of humans (and other mammals) is in the form of urea. In conditions of acidosis, urine ammonium ion increases but it does not exceed urea nitrogen. Uric acid is a normal nitrogen excretion product in humans and in higher primates but not in most other mammals, which have an active uricase. The amount of nitrogen excreted as urate is small compared to that excreted as urea. Creatinine is also a normal nitrogen excretion product in humans, and the relatively small but constant quantity is related to muscle mass. Urinary creatinine analysis is often performed to confirm completeness of 24-hour urine collections. Xanthine is found in the urine of humans in significant amounts only when inhibitors of xanthine dehydrogenase are administered in the treatment of hyperuricemia. *Biochemistry,* p. 217.
8. The answer is D: reactions I and III. Reaction I is catalyzed by carbamoyl-phosphate synthetase I and requires two molecules of ATP. Reaction III is catalyzed by argininosuccinate synthetase, and this condensation of aspartate and citrulline is driven by the cleavage of ATP to an adenylylated intermediate and pyrophosphate, followed by the displacement of AMP. Hydrolysis of PP_i is catalyzed by a separate pyrophosphatase, and the synthesis of argininosuccinate requires two high-energy bonds. *Biochemistry,* pp. 218, 219.
9. The answer is E: V (the arginine to ornithine conversion catalyzed by arginase). A specific protein is responsible for translocating ornithine, the regenerating substrate of the urea cycle and a product of reaction V, from the cytosol into the mitochondrion. A defect in this translocase results in hyperammonemia, and unmetabolized ornithine is released into the plasma. Carbamoyl phosphate is synthesized by synthetase I, but the amount of acceptor substrate (ornithine) is low. Ornithine transcarbamoylase catalyzes the adventitious reaction of carbamoyl phosphate with lysine (the higher homolog of ornithine) to produce homocitrulline. *Nelson,* p. 327.

10. The answer is A: reaction I, catalyzed by carbamoyl-phosphate synthetase I, is rate-limiting. Although the levels of enzyme activity for every step in the cycle can increase in response to a high-protein diet, it is this initial reaction that is accelerated by an allosteric modifier, *N*-acetylglutamate, and is rate-limiting. *N*-Acetylglutamate is formed from glutamate and acetyl-CoA as catalyzed by *N*-acetylglutamate synthase; this enzymatic activity is increased when arginine levels rise. *Biochemistry,* p. 218.
11. The answer is D: reaction IV, catalyzed by argininosuccinate lyase, cleaves argininosuccinate to arginine and fumarate. The net result of reactions III and IV is to convert the carbon chain of aspartate to fumarate, while contributing one of the two nitrogen atoms required for the formation of urea. Fumarate may then be reconverted to aspartate in a sequence of reactions catalyzed by fumarase (to form malate), malate dehydrogenase (to form oxaloacetate), and aspartate aminotransferase (to form aspartate). The latter reaction involves transfer of an amino group from glutamate, so both of the nitrogen atoms in urea can be derived from glutamate intermediates. *Biochemistry,* p. 219.
12. The answer is B: glutamate dehydrogenase. Glutamate dehydrogenase catalyzes a reversible oxidative deamination. All the other enzymes catalyze irreversible oxidative decarboxylations, involving thiamine pyrophosphate, lipoate, coenzyme A, FAD, NAD^+, and a complex of three different enzyme activities. The mechanism of these oxidative decarboxylations closely resembles that used in the pyruvate dehydrogenase reaction. *Biochemistry,* pp. 214, 215, 225, 227, 233, 237.
13. The answer is A: decreased methyltetrahydrofolate levels. Several steps are required to convert cobalamin to methylcobalamin, the cofactor of the methyltransferase reaction converting homocysteine to methionine, and adenosylcobalamin, the cofactor of the methylmalonyl-CoA mutase reaction. The deficiency of methylcobalamin leads to homocystinuria and hypomethioninemia. A deficiency of cellular cobalamin leads to a megaloblastic anemia as occurs in pernicious anemia. A deficiency of adenosylcobalamin leads to methylmalonic acidemia. Decreased transfer of the methyl group from methyltetrahydrofolate leads to an increase and NOT a decrease in tissue levels of this metabolite. *Biochemistry,* p. 227.
14. The answer is B: holocarboxylase synthetase deficiency. Biotin is a cofactor of acetyl-CoA carboxylase, 3-methylcrotonyl-CoA carboxylase, propionyl-CoA carboxylase, and pyruvate carboxylase. Deficiency of holoenzyme synthetase, which catalyzes the coupling of biotin to each of these enzymes, affects the metabolism of all of the substrates. Impaired ability to metabolize pyruvate leads to lactic aciduria, and the impaired ability to metabolize propionyl-CoA leads to propionic aciduria. Impaired ability to metabolize β-methylcrotonyl-CoA leads to excretion of the corresponding acid in the urine. Affected patients have a severe metabolic acidosis and ketosis. Symptoms become apparent immediately after birth. A similar clinical picture develops in biotinidase deficiency. This disease results from the impaired ability to hydrolytically cleave the bond between biotin and the ε-amino group of lysine in biotinyl-lysine peptide degradation products of the carboxylase enzymes. Symptoms of this disorder occur at about 6 weeks of age. Both holocarboxylase synthetase and biotinidase deficiency respond to biotin treatment. *Nelson,* p. 319.
15. The answer is A: a defect in urea synthesis. Urea is formed in liver from ammonia, aspartate, and bicarbonate. A defect in any enzyme of the urea cycle results in abnormally low amounts of urea. As a result, increased ammonium ion, glutamine, aspartate, and alanine are found in the blood. Seizures, mental retardation, and other neurological abnormalities are common in a wide variety of inborn metabolic diseases including urea cycle defects. The biochemical basis for neurological symptoms is complex. Krebs cycle metabolites are depleted. Moreover, glia in brain convert glutamate to glutamine as part of normal GABA metabolism. Excess glutamine synthesis in glia can result in cerebral edema (which can be observed by CT scanning) and bulging of the anterior fontanelles (observed in this patient). Hyperammonemia (not an absence of urea nitrogen) also occurs in metabolic disorders that do not involve urea cycle enzymes including ketothiolase deficiency, propionic acidemia, methylmalonic acidemia, and transient hyperammonemia of the newborn. *Biochemistry,* pp. 218–220; *Nelson,* p. 329.
16. The answer is D: glycine cleavage complex deficiency. Deficiency of the glycine cleavage complex results in nonketotic hyperglycinemia, and none of the traditional amino acidopathies result in hyperammonemia. Clinical manifestations of nonketotic hyperglycinemia begin during the first days of life, and death ensues rapidly. Ketotic hyperglycinemia is due to the organic acidopathies such as propionic acidemia or methylmalonic acidemia. Hyperammonemia without acidosis, as observed in this patient, can be due to deficiencies of any of the enzymes of the urea cycle including carbamoyl-phosphate synthetase I, ornithine transcarbamoylase, argininosuccinate synthetase, argininosuccinate lyase, and arginase. A deficiency of *N*-acetylglutamate synthase, which catalyzes the formation of an allosteric activator of carbamoyl-phosphate synthetase I, also results in hyperammonemia based on a deficiency of urea cycle activity. (There is only one documented case of *N*-acetylglutamate synthase deficiency.) Although the incidence of a given urea cycle defect is small, the overall incidence of this group of disorders is about 1/30,000 live births. Hyperammonemia with acidosis is caused by most, if not all, organic acidemias. It is postulated that carbamoyl-phosphate synthetase I is inhibited by the organic acids, leading to hyperammonemia. *Biochemistry,* p. 220. *Nelson,* p. 323.
17. The answer is D: carbamoyl-phosphate synthetase I. A deficiency of argininosuccinate synthetase is accompanied by increased circulating citrulline, and a deficiency of argininosuccinate lyase is accompanied by an elevation of circulating argininosuccinate. A deficiency of arginase is associated with increased circulating arginine. Hyperammonemia in the absence of elevations of these amino acids can be caused by carbamoyl-phosphate synthetase I or ornithine transcarbamoylase deficiency. Carbamoyl-phosphate synthetase I is activated allosterically by *N*-acetylglutamate, and a deficiency of *N*-acetylglutamate synthase could also explain the amino acid levels observed in this patient; only one patient has ever been described with such a deficiency. *Biochemistry,* p. 219. *Nelson,* p. 327.
18. The answer is C: ornithine transcarbamoylase. Argininosuccinate synthetase deficiency is associated with an elevation of citrulline (which is not present in this patient). Argininosuccinate lyase deficiency is associated with an elevation of argininosuccinate (which is not present in this patient). Ornithine transcarbamoylase defi-

ciency results in the levels of amino acids seen in this patient and accounts for the orotic acid in the urine. Excess carbamoyl phosphate, formed in the mitochondria, is translocated to the cytosol and reacts with aspartate in the pyrimidine biosynthetic pathway, resulting in orotic acid. *N*-Acetylglutamate deficiency is associated with decreased carbamoyl phosphate production; consequently, there is no excessive substrate to drive orotic acid production and orotic aciduria. *Biochemistry,* p. 219. *Nelson,* p. 327.

REFERENCES

Behrman, R. E. *Nelson Textbook of Pediatrics,* 14th ed. W. B. Saunders Company, Philadelphia, 1992.

Roskoski, R., Jr. *Biochemistry.* Philadelphia, W. B. Saunders Company, Philadelphia, 1996.

CHAPTER FOURTEEN

NUCLEOTIDE METABOLISM

SYNOPSIS

OBJECTIVES

1. To recognize the pyrimidine and purine bases and identify their precursors.
2. To depict the reaction for synthesis of deoxyribonucleotides.
3. To outline nucleotide catabolism, urate formation, and purine salvage.
4. To explain the control of purine and pyrimidine synthesis.
5. To describe the Lesch-Nyhan syndrome and explain the action of allopurinol.
6. To describe the actions of nucleotide antimetabolites.

Objective 1: To recognize the pyrimidine and purine bases and identify their precursors.

I. Nucleoside and nucleotide structure
   A. Nucleosides consist of a purine or pyrimidine base (Fig. 14–1) attached to a sugar (ribose or 2-deoxyribose) through an energy-poor β-glycosidic bond
   B. Nucleotides are nucleoside phosphate esters, and these esters are predominantly 5′ in nature
II. Nucleotide biosynthesis
   A. Pyrimidines
      1. The atoms of the pyrimidine ring are derived from carbamoyl phosphate and aspartate (Fig. 14–2)
      2. **Carbamoyl-phosphate synthatase II,** the rate-limiting enzyme for pyrimidine synthesis in humans, catalyzes a reaction between bicarbonate, glutamine (the amino group donor), and two molecules of ATP (2 ATP → 2 ADP + P_i) to form carbamoyl phosphate
      3. **Aspartate transcarbamoylase** catalyzes a reaction between carbamoyl phosphate and aspartate to produce carbamoylaspartate and phosphate
      4. Under the aegis of **dihydroorotase,** the adduct cyclizes to form dihydroorotate, and this is oxidized to form orotate as catalyzed by **dihydroorotate dehydrogenase,** an enzyme found in the inner mitochondrial membrane
      5. Orotate reacts with phosphoribosylpyrophosphate (PRPP) to form orotidine monophosphate, which undergoes an exergonic decarboxylation catalyzed by **OMP decarboxylase,** forming uridine monophosphate
      6. All but one of the enzymes of the pyrimidine pathway occur in the cytosol
         a. The first three enzymes of the pyrimidine pathway occur in the same cytosolic protein as a trifunctional protein, or polyprotein
         b. The initial letters of each enzyme activity of this trifunctional protein form the acronym CAD (*c*arbamoyl-phosphate synthetase II, *a*spartate transcarbamoylase, and *d*ihydroorotase), and the protein is called the CAD complex
         c. The dehydrogenase, a protein with one activity, is an integral inner mitochondrial membrane protein
            (1) The enzyme can interact with cytosolic dihydroorotate
            (2) This enzyme is a flavoprotein that transfers its electrons to coenzyme Q
         d. The last two enzymes of the pathway (orotate phosphoribosyltransferase and OMP decarboxylase) occur as a bifunctional protein in the cytosol called UMP synthase
      7. UTP reacts with glutamine in an ATP-dependent reaction to form cytidine triphosphate
      8. Orotic aciduria is caused by a deficiency of the UMP synthase complex
   B. Purines
      1. The source of the atoms of the purine ring is shown in Figure 14–3
      2. *The first and committed step in purine biosynthesis is catalyzed by glutamine-PRPP amidotransferase*
         a. PRPP activates this enzyme allosterically and serves as a substrate
         b. AMP and GMP, synthesized from IMP, inhibit the amidotransferase reaction
         c. The enzyme is also inhibited by derivatives of allopurinol, a drug used in the treatment of gout
      3. IMP is converted to AMP and GMP
         a. The addition of the 6-amino group to form AMP involves a two-step process
            (1) Aspartate serves as the source of the amino group attached to position 6 of the purine ring of AMP in a reaction that requires GTP, which is cleaved to form GDP and P_i
            (2) Fumarate is cleaved from the substrate, yielding AMP

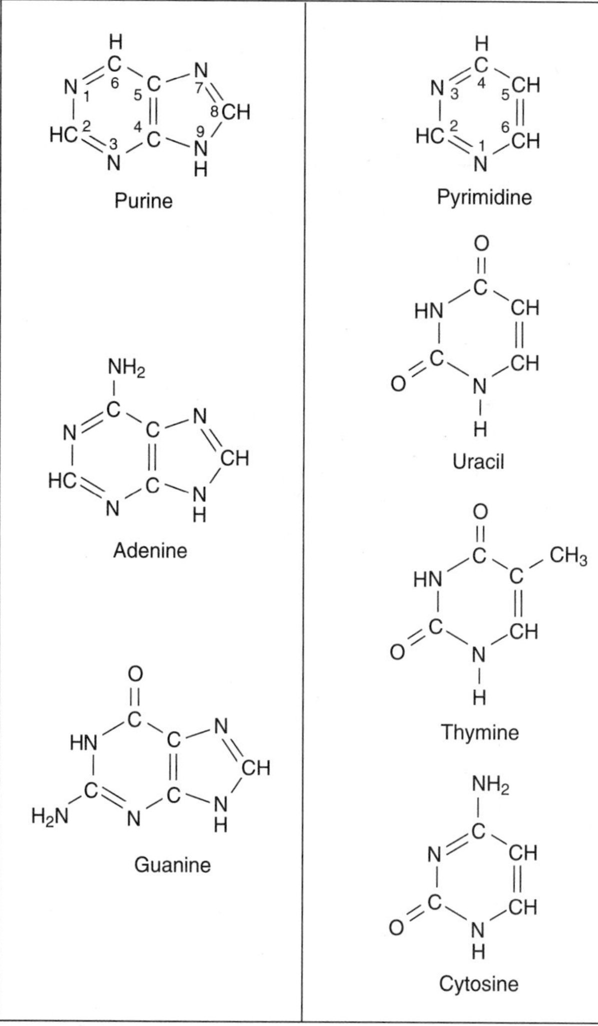

FIGURE 14-1. Structures of the purine and pyrimidine bases.

b. IMP is first oxidized to form xanthosine 5′-monophosphate (XMP)
   (1) XMP reacts with glutamine in an ATP-dependent reaction
   (2) GMP forms, and ATP yields AMP and PP_i

Objective 2: To depict the reaction for synthesis of deoxyribonucleotides.

III. Ribonucleotide reductase and deoxyribonucleotide synthesis
   A. **Ribonucleotide reductase** catalyzes a unidirectional reaction
      1. The enzyme catalyzes a reaction between various ribonucleoside diphosphates and reduced thioredoxin, yielding 2′-deoxyribonucleotide, oxidized thioredoxin, and water
      2. The enzyme is regulated allosterically by a variety of nucleotides, and dATP serves as an allosteric inhibitor for the reduction of all nucleoside diphosphates

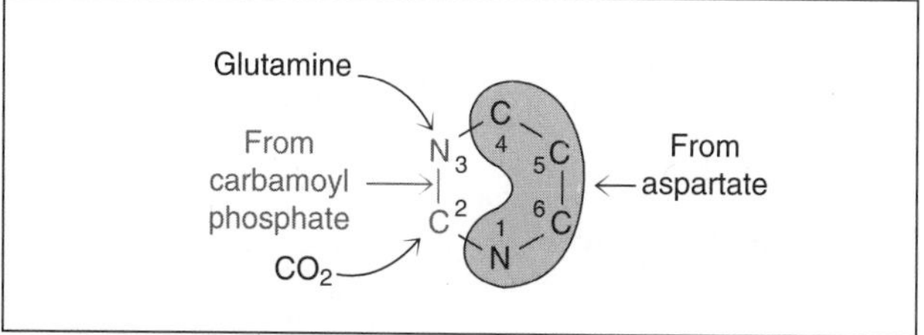

FIGURE 14-2. Sources of the atoms of the pyrimidine ring.

   B. **Thioredoxin reductase** restores thioredoxin to its reduced state using NADPH as reductant

IV. Thymidylate synthesis and the tetrahydrofolate cycle
   A. dUDP, formed via the ribonucleotide reductase reaction, is converted to dUTP, which is hydrolyzed to dUMP
   B. **Thymidylate synthase** catalyzes a reaction between dUMP and methylenetetrahydrofolate to yield dTMP (thymidylate) and dihydrofolate
      1. Methylene-THF acts as both a methyl donor and reductant
      2. The main source of one-carbon groups in metabolism is from the amino acid serine
      3. To participate in further reactions, DHF must be converted to tetrahydrofolate as catalyzed by **dihydrofolate reductase**

V. Antimetabolites and cancer chemotherapy
   A. Fluorouracil and thymidylate synthase
      1. Fluorouracil is converted to fluoro-2′-deoxyuridylate, a structural analogue of dUMP, which binds to the enzyme and undergoes a partial reaction
         a. Midway through the reaction, fluorodeoxyuridylate forms a covalent adduct that bridges thymidylate synthase and N^5,N^{10}-methylene-THF
         b. This process, which requires the enzyme as a catalytic participant, is an example of suicide inhibition
      2. The covalent attachment of fluorodeoxyuridylate to thymidylate synthase produces irreversible inhibition
   B. Methotrexate and dihydrofolate reductase
      1. Methotrexate is a potent competitive inhibitor of dihydrofolate reductase with respect to dihydrofolate as substrate
      2. Because of the reduction of the concentration of tetrahydrofolate resulting from methotrexate treatment, the synthesis of thymidylate and purines is inhibited

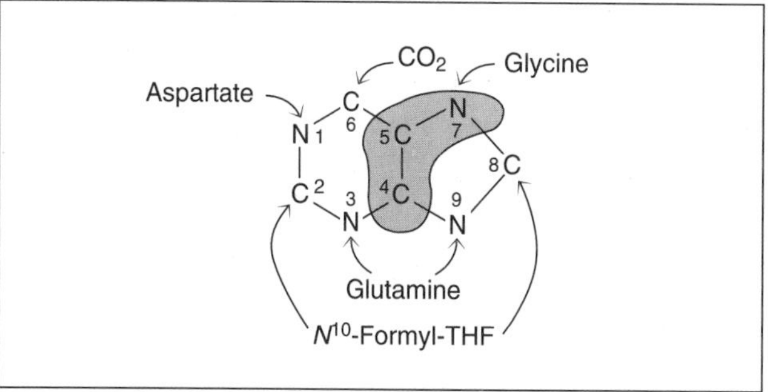

FIGURE 14-3. Sources of atoms of the purine ring.

Objective 3: To outline nucleotide catabolism, urate formation, and purine salvage.

VI. Nucleotide catabolism
- A. Pyrimidines
  1. Uracil is catabolized in a series of reactions to acetyl-CoA
  2. Thymine is catabolized in a series of reactions to propionyl-CoA
- B. Purines
  1. **Xanthine dehydrogenase** catalyzes the conversion of hypoxanthine to xanthine and xanthine to uric acid according to the following equations:

$$\text{Hypoxanthine} + NAD^+ + H_2O \rightarrow \text{Xanthine} + NADH + H^+ \quad (14.1)$$

$$\text{Xanthine} + NAD^+ + H_2O \rightarrow \text{Urate} + NADH + H^+ \quad (14.2)$$

  2. Xanthine dehydrogenase can be converted to xanthine oxidase by adventitious oxidation reactions; such reactions may occur following vascular occlusion
  3. Xanthine oxidase activity results in the production of hydrogen peroxide
- C. Disorders of purine catabolism
  1. **Adenosine deaminase** deficiency produces severe combined immunodeficiency disease (SCID) as a result of aberrant nucleotide metabolism affecting the immune system
  2. **Purine nucleoside phosphorylase** deficiency also produces an immunodeficiency

VII. Salvage pathways for purine nucleotide synthesis
- A. A salvage pathway is a process whereby a metabolite is reutilized for the biosynthesis of a compound from which the metabolite was derived
- B. **Adenine phosphoribosyltransferase** catalyzes the reaction between adenine and PRPP to form AMP and pyrophosphate
- C. **Hypoxanthine-guanine phosphoribosyltransferase** (HGPRT) catalyzes an analogous reaction

Objective 4: To explain the control of purine and pyrimidine synthesis.

VIII. Regulation of nucleotide synthesis
- A. Purines
  1. The committed and chief regulatory step in the pathway for purine biosynthesis *de novo* is catalyzed by glutamine PRPP amidotransferase
     - a. This reaction involves the conversion of PRPP to phosphoribosylamine (Fig. 14–4)
     - b. This enzyme is inhibited by IMP, AMP, GMP, and allopurinol ribonucleotide
  2. PRPP synthetase plays a secondary role in the regulation of purine nucleotide biosynthesis
     - a. PRPP synthetase is inhibited by purine nucleotides
     - b. PRPP, moreover, serves as a feed-forward activator of the PRPP amidotransferase reaction

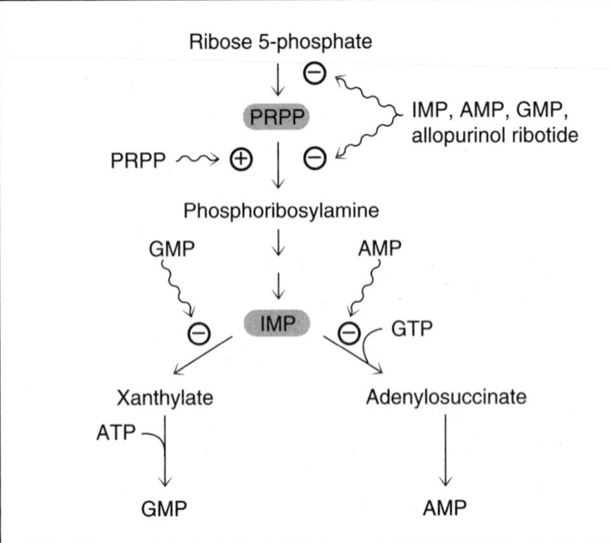

FIGURE 14–4. Regulation of purine biosynthesis.

  3. GMP inhibits its synthesis from IMP, and AMP inhibits its synthesis from IMP in secondary regulatory steps
- B. Pyrimidines
  1. The primary regulatory step in pyrimidine synthesis in humans is the formation of carbamoyl phosphate as catalyzed by carbamoyl-phosphate synthetase II
  2. Carbamoyl-phosphate synthetase II is inhibited by UDP and UTP; however, this enzyme is activated by ATP
  3. The primary regulatory step of pyrimidine biosynthesis in *Escherichia coli* and some other bacteria is catalyzed by aspartate transcarbamoylase (ATCase), a famous allosteric enzyme that is inhibited by CTP

Objective 5: To describe the Lesch-Nyhan syndrome and explain the action of allopurinol.

IX. Purine metabolism in the Lesch-Nyhan syndrome
- A. *The syndrome is caused by an absence of hypoxanthine-guanine phosphoribosyltransferase (HGPRT) activity*
- B. Three mechanisms account for the hyperuricemia of Lesch-Nyhan syndrome
  1. The inability to salvage hypoxanthine and guanine permits increased conversion of hypoxanthine and guanine to urate
  2. A deficiency in the salvage pathway leads to a decrease in IMP and GMP concentrations, which removes normal feedback inhibitors of the *de novo* pathway at the level of PRPP amidotransferase and PRPP synthetase
  3. PRPP's utilization decreases and its concentration increases because less is used by the salvage pathway; the elevation of PRPP and the decline in feedback inhibitors stimulates the PRPP amidotransferase reaction and leads to a 200-fold

increase in purine synthesis by the *de novo* pathway

X. Gout and the action of allopurinol
  A. Gout is the result of excess purine production
  B. The therapeutic effect of allopurinol results from three mechanisms
    1. Allopurinol is oxidized to alloxanthine by xanthine dehydrogenase, and allopurinol and alloxanthine are inhibitors of xanthine dehydrogenase
      a. Xanthine dehydrogenase inhibition decreases urate formation, and hypoxanthine and xanthine accumulate
      b. Allopurinol and alloxanthine are also substrates for HGPRT
      c. The products of the reaction are the corresponding ribonucleotides
    2. The production of allopurinol and alloxanthine ribonucleotides consumes and thereby decreases the concentration of PRPP, an activator of glutamine PRPP amidotransferase
    3. Allopurinol ribonucleotide and alloxanthine ribonucleotide are feedback inhibitors of PRPP amidotransferase

Objective 6: To describe the actions of nucleotide antimetabolites.

XI. Selected antimetabolites and nucleotide metabolism
  A. **Fluorouracil** (FU) interferes with thymidylate synthesis and is incorporated into RNA to produce dysfunctional RNA
  B. **Mercaptopurine** must first be converted to 6-thioinosine 5′-monophosphate, and this derivative, a potent inhibitor of purine nucleotide biosynthesis, inhibits adenylosuccinate synthetase and IMP dehydrogenase
  C. **Sulfonamide antibiotics** are used in the treatment of various infectious diseases
    1. These agents are structural analogues of *p*-aminobenzoate, a component of folate
    2. Sulfonamides inhibit competitively the incorporation of *p*-aminobenzoate into folate
    3. This family of antibiotics is effective in bacteria that synthesize their own folate; these bacteria are unable to transport folate or its analogues into their cells
  D. **Trimethoprim** is an antibiotic that inhibits dihydrofolate reductase in sensitive bacteria

QUESTIONS

DIRECTIONS. (Items 1–4): Each set of matching questions in this section consists of a list of several lettered options followed by several numbered items. For each numbered item, select the ONE lettered option that is most closely associated with it. Each lettered option may be selected once, more than once, or not at all. Correct answers and explanations are given at the end of the chapter.

Items 1–2

(A) Carbamoyl phosphate
(B) Inosine monophosphate
(C) Orotidine monophosphate
(D) 5-Phosphoribosyl-1-pyrophosphate (PRPP)
(E) 5-Phosphoribosylamine

For the given biochemical property, select the appropriate metabolite

1. The first pyrimidine nucleotide formed in *de novo* synthesis
2. The product formed at the major regulatory step in *de novo* purine nucleotide synthesis

Items 3–4

(A) Adenylosuccinate → adenosine monophosphate
(B) Inosine monophosphate → adenylosuccinate
(C) Inosine monophosphate → xanthosine monophosphate
(D) Xanthosine monophosphate → guanosine monophosphate
(E) Xanthine → urate

For each biochemical property given, select the correct biochemical reaction

3. Reaction inhibited by AMP and requiring GTP
4. Reaction requiring ATP

DIRECTIONS. (Items 5–18): Each of the numbered items or incomplete statements in this section is followed by answers or by completions of the statement. Select the ONE lettered answer or completion that is BEST in each case.

5. Which of the following is a true statement regarding cytosolic carbamoyl-phosphate synthetase II in humans?
   (A) It is one of three activities residing in a single polypeptide called the CAD complex
   (B) It is allosterically activated by *N*-acetylglutamate
   (C) It requires free ammonium ion as nitrogen donor
   (D) It catalyzes the rate-limiting reaction in *de novo* purine nucleotide synthesis
   (E) It cleaves ATP to AMP and PP_i during the reaction sequence

6. 5-Phosphoribosyl-1-pyrophosphate (PRPP) is an intermediate in all of the following pathways EXCEPT
   (A) *de novo* purine nucleotide synthesis
   (B) *de novo* pyrimidine nucleotide synthesis
   (C) the pentose phosphate pathway
   (D) purine salvage pathways
   (E) NAD^+ synthesis

7. A deficiency of orotate phosphoribosyltransferase can be associated with each of the following abnormalities EXCEPT

   (A) orotic aciduria
   (B) decreased activity of carbamoyl-phosphate synthetase II
   (C) a deficiency of orotidine 5′-phosphate decarboxylase
   (D) a megaloblastic anemia
   (E) decreased conversion of tryptophan to NAD^+

8. Treatment of leukemias and lymphomas with methotrexate can lead to decreased incorporation of one-carbon units from tetrahydrofolate derivatives into purines at which position(s) shown in the figure below?

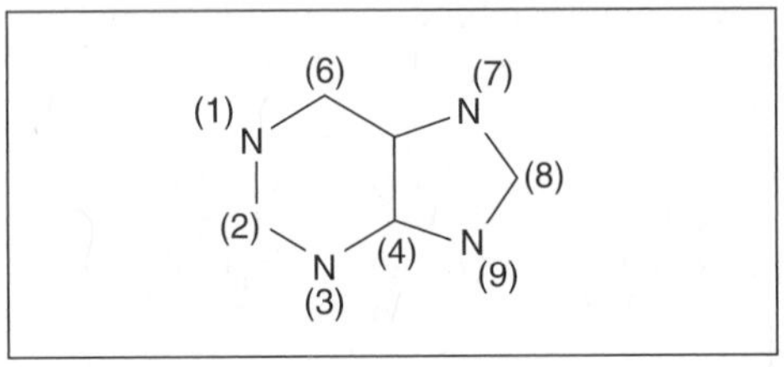

(6) (7)
(1) N N
(8)
(2) (4) N
N (9)
(3)

   (A) 2, 4, and 5
   (B) 3, 6, and 9
   (C) 4, 5, and 6
   (D) 2 and 8
   (E) 6 only

9. Which of the following is a true statement regarding ribonucleotide reductase, the activity of which is high in rapidly dividing tumor cells?

   (A) It converts the ribose moiety of a nucleotide to a 2′-deoxyribose moiety
   (B) It is allosterically activated by dATP
   (C) It acts exclusively on nucleoside monophosphates
   (D) It converts ribonucleotides to ribonucleosides
   (E) It converts oxidized thioredoxin to reduced thioredoxin

10. Thymidylate synthase, an enzyme whose activity is high in rapidly dividing tumor cells, performs all of the following functions EXCEPT

   (A) transferring a one-carbon group from N^5,N^{10}-methylene tetrahydrofolate to C^5 of dUMP
   (B) using the tetrahydrofolate one-carbon carrier as a reductant
   (C) undergoing inhibition by a derivative of 5-fluorouracil
   (D) providing pyrimidine nucleotides for mRNA synthesis

11. Methotrexate inhibits nucleotide synthesis via inhibition of which one of the following enzymes?

   (A) Thymidylate synthase
   (B) PRPP amidotransferase
   (C) Dihydrofolate reductase
   (D) Aspartate transcarbamoylase
   (E) Argininosuccinate synthetase

12. An inborn error of human metabolism that results in the inability to catalyze the final step in purine catabolism is caused by a deficiency of which one of the following enzymes?

   (A) Inosine triphosphatase (ITPase)
   (B) Pyrimidine 5′-nucleotidase
   (C) Purine nucleoside phosphorylase
   (D) Uricase
   (E) Xanthine dehydrogenase

13. Severe combined immunodeficiency disease (SCID) is a result of a genetic deficiency of which of the following enzyme activities?

   (A) Adenine phosphoribosyltransferase
   (B) Adenosine deaminase
   (C) Adenylate deaminase
   (D) Thymidine kinase
   (E) Hypoxanthine/guanine phosphoribosyl transferase

14. All of the following are true statements regarding Lesch-Nyhan syndrome EXCEPT

   (A) It is accompanied by a decrease in glutamine PRPP amidotransferase activity
   (B) It is a result of a genetic deficiency in a purine salvage pathway
   (C) It is a cause of hyperuricemia and gout
   (D) It is a cause of aggressive and self-mutilative behavior
   (E) It is associated with a lack of HGPRT activity

Items 15–18

History

A 53-year-old male realtor presents with a chief complaint of pain in the big toe of his left foot. The patient says that the pain began about 1:00 AM and became so severe that he could not bear to have the bed sheet touch his toe. He spent the previous day golfing, concluded by several cocktails, a large meal, and wine. The patient reports that several distant family members (both men and women) have arthritis. Several previous episodes of joint pain dissipated after a few hours, but the current pain has lasted more than 12 hours and gives no indication of subsiding. The patient denies taking medications or having severe abdominal pain, hematuria, hypertension, neoplastic disease, or radiation therapy.

Physical Examination

Physical examination reveals a hot, red, and sensitive metatarsophalangeal joint on the large toe on his left foot. Inspection of the external ears discloses multiple small tophi. His temperature is 38.4 °C (101.1 °F); pulse, 76/min; respiratory rate, 16/min; and blood pressure, 122/80 mm Hg.

Laboratory

Blood urea nitrogen (BUN), 16 mg/dL (normal, 7–18 mg/dL)
Creatinine, 0.8 mg/dL (normal, 0.7–1.3 mg/dL)
Uric acid, 10.2 mg/dL (normal, 3.5–7.2 mg/dL)
γ-Glutamyl transpeptidase, 40 U/L (normal ♂, 9–50 U/L)

Aspartate aminotransferase (AST, SGOT), 16 U/L (normal, 10–30 U/L)
Alkaline phosphatase, 60 U/L (normal ♂, 50–130 U/L)
Acid phosphatase, 8 U/dL (normal, 2.5–11.5 U/L)
Calcium, 9.2 mg/dL (normal, 8.4–10.2 mg/dL)
Phosphate, 4.0 mg/dL (normal, 2.7–4.5 mg/dL)
Oxalate, 140 μg/dL, normal, 100–240 μg/dL)
Glucose, 82 mg/dL (normal, 70–105 mg/dL)
Total cholesterol, 194 mg/dL; recommended, <200 mg/dL)

The red cell count, hematocrit, hemoglobin, white blood count, differential, and platelet counts were normal. Urinalysis revealed a specific gravity of 1.016; pH, 5.8, negative for protein, white blood cells, red blood cells, or crystals. The patient was treated with colchicine, and this provided substantial relief within 2 hours. Allopurinol was prescribed on an outpatient basis. A 24-hour urine sample, obtained after 3 days on a purine-restricted diet, contained 1.1 g of uric acid (normal, <0.6 g/d), and a creatinine clearance was 110 mL/min/1.73 m² (normal, 90–140).

15. The provisional diagnosis in this patient is
    (A) gout secondary to diuretic medication
    (B) gout secondary to renal disease
    (C) osteoarthritis
    (D) primary gout

16. Allopurinol is a both a substrate and inhibitor of
    (A) dihydrofolate reductase
    (B) glutamine PRPP amidotransferase
    (C) ribonucleotide reductase
    (D) thymidylate synthase
    (E) xanthine dehydrogenase

17. Allopurinol and alloxanthine are substrates for
    (A) adenine phosphoribosyltransferase
    (B) adenosine deaminase
    (C) AMP deaminase
    (D) glutamine PRPP amidotransferase
    (E) hypoxanthine/guanine phosphoribosyltransferase

18. Following treatment with allopurinol, which of the following is likely to be observed?
    (A) Decreased amounts of hypoxanthine and xanthine are excreted in the urine
    (B) Increased amounts of urate are excreted in the urine
    (C) The concentration of cellular PRPP is decreased because of the conversion of allopurinol and alloxanthine to their respective ribonucleotides
    (D) Decreased PRPP concentration results in increased activity of glutamine PRPP amidotransferase
    (E) Decreased conversion of hypoxanthine to IMP occurs because of decreased HGPRT activity

ANSWERS AND EXPLANATIONS

1. The answer is C: orotidine monophosphate is the first pyrimidine nucleotide formed in *de novo* synthesis. The first pyrimidine formed, however, is orotate, which adds phosphoribose and is decarboxylated in subsequent reactions. *Biochemistry,* p. 248.
2. The answer is E: 5-phosphoribosylamine is formed during the major regulatory step in *de novo* purine nucleotide synthesis. The reaction is catalyzed by glutamine PRPP amidotransferase, which replaces the pyrophosphate at C^1 of PRPP with the amide nitrogen of glutamine. In the process, the configuration at C^1 changes from α to β. The enzyme is subject to feedback inhibition by the end products of the pathway, AMP, GMP, and IMP. *Biochemistry,* pp. 253, 263.
3. The answer is B: the conversion of inosine monophosphate to adenylosuccinate requires GTP and is inhibited by AMP, the product formed in the following step. This is another example of feedback inhibition and represents a secondary level of regulation of purine nucleotide synthesis. *Biochemistry,* pp. 254, 263.
4. The answer is D: the conversion of xanthosine monophosphate to guanosine monophosphate involves the replacement of an oxygen atom attached at position 2 on the purine ring with the amide nitrogen of glutamine, and the process is driven by cleavage of ATP to AMP and PP_i, with subsequent cleavage of pyrophosphate to provide an additional energy differential between reactants and products. Note that synthesis of AMP from IMP requires GTP, and synthesis of GMP from IMP requires ATP, another subtle but effective mode of regulatory control ensuring the appropriate quantities of each purine nucleotide. *Biochemistry,* p. 254.
5. The answer is A: human *c*arbamoyl-phosphate synthetase II is one of three enzyme activities in the polyprotein CAD complex, the other two being *a*spartate transcarbamoylase and *d*ihydroorotase. Formation of carbamoyl phosphate is the rate-limiting step in *de novo* pyrimidine nucleotide synthesis in animals. In contrast to the mitochondrial carbamoyl-phosphate synthetase I used in the urea cycle, the cytosolic enzyme uses glutamine, not ammonium ion, as nitrogen donor, and the activity of the cytosolic enzyme is unaffected by *N*-acetylglutamate, an allosteric activator of the mitochondrial urea-cycle enzyme. Both the mitochondrial and the cytosolic reactions involve cleavage of two molecules of ATP to ADP (not AMP), and PP_i is not formed in either reaction. *Biochemistry,* p. 249.
6. The answer is C: the pentose phosphate pathway. Although PRPP is formed from ribose 5-phosphate, a product of the pentose phosphate pathway, PRPP is NOT an intermediate in the pathway. PRPP is used as an activated donor of the ribose 5-phosphate group in *de novo* purine and pyrimidine nucleotide synthesis, in the purine salvage reactions catalyzed by APRT and HGPRT, and in NAD^+ synthesis from quinolinate, nicotinate, or nicotinamide. *Biochemistry,* pp. 104, 235, 262, 263.
7. The answer is B: carbamoyl-phosphate synthetase II activity is increased, NOT decreased, in orotate phosphoribosyltransferase deficiency. Failure to form UMP prevents formation of UDP and UTP, which are allosteric inhibitors of carbamoyl-phosphate synthetase II. Orotate phosphoribosyltransferase is the first of two enzymatic activities carried by the dual-function protein known as UMP synthase. The second activity is orotidine 5′-phos-

phate decarboxylase, and since both activities are on the same polypeptide, a deficiency of one is usually associated with a deficiency of the other. The failure to add a phosphoribosyl group to orotate leads to a buildup of orotate in the blood and excretion in the urine. Lack of available pyrimidine nucleotides decreases synthesis of rapidly proliferating blood cells in the bone marrow and results in a megaloblastic anemia. UMP synthase deficiency decreases formation of NAD^+ from tryptophan, since these activities are also used in conversion of quinolinate to nicotinate ribonucleotide, a two-step reaction sequence in the tryptophan to NAD^+ pathway. *Biochemistry,* pp. 235, 263.

8. The answer is D: the carbon atoms at positions 2 and 8 are contributed by N^{10}-formyl tetrahydrofolate. Atoms 4, 5, and 7 are derived from glycine, atoms 3 and 9 from the amide nitrogen of glutamine, atom 6 from CO_2, and atom 1 from the α-amino group of aspartate. *Biochemistry,* p. 251.
9. The answer is A: ribonucleotide reductase converts the ribose moiety of a nucleotide to a 2′-deoxyribose moiety. The enzyme is subject to complicated allosteric regulation, but the overall activity is inhibited, not activated, by dATP. Nucleoside *diphosphates* are the substrates for the reaction that involves removal of the oxygen at C^2 of the ribose, reduction of the oxygen to water using hydrogen atoms derived from cysteinyl sulfhydryl groups of thioredoxin, with consequent formation of the oxidized thioredoxin containing a disulfide bond. Ribonucleosides are not involved in the reaction. *Biochemistry,* pp. 254–255.
10. The answer is D: provision of pyrimidine nucleotides for mRNA synthesis is NOT a function of thymidylate synthase. Since the thymine nucleotides are found almost exclusively in DNA, thymidylate synthase is used to form nucleotides for DNA, not RNA, synthesis. Thymidylate synthase converts dUMP to dTMP by addition of a methyl group to position five of the deoxyuridylate pyrimidine ring. N^5,N^{10}-Methylene tetrahydrofolate contributes both a methylene group and reducing equivalents in the form of hydrogen atoms from positions 5 and 6 of the pterin ring, resulting in the formation of dihydrofolate, which must then be reduced to regenerate the active tetrahydrofolate. The synthase is inhibited by 2′-deoxy-5-fluorouridine monophosphate, a derivative of 5-fluorouracil. *Biochemistry,* pp. 255–256, 306.
11. The answer is C: dihydrofolate reductase. The methotrexate structure is very similar to that of folate, one of the substrates of dihydrofolate reductase, which converts folate to dihydrofolate and then dihydrofolate to tetrahydrofolate. Tetrahydrofolate is the active form for the one-carbon carrier used in synthesis of thymidylate and in *de novo* purine synthesis. Any inhibition of the regeneration of tetrahydrofolate from the dihydrofolate formed in the thymidylate synthase reaction, or blockage in formation of tetrahydrofolate from dietary folate, will result in a failure to form sufficient purines and pyrimidines for cell proliferation. Although all cells must maintain an inventory of tetrahydrofolate to support normal function, rapidly proliferating cells require ample deoxyribonucleotides for DNA synthesis, and these cells thus convert substantial tetrahydrofolate into dihydrofolate in the thymidylate synthase reaction. Rapidly proliferating cells are most sensitive to the actions of methotrexate. Thymidylate synthase is not directly inhibited by methotrexate, even though it is one of the enzymes using a tetrahydrofolate derivative. PRPP amidotransferase, aspartate transcarbamoylase, and argininosuccinate synthetase are all sites of regulatory control, but none are inhibited by methotrexate. *Biochemistry,* p. 257.
12. The answer is E: xanthine dehydrogenase. This enzyme catalyzes the oxidation of xanthine to uric acid (and the oxidation of hypoxanthine to xanthine), and a deficiency of this enzyme leads to xanthinuria and hypouricemia. Xanthine is more soluble than urate, but urinary calculi composed of nearly pure xanthine can result from this uncommon metabolic defect. The enzyme uses NAD^+ as oxidant in normal tissues but is converted in hypoxic tissues to a slightly altered form that utilizes molecular oxygen as oxidant and produces hydrogen peroxide. The altered enzyme is given the name xanthine oxidase, and this is the name often used (incorrectly) in textbook discussions of purine catabolism. In most animals, uric acid is further degraded by the enzyme uricase, but humans lack this enzyme. Purine nucleoside phosphorylase is used in purine degradation but does not catalyze the final step. Pyrimidine 5′-nucleotidase is used in the degradation of pyrimidines, not purines. A deficiency of this enzyme causes a hemolytic anemia. ITPase deficiency results in the accumulation of ITP in red blood cells; however, this deficiency has no known clinical consequences. *Biochemistry,* pp. 259, 261.
13. The answer is B: adenosine deaminase. Deficiency in adenosine deaminase affects both B and T cells of the immune system, probably because of a buildup of dATP with resultant inhibition of ribonucleotide reductase. The level of adenine *ribo*nucleotides does not increase significantly, because an alternative pathway exists for their catabolism. AMP (but *not* dAMP) is converted by adenylate deaminase to inosine monophosphate, which is then catabolized normally. Deficiency of purine nucleoside phosphorylase also results in severe combined immunodeficiency disease (SCID), affecting primarily T cells, although the mechanism is more obscure. Defects in adenine phosphoribosyltransferase produce urinary calculi composed of 2,8-dihydroxyadenine, a metabolite resulting from aberrant adenine metabolism. Defects in adenylate deaminase, which lead to elevated ATP levels, have been reported, but they do not lead to any disease state. A deficiency of thymidine kinase has not been described. Deficiency of hypoxanthine/guanine phosphoribosyl transferase results in Lesch-Nyhan syndrome, the inborn error of metabolism that produces hyperuricemia and can produce a megaloblastic anemia but not SCID. Another inborn error of metabolism is due to a 100-fold increase of adenosine deaminase activity in red blood cells; enzyme activity in other cells is normal. High enzyme levels deplete red cell adenine nucleotides and ATP and produce a hemolytic anemia. The mechanism for the increased production of enzyme is an enigma. *Biochemistry,* pp. 259–260.
14. The answer is A: glutamine PRPP amidotransferase activity is increased, NOT decreased, in Lesch-Nyhan syndrome. Lesch-Nyhan syndrome results from a deficiency of hypoxanthine/guanine phosphoribosyltransferase, the salvage enzyme used to regenerate IMP and GMP from hypoxanthine and guanine, respectively. Lack of this enzyme results in lowered levels of IMP and GMP, two inhibitors of *de novo* purine nucleotide synthesis, and in elevated levels of PRPP, an activator of *de novo* purine nucleotide synthesis. The PRPP levels are thought to rise because less is being utilized in the salvage pathways. A combination of more activator and less inhibitor allows purine synthesis to run unchecked, producing very large amounts of purines and therefore uric acid. Hyperuricemia and gout follow. The marked aggressive-

ness and self-mutilative behavior is characteristic of the disease but is difficult to explain biochemically. It has been suggested that the brain is highly dependent on the salvage pathways, since the *de novo* pathway is relatively inactive in this tissue. *Biochemistry,* pp. 263–264.

15. The answer is D: primary gout. Primary gout results from the overproduction or underexcretion of uric acid for periods of 20–30 years. The cause of 99% of the cases of primary gout is unknown. Gout is more common in men (95% of cases) and becomes manifest during midlife. In this patient, urea nitrogen, creatinine, and creatinine clearance, which are tests of renal function, are normal, thereby indicating that hyperuricemia is not secondary to renal disease. Moreover, nephropathy is a common complication of gout but does not yet appear to be a problem in this patient. Urolithiasis (kidney stones) is a common complication of primary and secondary gout; lack of characteristic abdominal pain or hematuria indicate that this has not been a complication in this patient. The patient is not hypertensive and denied taking medication for hypertension. Diuretics, which can be used in the treatment of hypertension, can produce hyperuricemia and lead to, or precipitate, gout. Myeloproliferative disorders (myeloma, leukemia) that result in increased tissue turnover can also lead to gout, but there is no indication that this patient has this problem. Osteoarthritis, which is common in both men and women and increases with age, is a more chronic condition that does not lead to an acute (sudden onset) inflammatory condition as observed in this patient. Most mammals degrade urate to allantoin and avoid the effects of hyperuricemia and gout. Is there any advantage to having near-saturating concentrations of urate in body fluids? Urate is a reductant, and it may protect against the harmful effects of oxidizing agents and supplement the postulated antioxidant actions of ascorbate, β-carotene, and vitamin E. *Biochemistry,* p. 264; *Cecil,* p. 1107.
16. The answer is E: xanthine dehydrogenase. Xanthine dehydrogenase catalyzes the conversion of hypoxanthine to xanthine and xanthine to uric acid. Allopurinol, which resembles hypoxanthine, is a competitive inhibitor at low concentrations (but a noncompetitive inhibitor at high concentrations). Allopurinol is also a substrate of xanthine dehydrogenase and is converted to alloxanthine, an analogue of xanthine. Allopurinol does not mimic dihydrofolate, phosphoribosylpyrophosphate, ribonucleoside diphosphates, or thymidylate and is not an inhibitor of dihydrofolate reductase, PRPP amidotransferase, ribonucleotide reductase, or thymidylate synthase. *Biochemistry,* pp. 264, 265.
17. The answer is E: hypoxanthine/guanine phosphoribosyltransferase. This enzyme catalyzes the reaction of allopurinol and alloxanthine with PRPP to form allopurinol ribonucleotide and alloxanthine ribonucleotide, respectively. Allopurinol and alloxanthine, which contain an oxygen bound to the 6 position of the purine-like ring, are not recognized by enzymes that react with compounds that contain the adenine ring such as adenosine deaminase, AMP deaminase, or adenine phosphoribosyltransferase. *Biochemistry,* pp. 264, 265.
18. The answer is C: the concentration of PRPP is decreased because of the conversion of allopurinol and alloxanthine to ribonucleotides. PRPP is one of the substrates for the hypoxanthine/guanine phosphoribosyl transferase (HGPRT) reaction. As a result of the reaction of allopurinol and alloxanthine with PRPP, the concentration of PRPP is decreased. This removes a substrate and activator of the PRPP amidotransferase reactions and decreases the rate of purine biosynthesis. Following the administration of allopurinol and its inhibition of xanthine dehydrogenase, there is increased hypoxanthine and xanthine but decreased urate excretion in the urine. Elevation of cellular hypoxanthine levels leads to increased conversion to IMP via the salvage pathway. *Biochemistry,* p. 264.

REFERENCES

Roskoski, R., Jr. *Biochemistry.* Philadelphia, W. B. Saunders Company, 1996.

Wyngaarden, J. B., L. H. Smith, Jr., and J. C. Bennett (eds.). *Cecil Textbook of Medicine,* 19th ed. Philadelphia, W. B. Saunders Company, 1992.

CHAPTER FIFTEEN

DNA BIOSYNTHESIS AND REPLICATION

SYNOPSIS

OBJECTIVES

1. To describe DNA structure and function.
2. To describe DNA replication.
3. To describe DNA repair
4. To describe recombinant DNA technology and the diagnosis of genetic diseases.

Objective 1: To explain how the structure of DNA relates to the functioning of the gene.

I. Biological information
  A. **Crick's law** of molecular biology states that information is transferred from DNA to DNA (replication), from DNA to RNA (transcription), from RNA to DNA (reverse transcription), from RNA to protein (translation), but not from protein to nucleic acid
  B. DNA, RNA, and protein are informational macromolecules whose unique sequences correspond to information
    1. Inherited traits are passed from one generation to the next, and the gene, made up of a specific DNA sequence, is the unit of inheritance
    2. *The number of genes in humans is estimated to be between 50,000 and 100,000*
II. Structure of DNA
  A. DNA sequence
    1. The sequence of bases along the sugar-phosphate backbone makes up the primary structure of DNA, and the specific sequence distinguishes the DNA of one gene from that of another
    2. A phosphodiester bond joins the 5′-hydroxyl group of deoxyribose to a 3′-hydroxyl group of an adjacent deoxyribonucleotide to form a repeating backbone (Fig. 15–1)
  B. DNA double helix
    1. DNA exists as a duplex, i.e., two strands of polydeoxyribonucleotide that exhibit **Watson-Crick complementary base pairing:** cytosine forms three hydrogen bonds with guanine, and thymine forms two hydrogen bonds with adenine (Fig. 15–2)
    2. *If the sequence of bases of one strand of DNA is known, the sequence of the complementary strand can be derived by complementary base-pairing rules* (PRINCIPLE 23 OF BIOCHEMISTRY)
    3. The complementary chains of the double helix exhibit opposite polarity, and they are **antiparallel:** one strand progresses in the 5′ → 3′ direction, and the opposite strand progresses in the 3′ → 5′ direction
      a. PRINCIPLE 28 OF BIOCHEMISTRY states that complementary base pairing is antiparallel
      b. If we know that a given sequence occurs on one strand of the duplex, then we can immediately deduce the corresponding sequence of bases of its complementary strand by using the principles of Watson-Crick base pairing, as illustrated here:

        5′ ACGT 3′ original sequence
        3′ TGCA 5′ deduced complement

    4. The DNA of a bacterial cell such as *Escherichia coli* consists of a single, duplex (double-stranded) molecule that forms a covalently closed circle
III. The human nucleus and chromatin
  A. Chromosomes
    1. Human cells contain 46 chromosomes, each of which contains a single DNA molecule
    2. The main classes of DNA include nonrepetitive, or unique, DNA (75%) and repetitive DNA (25%)
  B. Nucleosomes
    1. Nucleosomes occur about every 200 base pairs and resemble a string of pearls
    2. Of these 200 base pairs, approximately 160 base pairs are wrapped around eight molecules of histones of a specific type (two each of histones H2A, H2B, H3, and H4)
    3. One molecule of histone H1 is associated with the DNA segments that link the nucleosomes together

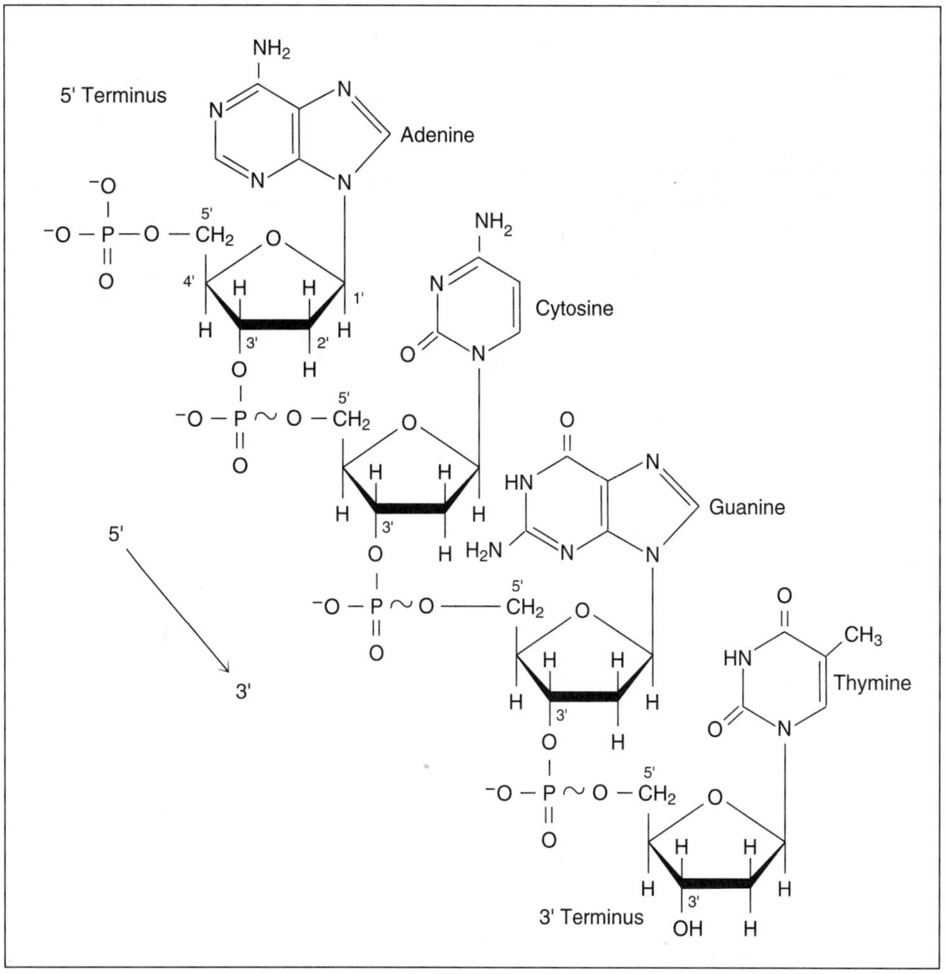

FIGURE 15-1. Structure of a tetranucleotide segment of DNA. An arrow paralleling the 5′ and 3′ carbon atoms of deoxyribose points in the 5′ to 3′ direction.

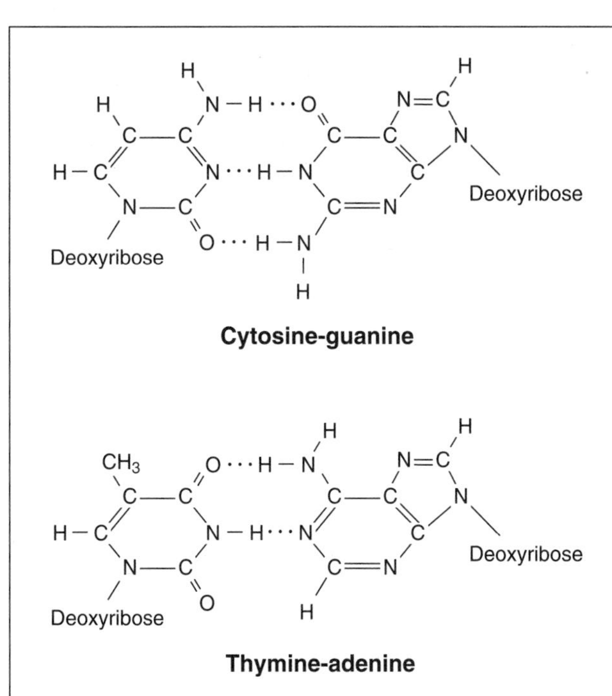

FIGURE 15-2. Watson-Crick base pairing.

Objective 2: To describe DNA replication.

IV. Overview of DNA replication
  A. Replication origins and replication forks
    1. Bacteria possess a single origin of replication per chromosome
    2. Humans possess about 40,000 replication origins among the 46 chromosomes
    3. The replication fork is the Y-shaped structure at which DNA elongation reactions and chain growth occur
  B. Semiconservative DNA replication
    1. Matthew **Meselson** and Franklin **Stahl** demonstrated that one strand of a parent duplex is associated with a newly synthesized strand in a daughter cell following replication, and the other strand is associated with a newly synthesized strand in the other daughter cell
    2. The two strands of DNA have opposite polarity
V. Enzymes of replication
  A. Bacterial enzymes
    1. *E. coli* possesses three **DNA polymerases** (**I, II,** and **III**)
      a. One strand of DNA serves as a template for the enzymes and directs the order of addition to the growing polynucleotide strand called the primer

b. The 3′ to 5′ hydrolase activity of polymerases I, II, and III performs a **proofreading** function, and the 5′ to 3′ hydrolase activity of polymerase I participates in DNA **repair**

c. *DNA polymerase III is the replication enzyme, and DNA polymerase I is the repair enzyme,* but the function of DNA polymerase II is a mystery

d. The phosphodiester bond of DNA is energy rich, and the incorporation of the deoxyribonucleotide into the strand is isoergonic, but the reaction is pulled forward by the hydrolysis of PP_i as catalyzed by inorganic pyrophosphatase

2. **DNA ligase** connects the 5′-phosphate to a free 3′ hydroxyl group and seals nicks or discontinuities in DNA
3. **DNA topoisomerases** catalyze reactions that alter supercoiling of DNA
   a. Type I enzymes cleave one strand, allow the intact strand to pass through the nick, and religate the DNA
   b. Type II enzymes cleave both strands, allow a portion of the intact duplex to pass through the nicks, and religate the DNA

B. Human enzymes
1. Human cells contain five DNA polymerases (α, β, γ, δ, and ε)
2. Human cells also contain DNA ligase and topoisomerases I and II

VI. DNA Replication in *E. coli*

A. Protein components
1. **Single-strand binding (SSB) protein** binds preferentially and cooperatively to single strands of DNA and thereby stabilizes the single-stranded state
2. **Helicase** possesses ATPase activity and opens the helix in the replication fork; two ATP molecules are expended for each base pair that is separated (one high-energy bond is expended by this process for each nucleotide incorporated into DNA)
3. DNA polymerases lack the ability to initiate DNA biosynthesis
   a. An essential protein called **primase** initiates the synthesis of short (≈5 nucleotides) strands of RNA
   b. These short strands of RNA serve as primers for deoxyribonucleotide elongation reactions
4. **DNA gyrase,** a topoisomerase II, catalyzes the ATP-dependent formation of negatively supertwisted DNA ahead of the replication fork

B. Replication of the leading and lagging strands
1. *Chain growth catalyzed by DNA polymerase occurs in the 5′ to 3′ direction* (Fig. 15–3)
2. Because the two strands of DNA are antiparallel and net replication occurs into the replication fork, different mechanisms must be responsible for synthesis of the two strands (Fig. 15–4)
   a. The leading strand is synthesized continuously

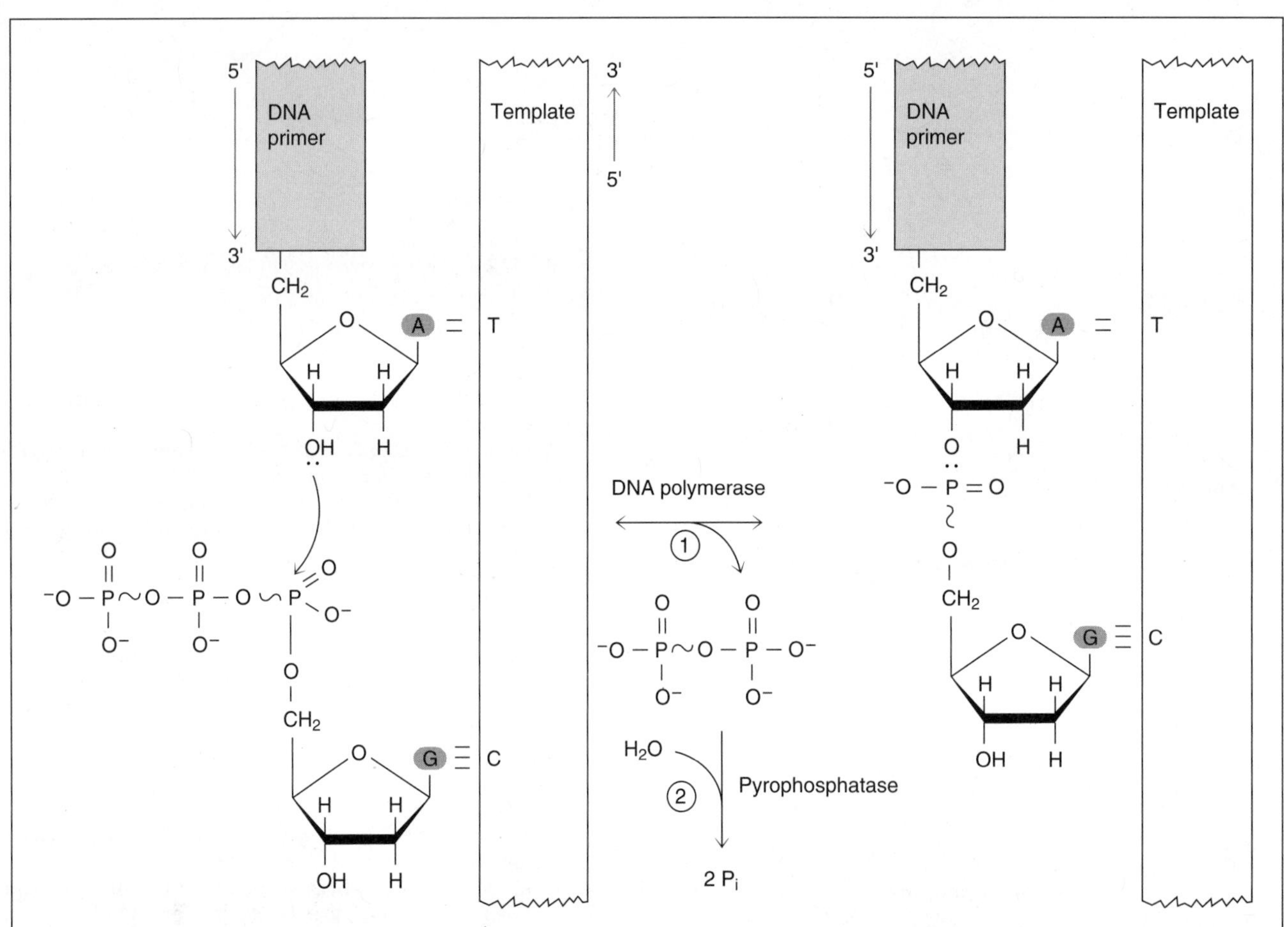

FIGURE 15-3. The elongation reaction of DNA synthesis. This diagram shows that chain growth is in the 5′ to 3′ direction.

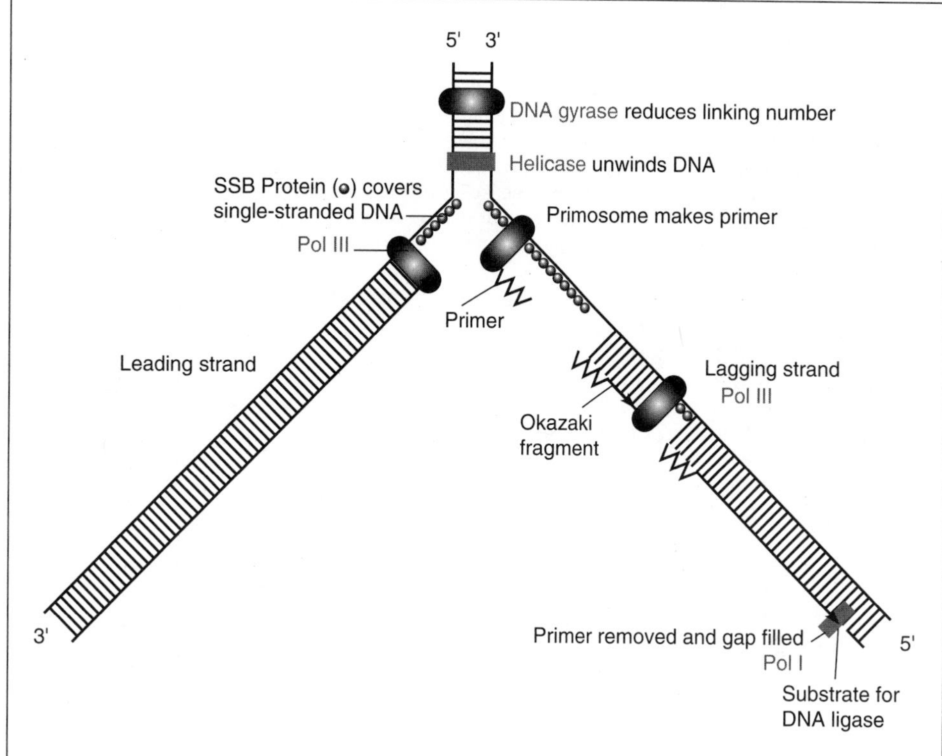

FIGURE 15-4. Diagram of the synthesis of the leading and lagging strand at the replication fork.

b. Although overall chain growth occurs into the intersection of the fork, synthesis of the lagging strand occurs discontinuously in the opposite direction but with exclusive $5' \rightarrow 3'$ polarity

c. Short (100–1000 nucleotides) DNA fragments that are made discontinuously are called **Okazaki fragments**

3. DNA polymerase I in *E. coli* removes the RNA primers with its 5′ to 3′ exonuclease activity and elongates primer strands through such discontinuities
4. DNA ligase seals the nicks between adjacent Okazaki fragments

VII. DNA replication in human cells

A. Initiation of DNA synthesis

1. Human chromosomes possess multiple origins of replication, and the origins are separated by about 150 kb
2. DNA polymerase α initiates both leading and lagging strand biosynthesis with its associated primase activity

B. Functions of the various replication enzymes

1. *DNA polymerase α is responsible for lagging strand biosynthesis*
2. *DNA polymerase δ and proliferating cell nuclear antigen (PCNA) are responsible for leading strand biosynthesis;* PCNA, an accessory protein, is necessary for DNA polymerase δ activity
3. *DNA polymerases β and ε function in nuclear repair synthesis, and DNA polymerase γ carries out replication within the mitochondrion*

C. Histones and nucleosomes

1. Histones that were present in the parental cell are distributed to the leading strand
2. Newly synthesized histones combine with the lagging strand
3. Nucleosomes are formed as a result of the association of histones with native DNA

VIII. Energy requirements for DNA replication

A. Two high-energy bonds are required to separate each base pair by the helicase in *E. coli*—this represents one high-energy bond per deoxyribonucleotide incorporated

B. Two high-energy bonds are used for each deoxyribonucleoside triphosphate substrate incorporated because of the pyrophosphate split

C. A total of three high energy bonds are required for the incorporation of each deoxyribonucleotide

Objective 3: To describe DNA repair.

IX. The four steps of nucleotide excision repair in humans

A. Repair nucleases catalyze the hydrolytic cleavage of the affected strand ≈22–24 phosphodiester bonds on the 5′ side of the molecular lesion and ≈5 phosphodiester bonds on the 3′ side of the lesion

B. A helicase promotes the release of the short DNA segment containing the molecular lesion

C. The 3′-hydroxyl group produced by endonuclease is used as a primer for repair synthesis to fill in the excised gap as catalyzed by repair polymerases (DNA polymerases β and ε)

D. DNA ligase activity seals the nick

X. The base excision repair system

A. Following spontaneous hydrolytic depurination, the most common insult suffered by DNA, an AP (apurinic) endonuclease cuts the DNA phosphodiester backbone on the 5′ side of the altered site

B. A family of DNA glycosylases also removes damaged bases (e.g., deaminated C and deaminated A residues), producing a substrate for AP endonuclease
C. After excision of the sugar phosphate residue by a phosphodiesterase, repair polymerases and DNA ligase restore the original sequence

XI. Mutations involving DNA repair
A. **Xeroderma pigmentosum,** a disease seen in children and young adults, is characterized by numerous pigmented spots and solar-induced circumscribed skin lesions
B. Xeroderma pigmentosum is due to mutation in enzymes required for nucleotide excision repair
1. Seven (A–G) genes have been described in this disorder, indicating that multiple proteins are required for nucleotide excision repair
2. Several lesions are not efficiently repaired as a result of the defects in the xeroderma pigmentosum repair system
a. Thymine dimers, the most common ultraviolet light–induced lesion, and other pyrimidine dimers (T–C, C–C) induced by ultraviolet light accumulate in xeroderma pigmentosum
b. Modifications induced by benzo[*a*]pyrene and other carcinogens also accumulate
c. Modifications produced by x-rays and by DNA alkylating agents do not accumulate in xeroderma pigmentosum and are repaired by the base excision repair process or other repair processes

Objective 4: To describe recombinant DNA technology and the diagnosis of genetic diseases.

XII. Preparation of recombinant DNA molecules
A. Restriction endonucleases
1. *Type II restriction endonucleases are sequence specific and cleave at palindromes;* a DNA palindrome occurs when the sequence on one strand of nucleic acid (from 5′ to 3′) is identical to that of its complementary strand (from 5′ to 3′):

5′ GGCC 3′
3′ CCGG 5′

2. The restriction enzymes are valuable because they cleave at specific and not random base sequences
B. Recombinant DNA and gene clones
1. **Vectors** are DNA molecules such as plasmids or viruses that replicate independently of the host chromosome and can carry (vector) DNA segments into host cells
2. **Plasmids** are DNA molecules that replicate independently of the chromosome; vectors such as pBR322, an *E. coli* plasmid, are used to produce clones or identical copies of DNA segments
3. Recombinant DNA is made naturally or in the laboratory by attaching segments of DNA to each other
a. Recombinant DNA molecules can be produced by ligating the cohesive ends of a plasmid and another DNA sample that have been treated with the same restriction enzyme
b. Total genomic DNA or DNA complementary to mRNA produced through the reaction of reverse transcriptase can be used to produce recombinant DNA molecules

XIII. Nucleic acid hybridization and electrophoretic blots
A. Hybridization
1. Single-stranded DNA, produced by alkali denaturation or by heating, can anneal with any complementary DNA or RNA, whatever the source, by a process called **hybridization**
a. Under stringent conditions, only perfectly matched Watson-Crick complementary structures can hybridize
b. Under less stringent conditions, complementary strands that contain some mismatches can hybridize
2. Labeled DNA or RNA, which can hybridize with complementary nucleic acid, is used as a **probe** to label nucleic acids
B. Electrophoresis and blotting
1. The distance that nucleic acids migrate in an electric field is inversely related to the molecular mass or number of monomeric residues in the polynucleotide
2. Several types of electrophoretic blots are useful in molecular medicine
a. The resolution of DNA by electrophoresis and transfer to nitrocellulose is called a **Southern blot** (named for Edwin Southern, the originator)
b. A similar analysis of RNA was dubbed a **Northern blot**
c. Electrophoresis and transfer of proteins are called a **Western blot**
3. Three steps are involved in electrophoretic blotting
a. The first step involves the electrophoretic resolution of macromolecules
b. The second step involves the transfer of the macromolecules to a bonding agent by a method that ensures that the spacial resolution is maintained
c. The third step involves the localization of the nucleic acid or protein with a nucleic acid probe or antibody, respectively

XIV. Polymerase chain reaction (PCR) technology
A. Amplification of DNA for study
B. Procedure
1. The chain reaction refers to the use of multiple cycles (25–35) of template- and primer-dependent DNA elongation reactions
2. The requirements include a target DNA (the template) for amplification, two DNA oligonucleotide primers complementary to the ends of each strand of the target DNA and extending toward the sequence that will bind the other primer, deoxynucleoside triphosphates, and heat-stable DNA polymerase obtained from *Thermus aquaticus* (*Taq* polymerase) or other heat-stable DNA polymerase

XV. DNA sequence analysis
A. Dideoxynucleotide chain termination
1. Chain terminators, which include ddATP, ddGTP, ddCTP, and ddTTP, are included in four independent reaction mixtures
2. When these dideoxynucleotides are incorporated into the growing chain at positions complementary to the cloned insert, elongation is impossible (there is no free 3′-hydroxyl group) and chain termination results
3. Each reaction produces a mixture of products that correspond to chain termination at each possible

location determined by complementary base pairing with the template of the DNA to be sequenced

B. Sequencing gels
   1. The products of the four independent reaction mixtures, which produce products that terminate at each nucleotide of the target DNA, are resolved by size by electrophoresis
   2. The sequence is read from the four parallel gels nucleotide by nucleotide

XVI. Genetic variation, polymorphism, and disease

A. **Restriction fragment length polymorphisms** (RFLPs)
   1. DNA samples are treated with restriction enzymes, electrophoresed, and probed
   2. The resulting Southern blots can exhibit different patterns (polymorphism), and the patterns can reflect specific genetic traits

B. **Allele-specific oligonucleotide** (ASO) analysis
   1. The use of oligonucleotide probes of about 12 nucleotides permits the identification of single base changes by allele-specific oligonucleotide probe analysis
   2. This procedure can be carried out directly on a nitrocellulose matrix and does not involve electrophoresis
   3. Single nucleotide changes can be detected directly, and the target sequence does not have to involve a restriction enzyme site

QUESTIONS

DIRECTIONS. (Items 1–18): Each of the numbered items or incomplete statements in this section is followed by answers or by completions of the statement. Select the ONE lettered answer or completion that is BEST in each case.

1. Which one of the following molecules consists of a linear duplex molecule with discrete 5′ and 3′ ends?

(A) *E. coli* DNA
(B) *E. coli* plasmid DNA
(C) human transfer RNA
(D) human mitochondrial DNA
(E) human nuclear DNA

2. Which one of the following molecules forms physiological complexes with histones H1, H2A, H2B, H3, and H4 *in vivo*?

(A) *E. coli* DNA
(B) *E. coli* plasmid DNA
(C) human transfer RNA
(D) human mitochondrial DNA
(E) human nuclear DNA

3. Leber's hereditary optic neuropathy (LHON) is transmitted maternally, and no affected males transmit the disease. Affected individuals may be male or female. The gene for this disorder occurs on

(A) an autosome
(B) mitochondrial DNA
(C) the X chromosome
(D) the Y chromosome

4. Which one of the following is a true statement regarding PCNA (proliferating cell nuclear antigen)?

(A) It forms a complex with DNA polymerase δ
(B) It participates in lagging strand biosynthesis
(C) It participates in ribosomal RNA transcription
(D) It is an RNA polymerase III transcription factor
(E) It functions in nuclear repair synthesis

5. Daunorubicin and doxorubicin are anthracycline antibiotics that are among the newer cancer chemotherapeutic agents used in the treatment of lymphomas and leukemias. These compounds inhibit which one of the following enzymes by destabilizing a protein-tyrosine phosphate intermediate?

(A) DNA polymerase α
(B) DNA polymerase β
(C) RNA polymerase II
(D) topoisomerase I
(E) topoisomerase II

6. Which one of the following enzymes catalyzes the elimination of nicks or discontinuities in DNA that occur during DNA repair or in the linking together of Okazaki fragments?

(A) AP exonuclease
(B) DNA gyrase
(C) DNA ligase
(D) topoisomerase I
(E) topoisomerase II

7. Which one of the following enzymes initiates synthesis of bacterial DNA?

(A) DNA polymerase α
(B) DNA polymerase I
(C) DNA polymerase II
(D) DNA polymerase III
(E) primase

8. The number of high-energy bonds that are required for the incorporation of a single deoxyribonucleotide into bacterial DNA is

(A) 0
(B) 1
(C) 2
(D) 3
(E) 4

9. All of the following are physiological substrates for DNA polymerase δ EXCEPT

(A) dUTP
(B) dATP
(C) dTTP
(D) dGTP
(E) dCTP

10. All of the following statements show biological information transfer occurring in a correct direction EXCEPT
    (A) DNA → RNA
    (B) RNA → DNA
    (C) RNA → protein
    (D) DNA → DNA
    (E) Protein → RNA

11. If one strand of DNA has the sequence 5′ GCAT 3′, what is the sequence of its complementary strand, written in the 5′ to 3′ direction?
    (A) CGTA
    (B) CGTU
    (C) ATGC
    (D) AUGC

12. Twenty percent of the bases of human DNA are cytosine. The adenine content of human DNA is therefore
    (A) 10%
    (B) 20%
    (C) 30%
    (D) 40%
    (E) 50%

13. Xeroderma pigmentosum, first described by Moritz Kaposi in 1863, is characterized by progressive degenerative changes of sun-exposed portions of the skin and eyes. There is a 200-fold increase in skin cancers, and a 20-fold increase in internal cancers. Affected individuals exhibit increased sensitivity to ultraviolet light but not to x-rays or DNA alkylating agents. Xeroderma pigmentosum is a result of a defect in
    (A) AP endonuclease
    (B) DNA ligase
    (C) DNA *N*-glycosylase
    (D) thymine dimer formation
    (E) nucleotide excision repair

14. Dideoxyinosine triphosphate, a compound derived from dideoxyinosine and used in the treatment of AIDS, inhibits DNA synthesis by
    (A) blocking the base pairing of cytidine with guanosine
    (B) failing to be incorporated into a DNA chain
    (C) forming a covalent complex with DNA polymerase δ
    (D) causing chain termination
    (E) promoting the cleavage of the DNA backbone

Items 15–18

History

A 29-year-old woman and her 32-year-old husband come to the obstetrics clinic for information and counseling concerning her pregnancy. They had previously had three children. Child I (a 7-year-old girl) and child II (a 4-year-old boy) are alive and healthy, and child III (a girl) died of cystic fibrosis at the age of 18 months, 1 year ago.

Physical Examination

An ultrasound examination during week 9 showed a dichorionic twin gestation with two placentas. The couple requested prenatal diagnosis. The crown-rump lengths of both fetuses were 27 mm, corresponding to 9.5 weeks.

Laboratory

Chorionic villus sampling was performed transabdominally under ultrasonic guidance with a linear 3.5-megahertz transducer with a puncture guide attached. Approximately 25 mg of tissue was obtained from each placenta. After DNA extraction, polymerase chain reactions were performed. The primers, which were designed to bracket the Δ508 mutation, led to the production of an 87-base-pair product from a normal CFTR gene and an 84-base-pair product from a Δ508 mutant gene. The products were subjected to polyacrylamide gel electrophoresis and localized by ethidium bromide staining. (Recall that smaller polynucleotides migrate faster than larger molecules.) Karyotypes reported 8 days after the procedure indicated that both fetuses had female karyotypes. The results for the PCR analysis of DNA from the parents, their children, the two fetuses, and an unaffected person and DNA containing a Δ508 mutation established by DNA sequence analysis are illustrated below.

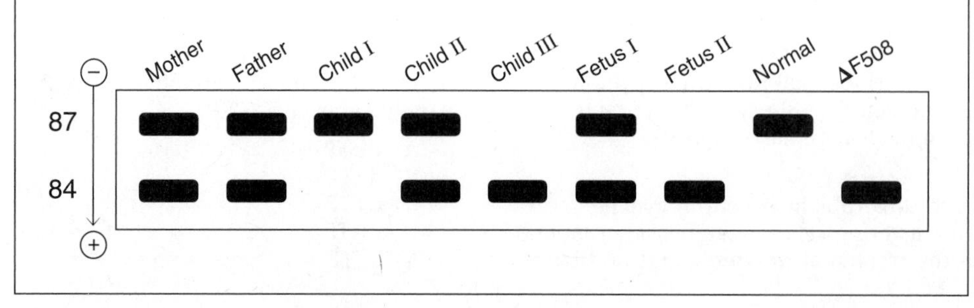

15. Which one of the following is NOT a true statement regarding these results?
    (A) Child I (♀) will be affected with cystic fibrosis
    (B) Child II (♂) was heterozygous for the Δ508 mutation
    (C) the father was heterozygous for the Δ508 mutation
    (D) the mother was heterozygous for the Δ508 mutation

16. Based upon the information provided in this case, cystic fibrosis is what class of genetic disease?
    (A) Autosomal dominant
    (B) Autosomal recessive
    (C) X-linked dominant
    (D) X-linked recessive

17. Which of the fetuses will be affected, according to the results from the polymerase chain reaction methodology?
    (A) Both fetus I and II will be affected

(B) Fetus I, but not fetus II, will be affected
(C) Neither fetus I nor II will be affected
(D) Fetus II, but not fetus I, will be affected

18. Cystic fibrosis in this family is a disease that results in the deletion of three nucleotides that do not form part of a palindrome. Methods that can be used to detect this type of mutation directly include each of the following EXCEPT

(A) allele-specific oligonucleotide analysis of a dot blot
(B) DNA sequence analysis
(C) altered electrophoretic migration of the complete cystic fibrosis gene
(D) single-stranded conformation polymorphism (SSCP)

ANSWERS AND EXPLANATIONS

1. The answer is E: human nuclear DNA. Human nuclear DNA is a linear duplex molecule. Although linear, chromosomal DNA exists in various topological isomers because portions of the DNA are tethered to proteins of the nuclear matrix. *E. coli* DNA, its plasmid DNA, and human mitochondrial DNA are covalently closed circular molecules. Human transfer RNA consists of a single strand that exists as an L-shaped molecule with some intrastrand double-stranded segments. *Biochemistry,* pp. 272, 275–276, 347, 349.
2. The answer is E: human nuclear DNA. Histones are basic proteins that occur in the nucleus of eukaryotic cells, and they form complexes with DNA and make up chromatin. Bacteria and mitochondria lack histones, and histones do not form functional complexes with RNA. *Biochemistry,* pp. 276–277, 278.
3. The answer is B: mitochondrial DNA. Mitochondrial DNA is derived from the egg, and none is contributed by the sperm. Mitochondrial diseases are transmitted maternally. Autosomal diseases are transmitted by both males and females, and both males and females can be affected. X-linked diseases are generally transmitted to male offspring (who contain a single X chromosome) from carrier mothers (who contain two X chromosomes). *Biochemistry,* pp. 360–361.
4. The answer is A: It forms a complex with DNA polymerase δ. DNA polymerase δ and proliferating cell nuclear antigen (PCNA) are responsible for leading strand biosynthesis. PCNA, an accessory protein, is necessary for DNA polymerase δ activity. DNA polymerases β and ε function in nuclear repair synthesis, and DNA polymerase γ carries out replication within the mitochondrion. RNA polymerase I catalyzes the synthesis of ribosomal RNA. RNA polymerase III transcription factors include TFIIIA, TFIIIB, and TFIIIC. *Biochemistry,* p. 281.
5. The answer is E: topoisomerase II. Topoisomerase II, an enzyme that interconverts topological isomers of DNA, makes nicks in both strands of a DNA duplex and allows a portion of the intact strand to pass through the discontinuities. Daunorubicin and doxorubicin interfere with the action of topoisomerase II at the nick-closing stage. As a result, these compounds produce strand scission. Actinomycin D, which is used in the treatment of a variety of cancers, is an antibiotic that inhibits both human and bacterial RNA synthesis. There are no compounds that are used clinically to inhibit DNA polymerases or topoisomerase I. *Biochemistry,* p. 453.
6. The answer is C: DNA ligase. After repair polymerases have filled in gaps, a free 3′-hydroxyl group and 5′-phosphate group make up the substrate for DNA ligase, an ATP-dependent enzyme that seals the nick or discontinuity. Topoisomerases catalyze the interconversion of topological isomers that differ in the degree of supercoiling. Topo I breaks one strand and alters the linking number by one; topo II breaks both strands and alters the linking number by two. DNA gyrase is an example of a bacterial DNA topoisomerase II; this enzyme alters the supercoiling preceding the replication fork and requires two ATP molecules for the separation of each base pair. An AP endonuclease catalyzes the hydrolysis of a phosphodiester on the 5′ side of a deoxyribosyl group that has lost its base. This hydrolysis leaves a free 3′-hydroxyl group. AP is an abbreviation for apurinic or apyrimidinic DNA. Exonuclease activity removes the defective region of the DNA by hydrolysis. *Biochemistry,* p. 282.
7. The answer is E: primase. All DNA polymerases, which lack the ability to initiate physiological DNA chain formation, are able to extend DNA or RNA primers. Primase is a specialized complex that synthesizes an RNA primer which can be elongated by DNA polymerase. The first few nucleotides are ribonucleotides, and these can be followed by ribo- or deoxyribonucleotides. Because primase is prone to incorporate noncomplementary bases, the primer is eliminated by exonuclease activity and deoxyribonucleotides are inserted by DNA polymerase I, the bacterial repair polymerase. *Biochemistry,* p. 284.
8. The answer is D: 3 high-energy bonds are required to form each phosphodiester bond in DNA. Two high-energy bonds correspond to the use of deoxyribonucleoside triphosphates, and the third high-energy bond is required for the action of DNA gyrase, a type II topoisomerase that expends two molecules of ATP (to 2 ADP and 2 P_i) for each base pair of the replication fork that is separated. *Biochemistry,* p. 286.
9. The answer is A: dUTP. Uracil is a component of RNA but NOT of DNA. dUTP is formed by phosphorylation after UDP is converted to dUDP by ribonucleotide reductase. Cells possess a powerful dUTPase that converts dUTP to dUMP, the substrate for thymidylate synthase. The four bases that are incorporated into DNA as the deoxyribonucleotide are adenine, thymine, guanine, and cytosine, and each of these is derived from the corresponding deoxyribonucleoside triphosphate. *Biochemistry,* p. 306.
10. The answer is E: Protein $\rightarrow$ RNA. The flow of information from DNA to DNA is replication, and from DNA to RNA is transcription. Both of these processes occur in the nucleus. RNA is transported from the nucleus to the cytosol, where it directs protein synthesis during translation. The flow of information from RNA to DNA is reverse transcription. It is a well documented process in retroviruses, and there are indications that such processes occur to a limited extent physiologically in noninfected cells. Information does NOT go from protein to RNA or from protein to DNA. *Biochemistry,* p. 270.

11. The answer is C: ATGC. The following illustrates Watson-Crick base pairing with a tetranucleotide 5′ GCAT 3′:

5′ GCAT 3′
3′ CGTA 5′

The complementary strand has the sequence, from 5′ to 3′, of ATGC. Answers B (CGTU) and D (AUGC) are incorrect because U does not occur in DNA. Answer A (CGTA) is incorrect because it has the incorrect polarity from the 5′ to 3′ end. *Biochemistry,* p. 272.
12. The answer is C: 30%. In duplex DNA, the molar fraction of C and G is the same, and the molar fraction of A and T is identical. Given a molar fraction of C equal to 20%, this indicates that the molar fraction of G is also 20%, for a total of 40%. The A and T content are 100%–40%, or 60%, or A + T = 60%. Since A = T, the content of A is one-half of 60%, or 30%. *Biochemistry,* p. 272.
13. The answer is E: a defect in nucleotide excision repair. In xeroderma pigmentosum, there is a defect in the intricate nucleotide excision–repair system. The repair system involves the interaction of at least seven gene products. This system is important for the removal of pyrimidine dimers that are induced by ultraviolet light (T-T, T-C, C-C), and a defect also results in a decrease in repair following the action of some carcinogens including benzo[*a*]pyrene. There is no defect in base excision repair indicating that DNA ligase, AP endonuclease, and DNA *N*-glycosylase are functional. Thymine dimers, which are unphysiological, are formed independently of the repair process. Their removal, however, is defective in xeroderma pigmentosum. *Biochemistry,* p. 289.
14. The answer is D: causing chain termination. Dideoxyinosine mononucleotide is incorporated into a DNA chain as catalyzed by DNA polymerase. The absence of a free 3′-hydroxyl group, however, does not permit chain extension. Dideoxyinosine triphosphate does not block G-C pairing, form a complex with DNA polymerase δ, or promote DNA backbone cleavage. *Biochemistry,* p. 340.
15. The answer is A: child I (♀) will be affected with cystic fibrosis is NOT true. Child I is homozygous for the slowly migrating PCR product that corresponds to the normal gene. Child II (♂), the father, and the mother possess both the normal (slowly migrating) and mutant gene (rapidly migrating) PCR products and are, therefore, heterozygotes. *Biochemistry,* p. 299.
16. The answer is B: autosomal recessive. The mother, father, and child II possess the mutant gene but are not affected. The disorder is therefore recessive, not dominant. When large populations are considered, cystic fibrosis occurs about equally in males and females and is therefore not X-linked. X-linked disorders, which are encoded by a mutant gene on the X chromosome, are carried by the mother and are expressed primarily in male children (possessing a single X chromosome). Females, however, can have a mild form of some X-linked diseases (e.g., nephrogenic diabetes insipidus) because of inactivation of one X chromosome (Lyon hypothesis). *Biochemistry,* p. 7.
17. The answer is D: fetus II, but not fetus I, will be affected. Fetus II contains the polymerase chain reaction product that corresponds to only the mutant gene; fetus II is therefore homozygous for this trait and will be affected. Fetus I contains the gene product that corresponds to the normal gene and will not be affected. *Biochemistry,* p. 7.
18. The answer is C: altered electrophoretic migration of the complete cystic fibrosis gene. More than 200 mutations have been described that result in cystic fibrosis. It is, therefore, NOT possible to design a simple genetic test that will detect all of them. The Δ508 deletion results from the deletion of a trinucleotide sequence and is responsible for about 70% of the mutations at the DNA level. This trinucleotide deletion is not large enough to detect by differences in electrophoretic migration of the entire gene. Allele-specific oligonucleotide analysis of dot blots and single-strand conformation polymorphism (SSCP) are commonly used to detect single base changes. DNA sequence analysis can detect single base changes, but it requires considerable work and is used by research teams to define the mutation in previously undefined cases. Because considerable detail about the cystic fibrosis gene and its sequence is available, it was possible to design primers for polymerase chain reaction that flanked the codon corresponding to phenylalanine 508 and to resolve the PCR products from the normal and mutant genes. The cystic fibrosis gene is linked to a particular DNA polymorphism that can be detected by restriction fragment length polymorphism. *Biochemistry,* pp. 299–303.

REFERENCE

Roskoski, R., Jr. *Biochemistry.* Philadelphia, W. B. Saunders Company, 1996.

CHAPTER SIXTEEN

RNA Biosynthesis and Processing

SYNOPSIS

OBJECTIVES

1. To recognize RNA and describe its synthesis in bacteria and in humans.
2. To outline the posttranscriptional processing of RNA.
3. To enumerate the five types of immunoglobulins.
4. To describe the life cycle of human immunodeficiency virus (HIV).
5. To outline the mechanisms of transcription inhibitors.

Objective 1: To recognize RNA and describe its synthesis in bacteria and in humans.

I. Structure and function of RNA
  A. RNA functions as an intermediary in the transfer of genetic information from DNA to protein as stated in Crick's law of molecular biology (PRINCIPLE 25 OF BIOCHEMISTRY)
  B. RNA is a polynucleotide with repeating 5′ to 3′ phosphodiester bonds linking adjacent ribose residues
  C. The bases that occur in RNA include adenine, uracil, guanine, and cytosine (Fig. 16–1) but not thymine

II. Synthesis of RNA by RNA polymerases
  A. DNA-dependent RNA polymerases function in both prokaryotes and eukaryotes
    1. RNA polymerase catalyzes the formation of phosphodiester bonds from a free 3′-hydroxyl group of an RNA strand and the activated α-phosphorus atom of an incoming ribonucleoside triphosphate
    2. Unlike DNA polymerases, RNA polymerases can initiate chain growth
    3. Chain growth occurs in the $5' \rightarrow 3'$ direction (PRINCIPLE 29 OF BIOCHEMISTRY), and chain polarity is antiparallel to that of the DNA template
    4. *The sequence of the synthesized polymer is directed by the DNA template according to Watson-Crick complementary base-pairing*
    5. Adenine in DNA specifies uracil in the RNA transcript, guanine specifies cytosine, cytosine specifies guanosine, and thymine specifies adenine
    6. Either strand of chromosomal DNA can be sense or antisense, depending upon whether or not it functions as template
      a. The DNA strand whose sequence corresponds to that of cellular RNA is called the **sense strand**
      b. The complementary strand, which serves as a template for RNA polymerase, is called the **antisense strand**
      c. Reported sequences corresponding to genetic and regulatory segments of a gene correspond to the sense strand
  B. *Escherichia coli* RNA polymerase is a single enzyme with variable promoter recognition subunits
    1. The protein subunit structure of the bacterial **holoenzyme** is $\alpha_2\beta\beta'\sigma$, and $\alpha_2\beta\beta'$ makes up the catalytic core
    2. *E. coli* RNA polymerase with a sigma (σ) subunit recognizes and binds to special sequences of DNA (**promoters**) that direct the initiation of gene transcription (Fig. 16–2)
    3. Five different sigma subunits recognize different promoters and are responsible for differential gene expression
    4. After chain initiation, the sigma subunit dissociates from the complex, and core polymerase completes the synthesis of the primary transcript
    5. A group of contiguous genes controlled by a single operator gene is called an **operon**
      a. A **cistron** is a unit of gene expression
      b. In prokaryotes, but not eukaryotes, the product of several contiguous genes may be transcribed to produce a **polycistronic message**
    6. Rifampin, a widely prescribed antibiotic, inhibits the initiation of bacterial RNA biosynthesis and interacts with the β-subunit

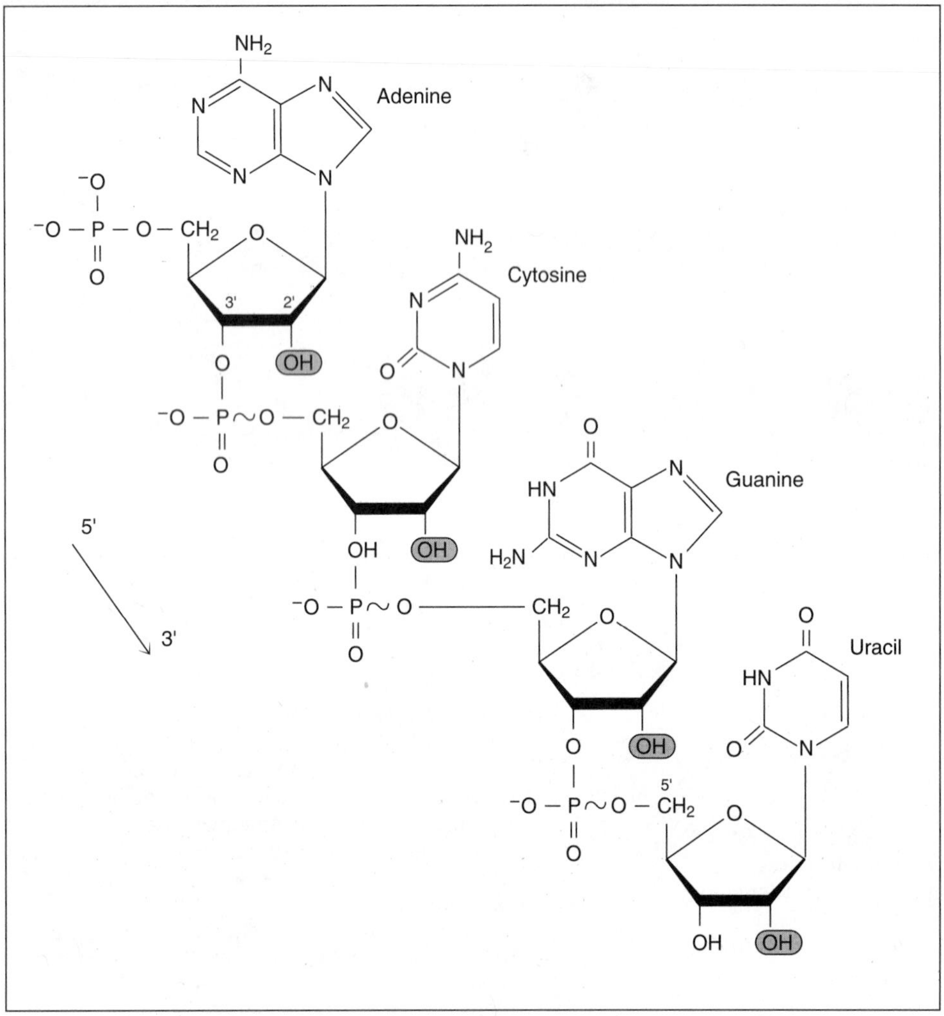

FIGURE 16-1. Structure of a segment of RNA. The arrow, which parallels the direction from the 5′ to 3′ carbon atoms of ribose, indicates the directionality of this RNA segment.

C. Human RNA polymerases have specialized functions
   1. RNA polymerase I is responsible for the production of a primary transcript corresponding to three (18S, 28S, and 5.8S RNA) of the four ribosomal RNA molecules in human cells
   2. RNA polymerase II is responsible for hnRNA/mRNA production
      a. Genes corresponding to hnRNA contain segments that are expressed in the mature mRNA (**exons**) and segments that are not expressed in mRNA (**introns**)
      b. **Promoters** determine the start sites for RNA synthesis, and **transcription elements** determine the frequency of transcription
         (1) Enhancers are DNA segments that increase transcription
         (2) Silencers are DNA segments that decrease transcription
         (3) Enhancers and silencers are active in either orientation (5′ to 3′ or vice versa)
         (4) Promoter elements for RNA polymerase II include TATA boxes, CAAT boxes, GC boxes, octomer sequences, and NF-κB sequences
      c. *TFIID, which recognizes the TATA box, recruits the basal transcription apparatus,* including RNA polymerase II and factors TFIIA, TFIIB, TFIIE, TFIIF, TFIIH, and TFIIJ
   3. RNA polymerase III is responsible for the synthesis of tRNA, 5S RNA, and other small RNA molecules

Objective 2: To outline the posttranscriptional processing of RNA.

III. Posttranscriptional RNA processing
   A. The newly synthesized RNA polymer is called the **primary transcript**
   B. A series of reactions may be required to convert the primary transcript into the functional RNA, and such processing reactions fall into a variety of classes
      1. The primary transcript may undergo partial degradation by a combination of exonucleases and endonucleases to yield a shorter polymer and fragments (which are degraded)
      2. The bases and sugars may undergo methylation, and the polynucleotide may undergo splicing
   C. The various primary transcripts of RNA in human cells can undergo a variety of processing reactions
      1. rRNA processing in human cells involves endonuclease, exonuclease, and methylation reactions

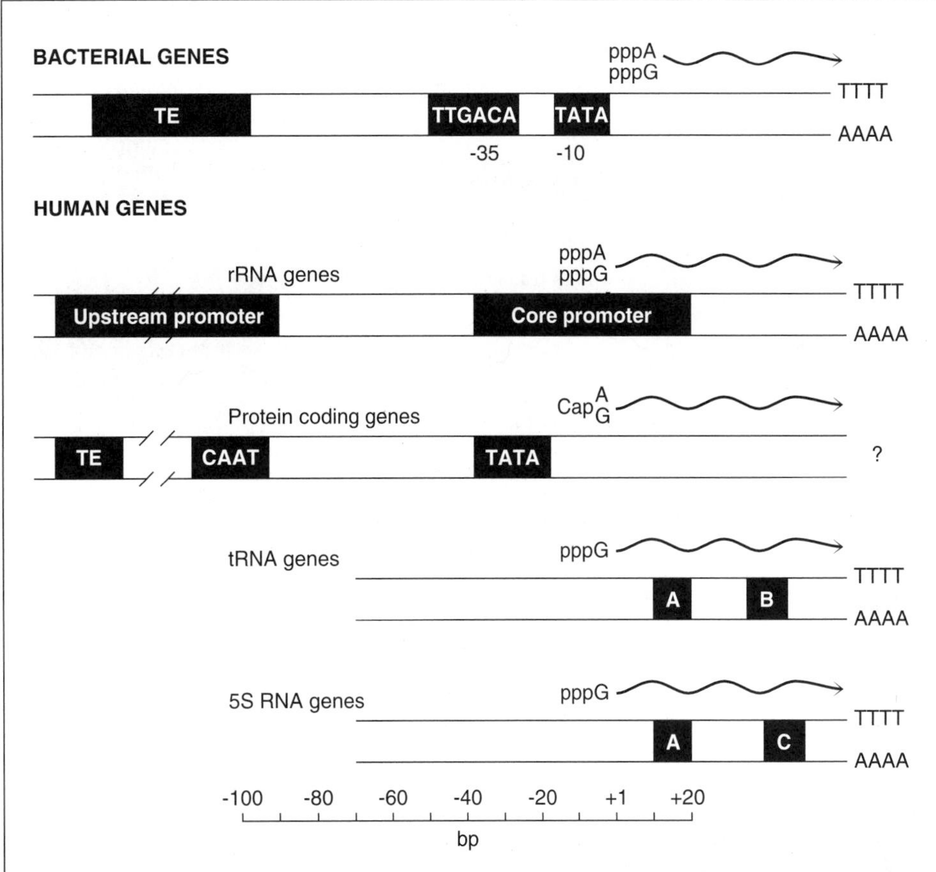

FIGURE 16-2. Diagram of promoter and transcription elements (TEs) of bacterial and human RNA polymerases. The promoters for RNA polymerase III transcripts include A, B, and C boxes that occur in the transcribed region. The sizes of the promoter and regulatory elements are not necessarily to scale.

2. hnRNA is processed to form mRNA
   a. Capping of hnRNA involves a reaction with GTP to produce a $5' \rightarrow 5'$ triphosphate cap that is methylated by *S*-adenosylmethionine
   b. A polyA tail is added on the 3′ end of hnRNA by serial reactions with ATP catalyzed by a polyA polymerase
   c. Nuclear mRNA splicing reactions are mediated by a spliceosome
      (1) The base sequence of an intron begins with GU and ends with AG
      (2) The stages of splicing include (1) transesterification with a branch-site adenosine, (2) displacement of the donor exon, (3) transesterification of the donor and acceptor exon, and (4) displacement of lariat RNA
      (3) Alternative splicing reactions can produce different mRNAs from the same primary transcript
      (4) Many people with systemic lupus erythematosus possess antibodies that inhibit splicing and a variety of other antinuclear antibodies
      (5) Abnormal splicing is one of the mechanisms responsible for β-thalassemia, a disease characterized by deficient β-globin synthesis
      (6) The mRNA corresponding to apo-B-48 is derived from the same hnRNA that leads to apo-B-100, the different gene products resulting from **RNA editing** that generates a stop codon by converting a site-specific cytosine of mRNA to uracil
      (7) Histone mRNA lacks introns, and it does not undergo splicing reactions
   d. A **tRNA nucleotidyl transferase** catalyzes the addition of CCA to substrate to produce the 3′ terminus that occurs in all mature tRNA molecules

Objective 3: To enumerate the five types of immunoglobulins.

IV. Antibody structure and formation
   A. Immunoglobulins share many common properties
      1. **Antibodies** are proteins that specifically recognize and bind to foreign, or nonself, molecules called **antigens**
      2. Antibodies, which are produced by B lymphocytes, are made up of two light chains and two heavy chains
         a. Light chains consist of a **variable region** (V_L) on the amino terminal half and a **constant region** (C_L) on the carboxyterminal half, and each of these segments is about 110 amino acid residues in length
         b. Heavy chains consist of a variable amino terminal portion (V_H) and three constant regions (C_H1, C_H2, C_H3), and each of these segments is also about 110 amino acids long
         c. Each antigen-binding site consists of residues derived from the variable region from one light and one heavy chain
         d. Two heavy chains are covalently attached by two disulfide bonds, and each of the variable and constant domains of the heavy and light chains contains intrachain disulfide bonds
         e. There are five major antibody isotypes, which are determined by the heavy chain: IgA, IgD, IgE, IgG, and IgM
            (1) *IgM and IgD are synthesized first*

TABLE 16–1. Steps in Antibody Formation

Process	Mechanism
Antigen independent	
Heavy chain production	
D-J joining	DNA rearrangement
V-D-J joining	DNA rearrangement
Expression of heavy chain	Transcription, processing, translation
Light chain production	
V-J joining	DNA rearrangement
Expression of light chain	Transcription, processing, translation
Expression of IgM (H and L chain) in the plasma membrane	
Isotype switching to IgD	Alternative splicing
Antigen dependent	
Secretion of IgM	Alternative splicing of the primary transcript
Isotype switching to IgA, IgG, and IgE	DNA rearrangement
Somatic rearrangement	Unknown

(2) IgG accounts for 80% of total circulating immunoglobulins

(3) IgA is the antibody that occurs in saliva, tears, milk, and intestinal secretions

B. The steps involving gene rearrangement and immunoglobulin production are outlined in Table 16–1

Objective 4: To describe the life cycle of human immunodeficiency virus (HIV).

V. HIV and reverse transcriptase

A. Retroviruses such as HIV and human T-cell lymphotropic virus contain reverse transcriptase

B. The term reverse signifies that biological information flows from RNA to DNA, opposite to the usual direction of transfer (PRINCIPLE 25 OF BIOCHEMISTRY)

C. Each AIDS retrovirus (HIV-1 and HIV-2) contains two identical single-stranded RNA genomes of about 9700 nucleotides, two molecules of lysine tRNA, reverse transcriptase, integrase, and a protease

D. The AIDS virus infects CD4-containing T cells, but the mechanism for viral invasion is unknown

E. **Reverse transcriptase** mediates the RNA template-dependent formation of double-stranded DNA from a single-stranded RNA by an intricate process

1. Reverse transcriptase possesses RNA-dependent DNA polymerase and DNA-dependent DNA polymerase activities at a single active site
2. Like other DNA-synthesizing enzymes, reverse transcriptase is unable to initiate DNA synthesis *de novo*, and it requires a primer (lysine tRNA)
3. Reverse transcriptase is accompanied by **RNAse H** activity, which degrades the RNA of an RNA-DNA complementary hybrid
4. The duplex DNA is integrated in the human genome as a provirus

Objective 5: To outline the mechanisms of transcription inhibitors.

VI. Inhibition of nucleic acid synthesis by drugs

A. Initiation of bacterial RNA polymerases is inhibited by rifampin

B. Actinomycin D is a peptide antibiotic that inhibits DNA-dependent RNA synthesis (both human and bacterial)

C. Azidothymidine (AZT) is a nucleoside analogue of thymidine in which the 3′-hydroxyl group is replaced by the azido group

1. It is used in the treatment of AIDS
2. It inhibits the elongation reactions by (a) inhibiting binding of thymidine triphosphate and by (b) causing chain termination after AZT is incorporated into the nucleotide chain

D. Acycloguanosine is used in the treatment of herpesvirus infection

1. This agent is phosphorylated by herpesvirus thymidine kinase but not by human thymidine kinase
2. This agent is thus effective only in cells that are infected by herpesvirus
   a. Its mechanism of action parallels that of AZT
   b. Acycloguanosine triphosphate is a competitive inhibitor with respect to deoxyguanosine triphosphate, and it causes chain termination after it is incorporated into DNA

E. Incorporation of cytosine arabinoside into DNA is deleterious to cell viability

VII. Bioenergetics of polynucleotide synthesis

A. The bioenergetics of DNA polymerases, RNA polymerases, polyA polymerase, tRNA nucleotidyl transferase (which adds CCA to the transcript), and primase is the same

B. The substrates are nucleoside or deoxyribonucleoside triphosphates, and the products are nucleotide polymers, with high-energy phosphodiester bonds, and inorganic pyrophosphate

C. The hydrolysis of pyrophosphate as catalyzed by pyrophosphatase is an exergonic process that pulls the nucleotidyl transferase reactions forward

QUESTIONS

DIRECTIONS. (Items 1–18): Each of the numbered items or incomplete statements in this section is followed by answers or by completions of the statement. Select the ONE lettered answer or completion that is BEST in each case. Correct answers and explanations are given at the end of the chapter.

1. Which one of the following enzymes is required for the synthesis of hnRNA/mRNA in humans?
   (A) RNA polymerase I
   (B) RNA polymerase II
   (C) RNA polymerase III
   (D) $\alpha_2\beta\beta'\sigma$

2. All of the following DNA sequences play an important role in mediating human gene expression EXCEPT
   (A) TATA box
   (B) CAAT box
   (C) GC box
   (D) Enhancers
   (E) *lac* Operon

3. Both DNA polymerases and RNA polymerases are able to
   (A) initiate polynucleotide synthesis
   (B) remove mononucleotides from the 3′ end
   (C) remove mononucleotides from the 5′ end
   (D) synthesize polynucleotides in the 5′ to 3′ direction
   (E) catalyze the hydrolysis of pyrophosphate (PP_i)

4. The posttranscriptional processing of rRNA involves which one of the following events?
   (A) Hydrolytic cleavage of portions of the primary transcript
   (B) Addition of a guanylate cap with a 5′ to 5′ triphosphate bridge
   (C) Addition of a polyA tail
   (D) Displacement of lariat RNA with a ribose moiety containing 2′, 3′, and 5′ phosphate linkages
   (E) Addition of CCA to the 3′ terminus

5. Which one of the following factors binds to the TATA box and sets the stage for the initiation of hnRNA/mRNA transcription?
   (A) Fos-Jun
   (B) Reverse transcriptase
   (C) TFID
   (D) TFIID
   (E) TFIIIA

6. Processes that are required for immunoglobulin synthesis are listed below. Which one is the first to occur?
   (A) Heavy chain V_H-D joining
   (B) Heavy chain D-J_H joining
   (C) Light chain V-J joining
   (D) Removal of the intervening sequences between V_κ and J_κ of the light chain
   (E) Recombination of DNA sequences in a switch (S) region upstream from the $C\mu$ gene to a downstream region that is 5′ to the C_H region

7. Which one of the following is the primer for human AIDS virus reverse transcriptase?
   (A) $CD4^+$ protein
   (B) gp120
   (C) TFIIIA
   (D) Lysine tRNA
   (E) Proviral DNA

8. Which one of the following enzymes is derived from HIV-1 virus particles and degrades RNA from an RNA-DNA hybrid?
   (A) DNA ligase
   (B) DNA polymerase δ exonuclease
   (C) *Eco*RI
   (D) Reverse transcriptase
   (E) RNAse H

9. Which one of the following human genes lacks introns?
   (A) Dystrophin
   (B) Immunoglobulin G
   (C) Histone
   (D) LDL receptor
   (E) Thyroglobulin

10. Which one of the following human mRNAs lacks a polyA tail?
   (A) Dystrophin
   (B) Immunoglobulin G
   (C) Histone
   (D) LDL receptor
   (E) Thyroglobulin

11. Which one of the following immunoglobulins occurs in saliva, tears, milk, and intestinal secretions?
   (A) IgA
   (B) IgD
   (C) IgE
   (D) IgG
   (E) IgM

12. All of the following enzymes require a DNA or RNA template EXCEPT
   (A) DNA polymerase
   (B) RNA polymerase
   (C) Reverse transcriptase
   (D) Deoxynucleotidyl terminal transferase
   (E) Primase

Items 13–17

History

The patient is a 35-year-old auto mechanic who presented with cough, fatigue, fever, and night sweats of 3 months' duration. Although he had a history of intravenous drug use intermittently for 17 years, he considered himself to be in good health. His cough was nonproductive (did not produce sputum). He denied hemoptysis (coughing blood), chest pain, headaches, jaundice, homosexual contacts, multiple sexual partners, and blood transfusions after 1977 and prior to blood screening for HIV in 1985. He knew of no one with pneumonia or tuberculosis. He had been imprisoned on several occasions during the previous 10 years and said that many of the inmates had chronic coughs that he attributed to cigarette smoking. The patient smoked more than a pack of cigarettes daily for 20 years. He had drunk about a liter of whiskey weekly for several years. He had decreased his intake greatly over the past 3 months because of his illness. He was not taking any prescription medication. The patient never weighed himself but stated that his clothes had become loose and baggy over the past 3 months.

Physical Examination

Physical examination revealed a thin man who appeared chronically ill. His pulse was 88/min; respirations, 18/min; temperature, 39.1 °C (102.4 °F); blood pressure, 118/68 mm Hg; mouth, no thrush; skin, clear without colored nodules but with numerous old needle marks on both forearms. There was no lymphadenopathy. Percussion of the chest revealed dullness on the left posterior basal area; no rales were heard by auscultation. Funduscopic and cardiac examinations were normal, and there was no hepatosplenomegaly or nuchal rigidity (a sign of meningitis).

Laboratory

Hematocrit, 36% (normal ♂, 39–49%)
White blood count, 6600/mL (normal, 4500–11,000/mL)
$CD4^+$ cell count, 420/μL (normal, >500/μL)
Polymorphonuclear leukocytes, 52% (normal, 54–64%)
Lymphocytes, 25% (normal, 23–33%)
Blood urea nitrogen (BUN), 12 mg/dL (normal, 7–18 mg/dL)
Creatinine, 0.8 mg/dL (normal, 0.7–1.3 mg/dL)
γ-Glutamyl transpeptidase, 24 U/L (normal ♂, 9–50 U/L)
Aspartate aminotransferase (AST, SGOT), 18 U/L (normal, 10–30 U/L)
Amylase, 104 U/L (normal, 25–125 U/L)
Total bilirubin, 0.4 mg/dL (normal, 0.2–1.0 mg/dL)
Cholesterol, 178 mg/dL (recommended, <200 mg/dL)
Electrolytes and venous pH, normal
Serum glucose, 84 mg/dL (normal, 70–105 mg/dL)
Lactate dehydrogenase (LDH), 180 U/L (normal, 210–380 U/L)
Serum albumin, 3.2 g/dL (normal, 3.5–5.0 g/dL)
Globulin, 3.4 g/dL (normal, 2.2–4.0 g/dL)

VDRL for syphilis was negative. The chest x-ray revealed hilar lymphadenopathy and a pleural effusion on the left side with diffuse interstitial infiltration. No cavitation was observed. The patient was positive for HIV by ELISA (enzyme-linked immunosorbent assay) and by Western blotting. A sputum specimen was negative for gram-positive, gram-negative, and acid-fast organisms. Blood and pleural effusion samples were taken for culture and for microbiological analysis for *Pneumocystis carinii, Mycobacterium tuberculosis, Mycobacterium avium-intracellulare, Cryptococcus neoformans,* and cytomegalovirus. Polymerase chain reaction analyses were positive for HIV and *M. tuberculosis* in the pleural effusion; PCR was negative for *P. carinii, M. avium-intracellulare, C. neoformans,* and cytomegalovirus. A tuberculin skin test revealed 10 mm of induration after 48 hours. Tests for mumps and *Candida* were also positive. The patient was started on isoniazid, rifampin, pyrazinamide, and AZT.

13. Besides HIV, as exhibited in this patient, hepatitis B can be transmitted by contaminated needles. Each of the following laboratory findings indicates that this patient does not have hepatitis EXCEPT

(A) Aspartate aminotransferase
(B) Total bilirubin
(C) Cholesterol
(d) γ-Glutamyl transpeptidase
(e) Lactate dehydrogenase

14. Which one of the following functions is inhibited by rifampin?

(A) Bacterial DNA polymerase
(B) Bacterial RNA chain elongation
(C) Human DNA polymerase
(D) Initiation of bacterial RNA synthesis
(E) HIV reverse transcriptase

15. The desired target of AZT in this patient is

(A) bacterial DNA polymerase
(B) bacterial RNA chain elongation
(C) human DNA polymerase
(D) HIV protease
(E) HIV reverse transcriptase

16. Pyrazinamide exhibits liver toxicity. To monitor for possible liver damage in this patient, the following analysis was planned on a periodic basis

(A) Amylase
(B) Aspartate aminotransferase and γ-glutamyl transpeptidase
(C) Cholesterol
(D) Serum glucose determinations
(E) White blood cell count

17. The target sequences for the AIDS virus that were employed for the polymerase chain reaction corresponded to the *gag, pol,* and *gp120* genes. The *pol* gene of AIDS encodes each of the following functions EXCEPT

(A) protease
(B) reverse transcriptase
(C) $CD4^+$
(D) integrase
(E) RNAse H

ANSWERS AND EXPLANATIONS

1. The answer is B: RNA polymerase II is required for the synthesis of hnRNA/mRNA in humans. RNA polymerase I is required for ribosomal RNA synthesis (the primary transcript that is processed to produce 18S, 28S, and 5.8S rRNA). RNA polymerase III catalyzes the synthesis of tRNA and small RNAs including the 5S RNA of the ribosome. $\alpha_2\beta\beta'\sigma$ is the *E. coli* RNA polymerase. *Biochemistry,* p. 310.
2. The answer is E: *lac* Operon. The *lac* operon is a 17-nucleotide sequence that regulates the transcription of three bacterial enzymes including galactose kinase, galactose acetyltransferase, and galactose permease. The single mRNA that encodes these proteins is a polycistronic messenger, not found in humans. The TATA box, CAAT box, GC box, and enhancers all play an important role in mediating human gene expression. Promoter elements (TATA, GC, and CAAT boxes) identify the start site for transcription, and transcription elements alter the frequency of gene transcription. Most promoters for RNA polymerase II transcripts exhibit a TATA box about 30 nucleotides upstream from the start site. Upstream promoter elements can include one or more GC boxes around −70 to −90 and a CAAT box (pronounced "cat") at −100. The TATA box is called a selector, and its function is to pinpoint the start site. Transcription elements include enhancers, silencers, and response elements. Enhancers are DNA sequences that increase the frequency of gene transcription. These can be located either upstream or downstream from the start site and may be in either orientation

and still be active (either 5′ → 3′ or 3′ → 5′). Silencers exhibit many of the same properties as enhancers except that they decrease the frequency of gene transcription. Often there are repeats of the same sequence, and the multiplicity yields more powerful regulatory effects. Response elements are target sequences for signaling molecules such as cyclic AMP. *Biochemistry*, pp. 309, 312.

3. The answer is D: synthesize polynucleotides in the 5′ to 3′ direction (PRINCIPLE 29 OF BIOCHEMISTRY). RNA but not DNA polymerases are able to initiate polynucleotide synthesis. Bacterial DNA polymerases are able to remove mononucleotides from the 3′ end (proofreading activity) and 5′ end (repair activity). Human DNA polymerases lack the 5′ to 3′ exonuclease activity; other proteins associated with the polymerases probably have this activity. RNA polymerases lack both nuclease activities. Pyrophosphatase, the enzyme that catalyzes the hydrolysis of pyrophosphate, is an independent enzyme and is not part of DNA or RNA polymerase. *Biochemistry*, pp. 306, 316.
4. The answer is A: hydrolytic cleavage of portions of the primary transcript. The RNA polymerase I primary transcript undergoes hydrolytic reactions to liberate 18S, 28S, and 5.8S RNA. These RNA molecules also undergo methylation reactions with *S*-adenosylmethionine as the activated methyl donor. Addition of a guanylate cap with a 5′ to 5′ triphosphate bridge and a polyA tail occurs in human mRNA synthesis. Displacement of lariat RNA with a ribose moiety containing 2′, 3′, and 5′ phosphate linkages occurs during intron removal as hnRNA is converted to mature mRNA. CCA is found universally at the 3′ end of tRNA, and a single enzyme catalyzes the addition of all three nucleotides to tRNAs that lack it. *Biochemistry*, pp. 316–325.
5. The answer is D: TFIID. Binding of TFIID is the primary interaction required for the expression of human genes that encode for proteins. The Fos-Jun complex interacts with AP1 sites corresponding to polymerase II transcripts. Reverse transcriptase is responsible for the synthesis of DNA directed by an RNA template (and DNA template). TFID participates in the expression of RNA polymerase I transcripts. TFIIIA binds to internal control regions of 5S rRNA genes and is a zinc finger protein (one of the first to be described). *Biochemistry*, p. 312.
6. The answer is B: heavy chain D-J_H joining. Following D-J_H joining, V-J joining and heavy chain expression occurs. This is followed by light chain production that involves V-J joining. IgM is expressed in the plasma membrane. Alternative splicing of the corresponding primary transcript is the isotype switching responsible for IgD synthesis. All these processes are antigen independent. Following antigenic stimulation, isotype switching to IgA, IgG, and IgE results from DNA rearrangement. *Biochemistry*, pp. 310, 312.
7. The answer is D: lysine tRNA. All DNA polymerases, including reverse transcriptase, require a primer. The primer for the AIDS virus reverse transcriptase is lysine tRNA which contains an 18-nucleotide segment that is complementary to 18 nucleotides of the viral RNA genome. Although tRNAs serve as primers for different retroviruses, their identity differs. Tryptophan tRNA, for example, serves as the primer for Rous sarcoma virus, the first retrovirus to be discovered. $CD4^+$ protein is not a primer but is the protein in lymphocytes that is recognized by the AIDS virus and promotes invasion (but the mechanism is unknown). gp120 Is a glycoprotein found in the AIDS virus envelope that is required for infection of target T cells. *Biochemistry*, p. 334.
8. The answer is E: RNAse H. This RNAse activity is unique in its ability to degrade RNA in an RNA-DNA hybrid. DNA ligase seals nicks in duplex DNA, and proofreading exonuclease catalyzes the 3′ to 5′ hydrolytic removal of a nucleotide that is mismatched with the base on the template. *Eco*RI is a bacterial restriction enzyme that catalyzes the site-specific cleavage of DNA at a GAATTC palindrome. Reverse transcriptase can synthesize DNA using an RNA and then a DNA template. *Biochemistry*, p. 334.
9. The answer is C: histone. Nearly all human genes that encode proteins contain introns. Interferon-α gene and histone genes lack introns, but this situation is rare. *Biochemistry*, pp. 311, 331.
10. The answer is C: histone. Nearly all human mRNAs possess a polyA tail. Histone mRNA is a commonly cited exception to this rule. *Biochemistry*, p. 319.
11. The answer is A: IgA. IgA is the antibody type that occurs in various secretions including tears, saliva, milk, and intestinal secretions. Newborns have the ability to absorb immunoglobulins intact from the colostrum of the mother's milk, and this provides passive immunity. IgG is the chief circulating antibody, and it can cross the placenta. IgM (a membrane–associated immunoglobulin) is the first antibody expressed by each B cell, and IgD is the second. The function of IgD is unclear. IgE is involved in allergic responses, and its levels increase with certain parasitic infections. *Biochemistry*, p. 326.
12. The answer is D: deoxynucleotidyl terminal transferase. This enzyme, along with polyA polymerase and tRNA nucleotidyl transferase, is able to catalyze polynucleotide elongation that is NOT directed by a template. Deoxynucleotidyl terminal transferase adds a few bases during D to J_H and V_H to D joining reactions of immunoglobulin rearrangement. Terminal transferase, one of the recombinases, is active in developing B lymphocytes. *Biochemistry*, p. 337.
13. The answer is C: cholesterol. Aspartate aminotransferase, bilirubin, γ-glutamyl transpeptidase, and lactate dehydrogenase are commonly elevated in patients with active hepatitis. Normal cholesterol levels are NOT diagnostic or helpful in making a diagnosis of hepatitis. *Biochemistry*, pp. 61–63.
14. The answer is D: initiation of bacterial RNA synthesis. Rifampin does not inhibit RNA polymerase elongation reactions, only the initiation process. Although the σ-subunit is uniquely associated with the initiation process, RNA polymerase mutants found in bacteria correspond to the β-subunit of the RNA polymerase holoenzyme. *M. tuberculosis* bacteria that are resistant to multiple drugs lack active catalase-peroxidase genes; how this relates to antibiotic resistance is unclear. The recommended treatment for tuberculosis includes isoniazid, rifampin, and pyrazinamide for at least 2 months. Continuation therapy should include isoniazid and rifampin for a minimum of 9 months. Ethambutol should be added for those with central nervous system involvement or when isoniazid resistance occurs. A lack of headaches and nuchal rigidity rules unlikely any central nervous system involvement in this patient. Symptoms of night sweats, cough, and fever are classical presenting symptoms of tuberculosis. Hemoptysis and cavitary lesions in the apex (superior portion) of the lung are also characteristic of uncomplicated tuberculosis, but they were not seen in this patient and are not seen in many other AIDS patients. This patient, an intravenous drug user, is in a high-risk category for AIDS. That the patient is infected by the AIDS virus is indicated by the ELISA test (enzyme-linked immunosorbent assay). The ELISA

test for AIDS, which is based upon the use of antigens corresponding to proteins of HIV that have been adsorbed to a solid surface and antibodies to which an enzyme has been linked, is used for screening. Because there are many false positives, it is necessary to confirm positive ELISA results by Western blotting. The diagnosis was further confirmed in this patient by polymerase chain reaction (PCR) methodology, currently a specialized test. Tuberculosis in AIDS patients can differ from the usual clinical picture of pulmonary tuberculosis in adults. The tuberculin test is negative in the majority of AIDS patients, but this patient responded. An AIDS patient may be infected with *M. tuberculosis* but may fail to respond to the antigenic stimulation of protein derived from the tubercle bacillus (purified protein derivative [PPD]) because of an impaired immune response. To assess the ability to respond to antigenic stimulation, mumps and *Candida* antigens are given as positive controls. Nearly all adults with normal immune responses will react with these antigens because of previous exposure. This patient reacted to all three tests, indicating that he was not yet severely immunocompromised. His $CD4^+$ count, which is almost normal, also indicates that he is not severely immunocompromised. It is not uncommon for an AIDS patient who is skin-test positive to become negative with progression of the disease. Sputum cultures are more often positive than sputum examinations for acid-fast bacilli, but these cultures may take 6 weeks before organisms begin to grow. The recent introduction of polymerase chain reaction technology for the diagnosis of infectious disease can decrease this time to a few days or less. PCR methods will detect fewer than 10 organisms, in comparison to the 10,000/mL necessary for a positive sputum smear. Besides tuberculosis, *Cryptococcus neoformans* and cytomegalovirus, which occur in individuals with AIDS, can cause meningitis. AIDS itself, moreover, can produce dementia. Patients that are HIV positive are generally treated prophylactically with isoniazid to prevent the development of tuberculosis. *Biochemistry*, pp. 337, 339–340; *Cecil*, p. 1734.

15. The answer is E: HIV reverse transcriptase. Azidothymidine is converted to AZT triphosphate, a competitive inhibitor *in vitro* of reverse transcriptase when the varied substrate is thymidine triphosphate. Moreover, AZT is incorporated into the DNA polynucleotide. Since the resulting DNA lacks a free 3′-hydroxyl group, chain termination occurs. Resistance to AZT that occurs in HIV infection is related to a mutation of codon 215 of reverse transcriptase. Resistance to ddI (dideoxyinosine) is associated with mutations involving codon 74. Several other mutations in reverse transcriptase have been described. There is a positive correlation between these mutations and a decline in $CD4^+$ cells. The development of inhibitors of HIV protease represents another avenue in the therapy for AIDS. *Biochemistry*, pp. 335, 340.
16. The answer is B: aspartate aminotransferase and γ-glutamyl transpeptidase. Aspartate aminotransferase, alanine aminotransferase, and γ-glutamyl transpeptidase are among serum enzymes that can be used to monitor hepatic dysfunction. Amylase is used to monitor pancreatic inflammation. Although glucose and cholesterol are liver metabolites, these are not sensitive indicators of liver function. Although this patient gave a history that suggests alcohol abuse, liver function tests including γ-glutamyl transpeptidase were normal, indicating that his alcohol intake has not produced liver disease. *Biochemistry*, pp. 61–63.
17. The answer is C: $CD4^+$. $CD4^+$ is encoded by the human host. Reverse transcriptase, RNAse H, and integrase are enzymes that are required for synthesis and integration of the virus into the host genome. An HIV protease is responsible for cleaving virally encoded polyproteins into the active functional units, and HIV protease represents a potential target for anti-AIDS drugs. *Biochemistry*, p. 334; *Cecil*, p. 1913.

REFERENCES

Roskoski, R., Jr. *Biochemistry*. Philadelphia, W. B. Saunders Company, 1996.

Wyngaarden, J. B., L. H. Smith, Jr., and J. C. Bennett (eds.). *Cecil Textbook of Medicine*, 19th ed. Philadelphia, W. B. Saunders Company, 1992.

CHAPTER SEVENTEEN

PROTEIN AND PEPTIDE BIOSYNTHESIS

SYNOPSIS

OBJECTIVES

1. To enumerate the salient aspects of the genetic code.
2. To describe the composition of the bacterial and human ribosomes.
3. To outline the reactions in the synthesis of aminoacyl-tRNA molecules.
4. To outline the steps of protein synthesis.
5. To compare bacterial and human protein synthesis.
6. To calculate the ATP requirement for peptide bond synthesis.
7. To depict mitochondrial DNA, RNA, and protein synthesis.

Objective 1: To enumerate the salient aspects of the genetic code.

I. mRNA-dependent protein synthesis
   A. The translation of the nucleic acid code of four letters to the protein code of 20 letters is an intricate process requiring more than 150 components
   B. The genetic code of nucleic acids specifies the amino acids found in proteins
      1. Each amino acid in a protein is encoded by three bases in RNA (PRINCIPLE 26 OF BIOCHEMISTRY)
      2. *AUG functions as the initiation codon, and methionine is the initiating amino acid for protein synthesis in humans, other animals, bacteria, and viruses*
      3. The genetic code is read triplet by triplet from the 5′ to 3′ direction of mRNA until a stop codon is reached
      4. Of the 64 possible codons of the standard genetic code, all but three—**UAG, UAA, UGA**—correspond to an amino acid (Table 17–1)
      5. For reading the biomedical literature, it is helpful to know that **AUG** corresponds to methionine and chain initiation and that **UAG, UAA,** and **UGA** produce chain termination
      6. Base pairing between the codon of mRNA and the anticodon in tRNA is antiparallel (PRINCIPLE 28 OF BIOCHEMISTRY)
         a. Nonstandard base pairing occurs between the 3′ position of the codon in mRNA and 5′ position of the anticodon in tRNA, and these sites are therefore designated as the wobble position
         b. Wobble base pairing allows one tRNA to interact with more than one codon

Objective 2: To describe the composition of the bacterial and human ribosomes.

II. Ribosomes: biochemical machines for protein synthesis
   A. Composition of *Escherichia coli* ribosomes
      1. The *E. coli* ribosome is a **70S** ribosome made up of one large and one small subunit
      2. The 30S subunit contains one molecule of rRNA (16S) and 21 proteins
      3. The 50S subunit contains 23S RNA, 5S RNA, and 35 proteins
      4. The 70S ribosome contains two functional sites termed the A site and the P site
         a. *A*minoacyl-tRNA binds at the **A site,** and *p*eptidyl-tRNA binds at the **P site**
         b. The activity that catalyzes peptide bond formation (**peptidyltransferase**) occurs in the large subunit
   B. Composition of eukaryotic ribosomes
      1. Human cytoplasmic ribosomes are larger with S values of **80S** for the whole ribosome and **60S** and **40S** for the large and small subunits, respectively
      2. The sedimentation coefficient of the mitochondrial ribosomes is about **60S**

Objective 3: To outline the reactions in the synthesis of aminoacyl-tRNA molecules.

III. Amino acid activation for protein biosynthesis
   A. Properties of aminoacyl-tRNA
      1. tRNA molecules are small RNA molecules consisting of 75–95 nucleotides

TABLE 17–1. The Standard Genetic Code

First letter (5′)	U		C		A		G		Third letter (3′)
	Second letter								
U	UUU	Phe	UCU	Ser	UAU	Tyr	UGU	Cys	U
	UUC	Phe	UCC	Ser	UAC	Tyr	UGC	Cys	C
	UUA	Leu	UCA	Ser	UAA	Stop	UGA	Stop	A
	UUG	Leu	UCG	Ser	UAG	Stop	UGG	Trp	G
C	CUU	Leu	CCU	Pro	CAU	His	CGU	Arg	U
	CUC	Leu	CCC	Pro	CAC	His	CGC	Arg	C
	CUA	Leu	CCA	Pro	CAA	Gln	CGA	Arg	A
	CUG	Leu	CCG	Pro	CAG	Gln	CGG	Arg	G
A	AUU	Ile	ACU	Thr	AAU	Asn	AGU	Ser	U
	AUC	Ile	ACC	Thr	AAC	Asn	AGC	Ser	C
	AUA	Ile	ACA	Thr	AAA	Lys	AGA	Arg	A
	AUG	Met	ACG	Thr	AAG	Lys	AGG	Arg	G
G	GUU	Val	GCU	Ala	GAU	Asp	GGU	Gly	U
	GUC	Val	GCC	Ala	GAC	Asp	GGC	Gly	C
	GUA	Val	GCA	Ala	GAA	Glu	GGA	Gly	A
	GUG	Val	GCG	Ala	GAG	Glu	GGG	Gly	G

2. Each amino acid is attached to the ribose of an adenosine residue via a high-energy bond at the 3′ end of tRNA, which ends with 5′. . .**CCA** 3′
3. tRNA can be represented as a two-dimensional cloverleaf structure with three loops, called (1) the **dihydrouridine loop,** (2) the **anticodon loop,** and (3) the **T loop** (for ribo*t*hymidine)

B. Formation of aminoacyl-tRNA
1. The enzymes that catalyze the activation of amino acids are called **amino acyl-tRNA synthetases—**one for each of the 20 standard amino acids used to make proteins
2. The following reaction is isoergonic, but it is pulled by PP_i hydrolysis in accordance with PRINCIPLE 14 OF BIOCHEMISTRY:

$$\text{ATP} + \text{tRNA} + \text{amino acid} \rightleftharpoons \text{AMP} + PP_i + \text{aminoacyl-tRNA}$$

IV. Components of protein synthesis

A. In bacteria, the *i*nitiation *f*actors are designated **IF,** the *e*longation *f*actors are designated **EF,** and the *r*elease *f*actors are designated **RF**

B. The factors in eukaryotes are similarly designated with an e prefix for *e*ukaryotic (for example, eIF for *e*ukaryotic *i*nitiation *f*actor)

C. Methionine-$tRNA_I^{Met}$ initiates protein synthesis in the cytosol of humans and other eukaryotes, and methionine-$tRNA^{Met}$ participates in the elongation reactions
1. In bacteria and in mitochondria, methionine-$tRNA_I^{Met}$ is converted to *N*-formyl-methionine $tRNA_I^{Met}$ prior to its use as the chain initiator
2. **IF2** (bacterial) and **eIF2** (eukaryotic) complex with aminoacylated initiator tRNA (*N*-formyl-Met-$tRNA_I^{Met}$ and Met-$tRNA_I^{Met}$, respectively) and GTP; these factors place initiator methionine-tRNA into the P site of the ribosome during chain initiation

D. Elongation factors are required for the synthesis of the multiple peptide bonds occurring in a polypeptide or protein
1. EF-T (elongation *f*actor-*t*ransfer) in bacteria consists of two components called **EF-Tu** (pronounced "ee eff tee you") and **EF-Ts** ("ee eff tee ess")
   a. The corresponding eEF1 in eukaryotes consists of α, β, and γ subunits
   b. EF-Tu or eEF1 each form **ternary complexes** consisting of (1) the protein factor, (2) aminoacyl-tRNA, and (3) GTP
   c. *Transfer factors deliver (transfer) the aminoacyl-tRNA to the A site of the ribosome;* the particular aminoacyl-tRNA that is placed in the A site is the one that is determined by specific codon-anticodon base pairing
   d. GTP is hydrolyzed to GDP and P_i, and Tu · GDP or eEF1α · GDP dissociates from the ribosome
2. The second class of elongation factor is EF-G (bacterial) and eEF2 (eukaryotic)
   a. These factors participate in the translocation of peptidyl-tRNA from the A site of the ribosome to the P site
   b. GTP is hydrolyzed to GDP and P_i during the process

E. Release factors recognize termination codons and promote the hydrolysis of peptidyl-tRNA

Objective 4: To outline the steps of protein synthesis.

V. Steps of protein biosynthesis

A. Formation of the initiation complex
1. Initiation factors, initiator methionine tRNA, mRNA, and the small ribosomal subunit interact
2. The large subunit combines with the complex, GTP is hydrolyzed, and methionine initiator tRNA is found in the P site
3. In prokaryotes, the Shine-Dalgarno sequence of rRNA interacts with a complementary region on mRNA to select the correct initiating AUG codon before *N*-formylmethionine tRNA binds to the complex
4. In eukaryotes, the 40S subunit and methionine initiator tRNA bind to the 5′ end of monocistronic mRNA and scan along the message until the first AUG is encountered

B. Elongation and translocation
1. An elongation factor delivers aminoacyl-tRNA to the A site based on specific codon-anticodon interaction, and GTP is hydrolyzed
2. Peptidyltransferase catalyzes peptide bond formation, and peptidyl-tRNA is found in the A site
3. The second elongation factor catalyzes the translocation of mRNA-peptidyl-RNA from the A site to the P site, and GTP is hydrolyzed

C. Release of polypeptides
1. When one of three termination codons occurs in the P site, release factors convert peptidyltransferase activity to hydrolase activity and peptidyl-tRNA is hydrolyzed
2. The ribosomes and mRNA dissociate

Objective 5: To compare bacterial and human protein synthesis.

VI. Comparison of bacterial and eukaryotic protein synthesis
  A. Bacteria use formylated Met-tRNA$_{I}^{Met}$ for initiation, and eukaryotes use unformylated Met-tRNA$_{I}^{Met}$
  B. Bacteria possess a sequence in mRNA near the initiating AUG codon that binds to a Shine-Dalgarno sequence in 16 S rRNA; eukaryotes lack the Shine-Dalgarno sequence
  C. The small ribosomal subunit and eIF4E of eukaryotes recognize the 7-methylguanine cap at the 5′ end of mRNA; the small ribosomal subunit with the attached initiator tRNA scans the mRNA from the 5′ end toward the 3′ end in search of the first AUG codon, which is then used to form the initiation complex
  D. Bacterial messenger RNAs can be either **monocistronic** or **polycistronic;** eukaryotic mRNAs are monocistronic

VII. The inhibitory action of antibiotics on bacterial protein synthesis is given in Table 17–2

Objective 6: To calculate the ATP requirement for peptide bond synthesis.

VIII. Bioenergetics of protein synthesis
  A. The activation of each amino acid as aminoacyl-tRNA requires the expenditure of two high-energy bonds (ATP → AMP + 2 P$_i$)
  B. Placement of aminoacyl-tRNA in the A site requires hydrolysis of GTP to GDP and P$_i$ (the expenditure of one high-energy bond)
  C. Similarly, translocation is also accompanied by the hydrolysis of GTP to GDP and P$_i$
  D. *A minimum of four high-energy bonds is thus required for the synthesis of each peptide bond during protein biosynthesis*
    1. The participation of chaperones in the formation of the active conformation of a protein results in the expenditure of additional ATP to form a functional protein
    2. The large amount of energy needed for peptide bond formation is the price required for converting the four-letter alphabet of nucleic acids to the 20-letter alphabet of proteins

Objective 7: To depict mitochondrial DNA, RNA, and protein synthesis.

IX. Mitochondrial DNA, RNA, and protein synthesis
  A. DNA synthesis
    1. Each mitochondrion contains between five and 10 copies of supercoiled circular DNA
    2. DNA polymerase γ is the mitochondrial polymerase
    3. Replication is bidirectional with unique origins of replication for the H strand and the L strand; each strand is synthesized continuously (no Okazaki fragments)
  B. RNA and protein synthesis
    1. Both strands of mitochondrial DNA are transcribed from a unique heavy and a unique light strand promoter that occurs in the D-loop region of the genome
    2. One strand is transcribed in the clockwise direction, and the other is transcribed in the counterclockwise direction
    3. mRNA molecules in mitochondria are not capped
    4. The first trinucleotide of each mRNA is an AUG that serves as the initiating codon for protein synthesis, and this is an unusual property
    5. The initiating amino acid in mitochondrial protein synthesis is *N*-formyl-Met-tRNA$_{I}^{Met}$ and thereby resembles the bacterial initiation process
    6. The mitochondrion contains all of the genes for mitochondrial tRNA molecules and rRNAs and about 20% of the genes for the proteins of the electron transport chain and ATP synthase; all other mitochondrial proteins are encoded by the nucleus

TABLE 17–2. Action of Antibiotics that Inhibit Bacterial Protein or Peptidoglycan Synthesis

Antibiotic	Site of Action	Mechanism	Use
Aminoglycosides (streptomycin, gentamicin)	30S subunit	Inhibit initiation, produce mistakes in translation	Gram negative
Cephalosporin	Cell wall	Inhibits transpeptidase cross-linking	Gram positive and gram negative
Chloramphenicol	50S subunit	Inhibits peptidyltransferase activity	Broad spectrum
Erythromycin	50S subunit	Inhibits translocation	Gram positive and gram negative
Penicillin	Cell wall	Inhibits transpeptidase cross-linking	Gram positive
Tetracycline	30S subunit	Inhibits aminoacyl-tRNA binding to the A site	Broad spectrum
Vancomycin	Cell wall	Blocks transfer of pentapeptide from cytoplasm to cell membrane	Gram positive

QUESTIONS

DIRECTIONS. (Items 1–6): Each set of matching questions in this section consists of a list of several lettered options followed by several numbered items. For each numbered item, select the ONE lettered option that is most closely associated with it. Each lettered option may be selected once, more than once, or not at all. Correct answers and explanations are given at the end of the chapter.

Items 1–3

(A) Initiation factor 1 (IF1)
(B) Initiation factor 2 (IF2)
(C) Initiation factor 3 (IF3)
(D) Elongation factor Tu (EF-Tu)
(E) Elongation factor Ts (EF-Ts)
(F) Elongation factor G (EF-G)
(G) Release factor 1 (RF1)
(H) Release factor 2 (RF2)

For each given characteristic, select the correct protein synthesis factor.

1. Binds *N*-formylmethionine $tRNA_{I}^{Met}$ and GTP
2. Binds methionine-tRNA and GTP
3. Mediates the exchange of GTP for GDP

Items 4–6

(A) Eukaryotic initiation factor 1 (eIF1)
(B) Eukaryotic initiation factor 2 (eIF2)
(C) Eukaryotic initiation factor 3 (eIF3)
(D) Eukaryotic initiation factor 4E (eIF4E)
(E) Eukaryotic elongation factor 1α (eEF1α)
(F) Eukaryotic elongation factor 1$\beta\gamma$ (eEF1$\beta\gamma$)
(G) Eukaryotic elongation factor (eEF2)
(H) Eukaryotic release factor (eRF)

For each biochemical description, select the correct protein synthesis factor

4. Recognizes the mRNA cap
5. Target of diphtheria toxin
6. Inserts aminoacyl-tRNA into the A site

DIRECTIONS. (Items 7–18): Each of the numbered items or incomplete statements in this section is followed by answers or by completions of the statement. Select the ONE lettered answer or completion that is BEST in each case.

7. Which one of the following bases, when it occurs in the wobble position in tRNA, can bind to three different bases (A, U, and C) in mRNA?

(A) Adenine
(B) Cytosine
(C) Guanosine
(D) Inosine
(E) Uracil

8. All of the following are intrinsic characteristics of the ribosome EXCEPT

(A) A site
(B) P site
(C) eEF-1 activity
(D) peptidyltransferase activity
(E) small and large subunit

9. The following equation shows the reaction for catalyzing aminoacyl-tRNA formation: ATP + tRNA + amino acid $\rightleftharpoons$ AMP + PP_i + aminoacyl-tRNA. All of the following are correct statements concerning the synthesis of aminoacyl-tRNA EXCEPT

(A) One enzyme catalyzes the formation of methionine tRNA and leucine tRNA from their reactants
(B) The amino acid forms a special oxygen ester with the 3′-terminal nucleotide of tRNA
(C) The products contain the same number of high-energy bonds as the reactants
(D) The reaction is functionally isoergonic
(E) A separate pyrophosphatase catalyzes the hydrolysis of pyrophosphate

10. GTP hydrolysis is required for each of the following activities EXCEPT

(A) chain initiation
(B) implanting aminoacyl-tRNA into the A site
(C) the peptidyltransferase reaction
(D) translocation
(E) chain termination and dissociation of the ribosomal subunits

11. Gelatin, a foodstuff that is derived from collagen, lacks tryptophan and cysteine. A diet that consists only of gelatin leads to a negative nitrogen balance (nitrogen excretion exceeds nitrogen intake) and decreased protein synthesis. The primary mechanism responsible for decreased protein synthesis in a diet lacking tryptophan is

(A) decreased ATP production
(B) failure to synthesize any aminoacyl-tRNA
(C) failure of mRNAs containing codons corresponding to tryptophan to bind to ribosomes
(D) failure to form an initiation complex
(E) failure to elongate polypeptides directed by mRNAs containing codons corresponding to tryptophan

12. Which of the following is a true statement regarding mitochondria?

(A) They contain their own unique DNA and RNA polymerases
(B) They contain linear DNA molecules
(C) They contain histones
(D) They divide at the same time as the cell
(E) They each contain one DNA molecule

13. The number of high-energy bonds required for the synthesis of each peptide bond during protein synthesis is
    (A) 0
    (B) 1
    (C) 2
    (D) 3
    (E) 4

14. Both prokaryotic and cytosolic eukaryotic protein synthesis involve which one of the following?
    (A) A Shine-Dalgarno sequence
    (B) A scanning mechanism for chain initiation
    (C) Unique methionine tRNAs for chain initiation and for chain elongation
    (D) Monocistronic and polycistronic mRNA molecules
    (E) Transfer of peptidyl-tRNA from the P site to the A site on the ribosome

Items 15–18

History

The patient is a 60-year-old woman who has severe bilateral low back pain, chills, fever to 40.0 °C (104 °F), and difficulty breathing of 2 days' duration. She has vomited after eating during this period. She notes that her urine was cloudy and had an unpleasant odor. The patient denies hematuria, dysuria (pain with urination), cough, chest pain, or diarrhea, nor has she experienced trauma to the back or physical exertion that might account for back pain. She denies knowing anyone with tuberculosis. She had a kidney infection 6 years previously, and kidney stones passed spontaneously. She says the pain from kidney stones was more severe than her present pain. The kidney infection was treated with sulfa drugs, which cured the infection but caused a skin rash and itching. She denies weight loss, abdominal pain, diarrhea, or blood in her stool.

Physical Examination

Physical examination reveals a temperature of 39.1 °C (102.5 °F); respiratory rate, 18/min; pulse, 90/min; blood pressure, 112/78 mm Hg; weight, 54 kg (118 lb); height 161 cm (5 ft, 3 in.). The patient appears to be in moderately acute distress with back pain. The results of the examination of the lungs and heart are unremarkable. Her abdomen is nontender with diminished bowel sounds. There is marked tenderness of both the right and left costovertebral angles to percussion. Results of pelvic and rectal examinations were normal.

Laboratory

Sodium, 128 mEq/L (normal, 135–145 mEq/L)
Potassium, 3.8 mEq/L (normal, 3.5–5.0 mEq/L)
Chloride, 93 mEq/L (normal, 100–110) mEq/L)
Carbon dioxide, 25 mEq/L (normal, 25–30 mEq/L)
Creatinine, 0.6 mg/dL (normal ♀, 0.6–1.1 mg/dL)
Blood urea nitrogen (BUN), 13 mg/dL (normal, 7–18 mg/dL)
Amylase, 37 U/L (normal, 25–125 U/L)
Lipase, 54 U/L (normal, 10–140 U/L)
Aspartate aminotransferase (AST, SGOT), 16 U/L (normal, 10–30 U/L)
Lactate dehydrogenase (LDH), 262 U/L (normal, 210–380 U/L)
Calcium, 9.8 mg/dL (normal, 8.4–10.2 mg/dL)
Phosphorus, 3.7 mg/dL (normal, 2.7–4.5 mg/dL)
Uric acid, 3.9 mg/dL (normal, 2.6–6.0 mg/dL)
Serum glucose, 72 mg/dL (normal, 70–105 mg/dL)
White blood cell count, 20,300/μL (normal, 4500–11,000/μL)
Hematocrit, 38.4% (normal ♀, 35–45%)
Neutrophils, 85% (normal, 54–62%)
Bands, 4% (normal, 3–5%)
Lymphocytes, 9% (normal, 23–33%)

Urinalysis showed a specific gravity of 1.022; many red and white blood cells were observed in an unspun specimen. The chest x-ray was normal. An ultrasound examination revealed several stones in the left calyx; the right kidney appeared normal. A specimen for a urine culture and antibiotic sensitivity was obtained, and the patient was immediately started on ampicillin and gentamicin.

15. The history, physical, and laboratory examination are consistent with a diagnosis of
    (A) gout
    (B) hepatitis
    (C) hyperparathyroidism
    (D) pancreatitis
    (E) pyelonephritis

16. *E. coli* infections are commonly treated with pyrimethamine and sulfoxazole. Because of the history of allergy to sulfa drugs, these were not used in this patient. Ampicillin, a penicillin analogue, exerts its antibacterial action by inhibiting
    (A) the extracytoplasmic transpeptidation at D-alanyl-D-alanine
    (B) ribosome-dependent chain initiation
    (C) peptidyl-tRNA translocation
    (D) glycine-tRNA synthesis
    (E) undecaprenyl phosphate synthesis

17. Gentamicin, an aminoglycoside with a mechanism of action similar to that of streptomycin, exerts its antibacterial effect by
    (A) inhibiting bacterial protein synthesis termination
    (B) inhibiting peptidyltransferase activity
    (C) inhibiting the implantation of aminoacyl-tRNA into the A site of the ribosome
    (D) causing misreading of the genetic code

18. The patient did not improve after 3 days of therapy. The urine culture showed *E. coli* that were not sensitive to ampicillin or gentamicin but were sensitive to tetracycline. She was switched to tetracycline, a drug that exerts its antibacterial effect by
    (A) inhibiting bacterial protein synthesis termination
    (B) inhibiting peptidyltransferase activity
    (C) inhibiting the implantation of aminoacyl-tRNA into the A site of the ribosome
    (D) causing misreading of the genetic code

ANSWERS AND EXPLANATIONS

1. The answer is B: initiation factor 2 (IF2). Initiation factor 2 (IF2) binds GTP and *N*-formylmethionine $tRNA_f^{Met}$; IF2 does not bind methionine $tRNA^{Met}$ and thus does not initiate bacterial protein synthesis with the incorrect form of the amino acid. *Biochemistry,* p. 350.
2. The answer is D: elongation factor Tu (EF-Tu). Elongation factor Tu (EF-Tu) binds methionine-tRNA and GTP; it does not bind *N*-formylmethionine $tRNA_f^{Met}$. If the formyl group were inadvertently placed in the A site, elongation could not occur. EF-Tu binds each of the aminoacyl-tRNAs that participate in protein synthesis. The release factors do not bind any form of aminoacyl-tRNA. *Biochemistry,* p. 350.
3. The answer is E: elongation factor Ts (EF-Ts). Elongation factor Ts (EF-Ts) mediates the exchange of GTP for GDP and readies EF-Tu for the next transferase reaction. *Biochemistry,* p. 350.
4. The answer is D: eukaryotic initiation factor 4E (eIF4E). eIF4E recognizes mRNA cap. eIF1 assists mRNA binding to the ribosome; eIF2 binds initiator Met-$tRNA_i^{Met}$ and GTP; eIF3 binds to 40S subunit prior to mRNA binding. *Biochemistry,* p. 351.
5. The answer is G: eukaryotic elongation factor (eEF2). *Corynebacterium diphtheriae,* the causative agent of diphtheria, contains a bacteriophage that encodes the gene for diphtheria toxin. The toxin binds to host cells and undergoes proteolytic cleavage to form an A and B chain. The A chain enters the cell by a process that requires the aid of the B chain. The A fragment catalyzes the ADP-ribosylation of eEF2 (NAD^+ is the donor). Following chemical modification, the elongation factor is inactivated. The site of ADP-ribosylation involves a posttranslationally modified histidine residue called diphthamide that occurs nearly exclusively in eEF2. *Biochemistry,* pp. 351, 359.
6. The answer is E: eukaryotic elongation factor 1α (eEF1α). This factor delivers aminoacyl-tRNA into the A site. After this occurs, GTP is hydrolyzed to GDP and P_i. eEF1$\beta\gamma$ mediates the exchange of GTP for GDP so that the factor can act again. *Biochemistry,* p. 353.
7. The answer is D: inosine. Inosine, which is a purine that does not occur in mRNA, contains a keto group on C^6. Inosine, which is derived from adenosine by hydrolytic deamination, resembles guanine in its base-pairing properties and readily pairs with cytosine. It has wider base-pairing potential and forms hydrogen bonds with both pyrimidines (uracil and cytosine) and with the opposite purine (adenine). It is unable to base pair with guanine, which it closely resembles. Cytosine in the anticodon can base pair only with guanine; this permits unique pairing of AUG (the unique initiating codon for methionine) with UAC in the anticodon. Uracil and guanosine can bind with two bases; uracil with two purines (A, G), and guanosine with two pyrimidines (U, C). Surprisingly, adenine does not occur in the wobble position of tRNA from any species. *Biochemistry,* p. 344.
8. The answer is C: eEF-1 activity. eEF-1 is a cytosolic and nonribosomal protein that carries aminoacyl-tRNA into the A (aminoacyl) site of the ribosome. The second ribosomal site is the P (peptidyl) site. The ribosome possesses peptidyltransferase activity. Ribosomes consist of a small and large subunit. These subunits dissociate when polypeptide synthesis is complete, and a small and large subunit reassociate during the protein synthesis initiation process. *Biochemistry,* pp. 346, 349.
9. The answer is A: one enzyme does NOT catalyze the formation of methionine-tRNA and leucine tRNA from their reactants. There is a single cytosolic amino acid tRNA synthetase for each of the 20 standard amino acids. Although there are two different tRNAs that correspond to methionine, a single methionine tRNA synthetase catalyzes the reaction between methionine and each of the tRNAs. Multiple tRNAs exist for most of the other amino acids, and a single amino acid tRNA synthetase catalyzes the combination of the specific amino acid with each one of them. The synthetase reaction is functionally isoergonic and proceeds without the loss of any high-energy bonds. Pyrophosphatase catalyzes the cleavage of pyrophosphate, a product of the amino acid tRNA synthetase reaction, to pull the reaction forward. *Biochemistry,* pp. 347, 349.
10. The answer is C: the peptidyltransferase reaction. GTP hydrolysis is required during chain initiation, implanting aminoacyl-tRNA into the A site, translocation, and chain termination. Only the peptidyltransferase reaction involving the reaction of aminoacyl-tRNA with peptidyl-tRNA does NOT directly require GTP. ATP is required for the synthesis of aminoacyl-tRNA. *Biochemistry,* pp. 350–355.
11. The answer is E: failure to elongate polypeptides directed by mRNAs containing codons corresponding to tryptophan. Tryptophan is an essential amino acid that cannot be synthesized from endogenous compounds and must be provided by the diet. There is diminished tryptophan-tRNA synthesis owing to a lack of substrate, but other aminoacyl-tRNAs can be synthesized from their corresponding tRNAs in reactions energized by ATP. Tryptophan is not required for the interaction of mRNA with the ribosome and formation of the initiation complex. A deficiency of methionine, however, would impair formation of the initiation complex. A paucity of tryptophan-tRNA diminishes elongation reactions at codons corresponding to tryptophan owing to the lack of substrate. *Biochemistry,* pp. 221, 349.
12. The answer is A: mitochondria contain their own unique DNA and RNA polymerases. DNA polymerase γ is the mitochondrial enzyme; mitochondrial RNA polymerase bears little resemblance to nuclear or bacterial enzymes, and its origin is obscure. Mitochondria contain several circular DNA molecules that lack histones. Mitochondrial DNA replication occurs throughout the cell cycle and is decoupled from that of the nucleus. *Biochemistry,* p. 358.
13. The answer is E: 4. Two high-energy bonds are required for the formation of each aminoacyl-tRNA ($ATP \rightarrow AMP + 2\ P_i$ or two high-energy bonds). A third high-energy bond is required for the insertion of amino-acyltRNA into the A site as $GTP \rightarrow GDP + P_i$. A fourth high-energy bond is required for translocation as $GTP \rightarrow GDP + P_i$. *Biochemistry,* p. 358.
14. The answer is C: unique methionine tRNAs for chain initiation and for chain elongation. The chain initiator in prokaryotes and in mitochondria is *N*-formyl-Met-$tRNA_f^{Met}$ and that for eukaryotes in the cytosol is Met-$tRNA_i^{Met}$ (lacking the formyl group). The elongation component is Met-$tRNA^{Met}$ for both prokaryotes and eukaryotes. Bacterial initiation involves the interaction of the Shine-Dalgarno sequence of rRNA by mRNA. Eukaryotes possess a scan-

ning mechanism for chain initiation. Prokaryotic mRNAs are monocistronic or polycistronic; those for eukaryotes are monocistronic. Some eukaryotic messengers encode for a single polypeptide with more than one activity, and these are called polyproteins. In some cases, for example, in fatty acid synthetase, the polyprotein persists as a polyprotein in the cell. In poliovirus and HIV, the polyprotein is cleaved by peptidases to yield the component activities. *Biochemistry,* pp. 349–356.

15. The answer is E: pyelonephritis. The patient's elevated white blood cell count with a high percentage of polymorphonuclear leukocytes and her elevated fever are evidence of a bacterial infection. The pain in the kidney area, cloudy urine (white cells in the urine or pyuria), and microscopic examination revealing red and white cells point to the urinary tract as the source of infection. Cystitis, which is common in women, is accompanied by dysuria, frequency, and sometimes hematuria (which this patient lacked). Cystitis is usually a low-grade infection without fever or leukocytosis. Pyelonephritis can be observed when the ureter is obstructed by kidney stones. The normal serum amylase and lipase rule pancreatitis unlikely; moreover, pancreatitis is more common in those with a history of high alcohol intake. The aspartate aminotransferase and lactate dehydrogenase and absence of jaundice rule hepatitis unlikely as a cause of her abdominal discomfort. Kidney stones occur in about 1% of the population, and the mechanism of causation is unknown. They can occur in gout (with elevated urate) or in hyperparathyroidism (with its elevated blood calcium and increased urinary calcium excretion). This patient had no evidence for these as causes of stones. *Cecil,* p. 593.
16. The answer is A: the extracytoplasmic transpeptidation at D-alanyl-D-alanine. Penicillin, ampicillin, cephalosporins, and their congeners react with a protein-cysteine of a bacterial transpeptidation enzyme and irreversibly inhibit the enzyme by covalent modification. These compounds do not affect the synthesis of glycine-tRNA that is involved in protein synthesis or the glycine-tRNA that adds the pentaglycine side chain to peptidoglycan. These antibiotics also lack an effect on undecaprenyl phosphate synthesis. *Biochemistry,* p. 369.
17. The answer is D: causing misreading of the genetic code. Aminoglycosides including gentamicin and streptomycin inhibit bacterial protein synthesis initiation (not chain termination) and cause misreading of the genetic code. *Biochemistry,* p. 357.
18. The answer is C: inhibiting the implantation of aminoacyl-tRNA into the A site of the ribosome. Tetracycline and its congeners inhibit the transfer reaction in bacterial protein synthesis. Chloramphenicol is an antibiotic that inhibits bacterial (and perhaps mitochondrial) peptidyltransferase activity. *Biochemistry,* p. 357.

REFERENCES

Roskoski, R., Jr. *Biochemistry.* Philadelphia, W. B. Saunders Company, 1996.

Wyngaarden, J. B., L. H. Smith, Jr., and J. C. Bennett (eds.). *Cecil Textbook of Medicine,* 19th ed. Philadelphia, W. B. Saunders Company, 1992.

CHAPTER EIGHTEEN

POSTTRANSLATIONAL MODIFICATION OF PROTEINS

SYNOPSIS

OBJECTIVES

1. To describe proteolytic processing and the signal peptide hypothesis.
2. To outline the steps involved in the covalent modification of proteins.
3. To compare the ubiquitin and the lysosomal pathways of protein degradation.

Objective 1: To describe proteolytic processing and the signal peptide hypothesis.

I. Overview of protein folding
   A. The primary structure of a protein determines its secondary, tertiary, and quaternary structure (PRINCIPLE 6 OF BIOCHEMISTRY)
   B. The following two enzyme systems accelerate the attainment of the final equilibrium conformation of proteins
      1. **Prolyl isomerase** catalyzes the *cis-trans* interconversions of polypeptidic prolines; proline occurs chiefly as the *trans* isomer in proteins but it can occur in selective positions as the *cis* isomer
      2. **Chaperones** are proteins that bind to hydrophobic regions of proteins and promote proper folding to the thermodynamically most stable protein conformations
         a. Many chaperones require ATP for their activity
         b. The amount of ATP expended to promote protein folding may approach one high-energy bond per peptide bond
II. Proteolytic processing
   A. The amino-terminal methionine residue that participates in the initiation process is removed from most proteins by a methionine-specific aminopeptidase
   B. Signal sequences, which target a protein to the plasma membrane for insertion or secretion, contain an amino-terminal **signal sequence** of 15–40 amino acid residues
      1. The signal contains at least one positively charged residue and a hydrophobic stretch of 10–15 residues
      2. A **signal recognition particle** (SRP), which is a G-protein that binds to the signal peptide, consists of several proteins and 7SL RNA (an RNA polymerase III transcript consisting of about 300 nucleotides)
      3. The signal recognition particle, nascent polypeptide, and ribosome diffuse to a **signal recognition particle receptor** on the endoplasmic reticulum, and polypeptide synthesis resumes
      4. A **signal peptidase** catalyzes the exergonic hydrolysis of the signal peptide from the nascent polypeptide chain in accordance with PRINCIPLE 5 OF BIOENERGETICS
   C. **Furin** is a proteolytic endopeptidase that participates in posttranslational processing
      1. It functions in the **unregulated** or **constitutive** secretory pathways for proteins such as serum albumin, synthesized by liver
      2. Furin catalyzes the hydrolysis of polypeptide substrates at paired basic residues such as Lys-Arg
III. Insulin biosynthesis
   A. Although insulin consists of two polypeptide chains, called A and B, that are linked by two disulfide bonds, insulin is first synthesized as a single polypeptide chain called preproinsulin
      1. **Preproinsulin,** which is the translation product of a single mRNA, contains a 24-residue signal peptide attached to an 86-residue **proinsulin** molecule
      2. After the initiation of its synthesis, preproinsulin is directed to the endoplasmic reticulum by the signal sequence
      3. A signal peptidase catalyzes the removal of the signal peptide
      4. The "pre" of preproinsulin and other prepropeptides refers to the polypeptide with the signal sequence

5. Cysteine residues undergo **protein disulfide isomerase**–catalyzed reactions, forming the disulfide bonds of proinsulin

B. Proinsulin is converted to insulin by specific proteolytic reactions
   1. Processing enzymes with trypsin-like specificity catalyze the hydrolytic removal of the connecting, or C, peptide
   2. The enzymes that catalyze the endoproteolytic cleavage of proinsulin are homologous to bacterial subtilisin (a serine protease) which contains the catalytic triad consisting of serine, histidine, and aspartate that is found in chymotrypsin (Chapter 4)
   3. Enzymes that participate in proinsulin processing include **prohormone convertase 2** (PC2) and **prohormone convertase 3/1** (PC3/1)
      a. The hydrolytic reactions catalyzed by these enzymes occur on the carboxyterminal side of paired basic residues
      b. Examples of paired basic residues include Lys-Arg and Arg-Arg
      c. The prohormone convertases participate in the synthesis of polypeptides that are secreted in **regulated** pathways, in contrast to furins that participate in unregulated pathways
   4. **Carboxypeptidase H,** an enzyme with the specificity of carboxypeptidase B, catalyzes the removal of basic residues from the carboxyl termini of the B–chain and C–peptide to form the mature protein hormone and connecting peptide

Objective 2: To outline the steps involved in the covalent modification of proteins.

IV. Covalent modification of proteins
   A. The amino terminus of selected proteins is acetylated (common) or myristoylated (uncommon) following a reaction with energy-rich acyl~CoA
   B. Protein phosphorylation by protein kinases is a frequent posttranslational modification
      1. Serine, threonine, and tyrosine are the residues in proteins that are phosphorylated
         a. Protein-serine or -threonine phosphate esters are energy poor, and such reactions are catalyzed by protein-serine/threonine kinases
         b. Protein-tyrosine phosphate esters are energy rich, and such reactions are catalyzed by protein-tyrosine kinases
      2. Regulation of protein kinases is intricate
         a. Families of protein kinases are regulated by several second messenger signaling molecules including cyclic AMP, cyclic GMP, diglyceride, and calcium
         b. Some protein kinases are regulated by their state of phosphorylation-dephosphorylation in serial reactions called protein kinase cascades
            (1) The protein kinase A–phosphorylase kinase–phosphorylase cascade was the first such cascade to be discovered
            (2) The Raf-Mek-Erk cascade is a second example
   C. Protein sulfation, a posttranslational modification that occurs in the Golgi, involves a reaction of the energy-rich phosphoadenosylphosphosulfate (PAPS) with the acceptor residue to form an energy-poor compound in a process that is exergonic according to PRINCIPLE 2 OF BIOENERGETICS
   D. Protein glycosylation is a specialized process that occurs in the endoplasmic reticulum and Golgi
      1. There are two varieties of glycoproteins in humans: *O*-linked and *N*-linked
         a. ***O*-Linked oligosaccharides** consist of carbohydrate bound to an oxygen derived from a polypeptidic serine or threonine
         b. ***N*-Linked oligosaccharides** consist of carbohydrate bound to the amide group of polypeptidic asparagine via a β-linkage, and these glycoproteins consist of three classes: **high mannose, complex,** and **hybrid**
         c. There are five main sugar donors in the biosynthesis of the oligosaccharides of glycoproteins: **uridine diphosphate sugars, guanosine diphosphate sugars, dolichol diphosphate sugars, dolichol monophosphate sugars,** and **CMP-*N*-acetylneuraminate**
      2. *N*-linked oligosaccharide synthesis is intricate
         a. The early steps in *N*-linked oligosaccharide synthesis involve the formation of a 14-membered core saccharide linked to dolichol diphosphate
         b. The 14-membered group is transferred *en bloc* to the acceptor protein-asparagine residue
            (1) This glycosyl transferase reaction proceeds with the loss of one high-energy bond and is exergonic
            (2) The acceptor asparagine is two residues on the carboxyterminal side of serine or threonine
         c. Following a series of hydrolytic reactions that remove several sugar residues, the product is a high-mannose *N*-linked oligosaccharide
         d. Additional steps are required for the formation of the *N*-linked complex or hybrid oligosaccharide
         e. The oligosaccharide-protein complex undergoes a series of condensation reactions catalyzed by glycosyltransferases and utilizing nucleotide sugar donors such as UDP-glucose, GDP-mannose, and CMP-*N*-acetylneuraminate
      3. *O*-linked oligosaccharide synthesis is simple
         a. Nucleoside diphosphate sugars serve as the activated donors
         b. Polypeptidic serine and threonine are the acceptors
   E. Prenylation: farnesylation and geranylgeranylation
      1. Prenylation modification occurs at a CAAX box at the carboxyl terminus of acceptor polypeptides, where C represents cysteine, A represents an aliphatic residue (not necessarily alanine), and X is leucine for geranylgeranylation and serine or methionine for farnesylation
      2. Farnesyl- or geranylgeranyl diphosphate are the prenyl donors
      3. Following prenylation of the cysteinyl sulfhydryl group, the AAX residues are removed by proteolysis and the carboxyl group of cysteine is methylated (AdoMet is the active donor)
   F. Vitamin K–dependent carboxylation
      1. Several calcium-binding proteins in the blood clotting cascade of reactions undergo a vitamin K–dependent carboxylation reaction
         a. Blood clotting involves a series of reactions in which the product of one process initiates a subsequent process, the product of which initiates still another—a cascade
         b. Blood clotting involves factors I–XIII (with the omission of VI)

c. Blood clotting involves at least six distinct proteases with a serine residue at the active site
   (1) These include factors II, VII, IX, X, XI, and XII
   (2) These serine proteases exhibit trypsin-like specificity (hydrolyzing a peptide bond on the carboxyl side of a basic amino acid residue)

d. During the proteolytic cascade, an inactive proenzyme (e.g., factor XII) is converted to an active enzyme, designated by an "a" following the factor number (e.g., XIIa)
   (1) At the end of the blood clotting cascade, prothrombin (II) is converted to thrombin (IIa)
   (2) The protein substrate for thrombin that results in clot formation is fibrinogen (factor I); fibrinogen is converted into a fibrin clot by proteolysis catalyzed by thrombin or factor IIa

e. Factors II, VII, IX, and X contain protein-γ-carboxyglutamate

2. The reactants for vitamin K–dependent carboxylation include a protein-glutamate, oxygen, carbon dioxide, and vitamin K
3. The products include protein γ-carboxyglutamate, water, and vitamin K 2,3-epoxide
4. The vitamin K epoxide is reconverted to reduced vitamin K by reduction with two moles of NADPH
5. Reactions of organic compounds with molecular oxygen are exergonic (PRINCIPLE 8 OF BIOENERGETICS), and this is the bioenergetic basis for protein carboxylation
6. Both exogenous and endogenous anticoagulants occur

a. Dicumarol and warfarin are vitamin K antagonists that function as anticoagulants and are used in the treatment of coronary thrombosis and pulmonary emboli
   (1) Because these agents inhibit posttranslational modification reactions, a few days' time is required to produce their therapeutic effect
   (2) The prothrombin time is the clinical test that is used to monitor the effect of vitamin K antagonists

b. Antithrombin III and protein C–protein S are natural anticoagulants in blood whose activity is modulated by exogenous compounds
   (1) Antithrombin III, activated by heparin, binds and inhibits many serine proteases including thrombin and Xa, accounting for the anticoagulant effects of heparin
   (2) Heparin increases the rate of formation of the antithrombin–protease complex by 1000-fold, and its effect occurs almost immediately
   (3) The activated partial thromboplastin time (aPTT) is used to monitor the effect of heparin

Objective 3: To compare the ubiquitin and the lysosomal pathways of protein degradation.

V. Protein degradation

A. Ubiquitin-mediated degradation
   1. The covalent attachment of ubiquitin is an ATP-dependent process that involves thioester intermediates and three enzyme components called E1, E2, and E3
   2. The covalent attachment of ubiquitin to target proteins involves the carboxyterminal glycine of the ubiquitin polypeptide with the ε-amino group of lysyl residues in the target
   3. Following ubiquitinylation, a multiprotein complex called **ubiquitin conjugate–degrading enzyme** catalyzes the hydrolysis of the targeted protein
   4. Cells contain **ubiquitin C-terminal hydrolase** activity, which catalyzes the hydrolysis of the linkage between the carboxyterminal glycine of ubiquitin and the ε-amide group, linking it to target proteins
   5. Free ubiquitin recycles to select other proteins for degradation

B. Lysosomes contain a variety of proteolytic enzymes called **cathepsins** that catalyze the hydrolysis of proteins

QUESTIONS

DIRECTIONS. (Items 1–3): The set of matching questions in this section consists of a list of several lettered options followed by several numbered items. For each numbered item, select the ONE lettered option that is most closely associated with it. Each lettered option may be selected once, more than once, or not at all. Correct answers and explanations are given at the end of the chapter.

Items 1–3

(A) Acetyl-CoA
(B) Myristoyl-CoA
(C) Palmitoyl-CoA
(D) *S*-Adenosylmethionine
(E) N^5-methyltetrahydrofolate
(F) Adenosine triphosphate
(G) CMP-*N*-acetylneuraminate
(H) UDP-glucose
(I) GDP-mannose
(J) Farnesyl pyrophosphate
(K) Phosphoadenosylphosphosulfate

For each biochemical property, select the correct metabolite.

1. Reacts with protein-cysteine residues to form a thioester
2. Reacts with CAAX box substrates
3. Reacts with protein-tyrosine residues but not protein-serine or protein-threonine

DIRECTIONS. (Items 4–17): Each of the numbered items or incomplete statements in this section is followed by answers or by completions of the statement. Select the ONE lettered answer or completion that is BEST in each case.

4. One cause of abnormal bleeding is failure to produce functional blood clotting factor X because of a mutation that converts glycine at position −3 to arginine. As a result of this mutation, the preproprotein cannot undergo which one of the following processing events?
   (A) Complex formation with the signal recognition particle
   (B) Cleavage by a signal peptidase
   (C) Physiological *O*-glycosylation
   (D) Phosphorylation
   (E) Formylation

5. A mutation in the insulin gene that involves the replacement of a Lys-Arg to a Lys-His results in a rare form of diabetes mellitus that is due to the failure to produce a functional insulin molecule because of inadequate
   (A) hydrolytic removal of a signal peptide
   (B) conversion of preproinsulin to proinsulin
   (C) *O*-linked glycosylation of a serine residue
   (D) protein sulfation
   (E) hydrolytic removal of the connecting peptide by prohormone convertase

6. Which one of the following enzymes is activated allosterically by diglyceride and by tumor promoters such as phorbol esters?
   (A) Calcium/calmodulin-dependent protein kinase
   (B) Protein kinase A
   (C) Protein kinase C
   (D) Protein kinase G
   (E) Pyruvate dehydrogenase kinase

7. All of the following enzymatic activities are regulated directly by calcium and calmodulin EXCEPT
   (A) calcium/calmodulin-dependent protein kinase
   (B) myosin light chain kinase
   (C) phosphorylase kinase
   (D) protein kinase C
   (E) type I cyclic nucleotide phosphodiesterase

8. In which one of the following enzymes does a hereditary deficiency of phosphatase leave the enzyme in a chronically active state?
   (A) Branched-chain keto acid dehydrogenase
   (B) Glycogen synthase
   (C) Liver pyruvate kinase
   (D) Phosphorylase kinase
   (E) Pyruvate dehydrogenase

9. Which one of the following chemical groups, which is lacking in I-cell disease, is responsible for targeting glycoproteins to the lysosome?
   (A) *N*-Acetylgalactosamine
   (B) *N*-Acetylglucosamine
   (C) *N*-Acetylneuraminate
   (D) Glucuronate
   (E) Mannose 6-phosphate

10. Which one of the following compounds is the lipid-soluble carrier of the oligosaccharide involved in *N*-linked glycoprotein synthesis?
    (A) Dolichol phosphate
    (B) Farnesyl pyrophosphate
    (C) Geranylgeranyl pyrophosphate
    (D) Ubiquinone
    (E) Undecaprenyl phosphate

11. The activity of which one of the following enzymes is decreased in scurvy
    (A) Acyl-CoA dehydrogenase
    (B) α-Ketoglutarate dehydrogenase
    (C) Lysyl hydroxylase
    (D) Prenyl-protein transferase
    (E) Vitamin K–epoxide reductase

12. All of the following are true statements regarding ATP in the ubiquitin system for degrading proteins EXCEPT
    (A) It is required for attaching ubiquitin to the target protein
    (B) It is required for importing the target protein into the lysosome
    (C) It is required for attaching the three conjugate factors (CF1, CF2, and CF3) of the conjugate-degrading enzyme to the target protein
    (D) It is degraded to AMP and pyrophosphate during the activation of ubiquitin

Items 13–17

History

The patient is a 34-year-old woman with the acute onset of severe right shoulder pain, dyspnea, cough, and hemoptysis that began 30 minutes before she was brought to the emergency clinic by her husband. Inspection revealed a woman who appeared anxious, in acute distress, and in a life-threatening situation. The patient has been followed in the renal clinic for 6 years with the nephrotic syndrome.

Physical Examination

Her temperature is 37.5 °C (99.6 °F); pulse, 120/min; respirations, 27/min; blood pressure, 110/66 mm Hg. She has a maculopapular erythematous (red) rash on her face and pedal edema. Examination of the thorax reveals diminished breath sounds bilaterally. Cardiac examination is normal except for tachycardia (increased heart rate).

Laboratory

Emergency laboratory studies revealed the following:
Hematocrit, 35% (normal ♂, 35–45%)
White blood count, 10,000/μL (normal, 4500–11,000/μL)
Platelets, 400,000/μL (normal, 150–450 10^3/μL)
Creatine phosphokinase (CPK), 62 U/L (normal, 26–140 U/L)
Lactate dehydrogenase (LDH), 274 U/L (normal, 208–378 U/L)
Aspartate aminotransferase (AST, SGOT), 12 U/L (normal, 10–30 U/L)
Serum glucose, 88 mg/dL (normal, 70–105 mg/dL)
Blood urea nitrogen (BUN), 35 mg/dL (normal, 7–18 mg/dL)
Electrolytes, normal

Arterial blood (while breathing room air) exhibited a pH of 7.42, pCO_2 of 35 mm Hg, and pO_2 of 77 mm Hg. An electrocardiogram showed a sinus tachycardia. A chest radiograph showed bilateral pleural effusion. Blood was drawn for prothrombin time, activated partial thromboplastin generation time, and blood chemistries. She was started on intravenous heparin.

The following laboratory studies were performed during the patient's hospital stay.

Serum albumin, 2.8 g/dL (normal, 3.5–5.0 g/dL)
Globulin, 4.2 g/dL (normal, 2.2–4.0 g/dL)
Cholesterol, 300 mg/dL (recommended, <200 mg/dL)
LDL cholesterol, 170 mg/dL (recommended, <130 mg/dL)
Triglyceride, 150 mg/dL (recommended 35–160 mg/dL)
Prothrombin time, 15 sec (control, 15 sec)
Blood urea nitrogen (BUN), 32 mg/dL (normal, 7–18 mg/dL)
Creatinine, 3.2 mg/dL (normal, 0.6–1.1 mg/dL)
Anti-DNA antibodies, positive (normal, negative)
Anti-small nuclear protein antibodies, positive (normal, negative)
VDRL, negative (normal, negative)
Urinalysis
- Birefringent particles by microscopic examination without red or white blood cells
- 24-hour urine protein, 9.6 g (normal, <0.2 g);
- Glucose, negative (normal, negative)
- Specific gravity, 1.020 (normal, 1.005–1.035)

13. Which one of the following conditions is most likely responsible for the sudden onset of chest pain in this patient?
    (A) Asthma
    (B) Myocardial infarction
    (C) Pneumonia
    (D) Pneumothorax
    (E) Pulmonary embolus

14. After 5 days of heparin treatment, the patient was started on warfarin. What is the mechanism of action of warfarin?
    (A) It blocks the reduction of vitamin K epoxide to vitamin K
    (B) It decreases albumin biosynthesis
    (C) It decreases fibrinogen biosynthesis
    (D) It inactivates factors VIII and Va by proteolysis
    (E) It inhibits many serine proteases including thrombin and Xa

15. Which one of the following laboratory tests monitors the effect of warfarin?
    (A) Activated partial thromboplastin time (aPTT)
    (B) Bleeding time
    (C) Platelet count
    (D) Prothrombin time
    (E) Serum fibrinogen

16. What is the physiological role of vitamin K?
    (A) It forms a complex with rhodopsin
    (B) It functions as an antioxidant
    (C) It mediates the conversion of protein-glutamates to protein-γ-carboxyglutamates
    (D) It mediates the hydroxylation of collagen-proline residues
    (E) It participates in the conversion of carboxyterminal glycine to an amide

17. This patient had the nephrotic syndrome based upon proteinuria of >3.5 g/d as well as hypoalbuminemia, hyperlipidemia, and lipiduria as indicated by birefringent particles by microscopic examination. Which one of the following disorders is a likely cause of nephrotic syndrome in this patient?
    (A) Diabetes mellitus
    (B) Essential hypertension
    (C) Lupus erythematosus
    (D) Myasthenia gravis
    (E) Syphilis

ANSWERS AND EXPLANATIONS

1. The answer is C: palmitoyl-CoA. The reaction of palmitoyl-CoA with protein-cysteine produces a hydrophobic tag that promotes association of polypeptides to membranes. Some forms of Ras protein, for example, are palmitoylated and bind to the plasma membrane. *Biochemistry,* p. 387.
2. The answer is J: farnesyl pyrophosphate. CAAX box substrates refer to proteins that end with cysteine–aliphatic-aliphatic-X residues. When X is methionine or serine, these proteins undergo reaction with farnesyl pyrophosphate to produce a derivative with a thioether bond connecting the isoprenoid farnesyl group with protein-cysteine. When X is leucine, these proteins undergo reaction with geranylgeranyl pyrophosphate to produce a derivative with a thioether bond connecting the geranylgeranyl group with protein-cysteine. *Biochemistry,* p. 387.
3. The answer is K: phosphoadenosylphosphosulfate (PAPS). This compound reacts with protein-tyrosine to form a sulfate ester. ATP reacts with protein-tyrosine, protein-serine, and protein-threonine to form phosphorylated products. *Biochemistry,* pp. 375, 378.
4. The answer is B: Cleavage by signal peptidase. An amino-terminal signal sequence consists of 15–40 amino acid residues. The signal contains at least one positively charged residue and a hydrophobic stretch of 10–15 residues. After the initiation of protein synthesis and about 70 elongation reactions, about 30 amino acid residues of the growing polypeptide extend from the ribosome. A signal recognition particle (SRP) binds to the signal peptide (the residue at position –3 does not extend from the ribosome and cannot be recognized by the signal recognition particle). The signal recognition particle consists of several proteins and 7SL RNA (an RNA polymerase III transcript consisting of about 300 nucleotides). The signal recognition particle requires GTP for activity and is a G-protein. The signal recognition particle, nascent polypeptide, and ribosome diffuse to a signal

recognition particle receptor on the endoplasmic reticulum. The ribosome also binds to two integral membrane ribosome receptors. GTP, which is bound to SRP, is hydrolyzed to GDP and P_i, and the signal recognition particle is released. Protein synthesis resumes. After transit through the endoplasmic reticulum membrane, a signal peptidase catalyzes the exergonic hydrolysis of the signal peptide from the nascent polypeptide chain. A mutation that changes the small, uncharged glycine with the larger, positively charged arginine at position −3 (three residues from +1, the first amino acid in the mature protein) renders the protein resistant to the action of signal peptidase; binding to the signal recognition particle and entry into the endoplasmic reticulum occur normally. The signal sequence is not a physiological substrate for glycosylation or phosphorylation. The amino terminus of nonmitochondrial eukaryotic proteins does not undergo formylation. *Biochemistry,* pp. 372–373.

5. The answer is E: hydrolytic removal of the connecting peptide by prohormone convertase. Prohormone convertases hydrolyze their substrates at paired basic residues (Lys-Arg and Arg-Arg are the preferred sequences). The mutation that results in the replacement of arginine 65 by histidine alters the C-peptide A-chain cleavage. As a result, there is diminished insulin production and increased circulation of a proinsulin intermediate. *Biochemistry,* p. 374.
6. The answer is C: protein kinase C. Diglyceride, a second messenger, is generated by the action of phospholipase C (this designation refers to one of four arbitrary Roman letters—A_1, A_2, C, and D). The C of protein kinase C refers to calcium (and not an arbitrary Roman letter) because most isoforms of this enzyme require calcium for expression of activity. Protein kinase C requires only basal amounts of calcium and is not regulated by calcium ion; rather, protein kinase C is controlled by alterations in the level of diglyceride. Protein kinase A is activated by cyclic AMP, the first of the second messengers to be described. Protein kinase G is regulated by cyclic GMP. There are three calcium/calmodulin-dependent protein kinases (I, II, and III) whose names are based upon the historical order of discovery. Calcium/calmodulin protein kinase II is a broad specificity protein kinase like protein kinase C and protein kinase A. Pyruvate dehydrogenase kinase, in contrast, is a narrow specificity protein kinase that is stimulated by NADH and acetyl-CoA; as a result of phosphorylation of pyruvate dehydrogenase, activity is diminished and this action follows the molecular logic of the cell (PRINCIPLE 9 OF BIOCHEMISTRY). *Biochemistry,* pp. 378, 439, 442.
7. The answer is D: protein kinase C. Protein kinase C requires calcium for expression of activity, but basal levels of calcium are sufficient when diglyceride is present. Myosin light chain kinase, calcium/calmodulin-dependent protein kinases (I, II, and III), and phosphorylase kinase are regulated by calcium and calmodulin. The δ-subunit of phosphorylase kinase is calmodulin. Of the five families of cyclic nucleotide phosphodiesterase that have been described, only the type I family is regulated by calcium/calmodulin. Of the eight or more families of adenylyl cyclase that have been described, types I, III, and VIII are stimulated by calcium/calmodulin. *Biochemistry,* pp. 146–147, 378, 416, 473.
8. The answer is D: phosphorylase kinase. Phosphorylation of phosphorylase kinase as catalyzed by protein kinase A (a cytosolic enzyme) increases its activity. Thus, the failure to remove the phosphoryl group results in a chronically active enzyme. In contrast, phosphorylation of branched-chain keto acid dehydrogenase by its specific protein kinase (a mitochondrial enzyme) is inhibitory. Phosphorylation of glycogen synthase and liver pyruvate kinase by protein kinase A also decreases their activities. *Biochemistry,* p. 504.
9. The answer is E: mannose 6-phosphate. The presence of mannose 6-phosphate on the exterior of a oligosaccharide chain targets the carbohydrate to the lysosome. The phosphorylation of mannose occurs by an unusual mechanism. An *N*-acetylglucosyl-1-phosphotransferase catalyzes a reaction between UDP-GlcNAc and a terminal mannose residue of the acceptor oligosaccharide (which is, in turn, covalently linked to protein). One product of the reaction is a phosphodiester between *N*-acetylglucosamine and the 6-hydroxyl group of mannose, and the other product is UMP. This reaction occurs with the loss of a high-energy bond and is exergonic (PRINCIPLE 2 OF BIOENERGETICS). Next, a phosphodiesterase catalyzes the hydrolytic removal of the terminal sugar (an exergonic process according to PRINCIPLE 5 OF BIOENERGETICS), leaving the 6-phosphomannosyl group linked to the oligosaccharide, the marker for lysosomal targeting. *Biochemistry,* pp. 383–385.
10. The answer is A: dolichol phosphate. Dolichol phosphate is an isoprenoid derivative that is responsible for the addition of oligosaccharides to protein-asparagine residues. Undecaprenyl phosphate is an isoprenoid group that participates in bacterial peptidoglycan biosynthesis. Ubiquinone is an electron carrier in the electron transport chain; it carries two electrons and two protons from complex II to complex III. Geranylgeranyl pyrophosphate and farnesyl pyrophosphate are isoprenoids that are added to the carboxyterminal CAAX box of acceptor proteins. The Ras protein accepts a farnesyl group, and the γ-subunit of heterotrimeric G-proteins accepts geranylgeranyl groups, to cite selected examples. *Biochemistry,* pp. 123, 126, 368, 387–388.
11. The answer is C: lysyl hydroxylase. Lysyl hydroxylase catalyzes the hydroxylation of lysine residues present in collagen using ascorbate, α-ketoglutarate, and oxygen as substrates. The products include succinate, carbon dioxide, dehydroascorbate, and the hydroxylated protein. This process is exergonic because of the decarboxylation (PRINCIPLE 6 OF BIOENERGETICS) and the reduction of molecular oxygen (PRINCIPLE 8 OF BIOENERGETICS). Prenyl-protein transferase is a generic name for the enzymes that add either farnesyl or geranylgeranyl groups to the carboxyterminal CAAX boxes of acceptor proteins. Acyl-CoA dehydrogenase of β-oxidation uses FAD as its oxidant, and enzyme activity is not directly affected by ascorbate. Vitamin K–epoxide reductase catalyzes the regeneration of vitamin K by reduction with NADPH; the epoxide is formed during the first step in the carboxylation of protein-glutamates in a process that requires carbon dioxide, vitamin K, and molecular oxygen as catalyzed by vitamin K–dependent carboxylase, which occurs in the Golgi. α-Ketoglutarate dehydrogenase is a Krebs cycle enzyme unrelated to posttranslational processing. *Biochemistry,* pp. 387–390.
12. The answer is B: ubiquitin is NOT required for importing the target protein into lysosomes. ATP is required for attaching ubiquitin to the target protein (ATP $\rightarrow$ AMP + 2 P_i) and for attaching the three conjugate factors (CF1, CF2, and CF3) of the conjugate-degrading enzyme to the target protein (ATP $\rightarrow$ ADP + P_i). *Biochemistry,* pp. 383–385, 392–393.
13. The answer is E: pulmonary embolus. A pulmonary embolus occurs after a deep vein thrombus is translocated to

the lungs. This results in acute shortness of breath, chest pain, hemoptysis (coughing blood), and hemodynamic collapse with decreased arterial oxygen. Chest pain can result from a myocardial infarction. This is often accompanied by electrocardiographic changes; an elevation of serum creatine phosphokinase occurs in 6–12 hours, and a normal level within the first hour in this patient is not helpful in ruling in or out a diagnosis of myocardial infarction. This patient, a female, would be very young to have a myocardial infarction in the absence of diabetes mellitus or familial hypercholesterolemia. Asthma can be diagnosed by characteristic wheezing that is audible by auscultation. Asthma is usually accompanied by eosinophilia because of an allergic component. Pneumonia can lead to chest pain and shortness of breath. Pneumonia is usually accompanied by a longer time of onset, fever, chills, and elevated white blood cell count. Pneumothorax or collapse of the lung is accompanied by the sudden onset of shortness of breath. Auscultation reveals an absence of breath sounds in the affected region; and radiolucency is observed by x-ray. *Cecil,* p. 421.

14. The answer is A: it blocks the reduction of vitamin K epoxide to vitamin K. Warfarin does not inhibit albumin synthesis; this patient's decrease in serum albumin is due to its massive loss in the urine. Fibrinogen posttranslational modification is not inhibited by warfarin. Plasmin, formed by the action of tissue plasminogen activator, inactivates factors VIII and Va by proteolysis. Heparin, and not warfarin, binds and inhibits many serine proteases including thrombin and Xa. *Biochemistry,* pp. 390, 496.
15. The answer is D: prothrombin time. A normal prothrombin time requires adequate fibrinogen, prothrombin, and factors V, VII, and X. Because the biosynthesis of prothrombin and factors VII, IX, and X requires vitamin K, the prothrombin time is used to monitor the effect of warfarin and other vitamin K antagonists. Activated partial thromboplastin time (aPTT) is the laboratory test used to determine the effectiveness of heparin treatment. The bleeding time is used in the assessment of von Willebrand factor. Bleeding disorders can occur when platelets are deficient; this can be assessed on a peripheral blood smear or by a platelet count. The final step in blood clotting is related to the conversion of fibrinogen to form a thrombus. With massive extracellular thrombus formation, the levels of fibrinogen can decline. *Biochemistry,* p. 497.
16. The answer is C: it mediates the conversion of protein-glutamates to protein-γ-carboxyglutamates. Vitamin A forms a complex with rhodopsin, and vitamins C, E, and β-carotene function as antioxidants. Vitamin C participates in the hydroxylation of collagen-prolines and the conversion of carboxyterminal glycine to an amide. *Biochemistry,* pp. 388–390.
17. The answer is C: lupus erythematosus. Lupus erythematosus is an autoimmune disease that characteristically occurs in premenopausal women. Affected individuals have a maculopapular erythematous rash on the face, and they have antibodies against DNA and small nuclear ribonucleoproteins. This disease has many manifestations, and the development of the nephrotic syndrome is one characteristic. The nephrotic syndrome also occurs in poststreptococcal glomerulonephritis and almost any disease, including diabetes mellitus, that can produce glomerular disease. Normal serum glucose and electrolytes render diabetes unlikely. The patient is normotensive, and the nephrotic syndrome is not a result of hypertension. Myasthenia gravis is an autoimmune disease where antibodies produced to the nicotinic cholinergic receptor at the neuromuscular junction lead to muscle weakness. Individuals with lupus and other autoimmune diseases often produce antibodies that also occur in response to infection by *Treponema pallidum* (a false-positive test). This patient, however, lacked a positive VDRL. *Cecil,* pp. 559 and 1522.

REFERENCES

Roskoski, R., Jr. *Biochemistry.* Philadelphia, W. B. Saunders Company, 1996.

Wyngaarden, J. B., L. H. Smith, Jr., and J. C. Bennett (eds.). *Cecil Textbook of Medicine,* 19th ed. Philadelphia, W. B. Saunders Company, 1992.

CHAPTER NINETEEN

NEUROTRANSMITTERS

SYNOPSIS

OBJECTIVES

1. To outline catecholamine metabolism.
2. To describe the metabolism of G-proteins.
3. To describe the metabolism of selected neurotransmitters.
4. To describe the metabolism and actions of opioid peptides.
5. To characterize the metabolism and actions of nitric oxide (NO).
6. To outline the rhodopsin-cyclic GMP cascade of the visual cycle.

Objective 1: To outline catecholamine metabolism.

I. First and second messengers
   A. Extracellular signaling molecules are called first messengers and include neurotransmitters, hormones, and growth factors
   B. Intracellular signaling molecules are called second messengers and include cyclic AMP, cyclic GMP, diglyceride, inositol trisphosphate, and calcium
II. Biologically active catecholamines—dopamine, norepinephrine, and epinephrine
   A. Catecholamines are synthesized by a common pathway
      1. Tyrosine hydroxylase catalyzes the first and rate-limiting reaction of the pathway
         a. Tyrosine hydroxylase is the main regulatory enzyme
         b. Tyrosine, oxygen, and tetrahydrobiopterin are substrates, and L-dopa, water, and dihydrobiopterin are products
         c. The oxidation of an organic compound by molecular oxygen is exergonic according to PRINCIPLE 8 OF BIOENERGETICS
      2. Aromatic amino acid decarboxylase catalyzes the conversion of L-dopa to dopamine
         a. This enzyme requires pyridoxal phosphate for activity
         b. The reaction, which is a decarboxylation reaction, is exergonic according to PRINCIPLE 6 OF BIOENERGETICS
      3. Dopamine β-hydroxylase catalyzes the conversion of dopamine to norepinephrine
         a. Ascorbate and oxygen are the other reactants, and water and oxidized ascorbate are the other products
         b. The reaction of molecular oxygen with an organic compound is exergonic according to PRINCIPLE 8 OF BIOENERGETICS
      4. Phenylethanolamine *N*-methyltransferase catalyzes the conversion of norepinephrine and *S*-adenosylmethionine to epinephrine and *S*-adenosylhomocysteine
         a. The reactants possess one more high-energy bond than the products
         b. The reaction is exergonic according to PRINCIPLE 2 OF BIOENERGETICS
   B. The pathway for the degradation of the catecholamines is intricate because it involves a network of reactions that uses four enzymes
      1. These enzymes are monoamine oxidase (MAO), catechol-*O*-methyltransferase (COMT), aldehyde reductase, and aldehyde oxidase
      2. The chief metabolite of dopamine is **homovanillate** (HVA), and the chief metabolite of norepinephrine is **vanillylmandelate** (VMA)
      3. Urinary VMA is commonly measured by the clinical chemistry laboratory as a diagnostic test for individuals who have a catecholamine-secreting tumor of the adrenal medulla called a pheochromocytoma

Objective 2: To describe the metabolism of G-proteins.

III. Adrenergic receptors and G-proteins
   A. The responses of various tissues to catecholamines are divided into two groups called α and β based upon the potency of a few adrenergic agents
      1. These receptors and all receptors that interact with heterotrimeric G-proteins contain seven transmembrane segments
         a. **G-proteins** bind and hydrolyze GTP
         b. Several classes of G-proteins have been described, including $\mathbf{G_s}$ (stimulatory) and $\mathbf{G_i}$ (inhibitory), proteins regulating adenylyl cyclase activity
         c. $\mathbf{G_P}$ activates phospholipase **C,** and $\mathbf{G_K}$ and $\mathbf{G_{Ca}}$ regulate potassium and calcium channels, respectively
      2. α_1-Receptors lead to the inhibition of adenylyl cyclase, and α_2-receptors lead to the activation of phospholipase C

3. β-Receptors lead to the activation of adenylyl cyclase

B. The activation of adenylyl cyclase by adrenergic receptors is intricate
   1. G-proteins consist of three polypeptide subunits named α, β, and γ
   2. Under basal conditions, the α-subunit contains bound GDP and exists in an inactive state
   3. Following the interaction of the activated receptor with the G-protein heterotrimer ($\alpha\beta\gamma$), GTP exchanges with GDP and the αG-GTP dissociates from the $\beta\gamma$-dimer and acts on its target protein
   4. αG-GTP has intrinsic GTPase activity, which leads to the formation of the inactive αG-GDP complex; this complex reassociates with the $\beta\gamma$-dimer to form inactive trimer that can be activated again
   5. The $\beta\gamma$-dimer has the potential to regulate cellular processes

C. Receptors that couple with G_i, which also contains α-, β-, and γ-subunits, inhibit adenylyl cyclase

D. Other receptors activate phospholipase C via G_p interaction
   1. Phospholipase C is responsible for the generation of two second messengers: diglyceride and inositol trisphosphate
   2. Diglyceride activates protein kinase C
   3. Inositol trisphosphate interacts with its receptor located on the endoplasmic reticulum and causes the release of calcium into the cytosol

E. The target of cholera toxin is αG_s
   1. The A_1 subunit of cholera toxin catalyzes the ADP-ribosylation of a specific arginine residue of αG_s proteins, and this modification inhibits the GTPase activity of αG_s; NAD^+ is the ADP-ribosyl donor
   2. As a result of inhibiting its GTPase activity, αG_s remains in its activated state and continuously stimulates adenylyl cyclase activity and elevates cellular cyclic AMP levels

F. The target of pertussis toxin is αG_i
   1. Pertussis toxin catalyzes the ADP-ribosylation of a specific cysteine in αG_i
   2. ADP-ribosylated αG_i cannot exchange GTP for bound GDP, and αG_i remains in a permanently inactivated state
   3. Cells thus lose the capability of inhibiting adenylyl cyclase under physiological conditions, and signal transduction is impaired

G. Dopamine receptors alter adenylyl cyclase activity
   1. D_1 receptors activate and D_2 receptors inhibit adenylyl cyclase activity
   2. Antischizophrenia drugs are characteristically D_2 receptor antagonists

H. Parkinson disease is due to the degeneration of the dopaminergic nigrostriatal pathway

Objective 3: To describe the metabolism of selected neurotransmitters.

IV. Acetylcholine

A. Metabolism
   1. Choline acetyltransferase catalyzes a reaction between choline and acetyl~CoA to produce acetylcholine and CoA according to PRINCIPLE 2 OF BIOENERGETICS
   2. Acetylcholinesterase is a ubiquitous extracellular enzyme that catalyzes the hydrolysis and inactivation of acetylcholine according to PRINCIPLE 5 OF BIOENERGETICS

B. Acetylcholine receptors
   1. **Muscarinic** receptors consist of a family of seven-transmembrane-segment receptors that inhibit adenylyl cyclase or that activate phospholipase C
   2. **Nicotinic** receptors are ligand-activated sodium channels
      a. The adult form consists of $\alpha_2\beta\varepsilon\delta$ subunits
      b. Each subunit possesses four transmembrane segments
      c. Acetylcholine binds to each of the two α-subunits to activate this receptor
      d. The formation of antibodies against the nicotinic receptor causes myasthenia gravis

V. Serotonin

A. Metabolism
   1. **Tryptophan hydroxylase** catalyzes a reaction of tryptophan, oxygen, and tetrahydrobiopterin to form 5-hydroxytryptophan, water, and *q*-dihydrobiopterin
   2. **Aromatic amino acid decarboxylase** (a pyridoxal phosphate–dependent enzyme) catalyzes the decarboxylation of 5-hydroxytryptophan to produce 5-hydroxytryptamine (serotonin) and carbon dioxide
   3. Serotonin is inactivated by sodium-dependent uptake into cells
   4. It is subsequently oxidized in a reaction catalyzed by MAO-A and aldehyde oxidase to produce 5-hydroxyindole acetate (5-HIAA)
   5. Urinary 5-HIAA can be measured to establish the diagnosis of carcinoid syndrome

B. Function
   1. Serotonin plays a role in sleep-wake cycles
   2. Reduced action of serotonin produces mental depression, and drugs that inhibit serotonin uptake from the synaptic region are used for the treatment of depression
   3. Several antiemetic drugs, which are important in patients undergoing cancer chemotherapy and radiation therapy, are serotonin antagonists

VI. GABA (γ-aminobutyric acid)

A. Metabolism
   1. **Glutamate decarboxylase** catalyzes the conversion of glutamate to GABA
      a. This enzyme requires pyridoxal phosphate for activity
      b. The reaction is exergonic in accordance with PRINCIPLE 6 OF BIOENERGETICS
   2. The action of GABA is terminated by sodium-dependent uptake
   3. GABA is metabolized by transamination to succinate semialdehyde and oxidized to succinate

B. Function
   1. GABA is the chief inhibitory neurotransmitter in brain
   2. GABA hyperpolarizes postsynaptic cells by increasing chloride conductance into the cell

C. Receptors
   1. The chief GABA receptor is a ligand-activated chloride channel
   2. Each receptor consists of several subunits, each of which has four transmembrane segments, like the nicotinic acetylcholine receptor

3. A quantitatively minor GABA receptor contains seven transmembrane segments and is coupled to G-proteins

VII. Glycine
  A. Glycine functions as an inhibitory neurotransmitter in the spinal cord
  B. The glycine receptor is a ligand-gated chloride channel, and each subunit of this receptor contains four transmembrane segments

VIII. Glutamate
  A. Function
    1. *Glutamate is the chief excitatory neurotransmitter in the human brain*
    2. Glutamate depolarizes postsynaptic cells by increasing sodium conductance
  B. Receptors
    1. The glutamate receptors are ligand-gated cation channels and are excitatory
    2. *The AMPA glutamate receptor is responsible for most "fast" synaptic transmission in the brain and spinal cord*
    3. The NMDA glutamate receptor may play a key role in memory

IX. Histamine
  A. Metabolism
    1. **Histidine decarboxylase,** a pyridoxal phosphate–dependent enzyme, catalyzes the conversion of histidine to histamine and carbon dioxide
    2. Histamine *N*-methyltransferase catalyzes a reaction between substrate and AdoMet to form *N*-methylhistamine, an inactive metabolite
  B. Receptors
    1. There are three subclasses of histamine receptor: H_1, H_2, and H_3
    2. H_1 receptor antagonists are used in the treatment of allergic responses, and many of these agents are over-the-counter medications
    3. H_2 receptor antagonists such as cimetidine are used in the treatment of peptic ulcers

Objective 4: To describe the metabolism and actions of opioid peptides.

X. Opioid peptide biosynthesis
  A. Opioids play a general role in pain perception and likely have other diverse actions
    1. Neuropeptides are synthesized by mRNA-dependent protein synthesis followed by proteolytic processing reactions
    2. Opioids are one class of neuropeptides, and this class of compounds has morphine-like actions; these substances include **β-endorphin, methionine-enkephalin, leucine-enkephalin,** and **dynorphin**
  B. The conversion of the propeptides to the final products is catalyzed by prohormone convertases and carboxypeptidase H, as described for insulin
    1. β-Endorphin is derived from **proopiomelanocortin** (POMC; pronounced "pom see")
    2. The **enkephalins** (the name means "in the head") are pentapeptides that are derived from preproenkephalin
    3. **Dynorphins** are opioid peptides that are synthesized from a third precursor called preprodynorphin
  C. These peptides are inactivated extracellularly by proteolytic cleavage and not by reuptake

Objective 5: To characterize the metabolism and actions of nitric oxide (NO).

XI. Nitric oxide and cyclic GMP
  A. **Nitric oxide synthase** is a P-450 type of heme protein that contains FAD and FMN and is activated by tetrahydrobiopterin
  B. Nitric oxide is derived from arginine and molecular oxygen in a reaction that involves NADPH, and the products include nitric oxide, citrulline, water, and $NADP^+$
  C. Nitric oxide is very unstable and breaks down spontaneously within a few seconds
  D. The inducible form of nitric oxide synthase, in contrast to the neuronal and constitutive enzymes, is active in the absence of calcium
  E. The action of nitric oxide is to stimulate the soluble form of guanylyl cyclase, and the resulting cyclic GMP activates its specific protein kinase

Objective 6: To illustrate the rhodopsin-cyclic GMP cascade of the visual cycle.

XII. The rhodopsin–cyclic GMP cascade
  A. The *cis* to *trans* isomerization of retinal, bound to opsin by a Schiff-base linkage, is the primary event in visual excitation
  B. Activated rhodopsin interacts with transducin, a G-protein
    1. Transducin consists of α-, β-, and γ-subunits that resemble those of G_s and G_i
    2. GTP exchanges for GDP, and αG_t activates cyclic GMP phosphodiesterase
  C. **Cyclic GMP phosphodiesterase** of the retina is a protein that consists of three subunits, also called α, β, and γ
    1. αG_t-GTP forms a complex with the γ-subunit of phosphodiesterase
    2. Dissociation of the γ-subunit leaves the $\alpha\beta$ heterodimer, the active form of the enzyme
  D. A cation channel is maintained in its open state by cyclic GMP
  E. Because of the rhodopsin-transducin mediated increase in phosphodiesterase activity, cyclic GMP levels fall and the cation channel is closed

QUESTIONS

DIRECTIONS. (Items 1–4): The set of matching questions in this section consists of a list of several lettered options followed by several numbered items. For each numbered item, select the ONE lettered option that is most closely associated with it. Each lettered option may be selected once, more than once, or not at all. Correct answers and explanations are given at the end of the chapter.

(A) Acetylcholine
(B) Dopamine
(C) Enkephalin
(D) Epinephrine
(E) GABA
(F) Glutamate
(G) Glycine
(H) Histamine
(I) Nitric oxide
(J) Norepinephrine
(K) Serotonin

For each description given, select the correct neurotransmitter.

1. Chief inhibitory neurotransmitter in the spinal cord
2. A diffusible gas
3. Its inactivation requires *N*-methylation
4. Deficient in Parkinson disease

DIRECTIONS. (Items 5–18): Each of the numbered items or incomplete statements in this section is followed by answers or by completions of the statement. Select the ONE lettered answer or completion that is BEST in each case.

5. Deprenyl, an agent that decreases dopamine catabolism and can be used in the treatment of Parkinson disease, is an inhibitor of which one of the following enzymes?
   (A) Aldehyde dehydrogenase
   (B) Aldehyde reductase
   (C) Catechol-*O*-methyltransferase
   (D) Monoamine oxidase–B
   (E) Phenylethanolamine *N*-methyltransferase

6. Which one of the following receptor types forms a cation channel?
   (A) α-Adrenergic
   (B) D_1 dopamine
   (C) H_1 histamine
   (D) Muscarinic acetylcholine
   (E) Nicotinic acetylcholine

7. Which one of the following receptor types interacts with a G-protein that alters adenylyl cyclase activity?
   (A) β-Adrenergic
   (B) $GABA_A$
   (C) AMPA glutamate
   (D) Kainate glutamate
   (E) NMDA glutamate

8. The action of which one of the following neurotransmitters is abolished by uptake into neuronal cells or glia?
   (A) Acetylcholine
   (B) γ-Aminobutyric acid (GABA)
   (C) Dynorphin
   (D) Enkephalin
   (E) Histamine

9. Which one of the following receptors is responsible for most of the "fast" synaptic transmission in the brain and spinal cord?
   (A) AMPA glutamate
   (B) NMDA glutamate
   (C) Glycine
   (D) Muscarinic acetylcholine
   (E) Nicotinic acetylcholine

10. Substrates for nitric oxide (NO) synthase include all of the following EXCEPT
    (A) arginine
    (B) NADPH + H^+
    (C) oxygen
    (D) urea

11. Which one of the following is a true statement regarding transducin?
    (A) It is a seven-transmembrane-segment protein
    (B) It consists of α-, β-, and γ-subunits that resemble those of G_s and G_i
    (C) It catalyzes the hydrolysis of cyclic GMP
    (D) It contains 11-*cis* retinal
    (E) It directly opens a cation channel

12. Seizures that are induced in infants owing to a deficiency of pyridoxine and thus pyridoxal phosphate are due to inadequate synthesis of which one of the following neurotransmitters?
    (A) Acetylcholine
    (B) Enkephalin
    (C) GABA (γ-aminobutyrate)
    (D) Glutamate
    (E) Glycine

13. Cholera toxin catalyzes the ADP-ribosylation of which one of the following proteins?
    (A) AB_5
    (B) $\beta\gamma G_i$
    (C) αG_i
    (D) αG_s
    (E) EF-2

14. Which one of the following substances can activate adenylyl cyclase in some of its target cells?
    (A) Dynorphin
    (B) β-Endorphin
    (C) Enkephalin
    (D) Epinephrine
    (E) Morphine

Items 15–18

History

The patient is a 26-year-old female attorney who developed fatigue during the previous 6 months. Her arms become tired while performing repetitive functions such as combing her hair, chasing after her 4-year-old boy, climbing stairs, or carrying books to her desk. She thought that this was part of normal aging, but she became alarmed when she began to see double. Diplopia occurs more in the evening when she is tired and can be relieved by closing her eyes and resting for 10 minutes. She says that her husband noted that she had slurred speech. She has no difficulty eating and denies shortness of breath, swollen joints, rashes, weight loss, dry mouth, abnormal bowel habits, and melena (blood in the stool). She is not aware of any relative who had any neuromuscular disease. Except for oral contraceptives, she takes no prescription medication.

Physical Examination

The patient does not appear to be in ill health. Her temperature is 37°C (98.6°F); pulse, 76/min; respirations, 14/min; blood pressure, 110/66 mm Hg; skin moisture, normal. The funduscopic examination was normal; there was bilateral ptosis of which the patient and her husband were unaware. She is unable to maintain an upward gaze for 90 seconds; one or the other eye returned to a horizontal position. Her hand grip is weak and becomes weaker as she tries to maintain a grip. Deep tendon reflexes are normal. Her general muscle strength seems normal. There are no joint abnormalities. The thyroid is not enlarged. Chest, cardiac, abdominal, and pelvic examinations were normal.

Laboratory

Hematocrit, white blood count and differential, sodium, potassium, chloride, glucose, calcium, phosphate, creatine phosphokinase, lactate dehydrogenase, aspartate aminotransferase, T_3, and T_4 were normal. Immunologic examination revealed antibodies to acetylcholine receptors. Antibodies to native DNA, denatured DNA, SSA/Ro and SSB/La (indicators of Sjögren syndrome), Scl-70 (an indicator of scleroderma), and thyroglobulin antibodies were negative. The injection of edrophonium, a short-acting anticholinesterase inhibitor, decreased ptosis, increased the range of ocular movement, and increased her hand grip. Chest x rays revealed an enlarged thymus.

15. The most likely cause of this patient's symptoms is
    (A) anemia
    (B) hypothyroidism
    (C) McArdle disease
    (D) myasthenia gravis
    (E) muscular dystrophy

16. Weakness is due to a deficiency of
    (A) red blood cells
    (B) thyroid hormone
    (C) glycogen phosphorylase
    (D) dystrophin
    (E) nicotinic acetylcholine receptor

17. This patient was treated with pyridostigmine (an inhibitor of acetylcholinesterase), prednisone (a glucocorticoid that suppresses the immune response), and azathioprine (an immunosuppressant). What is the function of pyridostigmine?
    (A) It increases the amount of acetylcholine that is released by exocytosis
    (B) It increases choline uptake at the neuromuscular junction
    (C) It increases the efficacy of acetylcholine that is released by exocytosis
    (D) It increases the activity of choline acetyltransferase
    (E) It increases the availability of acetyl-CoA

18. The nicotinic receptor at the neuromuscular junction consists of a pentamer composed of four different kinds of subunits. Which one of the following subunits binds acetylcholine?
    (A) α
    (B) β
    (C) γ
    (D) δ
    (E) ε

ANSWERS AND EXPLANATIONS

1. The answer is G: glycine. Glycine, one of the standard amino acids, is the chief inhibitory neurotransmitter in the spinal cord. It acts via a ligand-gated chloride channel and hyperpolarizes postsynaptic cells and is therefore inhibitory. *Biochemistry,* p. 411.
2. The answer is I: nitric oxide. This substance, which is derived from arginine, is a gas that diffuses from its site of synthesis and activates guanylyl cyclase. This is one of the few neurotransmitters that is not released from vesicles by a calcium-dependent process. Other extracellular signaling molecules such as prostaglandins, thromboxane, leukotrienes, steroid hormones, and platelet activating factor are also synthesized on demand, are not stored in vesicles, and are not released by calcium-dependent exocytosis. *Biochemistry,* p. 412.
3. The answer is H: histamine. Histamine is inactivated extracellularly by *N*-methylation with *S*-adenosylmethionine as methyl donor. Histamine and acetylcholine are the two low-molecular-mass compounds that are inactivated by metabolism and not by uptake. The neuropeptides are also inactivated by metabolism (hydrolysis) and not reuptake. *Biochemistry,* p. 412.
4. The answer is B: dopamine. Dopamine is the neurotransmitter of the nigrostriatal pathway that is deficient in Parkinson disease. This disorder is treated by the administration of oral L-dopa and an inhibitor of peripheral

aromatic amino acid decarboxylase. L-Dopa crosses the blood-brain barrier and is decarboxylated to form dopamine, a compound that does not cross the blood-brain barrier. *Biochemistry,* pp. 406–407.

5. The answer is D: Monoamine oxidase–B. Monoamine oxidase–B is the isozyme of monoamine oxidase that preferentially catalyzes the oxidation of dopamine; this enzyme is inhibited by deprenyl, which can be used in the treatment of Parkinson disease and mental depression. Monoamine oxidase–A, which preferentially catalyzes the oxidation of norepinephrine and serotonin, is inhibited by clorgyline, which has been used experimentally in the treatment of mental depression. Aldehyde dehydrogenase, aldehyde reductase, catechol-*O*-methyltransferase, and monoamine oxidase catalyze reactions that catabolize catecholamines. Phenylethanolamine *N*-methyltransferase catalyzes the conversion of norepinephrine to epinephrine. *Biochemistry,* p. 400.
6. The answer is E: nicotinic acetylcholine. The nicotinic acetylcholine receptor, which consists of five subunits, is a ligand-gated ion channel in which acetylcholine is the physiological ligand. Nicotinic receptors contain several subunits, each of which has four transmembrane segments, four transmembrane segments being characteristic of ligand-activated ion channel receptors. The second transmembrane segment (M_2) of the four transmembrane segments forms the ion channels. α-Adrenergic, D_1 dopamine receptors, H_1 histamine receptors, and muscarinic acetylcholine receptors are seven-transmembrane-segment receptors that interact with G-proteins. *Biochemistry,* p. 403.
7. The answer is A: β-adrenergic. β-Adrenergic receptors are seven-transmembrane-segment receptors that were the first receptors that were shown to activate adenylyl cyclase activity, and these receptors interact indirectly with adenylyl cyclase via G_s. In contrast, NMDA glutamate, AMPA glutamate, kainate glutamate, and $GABA_A$ receptors are ligand-gated ion channels. *Biochemistry,* p. 403.
8. The answer is B: γ-aminobutyric acid (GABA). γ-Aminobutyric acid (GABA), glutamate, glycine, the catecholamines, and serotonin are inactivated by transport from the synaptic region into cells (neurons or glia). The transmitters that are inactivated by hydrolytic metabolism include acetylcholine and neuropeptides such as enkephalin, dynorphin, and endorphin. Histamine is inactivated by a methylation reaction. *Biochemistry,* p. 410.
9. The answer is A: the AMPA glutamate receptor is responsible for most of the "fast" synaptic transmission in the brain and spinal cord. The NMDA glutamate receptor, which requires both glutamate and glycine for activation, is less prevalent than the AMPA receptor. Nicotinic acetylcholine and glycine responses are fast, but they represent a small portion of all fast neurotransmission. The muscarinic receptor, acting via G-proteins, promotes slow neurotransmission. *Biochemistry,* p. 412.
10. The answer is D: urea. Arginine is hydrolyzed to produce urea, the main nitrogen excretion product in humans. A nitrogen of arginine is also the precursor for NO (nitric oxide), an extracellular signaling molecule. Molecular oxygen and NADPH + H^+ are also required for NO synthesis. The action of NO is to activate the soluble form of guanylyl cyclase; this enzyme contains a heme group that binds NO. Cyclic GMP in nonretinal cells activates protein kinase G. *Biochemistry,* pp. 412, 415.
11. The answer is B: transducin consists of α-, β-, and γ-subunits that resemble those of G_s and G_i. Cyclic GMP in retina, in contrast to other cells, maintains a cation channel in its open state. Because of the rhodopsin-transducin mediated increase in phosphodiesterase activity, cyclic GMP levels fall and the cation channel is closed. This produces hyperpolarization of the plasma membrane of the rod cell. Rhodopsin is a seven-transmembrane-segment protein that contains 11-*cis* retinal. Cyclic GMP phosphodiesterase catalyzes the hydrolysis of cyclic GMP. Cyclic GMP directly opens a cation channel. *Biochemistry,* pp. 416–417.
12. The answer is C: GABA (γ-aminobutyrate). A deficiency of pyridoxine and thus pyridoxal phosphate in children leads to seizures, and this is thought to be related to a deficiency of GABA. Glutamate decarboxylase is most sensitive to pyridoxal phosphate deficiency despite the requirement for pyridoxal phosphate for other aspects of neurotransmitter metabolism. Aromatic amino acid decarboxylase, for example, requires pyridoxal phosphate as cofactor. Aromatic amino acid decarboxylase is required for dopamine, norepinephrine, epinephrine, and serotonin biosynthesis. Choline acetyltransferase, the enzyme that catalyzes the biosynthesis of acetylcholine, lacks pyridoxal phosphate. All eukaryotic transaminases, including GABA transaminase, contain pyridoxal phosphate. Glycine is the chief inhibitory neurotransmitter in the spinal cord, and aberrant glycine metabolism is not associated with seizures. *Biochemistry,* p. 412.
13. The answer is D: αG_s. As a result of the ADP-ribosylation of G_s, αG_s is locked into its activated state because it is unable to catalyze the hydrolysis of GTP. In turn, adenylyl cyclase activity is constantly stimulated. Besides explaining the mechanism of fluid loss from the intestine of people infected with cholera, this toxin is used experimentally in studies of G-protein action. AB_5 is the subunit structure of cholera toxin. $\beta\gamma G_i$ is not a target for cholera toxin. Pertussis toxin is a heterodimeric protein like cholera toxin. Pertussis toxin catalyzes the ADP-ribosylation of a specific cysteine in αG_i. ADP-ribosylated αG_i cannot exchange GTP for bound GDP, and αG_i remains in a permanently inactivated state. Cells thus lose the capability of inhibiting adenylyl cyclase under physiological conditions, and signal transduction is impaired. EF-2, the elongation factor, is a target for the ADP-ribosylation catalyzed by diphtheria toxin; the residue of EF-2 that is modified is diphthamide. *Biochemistry,* pp. 403, 406.
14. The answer is D: epinephrine. Acting via the β-adrenergic family of receptors, epinephrine can activate adenylyl cyclase in some of its target cells. Acting via the α-receptor, epinephrine can inhibit adenylyl cyclase via G_i. The opioids, including enkephalin, dynorphin, β-endorphin, and morphine, can only inhibit adenylate cyclase activity via G_i. *Biochemistry,* pp. 401, 403.
15. The answer is D: myasthenia gravis. Myasthenia gravis occurs most often in young women and is characterized by weakness and diplopia that is aggravated by activity and diminished by rest. Antibodies to the nicotinic acetylcholine receptor were also demonstrated in this patient. The fatigue was not due to anemia, because her hematocrit is reported as normal. Although hypothyroidism can produce fatigue, the T_3 and T_4 levels were normal. Anemias can also produce fatigue, but they do not produce muscle weakness and diplopia. McArdle disease is characterized by muscle weakness that is aggravated by activity, but antibodies to the nicotinic receptor do not characterize this disorder. Muscular dystrophy is usually a disease of boys. Carrier mothers are generally asymptomatic. There is generally an elevation of creatine phosphokinase in muscular dystrophy patients and in

asymptomatic carrier mothers. *Biochemistry,* p. 408; *Cecil,* p. 2265.

16. The answer is E: nicotinic acetylcholine receptor. The deficiency is a result of autoimmune antibodies directed against this receptor. The basis of the autoimmunity is not understood, and a significant fraction of such patients have an enlarged thymus. Thymectomy increases the remission rate and improves the clinical course of myasthenia gravis. The muscarinic acetylcholine receptor occurs in smooth muscle and not voluntary muscle. Thyroid hormone is decreased in myxedema. Glycogen phosphorylase is deficient in McArdle disease, and dystrophin is deficient in muscular dystrophy. *Biochemistry,* p. 408; *Cecil,* p. 2265.
17. The answer is C: It increases the efficacy of acetylcholine that is released by exocytosis. Pyridostigmine does not increase the amount of acetylcholine that is released by exocytosis, activate choline acetyltransferase, increase choline uptake, or increase the availability of acetyl-CoA. By inhibiting the breakdown of acetylcholine, pyridostigmine increases the effectiveness or efficacy of the acetylcholine that is released.
18. The answer is A: α. The adult neuromuscular junction consists of $\alpha_2\beta\varepsilon\delta$ subunits. It requires two molecules of acetylcholine to activate this receptor, one per each of the two α-subunits in the pentameric complex. *Biochemistry,* p. 408.

REFERENCES

Roskoski, R., Jr. *Biochemistry.* Philadelphia, W. B. Saunders Company, 1996.

Wyngaarden, J. B., L. H. Smith, Jr., and J. C. Bennett (eds.). *Cecil Textbook of Medicine,* 19th ed. Philadelphia, W. B. Saunders Company, 1992.

CHAPTER TWENTY

HORMONES AND GROWTH FACTORS

SYNOPSIS

OBJECTIVES

1. To describe hypothalamic and pituitary hormones.
2. To describe the hormonal regulation of calcium metabolism.
3. To compare signal transduction initiated by glucagon and insulin.
4. To describe the unique properties of atrial natriuretic factor.
5. To delineate the actions of the renin-angiotensin system.
6. To portray the actions of steroid hormones.

Objective 1: To describe hypothalamic and pituitary hormones.

I. Signal transduction
  A. Signal transduction is the process by which extracellular signals generate intracellular signals that mediate physiological responses
  B. Transduction refers to the conversion of one type of signal to another
II. Hypothalamic neurohormones
  A. Hormones secreted by the hypothalamus are carried by the hypophyseal portal venous system to the anterior pituitary, where they act by stimulating or inhibiting the secretion of anterior pituitary hormones
  B. Thyrotropin-releasing hormone, a tripeptide and the first hypothalamic hormone whose structure was determined, regulates thyrotropin (thyroid-stimulating hormone) secretion
III. Pituitary hormones
  A. Anterior pituitary hormones
    1. Growth hormone (pituitary), prolactin (pituitary), and chorionic somatomammotropin (placenta) are a family of homologous protein hormones that promote growth and are lactogenic
      a. The growth-promoting effects of growth hormone are mediated by insulin-like growth factor–1
      b. Growth hormone excess in children and adolescents results in **gigantism,** and growth hormone excess in adults results in **acromegaly**
      c. Growth hormone–deficient dwarfs respond to human growth hormone but not to that of other animals
    2. Thyrotropin, luteinizing hormone, follicle-stimulating hormone, and chorionic gonadotropin are glycoprotein hormones that consist of two subunits: the α-subunits are identical and the β-subunits differ
    3. Adrenocorticotropic hormone (ACTH, corticotropin) activates adenylyl cyclase in its target cells, and this leads to the increased rate of conversion of cholesterol (C_{27}) to pregnenolone (C_{21}), the rate-limiting step in steroid hormone biosynthesis
  B. Posterior pituitary hormones
    1. Vasopressin and oxytocin are nonapeptides produced in the posterior pituitary gland by mRNA-dependent protein synthesis and posttranslational processing
    2. Intravenous oxytocin is used in human therapeutics to induce labor in childbirth

Objective 2: To describe the hormonal regulation of calcium metabolism.

IV. Hormones and calcium metabolism
  A. The regulation of extracellular calcium is intricate and involves parathyroid hormone, calcitonin, and calcitriol
    1. Parathyroid hormone and calcitriol action increase plasma calcium
    2. Calcitonin decreases plasma calcium
  B. Organ systems that participate in calcium homeostasis include intestine, kidney, and bone
  C. Calcitriol metabolism involves the cooperation of three tissues
    1. Calcitriol is derived from 7-dehydrocholesterol in the skin by a photoactivation reaction
    2. This is followed by 25-hydroxylation in liver and 1-hydroxylation in kidney
    3. A 24-hydroxylation in kidney results in an inactive metabolite

Objective 3: To compare signal transduction initiated by glucagon and insulin.

V. Antagonistic effects of glucagon and insulin action
  A. Glucagon, which has a seven-transmembrane-segment receptor, operates through a cyclic AMP system via G-proteins
  B. Insulin's receptor, in contrast, contains two α-subunits (exterior) and two transmembrane β-subunits
    1. The β-subunits possess protein-tyrosine kinase activity
    2. Insulin and other hormones and growth factors activate Ras
      a. Grb2 and GEF (guanine nucleotide exchange factor) are required for Ras activation
      b. Ras is a G-protein
      c. Ras activates a Raf-Mek-Erk protein kinase cascade
      d. Mek is a dual-specificity protein kinase that phosphorylates both threonine and tyrosine Erk residues
      e. HVH1 is a dual-specificity protein-threonine and protein-tyrosine phosphatase that acts on Erk
    3. Protein kinase A, downstream from glucagon, catalyzes the phosphorylation and inactivation of Raf, which accounts in part for the antagonistic effects of glucagon and insulin
    4. Protein kinase C catalyzes the phosphorylation and activation of Raf

VI. Cytokine signal transduction
  A. Receptor and nonreceptor protein-tyrosine kinases
    1. Insulin and epidermal growth factor receptors are protein-tyrosine kinases
    2. Erythropoietin and other ligands activate their receptors, which then activate nonreceptor protein-tyrosine kinases
  B. Protein phosphatases
    1. The CD45 protein of immune cells is an example of a receptor protein-tyrosine phosphatase
    2. Other phosphatases are cytosolic, and still others are membrane-associated but do not possess ligand-recognition domains
  C. Receptor protein-serine kinases
    1. Transforming growth factor β receptors are transmembrane protein-serine/threonine kinases
    2. The substrates for such protein kinases have not been determined
    3. Protein-serine/threonine phosphatases described thus far are cytosolic

Objective 4: To describe the unique properties of atrial natriuretic factor.

VII. Atrial natriuretic peptide
  A. Atrial natriuretic peptide is synthesized, stored, and secreted by the atria
  B. The receptor for atrial natriuretic peptide is a protein of about 1000 amino acid residues and one transmembrane segment
    1. The extracellular domain recognizes atrial natriuretic peptide, and the intracellular domain of the atrial natriuretic peptide receptor possesses guanylyl cyclase activity
    2. The regulation of this membrane-associated guanylyl cyclase is controlled directly by the stimulatory ligand and does not involve G-proteins
    3. Cyclic GMP, the intracellular second messenger, activates protein kinase G to bring about its physiological actions

Objective 5: To delineate the actions of the renin-angiotensin system.

VIII. Renin and angiotensin
  A. Renin (active) and prorenin (inactive) are secreted from juxtaglomerular cells following the stimulation of β_1-adrenergic receptors by norepinephrine, which is released from sympathetic neurons
  B. Renin, a proteolytic enzyme, catalyzes the hydrolysis of angiotensinogen to produce angiotensin I, a decapeptide
  C. Angiotensin-converting enzyme (ACE) catalyzes the hydrolysis of angiotensin I (inactive) to angiotensin II (active), and a peptidase catalyzes the conversion of angiotensin II to angiotensin III (active)
  D. ACE inhibitors are widely used in the treatment of hypertension and congestive heart failure

Objective 6: To portray the actions of steroid hormones.

IX. Steroid hormone action
  A. The steroid hormone family includes calcitriol, thyroid hormones (T_3 and T_4), and retinoate
  B. The steroid hormone family of first messenger molecules acts by altering gene expression
    1. These hormones possess intracellular receptors
    2. Following the formation of the hormone-receptor complex, the activated receptor alters the transcription of target genes
    3. These genes contain hormone response elements that are recognized by the hormone-receptor complex
  C. The true steroid hormone receptors are located initially in the cytosol and move to the nucleus after binding to their hormone
    1. Each receptor possesses a ligand-recognition domain, a zinc-finger DNA binding domain, and a variable domain
    2. The receptor binds to DNA as a dimer
  D. Receptors for the other hormones of this family (thyroid hormone, retinoate, and vitamin D) are located initially in the nucleus, where they alter gene transcription after binding to their activating ligand

QUESTIONS

DIRECTIONS. (Items 1–10): Each set of matching questions in this section consists of a list of several lettered options followed by several numbered items. For each numbered item, select the ONE lettered option that is most closely associated with it. To avoid spending too much time on matching sets with large numbers of options, it is generally advisable to begin each set by reading the list of options. Then, for each item in the list, try to generate the correct answer and locate it in the option list, rather than evaluating each option individually. Each lettered option may be selected once, more than once, or not at all. Correct answers and explanations are given at the end of the chapter.

(A) Adrenocorticotropic hormone (ACTH)
(B) Aldosterone
(C) Angiotensin II
(D) Atrial natriuretic peptide
(E) Glucagon
(F) Insulin
(G) Insulin-like growth factor–1
(H) Melatonin
(I) Prolactin
(J) Renin
(K) Somatomammotropin
(L) Thyrotropin
(M) Thyrotropin-releasing hormone (TRH)
(N) Vasopressin

For each biochemical property given, select the correct hormone.

1. The level of this hormone is diminished in growth hormone–deficient dwarfs
2. An excessive amount of this hormone produces hypertension and hypokalemia (plasma potassium <4.0 mM) while there is suppressed plasma renin activity
3. This hormone is unique to pregnant women
4. This hormone is a glycoprotein that is made of an α-subunit and a β-subunit
5. This hormone is generated in the circulation
6. This hormone increases iodide transport in target cells
7. The prohormone for this substance is synthesized in the liver

(A) Acromegaly
(B) Addison disease
(C) Cushing syndrome
(D) Diabetes mellitus
(E) Diabetes insipidus
(F) Dwarfism
(G) Graves disease
(H) Pheochromocytoma

For each given characteristic, select the correct endocrine disease.

8. Increased skin pigmentation due to high levels of ACTH (adrenocorticotropin)
9. Can be treated with the recombinant human hormone but not with bovine or porcine hormones
10. Increased urinary 17-ketosteroid secretion

DIRECTIONS. (Items 11–18): Each of the numbered items or incomplete statements in this section is followed by answers or by completions of the statement. Select the ONE lettered answer or completion that is BEST in each case.

11. A patient who underwent partial thyroidectomy for the treatment of Graves disease developed hypocalcemia and a positive Chvostek sign. These conditions are due to a deficiency of

(A) calbindin
(B) calcitonin
(C) calcitriol
(D) calmodulin
(E) parathyroid hormone

12. The mechanism of insulin action involves each of the following steps EXCEPT

(A) interaction with a receptor that consists of two α-subunits and two β-subunits
(B) interaction with G_s, a guanine nucleotide heterotrimeric protein that activates adenylyl cyclase
(C) activation of protein-tyrosine kinase activity
(D) activation of Ras
(E) activation of the Raf-Mek-Erk protein kinase cascade

13. The mechanism of action of glucagon involves all of the following steps EXCEPT

(A) interaction with a seven-transmembrane-segment receptor
(B) activation of a G_s heterotrimeric protein
(C) generation of cyclic AMP as second messenger
(D) activation of protein kinase C
(E) activation of phosphorylase kinase and inhibition of glycogen synthase

14. Which one of the following substances possesses an intracellular receptor that functions in the nucleus?

(A) Adrenocorticotropic hormone
(B) Angiotensin
(C) Thyroid hormone (T_3 and T_4)
(D) Transforming growth factor β
(E) Vasopressin

Items 15–18

History

The patient is a 44-year-old female high school teacher who sought help for intermittent rapid heart rate (tachycardia) of 4 months' duration. She noted extreme mood variability, tremulousness, difficulty getting to sleep, and a 4.5-kg (10-lb) weight loss despite an increased appetite. She feels warm most of the time and sleeps without covers while her husband uses covers. She has noted burning, tearing, and itching of her eyes. Her eyes, moreover, appear to bulge.

Physical Examination

Her temperature is 37°C (98.6°F); pulse, 120/min; blood pressure, 150/70 mm Hg; height, 160 cm (5 ft, 3 in.); and weight, 49 kg (108 lb). The pupils are equal, react to light, and accommodate. She has bilateral lid lag (i.e., the upper lid lags behind the globe when the patient is asked to gaze slowly downward). Funduscopic examination is normal. She has bilateral proptosis, 22 mm on the right and 23 mm on the left (normal, <16 mm). Her thyroid is diffusely enlarged and estimated to be three times normal size. No thyroid nodules were palpated. Her heart rate is regular. Her skin is fine, warm, and moist. Knee and ankle reflexes are brisk bilaterally.

Laboratory

T_4, 21 μg/dL (normal, 5–12 μg/dL)
T_3, 1100 ng/dL (normal, 100–200 ng/dL)
Thyroid-stimulating hormone (TSH), <0.1 mU/L (normal, 2–10 mU/L)
Cholesterol, 162 mg/dL (recommended, <200 mg/dL)
Creatine phosphokinase (CPK), 32 U/L (normal ♀, 26–140 U/L)
Aspartate aminotransferase (AST, SGOT), 32 U/L (normal, 10–30 U/L)
Alkaline phosphatase, 124 U/L (normal, 42–98 U/L)
Total bilirubin, 0.6 mg/dL (normal, 0.2–1.0 mg/dL)
Serum glucose, 86 mg/dL (normal, 70–105 mg/dL)
Calcium, 10.2 mg/dL (normal, 8.4–10.2 mg/dL)
Phosphorus, 3.9 mg/dL (normal, 2.7–4.5 mg/dL)
Hematocrit, 38% (normal ♀, 35–45%)
White blood count, 6600/μL (normal, 4500–11,000/μL)
Polymorphonuclear leukocytes, 61% (normal, 54–62%)
Lymphocytes, 35% (normal, 23–33%)
Monocytes, 2% (normal, 3–7%)
Eosinophils, 2% (normal, 1–3%)

The patient was started on propranolol and propylthiouracil.

DIRECTIONS. (Items 15–18): Each of the numbered items or incomplete statements in this section is followed by answers or by completions of the statement. Select the ONE lettered answer or completion that is BEST in each case.

15. The most likely diagnosis in this patient is
    (A) adenoma of the thyroid gland
    (B) diabetes mellitus
    (C) Graves disease
    (D) hyperparathyroidism
    (E) pheochromocytoma

16. Which one of the following tests assesses the secretion of catecholamines from the adrenal medulla?
    (A) Measurement of monoamine oxidase in lymphocytes
    (B) Measurement of urinary 5-hydroxyindoleacetic acid
    (C) Measurement urinary 17-ketosteroids
    (D) Measurement of urinary homovanillate (HVA)
    (E) Measurement of urinary vanillylmandelic acid (VMA)

17. Which one of the following is a true statement regarding propranolol?
    (A) It inhibits the uptake of iodide by the thyroid gland
    (B) It inhibits the formation of protein-bound T_4 and T_3 in thyroglobulin
    (C) It inhibits oxidation and binding of iodine to thyroglobulin
    (D) It inhibits the proteolysis and release of thyroglobulin
    (E) It is a β-adrenergic antagonist

18. When cyclic AMP generation in normal thyroid plasma membrane fractions was measured under the following conditions, the following data were obtained:

Basal production	31 pmol
Propranolol, 1 μM	31 pmol
Normal human immunoglobulin fraction	31 pmol
TSH, 10 nM	540 pmol
TSH, 10 nM + 1 μM propranolol	540 pmol
TSH, 10 nM + normal human immunoglobulin fraction	540 pmol
Patient's immunoglobulin fraction	350 pmol
Patient's immunoglobulin fraction + 1 μM propranolol	350 pmol
TSH, 10 nM + patient's immunoglobulin fraction	350 pmol

From these data and the case history, the molecular basis for the development of this patient's elevated serum T_4 and T_3 is due to
    (A) stimulation of the TSH receptor by the patient's immunoglobulin but not by normal immunoglobulin
    (B) inhibition of adenylyl cyclase by TSH
    (C) failure to produce TSH
    (D) increased production of TSH
    (E) activation of the β-adrenergic receptor by the patient's immunoglobulin

ANSWERS AND EXPLANATIONS

1. The answer is G: insulin-like growth factor–1. Growth hormone is a major hormone produced by the anterior pituitary. This protein hormone has direct effects on target cells (glucose transport, differentiation of adipocytes, and cytochrome P-450 activity in liver cells), but its important physiological effects in promoting growth are mediated by insulin-like growth factor–1, a hormone produced by the liver. The secretion of insulin-like growth factor–2, another protein produced by the liver, is also stimulated by growth hormone. The effects of insulin-like growth factor–2 are unclear. *Biochemistry*, p. 421.
2. The answer is B: aldosterone. Aldosterone is a C_{21} steroid with a diagnostic C^{18} aldehyde group. This hormone promotes sodium retention and potassium and proton excretion from the kidney. Primary aldosteronism results in an excess of aldosterone production that causes hypertension and hypokalemia. This condition, which ac-

counts for less than 1% of all cases of hypertension, can be produced by an adrenal tumor or by adrenal hyperplasia. Surgical extirpation of the tumor is usually curative; medical therapy with spironolactone, an aldosterone antagonist, is used in patients with adrenal hyperplasia. In primary hyperaldosteronism, there is no increase in renin or angiotensin II, agents that lead to increased aldosterone production. The other steroid hormones include glucocorticoids, progestins, estradiol, and testosterone. These hormones have intracellular receptors that are initially located in the cytosol. After the hormone diffuses into the cell, the hormone binds to its corresponding receptor, and the receptor is converted to its activated form and moves into the nucleus. Each of the steroid hormone receptors is a dimer that is made up of monomers containing a hormone-binding domain, a DNA-binding domain, and a dimerization domain. The activated hormone binds to specific target sequences in the genome called steroid hormone response elements that either increase gene transcription (enhancers) or decrease gene transcription (silencers). *Biochemistry,* pp. 432–434.

3. The answer is K: somatomammotropin. This hormone, which is related to growth hormone and prolactin, is produced by the placenta. Although the placenta produces a prodigious amount of hormone ($\approx$1 g/d), the function of the hormone is unclear. Individuals who do not produce this hormone have normal pregnancies. *Biochemistry,* p. 422.
4. The answer is L: thyrotropin. Thyrotropin, luteinizing hormone, follicle-stimulating hormone, and chorionic gonadotropin are glycoprotein hormones that consist of two subunits: the α-subunits are identical and the β-subunits differ. *Biochemistry,* p. 421.
5. The answer is C: angiotensin II. Angiotensin II, an octapeptide, is formed from the hydrolysis of angiotensin I, a decapeptide. Angiotensin II stimulates the synthesis and secretion of aldosterone; angiotensin II is also a potent vasoconstrictor. *Biochemistry,* p. 431.
6. The answer is L: thyrotropin. Thyrotropin stimulates the synthesis and secretion of thyroid hormone (triiodothyronine and tetraiodothyronine). As part of this process, thyrotropin stimulates the transport of iodide into thyroid cells. *Biochemistry,* p. 422.
7. The answer is C: angiotensin II. Angiotensinogen, the precursor of angiotensin II, is synthesized and secreted by the liver. Insulin-like growth factor–1, which is a polypeptide that is synthesized by the liver, is a hormone, not a prohormone. *Biochemistry,* p. 431.
8. The answer is B: Addison disease. Addison disease results from a deficiency of the adrenal gland. As a result of hypoadrenocorticism, there is a compensatory increase in ACTH. ACTH is an analogue of melanocyte-stimulating hormone, and elevated levels of ACTH lead to increased melanin synthesis and skin pigmentation. *Biochemistry,* p. 423.
9. The answer is F: dwarfism. Children who produce inadequate growth hormone can be treated with human growth hormone; growth hormone from other sources is ineffective. In contrast, bovine and porcine hormones are effective in the treatment of diabetes mellitus. Growth hormone can be produced by modern biotechnology. This development has revolutionized the treatment of pituitary dwarfs because there is now an adequate supply of hormone without the risk of disease produced by growth hormone isolated from human cadavers. *Biochemistry,* p. 422.
10. The answer is C: Cushing syndrome. This disorder is the result of overproduction of glucocorticoids. These compounds are metabolized to form 17-ketosteroids, which are excreted in the urine. They can be measured to establish or confirm the diagnosis. *Biochemistry,* p. 423.
11. The answer is E: parathyroid hormone. All the parathyroid glands are occasionally removed inadvertently during subtotal thyroidectomy, and the action of parathyroid hormone is to increase serum calcium. A deficiency of parathyroid hormone leads to hypocalcemia, and this is associated with unilateral spasm being elicited by a slight tap over the facial nerve (Chvostek sign). Parathyroid hormone acts on osteoblasts (which then act on osteoclasts), and parathyroid hormone increases calcium reabsorption by the kidney. Calbindin is an intestinal protein that is induced by calcitriol and participates in calcium absorption. Calcitonin decreases serum calcium by decreasing bone and calcium resorption by inhibiting osteoclastic activity via the cyclic AMP second messenger system. Calcitriol increases calcium and phosphate reabsorption in the kidney and induces an intestinal calcium-transport protein. As a result of these actions, serum calcium is elevated. Calmodulin, which is a ubiquitous protein containing 148 amino acids, has four calcium-binding sites. After binding calcium, the protein undergoes a conformational change and can interact with and alter activity of target proteins including several protein kinases. *Biochemistry,* pp. 423–424.
12. The answer is B: interaction with G_s, a guanine nucleotide heterotrimeric protein that activates adenylyl cyclase. Insulin generally promotes a decrease in intracellular cyclic AMP and NOT an activation of adenylyl cyclase and generation of cyclic AMP. The insulin receptor consists of two α-subunits (which are on the cell exterior and bind to insulin) and two β-subunits that occur on the cell interior. The β-subunits possess protein-tyrosine kinase activity. Through the actions of Grb2 and GEF, insulin activates Ras. The Raf-Mek-Erk cascade is a downstream event in the insulin signal transduction process. *Biochemistry,* pp. 424–428.
13. The answer is D: the mechanism of action of glucagon does NOT involve activation of protein kinase C. Glucagon acts via the cyclic AMP second messenger system. Following the binding of glucagon to its seven-transmembrane-segment receptor, the complex interacts with a heterotrimeric G-protein called G_s (a guanine nucleotide-binding protein that stimulates adenylyl cyclase). As a result of activation of adenylyl cyclase, increased cyclic AMP is generated. The action of cyclic AMP is to activate its cognate protein kinase, called protein kinase A (protein kinase C is the enzyme that is activated by diglyceride and requires calcium for its activity). One action of protein kinase A is the phosphorylation and activation of phosphorylase kinase; another is phosphorylation and inhibition of glycogen synthase. *Biochemistry,* pp. 143–146, 424.
14. The answer is C: thyroid hormone (T_3 and T_4). Extracellular signals that possess intracellular receptors include the five classes of steroid hormones, thyroid hormone (T_3 and T_4), calcitriol (a vitamin D–derived substance), and retinoate. Other extracellular signals interact with receptors that are localized in the plasma membrane. *Biochemistry,* pp. 432–434.
15. The answer is C: Graves disease. Graves disease is characterized by an enlarged thyroid gland, oculopathy (lid lag and exophthalmus), and thyrotoxicosis. Symptoms of thyrotoxicosis in this patient include tachycardia, mood variability, tremulousness, weight loss, and heat intoler-

ance. Thyrotoxicosis can result from an adenoma of the thyroid, but physical examination revealed a diffusely enlarged thyroid lacking nodular enlargement. Hashimoto thyroiditis is another cause of thyrotoxicosis, but it is not accompanied by oculopathy. Weight loss and nervousness sometimes accompany diabetes mellitus; in this patient, the normal blood glucose makes this diagnosis unlikely. A small portion of patients with Graves disease have abnormalities of calcium metabolism; this patient's calcium and phosphate levels are normal, ruling hyperparathyroidism unlikely. One possible complication of subtotal thyroidectomy in the treatment of Graves disease is hypoparathyroidism in the event that all the parathyroid glands are inadvertently removed. Complete parathyroidectomy leads to hypocalcemia. Patients with Graves disease exhibit tachycardia, tremulousness, and lid lag, and such symptoms may be produced by a pheochromocytoma (a tumor of the adrenal medulla). In hyperthyroidism, these symptoms result from increased sensitivity to catecholamines and not sympathetic nervous system overactivity. The diastolic arterial pressure is normal in this patient, whereas it is generally elevated in pheochromocytoma. *Biochemistry,* p. 17; *Williams,* p. 419.

16. The answer is E: measurement of urinary vanillylmandelic acid (VMA). Such a test can be used to determine whether there is excessive catecholamine secretion by a pheochromocytoma. When the symptoms of thyrotoxicosis occur before the oculopathy and without thyroid enlargement, as is occasionally the case, then alternatives such as a pheochromocytoma have to be considered. Urinary 5-hydroxyindoleacetic acid is increased in carcinoid syndrome, and this is due to excessive production of serotonin. Symptoms include skin flushing. Urinary 17-ketosteroids are measured when adrenal cortical and not medullary disease is expected. Homovanillate (HVA) is the chief urinary metabolite of dopamine, and dopamine is not excreted in significant amounts by the adrenal medulla (dopamine is an intermediate in the synthesis of norepinephrine and epinephrine). *Biochemistry,* p. 401; *Williams,* p. 668.

17. The answer is E: propranolol is a β-adrenergic antagonist. Its purpose is to decrease the symptoms of sympathetic nervous system activity; it is not given to treat the primary disorder of hyperthyroidism. Thiocyanate and perchlorate inhibit the uptake of iodide by the thyroid gland and were formerly used in the treatment of hyperthyroidism. Propylthiouracil and related compounds are used in the treatment of hyperthyroidism, and they inhibit oxidation and binding of iodine to thyroglobulin and the formation of protein-bound T_4 and T_3 in thyroglobulin. Iodide, formerly used in the treatment of hyperthyroidism, inhibits the proteolysis and release of thyroglobulin. *Williams,* p. 419.

18. The answer is A: stimulation of the TSH receptor by the patient's immunoglobulin but not by normal immunoglobulin. The data also indicate that binding of the immunoglobulin blocks the binding of TSH to its receptors. Studies indicate that Graves disease is an autoimmune disease; the resulting antibodies are directed against and activate the TSH receptor. These studies also show that TSH acts via the cyclic AMP second messenger system. This activation is not inhibited by propranolol, a β-receptor antagonist, indicating that activation by immunoglobulin is not due to activation of the β-receptor. The decreased, and not increased, TSH present in this patient is due to feedback inhibition of TSH by T_3 and T_4. *Williams,* p. 419.

REFERENCES

Roskoski, R., Jr. *Biochemistry.* Philadelphia, W. B. Saunders Company, 1996.

Wilson, J. D., and D. W. Foster. *Williams Textbook of Endocrinology,* 8th ed. Philadelphia, W. B. Saunders Company, 1992.

CHAPTER TWENTY-ONE

CANCER, ONCOGENES, AND TUMOR SUPPRESSOR GENES

SYNOPSIS

OBJECTIVES

1. To outline the pathways of carcinogen metabolism.
2. To describe the main human carcinogens.
3. To describe the actions of protooncogenes, oncogenes, and tumor suppressors.
4. To outline the mechanisms of therapeutic agents used in the treatment of human neoplasia.
5. To outline the postulated relationships between diet and cancer.

Objective 1: To outline the pathways of carcinogen metabolism.

I. Biochemistry of cancer cells
   A. The development of cancer cells involves several steps that are incompletely understood
      1. *Several somatic mutations are required to produce cancer, and this concept is called the multistage theory of carcinogenesis*
      2. These steps involve mutations that produce growth-promoting cellular oncogenes (cancer-causing genes) and the inactivation of tumor suppressor genes
   B. The increased production of lactate by tumor cells is called the Warburg effect
II. Carcinogen metabolism
   A. Chemical carcinogens, which are compounds that produce cancer, are found in tobacco smoke, food contaminants (e.g, aflatoxin from *Aspergillus*), and solvents used in industry and manufacturing
   B. Chemical carcinogens are **direct** or **indirect acting**
      1. The direct-acting carcinogens react with nucleophilic groups in nucleic acids and produce mutations
      2. The indirect-acting carcinogens must be metabolized to **ultimate carcinogens** that are mutagenic
      3. The process for converting the indirect-acting agents to the ultimate carcinogen involves oxidations mediated by cytochrome P-450
   C. Carcinogens can be detected by the Ames test
      1. The Ames test is based on carcinogen mutagenicity, as detected in *Salmonella*
      2. Suspected compounds are first incubated with liver extracts, containing cytochrome P-450, to convert an indirect carcinogen to an ultimate carcinogen
      3. A carcinogen will cause a histidine-requiring *Salmonella* strain to grow in the absence of histidine
   D. The carcinogenic effects of tumor **initiators** (e.g., benzo[*a*]pyrene) are often enhanced by subsequent applications of tumor **promotors** (e.g., phorbol myristate)

Objective 2: To describe the main human carcinogens.

III. Causes of human neoplasia
   A. Environmental factors
      1. Tobacco smoke is the predominant cause of cancer mortality in the United States and many other nations
         a. Tobacco smoke contains several carcinogens, including polycyclic hydrocarbons
         b. Perhaps a third of all cancer deaths in the United States are directly attributable to tobacco use, and cigarette smoking is the largest single preventable cause of cancer
      2. Ionizing radiation from radioactive chemicals and x rays can produce cancer in humans
   B. DNA viruses
      1. Hepatitis B virus, which is responsible for serum hepatitis, is the virus most commonly linked to cancer in the United States
         a. Only a small fraction of carriers develop hepatomas, and this occurs many years (20–30) after the primary infection develops

b. The pathogenesis of hepatitis B–induced tumorigenesis is a mystery

2. Epstein-Barr virus is a herpes-like DNA virus that produces two types of neoplasm in humans, including Burkitt lymphoma (common in certain parts of Africa), a primary cancer in children, and nasopharyngeal carcinoma (common in southern China)
   a. Epstein-Barr virus is a causative agent of infectious mononucleosis in the United States
   b. The mechanism for the production of tumors is unknown

C. RNA viruses
1. Rous sarcoma virus was the first virus shown to produce tumors in animals
   a. This virus produces sarcomas in chickens and rodents
   b. The oncogene of Rous sarcoma virus is a protein-tyrosine kinase, the first protein-tyrosine kinase to be discovered
2. **Human T-cell lymphotropic virus** (HTLV), the only retrovirus that causes a neoplastic disorder in humans, is associated with a T-lymphocytic neoplasia seen in southern Japan

Objective 3: To describe the actions of protooncogenes, oncogenes, and tumor suppressors.

IV. Mechanisms of neoplastic transformation

A. Cellular oncogenes
1. Cellular oncogenes result from mutation, amplification (production of more copies of genetic DNA than are normally present), or overexpression (increased transcription and translation of existing genes) of normal cellular genes, but cellular oncogenes in humans are not the result of viral infection
2. Proteins that participate in controlling cell growth include (a) growth factors, (b) receptor protein-tyrosine kinases, (c) nonreceptor protein-tyrosine kinases, (d) Ras, (e) protein-serine/threonine kinases, (f) nuclear proteins and transcription factors, and (g) a mitochondrial protein
3. Ras is a GTP-binding protein that is implicated in several types of human cancers
   a. Oncogenic *ras* can be derived from the normal cellular protooncogene by a mutation of a single nucleotide
   b. *ras* Oncogenes occur in about 25% of all human neoplasms, but this association is neither necessary nor sufficient to produce a particular neoplasm
4. The receptor and nonreceptor protein-tyrosine kinases catalyze the phosphorylation of phospholipase C_γ, an isoenzyme of phospholipase C
   a. The stimulation of diglyceride and inositol trisphosphate formation catalyzed by phospholipase C represents one plausible mechanism for the effects of growth factors and oncogenes
   b. Protein-tyrosine kinases can activate the Raf-Mek-Erk signal transduction pathway to produce their growth stimulatory effects
   c. Downstream targets of this pathway include the AP-1 transcription factor that is made up of Fos and Jun

B. Protooncogene translocation and amplification
1. Malignant transformation in **chronic myelogenous leukemia** is related to the translocation of the *abl* protooncogene from its normal position on chromosome 9 to chromosome 22
   a. *abl* Encodes a protein-tyrosine kinase
   b. The **Philadelphia chromosome** (Ph^+) is an abbreviated chromosome 22 that results from a reciprocal translocation with chromosome 9
   c. The translocation of *abl* contributes to the malignant state and is a strong diagnostic indicator of chronic myelogenous leukemia
2. In **Burkitt lymphoma,** the *myc* protooncogene is translocated from chromosome 8 to chromosome 14, which carries the antibody heavy chain genes
   a. Burkitt lymphoma, which is associated with Epstein-Barr virus infection, is a neoplasm of B lymphocytes
   b. The antibody genes are actively transcribed in B cells

C. Tumor suppressor genes
1. The retinoblastoma (*RB1*) gene was discovered during the study of the pathogenesis of retinoblastoma, a childhood malignancy
   a. The *RB1* gene is entirely or largely deleted in many retinoblastoma tumors
   b. The retinoblastoma gene product is a nuclear protein with a molecular mass of 105 kDa
   c. RB1 protein becomes heavily phosphorylated as cells begin to duplicate their DNA in the S phase of the cell cycle; otherwise, the protein is lightly phosphorylated
      (1) The lightly phosphorylated retinoblastoma gene product inhibits cell division
      (2) The heavily phosphorylated form is less inhibitory
2. The *p53* gene was discovered during the study of virus-induced neoplasia
   a. p53 is a tumor suppressor with a molecular mass of 53 kDa (hence, its name)
   b. *Alteration of p53, which occurs in about half of all human neoplasms, is one of the most common biochemical findings in human neoplasia*
   c. p53 binds to DNA, and mutant forms fail to bind
      (1) Normal p53 can put the brakes on cell growth and division, prevent the unruly amplification and mutation of DNA, and push cells into a programmed self-destruction pathway called apoptosis
      (2) Mutant p53 fails to perform these functions and contributes to production of the neoplastic state

Objective 4: To outline the mechanisms of therapeutic agents used in the treatment of human neoplasia.

V. Cancer chemotherapy

A. Agents that modify DNA by alkylation include the nitrogen mustards and cisplatin

B. Antimetabolites that inhibit purine synthesis include mercaptopurine, thioguanine, and methotrexate

C. Agents that inhibit deoxyribonucleotide formation include hydroxyurea and fluorouracil
D. Incorporation of cytosine arabinoside into DNA produces abnormal DNA
E. Several enzymes are the targets of chemotherapeutic agents
   1. Methotrexate is a competitive inhibitor of dihydrofolate reductase, and fluorouracil is converted to an agent that is a suicide inhibitor of thymidylate synthase
   2. Agents that modify DNA by interacting with topoisomerase II include antibiotics (e.g., daunorubicin, doxorubicin) and plant alkaloids (e.g., etoposide, teniposide)
   3. Actinomycin D inhibits DNA-dependent RNA polymerase
F. Asparaginase inhibits protein biosynthesis indirectly
G. The *Vinca* alkaloids disrupt microtubule function and mitosis
H. Sex hormone antagonists are used in the treatment of cancer of the breast and prostate

Objective 5: To outline the postulated relationships between diet and cancer.

VI. Diet and cancer
A. Epidemiological studies indicate that high dietary fat increases the incidence of cancer of the colon, rectum, and breast
B. There is an inverse correlation between colorectal cancer and fiber intake
C. Some epidemiological studies suggest an inverse relationship between cancer incidence and intake of foods high in several antioxidant nutrients such as ascorbate, β-carotene, and vitamin E
   1. β-Carotene and vitamin E (tocopherol) are lipids that dissolve in membranes
   2. Ascorbate, in contrast, is a hydrophilic vitamin
   3. These antioxidants may function as scavengers of reactive oxygen intermediates that are generated from ionizing irradiation

QUESTIONS

DIRECTIONS. (Items 1–4): The set of matching questions in this section consists of a list of several lettered options followed by several numbered items. For each numbered item, select the ONE lettered option that is most closely associated with it. To avoid spending too much time on matching sets with large numbers of options, it is generally advisable to begin each set by reading the list of options. Then, for each item in the list, try to generate the correct answer and locate it in the option list, rather than evaluating each option individually. Each lettered option may be selected once, more than once, or not at all. Correct answers and explanations are given at the end of the chapter.

(A) Actinomycin D
(B) Asparaginase
(C) Bleomycin
(D) Cisplatin
(E) Chlorambucil
(F) Cytosine arabinoside
(G) Daunorubicin
(H) Diethylstilbestrol
(I) Fluorouracil
(J) Flutamide
(K) Hydroxyurea
(L) Interferon α
(M) Mercaptopurine
(N) Methotrexate
(O) Tamoxifen
(P) Thioguanine
(Q) Vinblastine

For each biochemical process, select the correct cancer chemotherapeutic agent.

1. An antibiotic that inhibits DNA-dependent RNA synthesis
2. An antibiotic that inhibits human topoisomerase II
3. A free radical scavenger that inhibits ribonucleoside diphosphate reductase
4. This substance decreases the extracellular levels of a protein precursor

DIRECTIONS. (Items 5–18): Each of the numbered items or incomplete statements in this section is followed by answers or by completions of the statement. Select the ONE lettered answer or completion that is BEST in each case.

5. The increased incidence of skin cancer and internal cancers in people with xeroderma pigmentosum is due to mutations that involve
   (A) nuclear receptors
   (B) nucleotide-excision repair
   (C) protein-tyrosine kinases
   (D) protooncogenes
   (E) tumor suppressor genes

6. Malignant transformation in chronic myelogenous leukemia is related to the translocation of which one of the following protooncogenes from its normal position on chromosome 9 to chromosome 22?
   (A) *abl*
   (B) *myc*
   (C) *p53*
   (D) *ras*
   (E) *RB1*

7. Phorbol esters, which activate protein kinase C, are examples of
   (A) direct carcinogens
   (B) indirect carcinogens
   (C) ultimate carcinogens
   (D) tumor promoters
   (E) tumor initiators

8. A chemical agent requires preincubation with a liver extract in order to cause the *Salmonella* test organism to grow in the absence of histidine. Which one of the following is a true statement regarding this chemical agent?
   (A) It is a tumor promoter
   (B) It is a direct-acting carcinogen
   (C) It is an indirect-acting carcinogen
   (D) It is an oncogene
   (E) It is a tumor suppressor gene

9. Which one of the following viruses has been shown to produce cancer directly in humans?
   (A) AIDS virus
   (B) HTLV (human T-cell lymphotropic virus)
   (C) Poliovirus
   (D) Rous sarcoma virus
   (E) Vaccinia virus

10. A mold that can contaminate food contains which one of the following carcinogens that produces liver cancer in humans?
   (A) Aflatoxin
   (B) Nitrite (NO_2^-)
   (C) Nitrosamine
   (D) Nitrosonornicotine
   (E) Phenol

11. Mutation of which one of the following tumor suppressor genes can lead to multiple eye tumors in children?
   (A) *bcl2*
   (B) *erb*B2/*neu*
   (C) RAR
   (D) *RB1*
   (E) *src*

12. Which one of the following tumor suppressor gene products, which plays a role in apoptosis and cell survival, is located in the inner mitochondrial membrane?
   (A) bcl2
   (B) NF1
   (C) p53
   (D) RB1
   (E) WT1

13. Which one of the following proteins plays a pivotal role in passing the checkpoint for initiation of cell division?
   (A) G_1 cyclin–dependent protein kinase
   (B) Histone H1
   (C) M cyclin–dependent protein kinase
   (D) Nuclear lamins
   (E) p54 phosphatase

Items 14–18

History

A 46-year-old female school teacher felt a lump in her left breast. Menses, which began at age 12, were regular until the past 18 months. She has one son and two daughters in good health. Her first child was born when the patient was 22 years old. There is no family history of breast or other cancers.

Physical Examination

Physical examination revealed a 2-cm, firm lesion in the upper outer quadrant of her left breast. The nipple appeared normal.

Laboratory

Laboratory examination revealed normal red and white blood cell counts, normal electrolytes, and normal kidney and liver function tests, including alkaline phosphatase. Urinalysis and chest x-ray were normal. Histological examination of the mass revealed a carcinoma, and the patient underwent a left radical mastectomy and node dissection. One of the 16 resected nodes showed metastasis. Microscopic examination revealed an infiltrating ductal carcinoma with a large proportion of cells in mitosis; the primary tumor was negative for estrogen receptor and progesterone receptor and positive for the *erb*B2/*neu* oncogene. The patient was started on chemotherapy consisting of cyclophosphamide, methotrexate, and fluorouracil.

14. It is unlikely that any residual tumor in this patient would respond to antiestrogen therapy or estrogen withdrawal because
   (A) a large proportion of cells were in mitosis
   (B) the tumor was positive for the *erb*B2/*neu* oncogene
   (C) the tumor was 2 cm in size
   (D) the tumor lacked estrogen receptor
   (E) the patient is perimenopausal

15. Which one of the following is a true statement regarding cyclophosphamide?
   (A) It is an alkylating agent
   (B) It inhibits dihydrofolate reductase
   (C) It inhibits human topoisomerase II
   (D) It is a hormone antagonist
   (E) It is an antimetabolite

16. Which one of the following is a true statement regarding methotrexate?
   (A) It aborts the catalytic cycle of human topoisomerase II
   (B) It is an alkylating agent
   (C) It inhibits dihydrofolate reductase
   (D) It is a hormone antagonist
   (E) It inhibits RNA polymerase

17. Which one of the following is a true statement regarding fluorouracil?
   (A) It is an alkylating agent
   (B) It inhibits human topoisomerase II
   (C) It inhibits dihydrofolate reductase
   (D) It is a hormone antagonist
   (E) It is incorporated into RNA and is also converted to an inhibitor of thymidylate synthase

18. Metastasis of a tumor to bone may be indicated by an elevation of which of the following serum enzymes?
   (A) Acid phosphatase
   (B) Alkaline phosphatase
   (C) Aspartate aminotransferase
   (D) γ-Glutamyl transpeptidase
   (E) Lactate dehydrogenase

ANSWERS AND EXPLANATIONS

1. The answer is A: actinomycin D. Actinomycin D, also called dactinomycin, is a peptide derivative that was one of the first antibiotics isolated from *Streptomyces* in the 1940s. Actinomycin D inhibits DNA-dependent RNA synthesis. This antibiotic, which intercalates with DNA between two adjacent G–C base pairs, binds to the DNA template and inhibits the elongation reactions of RNA, but not DNA, synthesis. *Biochemistry,* p. 453.
2. The answer is G: daunorubicin. Daunorubicin and doxorubicin produce breaks in DNA in a process that involves topoisomerase II. Topoisomerase II forms phosphodiesters through protein-tyrosine residues with the backbone of DNA during the catalytic cycle. Topoisomerase II thereby creates discontinuities in DNA during its catalytic cycle, and daunorubicin and doxorubicin abort complete catalysis and thereby produce aberrant DNA cleavage. Etoposide and teniposide also cause topoisomerase II to cleave DNA in an aberrant reaction. *Biochemistry,* p. 453.
3. The answer is K: hydroxyurea. Hydroxyurea, which is a chemical scavenger that destroys an active site protein-tyrosyl free radical intermediate, is an inhibitor of the ribonucleoside diphosphate reductase. Hydroxyurea decreases the formation of deoxyribonucleotide precursors of DNA. *Biochemistry,* p. 453.
4. The answer is B: asparaginase. Many normal cells synthesize asparagine in amounts sufficient for protein synthesis. Biosynthesis involves a reaction between aspartate, glutamine (the amide donor), and ATP (which undergoes a pyrophosphate split) as catalyzed by asparagine synthetase. Many neoplastic cells, however, require an exogenous source of asparagine for protein synthesis. Asparaginase catalyzes the hydrolysis of asparagine to aspartate and ammonia. This reaction is exergonic according to PRINCIPLE 5 OF BIOENERGETICS. Asparaginase, isolated and purified from *Escherichia coli* or from *Erwinia carotovora,* when injected, catalyzes the degradation of extracellular asparagine and thereby deprives cells of this amino acid. A deficiency of a single amino acid in a cell prevents protein synthesis and causes cell death. Since asparaginase is a foreign protein, it is antigenic, and allergic reactions can occur. The enzymes from *E. coli* and *E. carotovora* are not immunologically cross-reactive. The *Erwinia* enzyme is used in individuals who develop antibodies to the *E. coli* enzyme. *Biochemistry,* p. 455.
5. The answer is B: nucleotide-excision repair. Several gene defects have been described in patients with xeroderma pigmentosum, and 10 or more proteins may be required for nucleotide-excision repair. In xeroderma pigmentosum, substrates that are not efficiently restored as a result of defects in the repair system include thymine dimers, the most common ultraviolet light–induced lesion, and other pyrimidine dimers (T–C, C–C) introduced by ultraviolet light. Moreover, modifications induced by benzo[*a*]pyrene and other carcinogens also accumulate. On the other hand, modifications produced by x-ray and by DNA alkylating agents do not accumulate in xeroderma pigmentosum, and these are repaired by other processes. *Biochemistry,* pp. 288–289.
6. The answer is A: the *abl* protooncogene. Malignant transformation in chronic myelogenous leukemia is related to the translocation of the *abl* protooncogene, which encodes a protein-tyrosine kinase, from its normal position on chromosome 9 to chromosome 22 to produce the Philadelphia chromosome. The translocation contributes to the malignant state and is a strong diagnostic indicator of chronic myelogenous leukemia. In Burkitt lymphoma, the *myc* protooncogene is translocated from chromosome 8 to chromosome 14, which carries the antibody heavy chain genes. Burkitt lymphoma, which is associated with Epstein-Barr virus infection, is a neoplasm of B lymphocytes. The antibody genes are actively transcribed in B cells. The *ras* gene, which encodes a G-protein, undergoes mutation in about 25% of all human cancers. *RB1* and *p53* are tumor suppressor genes and not oncogenes. *Biochemistry,* pp. 445–446.
7. The answer is D: tumor promoters. In a two-stage model for producing tumors in animals, the single application of a tumor initiator such as benzo[*a*]pyrene must be followed by the application of a tumor promoter before neoplastic transformation occurs. One type of tumor promoter is phorbol ester, an activator of protein kinase C. This agent will not produce neoplasia when it is applied alone. Activation of protein kinase C may facilitate tumorigenesis by activating the Raf-Mek-Erk signal transduction cascade. Direct carcinogens are capable of producing neoplastic transformation without undergoing metabolic change. Indirect carcinogens must be metabolized by the cytochrome P-450 electron transport system to form the active agent called the ultimate carcinogen. *Biochemistry,* p. 439.
8. The answer is C: an indirect-acting carcinogen. The cytochrome P-450 system mediates the oxidation of indirect carcinogens to hydroxylated compounds that are the ultimate carcinogens. This provides the rationale for treating compounds with liver extracts prior to testing their mutagenicity based upon the Ames test using histidine-requiring strains of *Salmonella.* A direct-acting carcinogen does not require chemical conversion to be mutagenic or carcinogenic. Tumor promoters *per se* are not carcinogenic. Oncogenes and tumor suppressor genes occur in the host cell. *Biochemistry,* p. 439.
9. The answer is B: HTLV (human T-cell lymphotropic virus). HTLV is an RNA retrovirus that produces a T-cell leukemia in humans. The number of viruses that produce cancer in humans is small. The AIDS virus *per se* does not produce malignancies in humans. The tumors that develop, such as Kaposi sarcoma, arise secondary to immunosuppression. Vaccinia virus and poliovirus do not produce tumors in humans. Rous sarcoma virus produces sarcomas in chickens and some rodents but not in humans. Epstein-Barr virus is a DNA virus that can cause malignancy in susceptible humans. Herpesvirus and hepatitis B virus are associated with certain types of tumors in humans, but the mechanism of tumorigenesis is unknown. *Biochemistry,* p. 443.
10. The answer is A: aflatoxin. Aflatoxin is a procarcinogen that is produced by *Aspergillus flavus,* a mold that can contaminate peanuts and other foods. Aflatoxin is metabolized to an ultimate carcinogen that produces hepatomas in humans. Nitrites, which occur in smoked foods, are metabolized to carcinogenic nitrosamines. Nitrosonornicotine is a nitrosamine metabolite that occurs in cigarette smoke. Phenol is a weak carcinogen, but it oc-

curs in relatively large amounts in cigarette smoke. *Biochemistry,* pp. 438, 440.

11. The answer is D: *RB1.* The retinoblastoma tumor suppressor gene was discovered during the analysis of the pathogenesis of retinoblastoma, a childhood malignancy of the retina. Tumor suppressor genes block abnormal growth and malignant transformation. The retinoblastoma gene product is a nuclear protein with a molecular mass of 105 kDa. The protein becomes heavily phosphorylated as cells begin to duplicate their DNA in the S phase of the cell cycle; otherwise, the protein is lightly phosphorylated. The lightly phosphorylated retinoblastoma gene product inhibits cell division, and the heavily phosphorylated form is less inhibitory. The most likely point at which the retinoblastoma gene protein exerts its effect is the G_1–S transition in the cell cycle. Unphosphorylated retinoblastoma gene protein binds to transcription factors and may alter the expression of genes involved in cell cycle regulation. Active retinoblastoma gene protein turns off the expression of the nuclear protooncogene *myc,* and this may be one mechanism for inhibiting cell division. In contrast, *bcl2, erb*B2/*neu,* and *src* are protooncogenes. RAR refers to the retinoate receptor. *Biochemistry,* pp. 446–447.

12. The answer is A: bcl2. Apoptosis (Greek "dropping off") is the normal and programmed destruction of cells during embryogenesis, development, and adult life. Disruption of apoptosis can promote inappropriate cell survival and the development of cancer and is yet another mechanism for neoplastic transformation. The bcl2 gene product resides in the inner mitochondrial membrane. How it participates in normal apoptosis is a mystery. p53 is a tumor suppressor with a molecular mass of 53 kDa, hence its name. The *p53* gene is inactivated by point mutations, and normal p53 protein can be inactivated by forming complexes with cellular proteins or by proteolysis. Oncoproteins produced by human papillomavirus, for example, trigger degradation of p53. Loss of p53 function occurs in 70% of colorectal cancers, 50% of lung cancers, and 40% of breast cancers. *Alteration of p53, which occurs in about half of all human neoplasms, is one of the most common biochemical findings in human neoplasia.* (Alteration of Ras, which occurs in about 25% of all human tumors, also is common.) p53 is usually localized in the nucleus and can be phosphorylated. p53 binds to DNA, and mutant forms fail to bind. p53 can put the brakes on cell growth and division, prevent the unruly amplification and mutation of DNA, and push cells into apoptosis. The suppression of cell death by mutant *p53* can lead to cancer. p53 can also turn on the synthesis of p21, a protein that inhibits cyclin-dependent protein kinase. As a result of inhibition of this kinase, the cell is unable to pass a checkpoint in the cell division cycle. Wilms tumor is a kidney tumor involving tumor suppressor genes. This tumor, like retinoblastoma, is expressed during childhood and occurs in sporadic (90%) and hereditary (10%) forms. One gene product, from the *WT1* locus, functions in the regulation of kidney and gonadal development and in the genesis of Wilms tumor. WT1, which contains four zinc-finger motifs, binds to DNA at target sequences and regulates the transcription of specific genes. This factor can suppress the transcription of the platelet-derived growth factor A chain, and this action may account, in part, for its tumor suppressor activity. The *NF1* gene is altered in von Recklinghausen neurofibromatosis, which occurs with a frequency of 1 in 3000 births. Half of these represent new mutations, making this one of the most commonly mutated alleles in the general population. Multiple tumors occur in affected individuals, the most common being the subcutaneous neurofibromas that are composed of proliferating neurites, Schwann cells, and fibroblasts. The tumors in 97% of affected individuals are benign. Analysis of the coding region of *NF1* has revealed significant homology to GAP, the GTPase activating protein that converts active Ras to its inactive form. The *NF1* gene product activates Ras-dependent GTP hydrolysis. A decline in GTPase activity of NF1 in neurofibromatosis may lead to increased Ras activity, and this can lead to neoplastic transformation via the downstream Raf signal transduction pathway. *Biochemistry,* p. 444.

13. The answer is A: G_1 cyclin–dependent protein kinase. The cell cycle consists of four phases (G_1, S, G_2, and M). Quiescent cells are considered to be in G_0 phase. During the cell division cycle, the cell passes through a number of checkpoints, or transition points, at which progression to the next stage can be promoted or halted. Checkpoints make cell division responsive to external conditions such as nutrients and growth factors. An orderly progression through the cell cycle ensures that mitosis, for example, starts only after all of the DNA has been replicated. The most important checkpoint in the cell cycle occurs at the initiation of DNA replication. If the conditions for cell division are unfavorable, the cell becomes arrested in G_1. A group of proteins called G_1 cyclins accumulate during G_1 and participate in the pathway to initiate DNA synthesis, and these proteins control the activity of their cognate G_1 cyclin–dependent protein kinase. This enzyme catalyzes the phosphorylation of proteins that initiate the S phase of the cell cycle. After this checkpoint is passed, proteases destroy the activating cyclins, and G_1 cyclin–dependent protein kinase activity declines. A second group, called M cyclins, participate in the pathway to initiate mitosis, and this is an important secondary checkpoint in the cell cycle. A different protein kinase, M cyclin–dependent protein kinase, is responsible for traversing the G_2–M checkpoint. There is an increased synthesis of cyclin M before M phase. Cyclin M associates with its kinase, but the latter becomes phosphorylated at specific tyrosine and threonine residues by other protein kinases that maintain inhibition, even in the presence of activating cyclins. To pass this checkpoint, p54 phosphatase catalyzes the dephosphorylation of threonine and tyrosine and the activation M cyclin–dependent protein kinase. The activated kinase initiates mitosis by catalyzing the phosphorylation of acceptor proteins. Cyclin M is degraded by proteolysis, and the kinase is thereby inactivated following destruction of the activator. The process is repeated during the next cell division. The substrates for M cyclin–dependent protein kinase include (1) histone H1, promoting chromosomal condensation, (2) nuclear lamins, causing dispersal of the nuclear membrane, (3) nucleolin, arresting ribosome synthesis, and (4) myosin light chain kinase, promoting cytokinesis. *Biochemistry,* pp. 448–449.

14. The answer is D: the tumor lacked estrogen receptor. Estrogens interact with intracellular receptors to bring about their physiological responses. Cells lacking this receptor are unlikely to respond to estrogen antagonists. Tumors that contain receptor may be stimulated by estrogens, and blockade of the receptor by antagonists such as tamoxifen is inhibitory. That a large portion of cells were in mitosis and are positive for the *erb*B2/*neu* oncogene indicates that the tumor is aggressive. *Biochemistry,* p. 455.

15. The answer is A: cyclophosphamide is an alkylating agent. The reaction of alkylating agents with the N^7 of guanine is prevalent. The modified base can pair abnormally during replication and lead to mutation, or it can be eliminated from DNA, leading to chain scission or DNA fragmentation. Cross-linking of DNA chains can also occur. Alkylating agents disturb cell growth, mitosis, differentiation, and cell function. More rapidly dividing cells are susceptible to the action of these agents. In slowly dividing cells, DNA repair processes can reverse the effects of DNA modification. *Biochemistry,* pp. 449–451.
16. The answer is C: methotrexate inhibits dihydrofolate reductase. Tetrahydrofolate derivatives are required for purine and thymidylate biosynthesis. Dietary folate must be converted to dihydrofolate and tetrahydrofolate in reactions catalyzed by dihydrofolate reductase prior to their participation in nucleotide metabolism. Dihydrofolate is also generated in the thymidylate synthetase reaction where methylenetetrahydrofolate acts as a reductant and methyl group donor. Methotrexate prevents the regeneration of tetrahydrofolate from dihydrofolate. Thymidylate synthesis is more sensitive to tetrahydrofolate depletion than is purine synthesis. Cell killing, however, proceeds more efficiently when both thymidylate and purine synthesis are inhibited. Doxorubicin, an inhibitor of human topoisomerase II, is also used frequently in the treatment of breast cancer. Actinomycin D but not methotrexate is an inhibitor of RNA polymerase. *Biochemistry,* p. 453; *Sabiston,* p. 543.
17. The answer is E: fluorouracil is incorporated into RNA and is also converted to an inhibitor of thymidylate synthase. Orotate phosphoribosyltransferase, one of the two activities of the UMP synthase complex of pyrimidine synthesis, catalyzes the reaction of PRPP with fluorouracil. Fluorouridine monophosphate can be converted sequentially to the di- and triphosphates in reactions involving ATP. Fluorouridine triphosphate can be incorporated into RNA, and this incorporation diminishes the posttranscriptional processing and physiological activity of RNA. Fluorouridine diphosphate can be converted to fluorodeoxyuridine diphosphate as catalyzed by ribonucleotide reductase. Fluorodeoxyuridine monophosphate, derived from precursors, is a suicide inhibitor of thymidylate synthase. Suicide inhibition requires the generation of an active species, during an abortive catalytic cycle, that reacts with and inactivates the enzyme. The clinical efficacy of fluorouracil is due to its incorporation into RNA and to inhibition of thymidylate synthase. *Biochemistry,* pp. 450, 453.
18. The answer is B: alkaline phosphatase. The metastasis of tumors to bone initiates a reactive process in bone that is accompanied by elevated serum alkaline phosphatase. This enzyme appears to be related to the deposition of calcium phosphate and formation of hydroxyapatite $[Ca_{10}(PO_4)_6(OH)_2]$ during osteoblastic activity. Alkaline phosphatase is also elevated in liver disease. *Biochemistry,* p. 62.

REFERENCES

Roskoski, R., Jr. *Biochemistry.* Philadelphia, W. B. Saunders Company, 1996.

Sabiston, D. C. (ed.). *Textbook of Surgery,* 14th ed. Philadelphia, W. B. Saunders Company, 1991.

CHAPTER TWENTY-TWO

MEMBRANE TRANSPORT

SYNOPSIS

OBJECTIVES

1. To compare diffusion, transport, and facilitated diffusion.
2. To note the mechanism for the primary active transport of ions.
3. To compare the class P, V, and F ATPases.
4. To describe secondary active transport.
5. To outline the γ-glutamyl cycle for amino acid transport.
6. To describe the cystic fibrosis transmembrane conductance regulator.

Objective 1: To compare diffusion, transport, and facilitated diffusion.

I. Diffusion and transport through membranes
   A. Oxygen, carbon dioxide, urea, and ethanol are among the few biologically important substances that can diffuse through membranes
   B. For larger polar molecules such as glucose, ions, and charged molecules such as amino acids, glucose 6-phosphate, and ATP, special transport systems effect translocation
   C. The rate of transport by simple diffusion is a linear function of the solute concentration and does not exhibit saturation
   D. In contrast, transport that is mediated by protein translocases exhibits saturation, and the initial rate of transport is a hyperbolic function of solute concentration

II. Facilitated diffusion
   A. Facilitated diffusion involves protein-mediated translocation without an external source of energy such as ATP (primary active transport) or a sodium gradient (secondary active transport)
   B. Transport of glucose into the erythrocyte is ATP- and sodium ion–independent
      1. The source of energy for transport is a glucose gradient
      2. The glucose translocase transports glucose down its concentration gradient until equilibrium is reached
      3. The glucose translocase of the erythrocyte is an integral membrane protein with a molecular mass of 45 kDa
   C. Seven subclasses of sodium-independent glucose transporter have been studied by cDNA analysis, called GLUT1 through GLUT7, based upon the order of discovery (GLUT, *glu*cose *t*ransporter)
      1. GLUT1 is the erythrocyte glucose transporter, and GLUT4, which occurs in muscle and adipocytes, is insulin responsive
      2. The GLUT family of transporters possess 12 transmembrane segments

Objective 2: To note the mechanism for the primary active transport of ions.

III. Primary active transport
   A. Sodium/potassium-ATPase
      1. The sodium/potassium-ATPase is a tetramer consisting of two dissimilar subunits
         a. Its composition is $\alpha_2\beta_2$, and its total molecular mass is 270 kDa
         b. Both subunits are transmembrane proteins
         c. The small β-subunit (40 kDa) is a glycoprotein with one transmembrane segment, and its function is unknown
         d. The large α-subunit (95 kDa), which contains eight transmembrane segments, reacts with ATP and contains the binding sites for sodium, potassium, ouabain, and the other cardiotonic steroids including digitalis
         e. Ouabain is a specific inhibitor of the sodium/potassium-ATPase
      2. The sodium/potassium-ATPase exists in two functionally distinct conformations called E_1 and E_2
         a. Three sodium ions in the cell interior bind to the enzyme (E_1), and ATP phosphorylates the α-subunit of the enzyme in a functionally isoergonic process (PRINCIPLE 1 OF BIOENERGETICS)
         b. The enzymic aspartyl-phosphate bond is initially energy rich
         c. The enzyme, which undergoes a conformational change to form E_2, delivers the three sodium ions to the exterior of the cell
         d. The phosphate remains linked to the same aspartyl group, but its standard free energy of hydrolysis is converted to an energy-poor variety ($E_1{\sim}P \rightarrow E_2{-}P$); the protein ($E_2$) alters the stan-

dard free energy of hydrolysis of the acylphosphate

e. Potassium binds to the exterior of the sodium/potassium-ATPase and is transported to the interior

f. The enzyme undergoes an exergonic hydrolytic dephosphorylation reaction (PRINCIPLE 5 OF BIOENERGETICS), and two potassium ions are released inside the cell

g. The enzyme reverts to the original E_1 conformation

B. Calcium-ATPase

1. The relaxation of skeletal muscle, which is mediated by a calcium-ATPase, requires the transport of calcium from the cytoplasm of muscle cells (sarcoplasm) into a specialized and abundant sarcoplasmic reticulum membrane system
2. Calcium-ATPase consists of a single polypeptide with 10 transmembrane segments
3. For each mole of ATP hydrolyzed, two moles of calcium are transported into the sarcoplasmic reticulum
4. The mechanism for transport is similar to that proposed for the sodium/potassium-ATPase

Objective 3: To compare the class P, V, and F ATPases.

C. Class P, V, and F ATPases

1. The ion-related ATPases are called **class P ATPases** because this group of enzymes proceeds through a *p*hosphorylated (**phospho-aspartyl**) covalent intermediate
2. The **class V** (for *v*esicle) **ATPases** transport protons and acidify intracellular organelles such as lysosomes by pumping protons against a concentration gradient of two or more pH units
3. The **class F ATPases** are the familiar F_oF_1 synthases that play a central role in the generation of ATP by oxidative phosphorylation

Objective 4: To describe secondary active transport.

IV. Secondary active transport

A. In secondary active transport, ATP provides the energy for transport indirectly (PRINCIPLE 13 OF BIOCHEMISTRY)

B. One mechanism for performing this function is to use the energy of an ion gradient to energize transport

C. The sodium/potassium-ATPase uses the energy of ATP to establish a sodium gradient

1. The concentration of sodium exterior to the cell is high, and that in the interior of cells is low
2. Sodium can move down its electrochemical gradient in an exergonic process, and sodium can drive the cotransport of glucose or other metabolites in an endergonic direction

D. Sodium-dependent (11 transmembrane segments) and sodium-independent (12 transmembrane segments) glucose translocases are not homologous

V. Secretion of acidic gastric juice

A. Four protein components are required for the generation of hydrochloric acid from parietal cells, including (1) a chloride-bicarbonate antiport protein, (2) a chloride channel protein, (3) a potassium channel protein, and (4) a proton/potassium-ATPase

B. The main source of energy for the secretion of protons is the ATP that sustains the activity of a proton/potassium-ATPase, a class P enzyme

1. The proton/potassium-ATPase pumps two protons in exchange for one potassium ion
2. This pump is electrogenic (more positive charges are pumped out of than into the cell)

Objective 5: To outline the γ-glutamyl cycle for amino acid transport.

VI. γ-Glutamyl cycle for amino acid transport

A. Glutathione, γ-glutamylcysteinylglycine, plays a role in amino acid transport in the nephron and jejunum

B. The amino acid is modified as a result of translocation across a membrane, and this process is classified as a **group translocation** reaction

C. Glutathione reacts with the amino acid to be transported to form a γ-glutamyl amino acid that is translocated into the cell

1. The amino acid is displaced, and 5-oxoproline forms simultaneously
2. 5-Oxoproline is converted to glutamate in an ATP-dependent process
3. Cysteinylglycine is hydrolyzed into the two constituent amino acids

D. Glutathione biosynthesis

1. γ-Glutamylcysteine forms from the two amino acids in a process driven by ATP (ADP and P_i result) and the concomitant loss of one high-energy bond (PRINCIPLE 2 OF BIOENERGETICS)
2. Glycine is linked to the dipeptide in a second ATP-requiring reaction (ADP and P_i result)

Objective 6: To describe the cystic fibrosis transmembrane conductance regulator.

VII. Chloride transport and cystic fibrosis

A. Cystic fibrosis is accompanied by an increase in sweat chloride concentration

B. The gene product is called CFTR (for *c*ystic *f*ibrosis *t*ransmembrane conductance *r*egulator)

1. The cystic fibrosis gene spans about 230 kilobases on chromosome 7q31 and contains 27 exons
2. The highest mRNA levels for CFTR occur in the pancreas, salivary glands, sweat glands, gut, and reproductive tract

a. The gene product is a large integral membrane protein of 170 kDa

b. The protein has 12 transmembrane segments, a regulatory (R) domain that contains sites for phosphorylation by protein kinase A (PKA), and two intracellular ATP-binding domains called nucleotide-binding folds (NBF-1 and NBF-2)

C. The most common mutation (70% of all cases) responsible for cystic fibrosis results in the deletion of phenylalanine 508, abbreviated ΔF508

QUESTIONS

DIRECTIONS. (Items 1–16): Each of the numbered items or incomplete statements in this section is followed by answers or by completions of the statement. Select the ONE lettered answer or completion that is BEST in each case. Correct answers and explanations are given at the end of the chapter.

1. All of the following substances freely diffuse across biological lipid bilayer membranes EXCEPT
   (A) carbon dioxide
   (B) malate
   (C) nitric oxide
   (D) oxygen
   (E) urea

2. The sodium-dependent transport of glucose in the kidney is an example of
   (A) antiport
   (B) group translocation
   (C) passive diffusion
   (D) primary active transport
   (E) secondary active transport

3. What type of plot represents substrate concentration versus rate of transport by simple diffusion?
   (A) Bell-shaped curve
   (B) Rectangular hyperbola
   (C) Sigmoidal curve
   (D) Straight line

4. Which one of the following glucose transporters is regulated by insulin?
   (A) GLUT1
   (B) GLUT2
   (C) GLUT3
   (D) GLUT4
   (E) GLUT5

5. All of the following are true statements regarding the sodium/potassium-ATPase EXCEPT
   (A) It consists of two α-subunits and two β-subunits
   (B) It forms an aspartyl-phosphate high-energy bond during translocation
   (C) It forms an aspartyl-phosphate low-energy bond during translocation
   (D) It translocates three sodium ions per ATP
   (E) It translocates three potassium ions per ATP

6. Which of the following is a true statement regarding cardiac glycosides such as digitalis, which are used in the treatment of heart failure?
   (A) They inhibit calcium-ATPase
   (B) They activate calcium-ATPase
   (C) They inhibit sodium/potassium-ATPase
   (D) They activate sodium/potassium-ATPase
   (E) They inhibit translocation by the plasma membrane sodium-calcium antiport protein

7. The enzyme responsible for maintaining the pH inside of lysosomes is a class
   (A) P ATPase
   (B) V ATPase
   (C) F ATPase
   (D) M ATPase

8. An inability to synthesize glutathione results from a deficiency of each of the following enzymes EXCEPT
   (A) γ-glutamylcysteine synthetase
   (B) glutathione reductase
   (C) glutathione synthetase
   (D) 5-oxoprolinase

9. In resting humans, the transport of ions accounts for approximately what percent of total ATP expenditure?
   (A) 1%
   (B) 2%
   (C) 5%
   (D) 25%
   (E) 75%

10. What is the number of high-energy bonds required for the translocation of a single amino acid by the γ-glutamyl transpeptidation cycle?
   (A) 0
   (B) 1
   (C) 2
   (D) 3
   (E) 4

11. Patients with mental retardation, glutathionemia, and glutathionuria have a defect in which one of the following enzymes?
   (A) Glutamine synthetase
   (B) γ-Glutamyl transpeptidase
   (C) γ-Glutamylcysteine synthetase
   (D) Glutathione synthetase
   (E) 5-Oxoprolinase

Items 12–16

History

The patient, a 9-year-old boy, was brought to the pediatric clinic because of a worsening chronic cough, expectoration, and wheezing. The patient had been followed since birth with a diagnosis of cystic fibrosis. The patient has a sister (14 years of age) and brother (17 years of age) who are in good health. The extended family history did not reveal relatives who had lung disease. The patient has had recurrent pneumonia that has been treated with antibiotics. Current management includes chest percussion to promote mucus drainage, DNAse treatment by aerosol to decrease the viscosity of pulmonary mucus, antibiotic treatment, and pancreatic enzyme replacement. Although peripheral to the main concern of this visit, the parents noted that his stools have become frequent, bulky, and greasy, and suggest that a change in dosage of pancreatic enzymes is in order. Previous polymerase chain reaction analysis of the patient's DNA was consistent with a ΔF508 mutation; sweat chloride values performed several years earlier were 70 mEq/L. The patient has never been jaundiced or experienced excessive bleeding.

Physical Examination

Physical examination revealed a patient not in apparent distress. His temperature is 37.4°C (99.4°F); pulse, 96/min; respirations, 20/min; and blood pressure, 118/76 mm Hg. The throat is red. Expiratory wheezes are heard bilaterally. The heart and abdomen are normal.

Laboratory

The hematocrit is normal. The white blood count is 23,600/μL (normal, 4500–13,500/μL) with 85% polymorphonuclear leukocytes (normal, 54–62%). Serum electrolytes are normal. A sputum culture revealed *Pseudomonas aeruginosa.* Chest x-ray shows hyperinflation of the lungs with lobar atelectasis. Chest percussion, recombinant DNAse, β-adrenergic agonists for bronchodilatation, pancreatic enzyme replacement, and fat-soluble vitamins were continued. The patient was started on oral ciprofloxacin (a nalidixic acid analogue).

12. Cystic fibrosis is what type of genetic disease?
    (A) Autosomal recessive
    (B) Autosomal dominant
    (C) X-linked recessive
    (D) X-linked dominant

13. What type of protein is the cystic fibrosis gene product?
    (A) Cytosolic
    (B) Mitochondrial
    (C) Integral plasma membrane
    (D) Lysosomal
    (E) Nuclear

14. The mechanism of the antibacterial action of ciprofloxacin, which is a congener of nalidixic acid, is based upon its inhibition of the
    (A) initiation of RNA synthesis
    (B) initiation of bacterial protein synthesis
    (C) insertion of aminoacyl-tRNA into the A site of the bacterial ribosome
    (D) peptidyltransferase reaction
    (E) topoisomerase reaction

15. Pancreatic enzyme replacement includes all of the following EXCEPT
    (A) trypsin
    (B) amylase
    (C) lipase
    (D) pepsin

16. What is the therapeutic mechanism of recombinant DNAse aerosol?
    (A) Bronchodilatation
    (B) Digestion of viscous DNA debris
    (C) Digestion of viscous mucin
    (D) Increasing chloride conductance
    (E) Stimulation of the immune system

ANSWERS AND EXPLANATIONS

1. The answer is B: malate. Malate is a polar compound that does NOT cross biological lipid bilayers by simple diffusion. The inner mitochondrial membrane contains several specific transport proteins that translocate this substance. In contrast, small nonpolar substances such as carbon dioxide, nitric oxide, and oxygen diffuse through membranes. Ethanol and water are also able to diffuse across lipid bilayers. Protons and hydroxide ions, in contrast, are unable to diffuse across lipid bilayers. *Biochemistry,* p. 122.
2. The answer is E: secondary active transport. Secondary active transport uses a source of chemical energy such as a sodium gradient that is produced by primary active transport. The cotransport of sodium and glucose in the same direction is called symport; this is an example of secondary active transport. Antiport refers to the exchange of a metabolite in one compartment for a metabolite in another compartment; the sodium/calcium exchange protein mediates such a process. Passive diffusion is independent of a saturable translocase. Primary active transport involves the direct coupling of translocation with a direct source of chemical energy such as ATP; the reaction catalyzed by the sodium/potassium-ATPase is an example. In group translocation, the chemical composition of the transferred metabolite is altered during translocation. *Biochemistry,* p. 458.
3. The answer is D: straight line. The rate of simple diffusion is a linear function of the substrate concentration. When transport is mediated by a finite number of translocation proteins, the process exhibits saturation and is represented by a rectangular hyperbola. When a process exhibits positive cooperativity, the response is a sigmoidal function of the substrate concentration. Bell-shaped curves represent a Poisson distribution of a given characteristic. *Biochemistry,* p. 458.
4. The answer is D: GLUT4. The GLUT4 translocase, which occurs in skeletal muscle and adipose tissue, is activated by insulin by a process that does not require protein synthesis. The GLUT4 receptor occurs in the plasma membrane and in intracellular membrane vesicles. In

response to insulin, GLUT4 translocation proteins are recruited to the plasma membrane and increase the quantity of glucose that can be transported. Altered glucose transport is reflected by an increase in velocity but not in concentration dependence at half-saturation. A notable property of liver is that glucose transport is insulin independent, and liver does not express the GLUT4 translocation protein. Other metabolic activities of liver are affected by insulin. *Biochemistry,* p. 459.

5. The answer is E: three potassium ions are NOT translocated per ATP. The sodium/potassium-ATPase consists of two α-subunits and two β-subunits, and it transports three sodium ions per ATP. Since it translocates only two potassium ions in the opposite direction, the sodium pump is electrogenic (produces a charge differential). The α-subunits first form an energy-rich aspartyl-phosphate bond; after translocation of three sodium ions to the exterior, the aspartyl-phosphate bond becomes a low-energy bond. A free aspartyl-phosphate group possesses a high-energy bond; proteins can alter the standard free energy of hydrolysis of such bonds. Proteins can also alter the pK_a of side chains of the constituent amino acids. *Biochemistry,* pp. 460–461.
6. The answer is C: they inhibit the sodium/potassium-ATPase. Cardiac glycosides bind to the exterior surface of the sodium/potassium-ATPase and inhibit the enzyme. As a result, the intracellular concentration of sodium is increased somewhat. This intracellular sodium exchanges for extracellular calcium by a process that is mediated by an antiport protein. The higher intracellular calcium ion concentration resulting from this process is thought to augment cardiac muscle contraction. *Biochemistry,* p. 461.
7. The answer is B: V ATPase. This class of enzyme is responsible for maintaining the pH inside of lysosomes and secretory vesicles. These enzymes lack a phosphorylated enzyme intermediate. The class V enzymes are composed of from three to five different polypeptide subunits. *Biochemistry,* p. 462.
8. The answer is B: glutathione reductase. Glutathione is γ-glutamylcysteinylglycine. The first step in its synthesis is catalyzed by γ-glutamylcysteine synthetase in an ATP-dependent process. Glutathione synthetase catalyzes the synthesis of the tripeptide. 5-Oxoproline is derived from the γ-glutamyl group of the translocated γ-glutamyl-amino acid. An ATP-dependent process is required to open the ring of 5-oxoproline to produce glutamate. Glutathione, which is a substrate for the γ-glutamyl transport cycle, is also a general reductant. Glutathione reductase catalyzes the conversion of oxidized glutathione (GSSG) to reduced glutathione (GSH). *Biochemistry,* pp. 464–465.
9. The answer is D: 25%. The generation and maintenance of ion gradients are energetically expensive, and this expenditure amounts to about one-quarter of total energy consumed during rest. *Biochemistry,* p. 458.
10. The answer is D: 3. Two molecules of ATP (two high-energy bonds) are required for the synthesis of glutathione; one ATP is required for the formation of γ-glutamylcysteine, and another is required to convert γ-glutamylcysteine to glutathione. A third ATP is required to convert 5-oxoproline to glutamate in a ring-opening process. *Biochemistry,* pp. 463–465.
11. The answer is B: γ-glutamyl transpeptidase. In this disorder, glutathione is synthesized normally and released into the extracellular compartment. It is not metabolized in the γ-glutamyl transpeptidase cycle, and it accumulates in the extracellular space, giving rise to glutathionemia and glutathionuria. γ-Glutamylcysteine synthetase deficiency produces a chronic hemolytic anemia and generalized aminoacidemia. There is impaired amino acid transport in renal tubules and aminoaciduria. 5-Oxoprolinase deficiency results in the excretion of moderate amounts of 5-oxoproline in the urine. Glutathione synthetase deficiency produces neurological deficits, metabolic acidosis, and 5-oxoprolinuria. In this case, 5-oxoproline is derived from γ-glutamylcysteine, the substrate for glutathione synthetase. *Biochemistry,* p. 464; *Nelson,* p. 325.
12. The answer is A: cystic fibrosis is an autosomal recessive disorder. The disease is not transmitted exclusively by the mother, and it is therefore not X-linked. An individual must receive the mutant gene from both parents to be affected, and the disorder is therefore recessive. Cystic fibrosis is the most common autosomal recessive disease in Caucasians, with a frequency of about 1 in 2000 live births, or 0.0005. The frequency of the gene is $(0.0005)^{1/2}$ or 0.022 (about 1 in 45). *Biochemistry,* p. 466.
13. The answer is C: integral plasma membrane. The gene product, a large integral membrane protein of 170 kDa, is called CFTR (for *c*ystic *f*ibrosis *t*ransmembrane conductance *r*egulator). The protein has 12 transmembrane segments, a regulatory (R) domain that contains sites for phosphorylation by protein kinase A (PKA), and two intracellular ATP-binding domains called nucleotide-binding folds (NBF-1 and NBF-2). The channels that conduct sodium and chloride ions across the apical membrane of the respiratory epithelia in people with cystic fibrosis are present and functional, but there is altered regulation of their activity. There is impaired ability to secrete chloride, and, secondarily, sodium and water, onto the epithelial surface. The impaired ability of CFTR to increase chloride channel activity leads to the paucity of water in mucous secretions, leading to pulmonary infection, pancreatic duct obstruction, and abnormally viscous gastrointestinal secretions called meconium. The direction of ion transport works in the reverse direction in the sweat glands, leading to elevated sweat chloride. *Biochemistry,* p. 466.
14. The answer is E: topoisomerase reaction. These compounds inhibit bacterial DNA gyrase, a type II topoisomerase, by inhibiting the strand-cutting reaction. Rifamycin is an inhibitor of the initiation of RNA synthesis, streptomycin and gentamicin inhibit initiation of bacterial protein synthesis, tetracyclines inhibit the insertion of aminoacyl-tRNA into the A site of the bacterial ribosome, and chloramphenicol inhibits the peptidyltransferase reaction. Tetracycline should not be given to children because it produces permanent brown discoloration of teeth. Discoloration of the permanent dentition occurs when it is given between 2 months and 5 years of age, but children up to 8 years of age may be affected. This discoloration is due to formation of tetracycline–calcium phosphate complexes that decompose. Treatment of pregnant women can produce discoloration of the teeth in their children, and it may depress bone growth during gestation. *Biochemistry,* p. 284.
15. The answer is D: pepsin. Pepsin, a digestive enzyme produced by the stomach, is NOT present in commercial pancreatic enzyme preparations. Such preparations include trypsin, amylase, and lipase. These are prepared from bovine and porcine sources. These pancreatic enzymes are sometimes packaged in enteric-coated tablets or capsules to maintain activity during passage through the acidic stomach milieu. The enzymes decrease the lipid and nitrogen content of the feces, and the appropriate dosage can be adjusted based upon such studies.

The dosage for children has to be gradually increased with age, and the parents were familiar with this procedure as elicited during the history (they probably knew more about this than the resident physician who cared for the patient). *Biochemistry,* p. 213.

16. The answer is B: digestion of viscous DNA debris. The pulmonary infections in cystic fibrosis result from the inability of patients to clear viscous mucus. The inflammatory reaction causes an accumulation of viscous DNA from bacteria and white blood cells (DNA was isolated initially from the pus of bandages in the 19th century). Recombinant human DNAse is given by aerosol in an effort to decrease the contribution of DNA to the viscosity of the mucous secretions. Human enzyme is used to avoid an immunogenic response. Human DNAse is not an immune system stimulant, nor does it alter chloride conductance. *Biochemistry,* pp. 298–299.

REFERENCES

Behrman, R. E. *Nelson Textbook of Pediatrics,* 14th ed. Philadelphia, W. B. Saunders Company, 1992.

Roskoski, R., Jr. *Biochemistry.* Philadelphia, W. B. Saunders Company, 1996.

CHAPTER TWENTY-THREE

MUSCLE AND CONNECTIVE TISSUE

SYNOPSIS

OBJECTIVES

1. To describe the sliding filament model of muscle contraction.
2. To outline high-energy phosphate metabolism of muscle.
3. To characterize the genetic defect responsible for muscular dystrophy.
4. To describe collagen and elastin.
5. To depict the structure and metabolism of proteoglycans.

Objective 1: To describe the sliding filament model of muscle contraction.

I. Muscle
  A. Ultrastructure
    1. The striations of skeletal muscle appear as alternating light and dark bands
      a. The dark bands are the **A bands** (*a*nisotropic) and contain the thick filaments of myosin; the A bands also contain the thin filaments that overlap the thick filaments
      b. The light bands are the **I bands** (*i*sotropic) and contain thin filaments
    2. Sarcomeres extend from one Z disk to the next
  B. Proteins
    1. Myosin makes up about 60% of the total protein in skeletal muscle
      a. It consists of two identical heavy chains, two essential light chains, and two regulatory light chains
      b. Myosin possesses ATPase activity, and *myosin is the site of energy transduction where the chemical energy of ATP* (the common currency of energy exchange, PRINCIPLE 10 OF BIOCHEMISTRY) *is converted into mechanical energy*
    2. **Actin** is the second major protein of muscle
      a. Several globular actin (G-actin) monomers form helical actin filaments (F-actin) and occur as such in the thin filaments of skeletal muscle
      b. The interaction of the myosin heads and actin filaments is responsible for the generation of force
    3. **Tropomyosin** is a long, thin molecule that blocks the interaction of actin and myosin in the resting state
    4. **Troponin,** which interacts with tropomyosin, is made of three different types of subunit
      a. **Troponin I** *i*nhibits the interaction of actin and myosin through the action of tropomyosin
      b. **Troponin C** binds *c*alcium reversibly
      c. **Troponin T** interacts with *t*ropomyosin
  C. Contraction
    1. Striated muscle contraction involves the troponin system
      a. Elevated sarcoplasmic calcium, produced after neuronal depolarization resulting from the action of acetylcholine at the nicotinic receptor, interacts with troponin
      b. Troponin moves tropomyosin and allows interaction of actin and myosin
      c. The ATPase activity of myosin generates an energized myosin that moves along actin by a ratchet-like process and generates force by the sliding filament mechanism
    2. Smooth muscle contraction does not involve the troponin system
      a. Smooth muscle cell contraction, like that of striated muscle, is regulated by alterations in the levels of intracellular calcium
      b. Following phosphorylation of the myosin light chains, catalyzed by **myosin light chain kinase,** myosin can interact with actin and generate force
      c. Following dephosphorylation of the regulatory myosin light chain, catalyzed by **phosphoprotein phosphatase,** interaction between actin and myosin is inhibited and contraction ceases

Objective 2: To outline high-energy phosphate metabolism of muscle.

II. High-energy phosphates
  A. Skeletal and cardiac muscle (and brain) contain significant amounts of phosphocreatine, a phosphoramidate (P~N) that serves as a storage form of high-energy phosphate
  B. Muscle and other tissues can regenerate ATP from ADP by the **adenylate kinase** reaction; this enzyme catalyzes a reaction between two molecules of ADP to yield ATP and AMP in an isoergonic process according to PRINCIPLE 1 OF BIOENERGETICS

C. The metabolism of red and white muscle differs
  1. White muscle uses glycolysis for most of its energy production
  2. Red muscle uses fatty acids as a major fuel
    a. Fatty acids are metabolized by β-oxidation to acetyl-CoA
    b. Acetyl-CoA metabolism via the Krebs cycle and oxidative phosphorylation yields substantial energy
  3. Some muscles such as the gastrocnemius contain both red and white muscle fibers

Objective 3: To characterize the genetic defect responsible for muscular dystrophy.

III. Duchenne muscular dystrophy
  A. Muscular dystrophy is due to an abnormality of the structural gene for **dystrophin** that results in reduced levels or absence of this protein
  B. Dystrophin helps maintain the integrity of muscle fibers
  C. The dystrophin gene is extremely large (2300 kb) and spans 1.5% of the X chromosome
    1. The 100-fold higher mutation rate of this gene when compared with most other genes may be related to this large size
    2. One-third of those with muscular dystrophy have new mutations, and two-thirds have carrier mothers
    3. Two-thirds of the mutations are deletions, and 5% involve duplications
    4. The gene has 79 exons, and dystrophin is a 430-kDa protein

Objective 4: To describe collagen and elastin.

IV. Collagen
  A. Structure and function
    1. *Collagen, which is the major macromolecule of connective tissue, is the predominant human protein and accounts for one-third of all protein by mass*
    2. Human collagen consists of more than one dozen different types of molecules composed of more than two dozen genetically distinct α-chains
      a. Type I collagen, a fibrillar collagen, accounts for 90% of all collagen by mass
      b. Type IV collagen, which forms meshes and not fibrils, is important because it forms basement membranes
    3. The most distinguishing property of collagen is that each α-chain forms a **left-handed helix** with three amino acid residues per turn
    4. Three left-handed helical polypeptides combine to form a **right-handed triple helical molecule**
    5. *Every third residue of collagen is glycine,* another distinguishing feature
    6. Glycine is the only amino acid small enough to exist at the central core of a triple helix
  B. Synthesis
    1. Collagen is synthesized as **preprocollagen α-chains** in the rough endoplasmic reticulum
    2. The signal peptide, which is remarkably long (about 100 amino acids), is cleaved by hydrolysis, yielding **procollagen α-chains**
    3. Prolyl and lysyl hydroxylation require oxygen, α-ketoglutarate, and ascorbate substrates; the hydroxylated prolyl or lysyl side chain, succinate, carbon dioxide, and oxidized ascorbate are the products
    4. Intrachain disulfide bonds connect carboxyterminal portions of three chains together for proper alignment prior to triple helix formation in the Golgi
    5. *Triple helix formation begins at the carboxyl terminus and extends to the amino terminus in a zipper-like process*
    6. *Procollagen is secreted from the fibroblast*
    7. **Procollagen amino terminal protease** and **procollagen carboxyterminal protease** are extracellular enzymes that catalyze the hydrolytic removal of amino and carboxyterminal fragments of the nascent triple helix, yielding tropocollagen
    8. **Tropocollagen** is the mature building block of **collagen**
      a. Cross-links form from ε-aldehyde groups derived from lysine and hydroxylysine residues and ε-amino groups of other lysine or hydroxylysine residues in tropocollagen
      b. Tropocollagen that has combined into fibrils is the substrate for lysyl oxidase, an enzyme that operates extracellularly
        (1) **Lysyl oxidase** requires pyridoxal phosphate and copper for activity
        (2) The products of the reaction include the aldehyde derivative of lysine or hydroxylysine
      c. The main cross-links in collagen include **hydroxylysyl pyridinoline** and **hydroxylysinonorleucine**
  C. Collagenopathies
    1. **Osteogenesis imperfecta** (brittle bone disease) is characterized by bone fragility that results from various mutations of **type I collagen**
    2. **Ehlers-Danlos syndrome** is a group of 10 generalized connective tissue disorders characterized by skin fragility, skin hyperextensibility, and joint hypermobility
    3. The genetic basis of these collagenopathies is heterogeneous

V. Elastin
  A. Elastin is the connective tissue protein responsible for the extensibility of lung, large arterial blood vessels, and some ligaments
  B. Elastin is synthesized as a soluble monomer of about 700 amino acids called **tropoelastin**
  C. Tropoelastin is secreted from fibroblasts and other connective tissue cells
    1. Specific lysine residues are deaminated to aldehydes in a reaction catalyzed by **lysyl *oxidase*,** the same copper-containing enzyme that acts on collagen
    2. The resulting aldehyde groups participate in **desmosine** and **isodesmosine** formation, hallmarks of elastin

Objective 5: To depict the structure and metabolism of proteoglycans.

VI. Proteoglycans have a widespread distribution in bone, cartilage, cornea, synovial fluid, teeth, and the vitreous of the eye
  A. Structure
    1. Proteoglycans consist of negatively charged polysaccharides (95% by mass) and proteins (5%)
      a. That carbohydrate is the main component is indi-

cated by naming them as protein derivatives (proteo) of carbohydrate (glycans)
   b. The carbohydrate portion is composed of glycosaminoglycans (GAGs; formerly called mucopolysaccharides)
2. Proteoglycans are built on a polysaccharide axis of hyaluronate
3. Hyaluronate is unusual because it is not covalently linked to protein as are the other glycosaminoglycans
4. Many core proteins, which emanate laterally from the long, thin hyaluronate axis, are bonded to the axis by a **link protein**
5. Link proteins stabilize the **noncovalent** attachment of hyaluronate to core proteins
6. Many chondroitin sulfate and keratan sulfate chains are covalently attached to the core proteins, and the carbohydrates constitute the major mass of the molecule
7. Linkage regions contain three or four carbohydrate residues to which the repeating units of disaccharides are attached

B. Synthesis
1. **Chondroitin sulfates** are the most abundant proteoglycans in humans, and the pathway for their biosynthesis illustrates the important principles for all classes of proteoglycans
2. The core protein is synthesized in the rough endoplasmic reticulum in an mRNA-dependent fashion
3. The three linking carbohydrates are added sequentially from activated UDP precursors in three sequential steps, and each step is catalyzed by a different transglycosylase
4. The repeating disaccharide is made of glucuronate and *N*-acetylgalactosamine
   a. The activated biosynthetic donors are UDP-glucuronate and UDP-GalNAc, according to PRINCIPLE 17 OF BIOCHEMISTRY
   b. Glucuronate transferase catalyzes the addition of glucuronate to the terminal galactosyl residue of the linkage region
   c. Next, a galactosyltransferase catalyzes the addition of GalNAc
   d. This process recurs many times to produce a chain of the repeating disaccharide
5. A sulfotransferase catalyzes a reaction between the 4-hydroxyl group of the *N*-acetylgalactosamine of the repeating disaccharide and phosphoadenosylphosphosulfate (PAPS)
   a. Active sulfate (PAPS) is an energy-rich compound, and the products are energy poor
   b. The reaction is exergonic in accordance with PRINCIPLE 2 OF BIOENERGETICS

QUESTIONS

DIRECTIONS. (Items 1–17): Each of the numbered items or incomplete statements in this section is followed by answers or by completions of the statement. Select the ONE lettered answer or completion that is BEST in each case. Correct answers and explanations are given at the end of the chapter.

1. Which of the following is a true statement regarding actin?
   (A) It forms cross-bridges with myosin
   (B) It contains two identical heavy chains (230-kDa molecular mass each)
   (C) It contains two essential light chains (16- to 20-kDa molecular mass each)
   (D) It contains two regulatory light chains (16- to 20-kDa molecular mass each)
   (E) It possesses ATPase activity

2. Which one of the following binds calcium and then undergoes a conformational change that triggers striated muscle contraction?
   (A) Calsequestrin
   (B) Tropomyosin
   (C) Troponin I
   (D) Troponin C
   (E) Troponin T

3. Smooth muscle lacks which of the following components?
   (A) Actin
   (B) Calcium
   (C) Calmodulin
   (D) Myosin
   (E) Troponin

4. What is the chief regulator of muscle contraction?
   (A) ATP
   (B) Calcium ion
   (C) Cyclic AMP
   (D) Cyclic GMP
   (E) Phosphatidylinositol 4,5-bisphosphate

5. Several types of osteogenesis imperfecta (brittle bone disease) are due to point mutations involving which one of the following amino acids?
   (A) Alanine
   (B) Glycine
   (C) Hydroxylysine
   (D) Hydroxyproline
   (E) Proline

6. Procollagen amino terminal protease and procollagen carboxyterminal protease function in which one of the following locations?
   (A) Endoplasmic reticulum
   (B) Extracellular space
   (C) Golgi
   (D) Mitochondrion
   (E) Plasma membrane

7. Lysyl oxidase, the extracellular enzyme that catalyzes the conversion of ε-amino groups of collagen-lysines to

aldehydes and is deficient in type VI Ehlers-Danlos syndrome, requires which one of the following substrates?

(A) Ascorbate
(B) α-Ketoglutarate
(C) Oxygen
(D) NADH
(E) Vitamin K

8. The repeating structure of chondroitin is shown in the following diagram. What are the constituents of chondroitin?

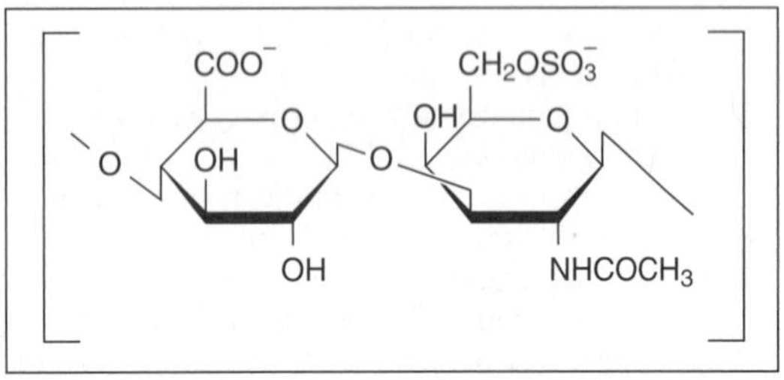

(A) L-Iduronate and *N*-acetylglucosamine 4-sulfate
(B) D-Galactose and *N*-acetylglucosamine 6-sulfate
(C) D-Glucuronate and *N*-acetylglucosamine
(D) D-Glucuronate 2-sulfate and *N*-sulfo-D-glucosamine 6-sulfate
(E) D-Glucuronate and *N*-acetylgalactosamine 6-sulfate

9. Proteoglycans consist of proteins and negatively charged polysaccharides. What percentage is the proportion of protein by mass?

(A) 5%
(B) 25%
(C) 50%
(D) 75%
(E) 95%

10. The sliding filament hypothesis for skeletal muscle contraction explains which one of the following statements?

(A) The A band length decreases during contraction
(B) The I band length is constant in the contracted and relaxed state
(C) The lengths of the thin filaments increase during contraction and decrease during relaxation
(D) The lengths of the thick filaments remain constant while the sarcomere length is shortened during contraction
(E) The fibers of the thick filaments, attached to the Z-disk structure at each end of a sarcomere, are pulled toward the center of the sarcomere by the thin filaments of the A band

11. The major protein of the A band of striated muscle is

(A) actin
(B) core protein
(C) link protein
(D) myosin
(E) troponin

Items 12–17

History

The patient is a 4-year-old boy who was brought to the pediatrics clinic for evaluation of clumsiness. Although the patient began walking by 12 months of age (within normal limits), the parents noticed that he had a broad-based waddling gait. The patient has two sisters (sister II-1, 7 years old; sister II-3, 10 years old) who are in good health. He began talking by 14 months and all of his developmental milestones were normal. The mother thought, however, that he was somewhat behind the developmental rate of his two sisters. The patient's mother has two sisters and one brother who are alive; she had a second brother who died of pneumonia at 13 years of age. This brother was confined to a wheelchair for the last 3 years of his life.

Physical Examination

Physical examination reveals an active boy not in acute distress. When he rose from the floor, his legs were spread, and he climbed up his thighs with his hands to right himself (Gowers sign). Muscles are firm. The calf muscles appear more prominent than normal. The patient is unable to lift his head against the force of gravity. Deep tendon reflexes are normal; there is no Babinski sign (normal).

Laboratory

Laboratory examination revealed a normal red and white blood cell count, normal hemoglobin, normal electrolytes including calcium, magnesium, and phosphate, and normal blood glucose. Blood lactate was normal, and the blood lactate increased normally following exercise. The serum creatine phosphokinase levels were 100 times normal. The urinalysis was normal. Muscle biopsy showed increased variability in fiber size with both small round fibers and hypertrophied ones. Necrotic fibers and mononuclear cells were seen, and connective tissue proliferation (fibrosis) was also present. Western blot analysis was negative for dystrophin. The mother and one sister (II-1) exhibited creatine phosphokinase values that are three to five times normal. The serum creatine phosphokinase value of sister II-3 was normal.

12. The likely inheritance of this disorder is

(A) autosomal dominant
(B) autosomal recessive
(C) X-linked dominant
(D) X-linked recessive
(E) a new mutation

13. The likely diagnosis is

(A) Duchenne muscular dystrophy
(B) McArdle disease (muscle phosphorylase deficiency)
(C) myasthenia gravis
(D) hypothyroidism

14. The isozyme form of creatine phosphokinase in skeletal muscle is

(A) B_4
(B) M_4
(C) BB
(D) MB
(E) MM

15. The dystrophin gene has all of the following characteristics EXCEPT

(A) it is large (2.3 million nucleotides)
(B) it contains only three introns

(C) it has a relatively high frequency of mutation
(D) it is allelic with that for Becker muscular dystrophy
(E) it can be studied by samples obtained by amniocentesis or chorionic villus sampling

Items 16–17

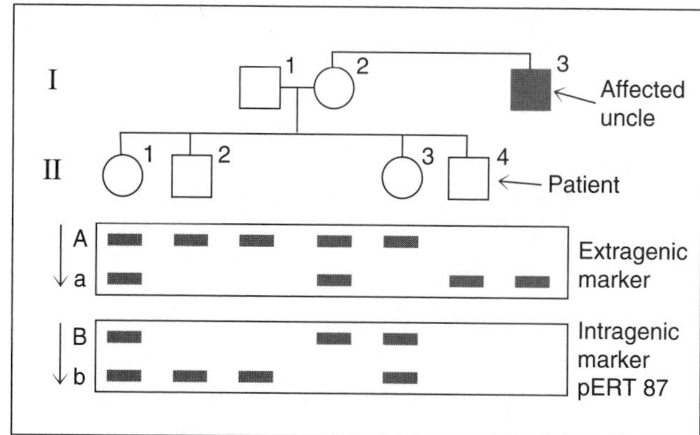

16. Restriction fragment analysis of DNA obtained from the lymphocytes of the patient (II-4), his two sisters (II-1 and II-3), brother (II-2), father (I-1), mother (I-2), and his deceased and affected uncle (I-3) appears above. A probe from outside of the gene was used in the analysis illustrated in the upper panel, and an intragenic probe corresponding to a segment near the 5′ end of the dystrophin gene (pERT87) was used in the analysis in the lower panel. Analysis of the upper panel in the accompanying diagram, corresponding to the extragenic marker, indicates that

(A) the A allele is associated with the disorder
(B) the mother carries one allele
(C) sister II-1 is a probable carrier
(D) sister II-3 is a probable carrier
(E) the father is a probable carrier

17. Analysis of the lower panel in the accompanying diagram, corresponding to the intragenic marker, indicates that

(A) the father contains the B allele
(B) the mother contains the b allele
(C) both daughters contain each allele
(D) the uncle and patient express the DNA corresponding to pERT87

ANSWERS AND EXPLANATIONS

1. The answer is A: actin forms cross-bridges with myosin. Myosin is the most abundant protein by mass in muscle. Myosin contains two identical heavy chains (230-kDa molecular mass each), two essential light chains (16- to 20-kDa molecular mass each), and two regulatory light chains (also 16- to 20-kDa molecular mass each) and possesses ATPase activity. *Biochemistry,* p. 472.
2. The answer is D: troponin C. Troponin consists of a complex of three proteins: troponins I, C, and T. Troponin C binds calcium and undergoes a conformational change that results in the rearrangement of troponin, tropomyosin, actin, and myosin. As a result of the displacement of tropomyosin by troponin, actin can interact with myosin and force is generated. Calsequestrin is a calcium-binding protein that occurs in the sarcoplasmic reticulum; it can bind up to 40 calcium ions. Calsequestrin serves as a repository for calcium transported into the sarcoplasmic reticulum. *Biochemistry,* p. 471.
3. The answer is E: troponin. Smooth muscle, which contains actin and myosin, lacks both troponin and a sarcoplasmic reticulum. As a result, the mechanism for triggering smooth muscle contraction differs from that of striated muscle. Calcium is derived from the extracellular space and the endoplasmic reticulum following the interaction with signaling molecules, binds with calmodulin, and activates myosin light-chain kinase, which initiates contraction by catalyzing the phosphorylation of regulatory myosin light chains. Cessation of contraction is the result of the dephosphorylation of these myosin light chains as catalyzed by phosphoprotein phosphatase. Following phosphorylation of the myosin light chains, myosin can interact with actin and generate force. Following dephosphorylation of the regulatory myosin light chain, interaction between actin and myosin is inhibited, and contraction ceases. *Biochemistry,* p. 472.
4. The answer is B: calcium ion. Calcium triggers striated muscle contraction by activating the troponin system. Calcium triggers smooth muscle contraction by interacting with calmodulin and activating myosin light-chain kinase. Cyclic AMP, cyclic GMP, and phosphatidylinositol 4,5-bisphosphate play ancillary regulatory roles in controlling muscle metabolism. *Biochemistry,* p. 471.
5. The answer is B: glycine. Every third amino acid in the triple helical region of collagen is glycine; mutations that change glycine to any other residue in these positions are deleterious and produce osteogenesis imperfecta (brittle bone disease). The collagen helix forms in the Golgi, and the direction of helix formation is from the carboxyl terminus to the amino terminus. Glycine mutations that are toward the carboxyl terminus usually produce more severe disease. *Biochemistry,* pp. 476, 478.
6. The answer is B: extracellular space. Collagen is synthesized as preprocollagen α-chains in the rough endoplasmic reticulum. The signal peptide, which is remarkably long ($\approx$100 amino acids) is cleaved by hydrolysis, yielding procollagen α-chains. Prolyl and lysyl hydroxylation occurs in the Golgi. A few hydroxylysine residues of each chain are glycosylated. Intrachain disulfide bonds form that connect carboxyterminal portions of three chains together. Disulfide bond formation aligns the three chains so that the physiological triple helix forms. Without proper alignment, abnormal triple helix formation can occur. The procollagen triple helix is formed in the Golgi. Triple helix formation begins at the carboxyl terminus and extends to the amino terminus in a zipper-like process. Procollagen has a central region of triple helix surrounded by nonhelical amino-terminal and carboxyterminal extensions, or propeptides. Procollagen is secreted from fibroblasts. Procollagen amino-terminal protease and procollagen carboxyterminal protease are

extracellular enzymes that catalyze the hydrolytic removal of amino- and carboxyterminal fragments of the nascent triple helix, yielding tropocollagen. Tropocollagen is the mature building block of collagen. *Biochemistry,* p. 477.

7. The answer is C: oxygen. The conversion of an amino group to an aldehyde requires oxygen. This is an extracellular reaction, and NADH would not be available. Lysyl hydroxylase and prolyl hydroxylase, which are present in the Golgi, use α-ketoglutarate, ascorbate, and the protein as substrates. Vitamin K is required for the conversion of protein-glutamate to protein γ-carboxyglutamate. These reactions, which involve the reaction of molecular oxygen with an organic molecule, are exergonic according to PRINCIPLE 8 OF BIOENERGETICS. *Biochemistry,* p. 478.
8. The answer is E: D-Glucuronate and *N*-acetylgalactosamine 6-sulfate are constituents of chondroitin. The sulfate can occur on the 6-hydroxyl group, shown here, or on the 4-hydroxyl group, forming chondroitin 6-sulfate or chondroitin 4-sulfate, respectively. L-Iduronate and *N*-acetylglucosamine 4-sulfate are components of dermatan sulfate; D-galactose and *N*-acetylglucosamine 6-sulfate are components of keratan sulfate. D-Glucuronate and *N*-acetylglucosamine are constituents of hyaluronate; D-glucuronate 2-sulfate and *N*-sulfo-D-glucosamine 6-sulfate are components of heparin. *Biochemistry,* p. 480.
9. The answer is A: 5%. Proteoglycans are named as derivatives of carbohydrate (glycans) because they consist of about 95% carbohydrate and only 5% protein. Glycoproteins are named as derivatives of protein and consist predominantly of protein. *Biochemistry,* p. 479.
10. The answer is D: the lengths of the thick filaments remain constant while the sarcomere length is shortened during contraction. During contraction it is the fibers of the thin filaments, attached to the Z-disk structure at each end of a sarcomere, that are pulled toward the center of the sarcomere by the thick filaments that make up the A band. Another aspect of the sliding filament hypothesis of muscle contraction is that the A band remains constant in length in the relaxed and contracted state while the I band decreases in length with contraction. The lengths of the filaments remain constant; shortening of the sarcomere is a result of one filament sliding past adjacent filaments and is not due to the contraction of either filament. *Biochemistry,* pp. 469–470.
11. The answer is D: myosin. Myosin, the ATPase and energy transducing protein of muscle, is the main protein of the A band. A stands for anisotropic, where the properties depend upon the direction from which they are observed. Myosin is a long, asymmetric protein, and its optical properties vary with direction. Actin occurs in the I band with the three troponins (I, C, and T) and tropomyosin. Link protein occurs in proteoglycans. Link proteins stabilize the noncovalent attachment of hyaluronate to core proteins. Core proteins of proteoglycans contain covalently attached carbohydrate chains made of repeating disaccharide units; such carbohydrates include chondroitin sulfate, keratan sulfate, dermatan sulfate, and others. *Biochemistry,* p. 470.
12. The answer is D: X-linked recessive. X-linked recessive diseases are characterized by phenotypic expression in males who obtain the disorder from carrier mothers. Women who are affected must receive an abnormal gene from both parents, or one of the X chromosomes undergoes translocation with an autosome. In the case of Duchenne muscular dystrophy, males rarely, if ever, reproduce, and homozygous females have not been seen. A few cases of Duchenne muscular dystrophy have occurred in women who have had a translocation of one of the X chromosomes or have an XO genotype (Turner syndrome). *Biochemistry,* p. 474.
13. The answer is A: Duchenne muscular dystrophy. The history and clinical findings correspond to Duchenne muscular dystrophy. This includes the waddling gait, Gowers sign, proximal muscle weakness, and a family history of a maternal male relative confined to a wheelchair who succumbs before 20 years of age. Myasthenia gravis is an autoimmune disorder that usually occurs in women in their third decade and men in the sixth decade of life. Although there can be proximal muscle weakness in hypothyroidism, there is no enlargement of the calf and no elevation of creatine phosphokinase. Moreover, deep tendon reflexes are diminished in hypothyroidism. McArdle syndrome usually presents in young adulthood, and there is a failure to produce lactic acid with exercise. Addison disease (hypoadrenocorticism), Cushing disease (hyperadrenocorticism), viral infection, and carnitine deficiency can also produce muscle weakness. *Biochemistry,* pp. 474–475; *Nelson,* p. 1544.
14. The answer is E: MM. Creatine phosphokinase is a dimer, excluding B_4 and M_4 as possibilities. There are M isozyme forms, which are expressed in muscle (MM), and B forms, which are expressed in brain (BB). Cardiac muscle expresses the hybrid form (MB), and this is the isozyme that is elevated following a myocardial infarction. Serum creatine phosphokinase determination has been proposed as a means of identifying carriers of Duchenne muscular dystrophy. When elevated, it provides strong evidence in support of the carrier state, but it will not identify all, or probably even most, carriers. Creatine phosphokinase values vary with age, falling early in life and rising after the fifth decade. About half the obligate carriers can be identified by means of this enzyme; however, false-positives occur in about 2.5% of tests. Advice to potential carriers should be based on controlled creatine phosphokinase levels from laboratories that consider age-related adjustments. Moreover, testing fetal blood is not a reliable means of identifying affected males *in utero. Biochemistry,* p. 64.
15. The answer is B: the dystrophin gene, having at least 70 exons, contains many more than three introns. The dystrophin gene, which is large (2.3 million nucleotides), has a high frequency of mutation, in part because of its large size. This gene is mutated in both Duchenne and Becker muscular dystrophy. Becker muscular dystrophy is milder, it has a later age of onset, and affected individuals live longer. It is also an X-linked disease and is characterized by elevated creatine phosphokinase levels in the serum. Most males are fertile, and affected women have been described. Both Becker muscular dystrophy and Duchenne muscular dystrophy are due to a variety of mutations. In Duchenne muscular dystrophy, there is little or no expression of dystrophin. In Becker muscular dystrophy, mutant dystrophin is expressed and is partially functional. Treatment of Duchenne muscular dystrophy is symptomatic, and affected individuals rarely survive to age 20 years. They generally succumb to respiratory failure. Cardiac muscle is usually affected. Since they are confined to a wheelchair by age 10–12 years, they rarely develop symptoms of heart failure because of their sedentary status.
16. The answer is C: sister II-1 is a probable carrier. The mother's genome contains two forms of restriction fragment lengths of DNA that hybridize to an extragenic marker corresponding to muscular dystrophy. Allele a, which is present in the affected uncle, represents the

probable allele corresponding to the disorder. The genome of sister II-1 contains this allele, but that from sister II-3, brother II-2, and the father lack this allele. The father possesses only one X chromosome, and men with Duchenne muscular dystrophy rarely, if ever, reproduce. Based upon genetic and historical grounds, the father could not be a carrier. Based upon the analysis of linked markers, genotype predictions are always less than 100% because one must consider that meiotic recombination could have disturbed the relationship between the disease and marker loci. The results of deletional analysis are more definitive, as noted in the answer to item 17.

17. The answer is C: both daughters contain each allele. The father contains the b allele, the mother contains the B allele, and both daughters contain each allele (one from the mother and the other from the father). Both alleles correspond to a segment of DNA within the dystrophin gene, and a positive signal indicates that a deletion has not occurred. The uncle and patient do not express the DNA corresponding to pERT87, indicating that a large deletion has occurred. About two-thirds of patients with muscular dystrophy contain deletions. The remainder include a variety of point mutations that are much more difficult to characterize.

REFERENCES

Roskoski, R., Jr. *Biochemistry.* Philadelphia, W. B. Saunders Company, 1996.

Behrman, R. E. *Nelson Textbook of Pediatrics,* 14th ed. Philadelphia, W. B. Saunders Company, 1992.

CHAPTER TWENTY-FOUR

HEMOGLOBIN, HEME, AND BLOOD COAGULATION

SYNOPSIS

OBJECTIVES

1. To describe the structure and function of hemoglobin.
2. To describe sickle cell anemia and the thalassemias.
3. To outline the pathway for heme synthesis and catabolism.
4. To describe blood clotting and the mechanisms of anticoagulants.
5. To describe the genetics of various coagulopathies.

Objective 1: To describe the structure and function of hemoglobin.

I. Properties of hemoglobin
  A. Structure
    1. Hemoglobin consists of four polypeptide chains and four heme groups; hemoglobin is a dimer of dimers with two chains from the α-family and two chains from the β-family
    2. Hemoglobin A, the principal hemoglobin in adults, consists of two α-chains and two β-chains as $\alpha_2\beta_2$
    3. The α- and β-chains of hemoglobin consist of helical regions (from A through H) and bends
      a. An invariant histidine in all hemoglobins, called F8 or the proximal histidine, binds heme
      b. F8 refers to the eighth residue of the F helix
  B. Cooperative oxygen binding
    1. The concentration dependence of oxygen binding to hemoglobin is expressed by a **sigmoidal curve;** *the sigmoidal curve is diagnostic of positive cooperativity*
    2. The quaternary structure of oxygenated hemoglobin is called the **R state** (for relaxed), and the conformation of the deoxygenated state is called the **T state** (for tense)
    3. Deoxyhemoglobin is tauter and more constrained than oxyhemoglobin because the T form contains eight more salt bridges between subunits than does the R form
    4. The ability of hemoglobin to bind oxygen decreases with an increase in acidity; protons make hemoglobin dump oxygen, and this is called the Bohr effect
      a. The difference in acidity between oxy- and deoxyhemoglobin is due to a difference in the pK_a values of the imidazole side chain of histidine 87 of the α-chains and histidine 92 of the β-chains
      b. The average pK_a of these histidines of deoxyhemoglobin is slightly basic (7.9) and that for oxyhemoglobin is slightly acidic (6.7)
      c. A decreased pH promotes a change in conformation of hemoglobin to a form (deoxyhemoglobin) better able to bind protons
    5. **2,3-Bisphosphoglycerate** (2,3-BPG), which occurs in the red cell, binds preferentially to the β-chains of deoxyhemoglobin and therefore promotes the release of oxygen from hemoglobin (2,3-BPG makes hemoglobin dump oxygen)
  C. Isohydric transport of carbon dioxide
    1. The term isohydric refers to a lack of change of hydrogen ion concentration (pH) during this process
    2. Deoxyhemoglobin carries protons (Bohr effect) and accounts for isohydric transport
    3. Carbon dioxide diffuses from respiring cells and combines with water within the red blood cell to form carbonic acid in a reaction catalyzed by **carbonic anhydrase** (a zinc-containing enzyme)
      a. Carbonic acid dissociates to form a proton and bicarbonate
      b. Consider the transport of bicarbonate and the hydrogen ion separately
        (1) Bicarbonate from the red cell enters the plasma through the **anion exchange protein** (band 3 protein) of the red cell membrane in exchange for plasma chloride
        (2) The hydrogen ion binds to deoxyhemoglobin (a weaker acid) that is formed after oxyhemoglobin (a stronger acid) releases oxygen
    4. The process reverses in the red blood cells in the lungs
      a. Deoxyhemoglobin binds oxygen and liberates a proton

b. Bicarbonate enters the red cell in exchange for chloride via the anion change protein
c. Bicarbonate and the proton combine to form carbonic acid, which then decomposes into carbon dioxide and water as catalyzed by carbonic hydrase
d. Carbon dioxide diffuses from the red cell and is expired

D. Another mechanism for carbon dioxide transport involves its reaction with the amino terminal residues of hemoglobin to form **carbaminohemoglobin**

Objective 2: To describe sickle cell anemia and the thalassemias.

E. Hemoglobinopathies
1. Sickle cell anemia
a. *Hemoglobin S differs from hemoglobin A by the conversion of β6 Glu → Val*
b. This alteration is due to an A → T transversion in the triplet codon for the sixth residue of the β-globin chain (transversions refer to the mutation of a purine to pyrimidine or vice versa; transitions refer to mutation of a purine to purine or pyrimidine to pyrimidine)
c. The subunit composition of sickle cell hemoglobin is $\alpha_2^A\beta_2^S$
d. In concentrated hemoglobin solutions that are partially or fully deoxygenated, this mutation leads to the aggregation of hemoglobin, which causes cell deformity
e. A heterozygote with sickle cell trait is asymptomatic, accounting for the designation of the disease as autosomal recessive
f. A single blood cell of a heterozygote contains 60% $\alpha_2^A\beta_2^A$ and 40% $\alpha_2^A\beta_2^S$

2. Thalassemias
a. Thalassemias are a heterogeneous group of hemoglobinopathies in which the mutation reduces the level of synthesis of the α- or β-chains
b. *The main groups are the α-thalassemias, in which α-chain synthesis is impaired, and the β-thalassemias, in which β-chain synthesis is impaired*
(1) The most common forms of α-thalassemias are due to gene deletions, and these deletions are produced by unequal crossing-over during meiosis
(2) β-Thalassemias are usually due to single nucleotide substitutions rather than deletions
(a) More than 80 different mutations produce β-thalassemia
(b) Mutations include almost every conceivable type of abnormality that can reduce the synthesis of an mRNA or protein
(c) These include promoter mutations that decrease transcription, cap site and initiator codon mutations, splicing mutations, frameshift mutations, nonsense mutations, and point mutations that produce unstable hemoglobin

Objective 3: To outline the pathway for heme synthesis and catabolism.

II. Heme
A. Function
1. Heme is an iron-containing tetrapyrrole that binds oxygen or participates in oxidation-reduction reactions
2. Heme occurs in hemoglobin, myoglobin, and mitochondrial cytochromes, cytochrome P-450, catalase, peroxidase, and the soluble form of guanylate cyclase

B. Biosynthesis
1. Protoporphyrin IX is derived from eight molecules each of **succinyl-CoA** and **glycine**
2. *The first and rate-limiting step in the biosynthesis of heme is catalyzed by* ***δ-aminolevulinic acid synthase*** *(ALA synthase), a pyridoxal phosphate enzyme*
3. Heme synthesis is diminished by lead
a. Children are more susceptible to lead toxicity than are adults
b. ALA dehydratase is the enzyme that is most sensitive to lead, followed by ferrochelatase

C. Catabolism
1. The first step in heme degradation is catalyzed by **heme oxygenase,** an enzyme of the endoplasmic reticulum
2. The reactants include two moles of oxygen, one mole of NADPH, and one mole of heme
3. Besides playing a role in heme degradation, this process generates carbon monoxide (**carbon monoxide** may serve as a second messenger in brain, thus resembling nitric oxide)
4. Heme is cleaved between the A and B rings to produce **biliverdin** (verdin, green), ferric iron, carbon monoxide, and water
5. Biliverdin reacts with NADPH in a reaction catalyzed by **biliverdin reductase** to form **bilirubin** (Latin *ruber* "red"); bilirubin is a bile pigment
6. Bilirubin, a lipophilic substance, is transported to the liver as a complex with albumin
a. Bilirubin reacts with two molecules of energy-rich UDP~glucuronate to form **bilirubin diglucuronide,** a hydrophilic energy-poor substance in accordance with PRINCIPLE 2 OF BIOENERGETICS
b. Bilirubin diglucuronide is direct bilirubin (referring to the van den Bergh reaction), and unconjugated bilirubin is indirect bilirubin

Objective 4: To describe blood clotting and the mechanisms of anticoagulants.

III. Blood clotting
A. Two pathways initiate blood clotting: intrinsic (simple) and extrinsic (complicated)
1. The **intrinsic pathway,** which may be initiated by an abnormal surface provided by damaged endothelium *in vivo* or glass *in vitro,* is so named because all components are present in blood; no exogenous component is required to initiate or propagate the reaction
2. The **extrinsic pathway** requires an extravascular component (**thromboplastin** or **factor III**), which results when blood contacts any tissue because of injury; many tissues express factor III
3. Both pathways merge at the common pathway
a. The **common pathway** involves the conversion of prothrombin to active thrombin, a serine protease

b. Thrombin catalyzes the conversion of fibrinogen to fibrin
c. The activation of prothrombin and the formation of fibrin are the two most important steps of blood clotting

B. Blood clotting involves a series of reactions in which the product of one process initiates a subsequent process, the product of which initiates still another—a **cascade**

C. Blood clotting involves at least six distinct proteases with a serine residue at the active site (the activated forms of factors II, VII, IX, X, XI, and XII)

D. These serine proteases exhibit trypsin-like specificity (hydrolyzing a peptide bond on the carboxyl side of a basic amino acid residue)

E. Factor VIII is the famous **antihemophilic factor** associated with hemophilia A

F. Factor IX is called **Christmas factor**
1. The factor is named for a person who had a disease resembling classic hemophilia but whose biochemical lesion was shown to be different
2. Christmas disease is hemophilia B

G. Von Willebrand factor performs two functions
1. It binds to receptors on the platelet surface and forms a bridge between the platelet and areas of vascular damage
2. Von Willebrand factor also binds to and stabilizes factor VIII
3. That a deficiency of any of these three factors produces the same clinical manifestations illustrates that the three factors interact during blood clotting

IV. Anticoagulants and fibrinolysis

A. Antithrombin III and protein C–protein S are natural anticoagulants in blood
1. **Antithrombin III,** activated by heparin, binds and inhibits many serine proteases including thrombin and Xa, accounting for the anticoagulant effects of heparin
2. **Protein C,** together with **protein S,** shuts off the coagulation pathway by inactivating factors VIII and Va by proteolysis

B. **Plasmin,** a serine protease formed from plasminogen, is responsible for fibrinolysis
1. **Tissue plasminogen activator** (tPA) is a serine protease that catalyzes the conversion of plasminogen to plasmin by hydrolyzing a single peptide bond
2. Soluble plasmin is inhibited by α_2-plasmin inhibitor
3. **Urokinase,** which is a family of serine proteases produced by the kidney, functions as a plasminogen activator

V. Laboratory tests for disorders of hemostasis

A. Measurement of the **bleeding time** is a sensitive laboratory index of primary hemostatic function
1. Bleeding time is elevated in people with von Willebrand disease
2. Thrombocytopenia (low platelet count) is a common cause of elevated bleeding time and abnormal bleeding
3. People with hemophilia have a normal bleeding time

B. **Activated partial thromboplastin time** (aPTT) reflects the functional state of the intrinsic pathway
1. Therapeutic heparin treatment increases aPTT
2. Elevated aPTT occurs in hemophilias A and B

C. **Prothrombin time** reflects the functional state of both the extrinsic and the intrinsic pathways
1. A normal result requires adequate fibrinogen, prothrombin, and factors V, VII, and X
2. Because the biosynthesis of prothrombin and factors VII, IX, and X requires vitamin K, the prothrombin time is used to monitor vitamin K antagonist (warfarin, dicumarol) therapy

Objective 5: To describe the genetics of various coagulopathies.

VI. Genetics of coagulopathies

A. Hemophilia A (factor VIII deficiency) and hemophilia B (Christmas disease or factor IX deficiency) are X-linked bleeding disorders
1. The human factor VIII gene contains two notable features
a. It contains an unusually large exon of 3106 base pairs (average size for exons is 75 to 200 base pairs)
b. The factor VIII gene contains an extremely large intron of 32,000 base pairs between exons 22 and 23
2. A variety of mutations in their corresponding genes can cause either hemophilia A or B

B. **Von Willebrand disease** is due to a mutation of the factor gene that is located on or near the tip of the short arm of chromosome 12

QUESTIONS

DIRECTIONS. (Items 1–18): Each of the numbered items or incomplete statements in this section is followed by answers or by completions of the statement. Select the ONE lettered answer or completion that is BEST in each case. Correct answers and explanations are given at the end of the chapter.

1. The transition from the R to T state involves large structural changes at which one of the following contacts?

(A) $\alpha_1\alpha_2$
(B) $\alpha_1\beta_1$
(C) $\alpha_1\beta_2$
(D) $\beta_1\beta_2$

2. Protons are able to promote oxygen dissociation (dumping) from normal adult hemoglobin. This process, which is responsible for the isohydric transport of carbon dioxide, is called

(A) the R state
(B) the T state
(C) positive cooperativity
(D) negative cooperativity
(E) the Bohr effect

3. The mutation that is responsible for the formation of sickle cell hemoglobin is

(A) conversion of a glutamate to valine in the β-chain
(B) conversion of a histidine to alanine in the F8 helix

(C) elimination of a stop codon
(D) a result of aberrant splicing
(E) deletion of the α-chain gene

4. The rate-limiting reaction in protoporphyrin IX synthesis is catalyzed by
   (A) δ-aminolevulinic acid (ALA) dehydratase
   (B) δ-aminolevulinic acid (ALA) synthase
   (C) coproporphyrinogen oxidase
   (D) ferrochelatase
   (E) protoporphyrinogen oxidase

5. The enzyme in the heme biosynthetic pathway that is most sensitive to lead is
   (A) δ-aminolevulinic acid (ALA) dehydratase
   (B) δ-aminolevulinic acid (ALA) synthase
   (C) coproporphyrinogen oxidase
   (D) ferrochelatase
   (E) protoporphyrinogen oxidase

6. The first step in heme catabolism is catalyzed by
   (A) bilirubin glucuronyltransferase
   (B) biliverdin reductase
   (C) coproporphyrinogen oxidase
   (D) β-glucuronidase
   (E) heme oxygenase

7. Patients with an obstruction of the bile duct exhibit primarily an increase in which one of the following tetrapyrrole derivatives?
   (A) Direct bilirubin
   (B) Indirect bilirubin
   (C) Stercobilin
   (D) Urobilin
   (E) Urobilinogen

8. The activated forms of all of the following factors are serine proteases EXCEPT
   (A) factor II (prothrombin)
   (B) factor VIII (antihemophilic factor)
   (C) factor IX (Christmas factor)
   (D) factor XI (thromboplastin antecedent)
   (E) factor XII (Hageman factor)

9. Which one of the following tests is used to establish the diagnosis of von Willebrand disease?
   (A) Activated partial thromboplastin time (aPTT)
   (B) Bleeding time
   (C) Platelet count
   (D) Prothrombin time
   (E) Vitamin K levels in serum

10. Which one of the following substances activates plasminogen without catalyzing the hydrolysis of a peptide bond?
   (A) α_2-Antiplasmin
   (B) Protein C–protein S complex
   (C) Streptokinase
   (D) Tissue plasminogen activator
   (E) Urokinase

11. The posttranslational modification of which one of the following substances, which lacks γ-carboxyglutamate, is NOT affected by vitamin K antagonists such as warfarin or dicumarol?
   (A) Factor II (prothrombin)
   (B) Factor VII (proconvertin)
   (C) Factor VIII (antihemophilic factor)
   (D) Factor IX (Christmas factor)
   (E) Protein S

Items 12–18

History

The patient is an 8-year-old boy with a chief complaint of fever, headache, and abdominal pain. The fever and headache began 48 hours prior to admission. His appetite was greatly decreased, and the parents had forced fluids. This is the fifth hospitalization for this patient; a diagnosis of sickle cell anemia was made at 7 months of age. He has been hospitalized with sickle cell crises several times; he had pneumonia twice and osteomyelitis once.

Physical Examination

The patient weighs 20 kg (5th percentile) and has a height of 125 cm (50th percentile). He appears lethargic and seriously ill. His temperature is 39.7°C (103.4°F); pulse, 122/min; respirations, 18/min; blood pressure, 110/66 mm Hg. He has scleral icterus. The throat is red and appears inflamed; the eardrums are normal. No adventitious sounds were heard in the thorax; bowel sounds were present but hypoactive. The spleen is enlarged and tender to palpation. Deep tendon reflexes are normal, and there was a positive Brudzinski sign (involuntary flexion of the knees and hips following flexion of the neck while supine) but no Babinski sign (extension of the great toe following stimulation of the plantar surface as opposed to the normal flexion of the great toe). There is nuchal rigidity.

Laboratory

Hematocrit, 26% (normal, 37–49%)
Hemoglobin, 8.2 g/dL (normal, 13–16 g/dL)
White blood count, 22,400/μL (normal, 5000–15,000/μL)
Polymorphonuclear leukocytes, 88% (normal, 54–62%)
Lymphocytes, 7% (normal, 25–33%)
Monocytes, 3% (normal, 3–7%)
Corrected reticulocyte count, 8% (normal, 1%)
Platelet count, 360,000/μL (normal, 150–400 $\times$ $10^3/\mu$L)
Total bilirubin, 2.1 mg/dL (normal, 0.1–1.0 mg/dL)
Direct bilirubin, 0.4 mg/dL (normal, 0.0–0.3 mg/dL)
Lactate dehydrogenase (LDH), 1560 U/L (normal, 150–500 U/L)
Serum glucose, 92 mg/dL (normal, 70–105 mg/dL)
Blood urea nitrogen (BUN), 16 mg/dL (normal, 7–18 mg/dL)
Creatinine, 0.5 mg/dL (normal, 0.3–0.7 mg/dL)

A lumbar puncture was performed, and the opening spinal fluid pressure was 310 mm H_2O (normal, 70–180). Examination of the cerebrospinal fluid revealed a white cell count of 3400 cells/μL (normal, $<0.5/\mu$L) with 92% polymorphonuclear leukocytes; glucose, 36 mg/dL (normal, $\approx$75% of serum glucose, or 70 mg/dL to correspond to the serum glucose); protein, 210 mg/dL (normal, <40 mg/dL).

Examination of the cerebrospinal fluid revealed gram-positive diplococci. Urinalysis and chest x-rays were normal. The patient was immediately started on ceftriaxone (a third-generation cephalosporin with a mechanism of action similar to that of penicillin). One day later, *Streptococcus pneumoniae* grew from the cerebrospinal fluid culture, and it was sensitive to penicillin, oxacillin, vancomycin, and a variety of cephalosporins including ceftriaxone.

12. The low concentration of cerebrospinal fluid glucose is related to which one of the following metabolic properties?
    (A) failure of glucose to cross the blood-brain barrier
    (B) decreased metabolism of glucose by the brain as a result of infection
    (C) metabolism of glucose by bacteria
    (D) hypoglycemia
    (E) decreased integrity of the blood-brain barrier for glucose

13. The mechanism of action of ceftriaxone, which has a mechanism of action similar to that of penicillin, is due to
    (A) inhibition of the initiation of bacterial protein synthesis
    (B) drug-induced misreading of the bacterial genetic code
    (C) inhibition of bacterial cell wall synthesis
    (D) inhibition of aminoacyl-tRNA transfer to the A site
    (E) inhibition of the bacterial peptidyltransferase reaction

Use the following electropherogram of the patient's hemoglobin, which was obtained at 7 months of age, for items 14–15.

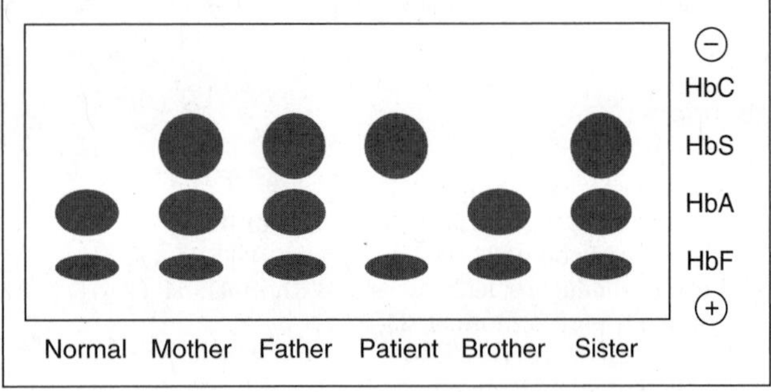

14. What does the electropherogram indicate regarding sickle cell anemia in the patient's family?
    (A) the mother lacks sickle cell trait
    (B) the father lacks sickle cell trait
    (C) the patient's brother is a carrier of the sickle cell gene
    (D) the patient's sister has sickle cell trait

15. Besides sickle cell disease, hemoglobin S/C disease is a hemolytic anemia that is characterized by erythrocytes that form sickle-shaped cells. The electropherogram indicates that the patient does not have hemoglobin S/C disease. Hemoglobin C, like sickle cell hemoglobin, involves a mutation at position 6 of the β-chain. Based upon the analysis of the electropherogram and a knowledge of the structures of hemoglobin A and hemoglobin S, hemoglobin C contains which one of the following amino acids in position 6 of the β-chain?
    (A) Alanine
    (B) Glycine
    (C) Leucine
    (D) Aspartate
    (E) Lysine

16. Splenomegaly in patients with sickle cell anemia is due to
    (A) bacterial inflammation
    (B) sickle cell aggregation and hemolysis
    (C) decreased white blood cell production
    (D) decreased platelet production
    (E) decreased red blood cell production

17. The pattern of bilirubin elevation observed in this patient is
    (A) prehepatic
    (B) due to inflammation of the liver (hepatic)
    (C) posthepatic (due to obstruction of the bile ducts)
    (D) due to a primary defect in bilirubin synthesis
    (E) due to a defect in bilirubin catabolism

18. The elevated lactate dehydrogenase is a result of which one of the following disorders?
    (A) Primary liver disease
    (B) Meningitis
    (C) Red cell hemolysis
    (D) Pneumonia
    (E) Myocardial infarction

ANSWERS AND EXPLANATIONS

1. The answer is C: $\alpha_1\beta_2$. Hemoglobin is a tetramer that consists of an $\alpha_2\beta_2$ structure. It consists of a dimer of $\alpha1\beta1$ and $\alpha2\beta2$ dimers. The transition from the R (relaxed) to the T (taut) state involves changes in the $\alpha_1\beta_2$ (and $\alpha_2\beta_1$) contacts; the T state has an increased number of ionic bonds between these contacts. The R state has greater affinity for oxygen, and the T state has less affinity. *Biochemistry,* pp. 486–487.
2. The answer is E: the Bohr effect. The acidification of oxyhemoglobin (in the R state), which occurs in active tissues, promotes oxygen release to these active tissues with the concomitant formation of deoxyhemoglobin (in the T state). This so-called Bohr effect is consonant with the molecular logic of metabolism (PRINCIPLE 9 OF BIOCHEMISTRY). Deoxyhemoglobin has a stronger affinity for protons than oxyhemoglobin, and deoxyhemoglobin is able to transport protons from the periphery to the lung in the absence of a pH change (this is called isohydric transport owing to the minimal change in hydrogen ion concentration because protons are bound to hemoglobin and are not free). Hemoglobin exhibits positive cooperativity; binding the first molecule of oxygen increases the

affinity for the second, which increases affinity for the third and fourth molecules. The *sine qua non* of positive cooperativity is a sigmoidal concentration-response curve. *Biochemistry,* p. 486.

3. The answer is A: a conversion of glutamate to valine at position 6 of the β-chain. This mutation involves the conversion of a hydrophilic and negatively charged residue to a hydrophobic and uncharged residue. Hemoglobin S can be distinguished from hemoglobin A by electrophoresis because of the difference in charge. It is postulated that the introduction of a hydrophobic group promotes abnormal association of neighboring molecules and the formation of aggregates that accounts for the gelation of deoxyhemoglobin S. Deficiency of α-chains results in α-thalassemia, and deficiency of β-chains produces β-thalassemia. Aberrant splicing, deletion of the α-chain genes, and a variety of other mutations produce thalassemia. Hemoglobin Constant Spring has a 31-residue extension that results from a mutation in the normal stop codon. Translation continues downstream to the next stop codon at position 173. Because hemoglobin Constant Spring mRNA is unstable, decreased formation of α-chains leads to one form of α-thalassemia. *Biochemistry,* p. 488.
4. The answer is B: δ-aminolevulinic acid synthase (ALA synthase). ALA synthase, which catalyzes the first and rate-limiting step in heme synthesis, catalyzes a unidirectional reaction. ALA synthase uses pyridoxal phosphate as cofactor. *Biochemistry,* p. 490.
5. The answer is A: δ-aminolevulinic acid (ALA) dehydratase. ALA dehydratase is most sensitive to lead, followed by ferrochelatase. For reasons unknown, children with lead poisoning typically present in the spring of the year. *Biochemistry,* p. 494.
6. The answer is E: heme oxygenase. Heme oxygenase, an enzyme of the endoplasmic reticulum, catalyzes a reaction of heme, two moles of oxygen, and one mole of NADPH. Besides playing a role in heme degradation, this process generates carbon monoxide and biliverdin, a green pigment. Carbon monoxide may serve as a second messenger in brain analogous to nitric oxide. *Biochemistry,* p. 491.
7. The answer is A: direct bilirubin. Biliverdin, formed from heme, reacts with NADPH in a reaction catalyzed by biliverdin reductase to form bilirubin. Bilirubin, a hydrophobic substance, is transported to the liver as a complex with albumin. Bilirubin reacts with two molecules of energy-rich UDP~glucuronate to form bilirubin diglucuronide, a hydrophilic energy-poor substance. Bilirubin diglucuronide is excreted in the bile. Hydrophobic bilirubin reacts slowly in the van den Bergh reaction and is called indirect bilirubin; hydrophilic bilirubin diglucuronide reacts rapidly and is called direct bilirubin. Direct bilirubin can be formed in liver cells, but in the presence of an obstructed bile duct (because of gallstones or a tumor), direct bilirubin cannot be transported into the gut where urobilinogen, stercobilin, and urobilin form. With hemolytic anemias and primary liver disease, there is generally a greater increase in indirect bilirubin than in direct bilirubin. *Biochemistry,* p. 491.
8. The answer is B: factor VIII (antihemophilic factor). Antihemophilic factor is a component that interacts with activated Christmas factor, a serine protease, and Ca^{2+} to catalyze the proteolytic conversion of X to Xa. The serine proteases of the blood clotting scheme each possess a catalytic triad consisting of serine, histidine, and aspartate, which is similar to the catalytic triad of chymotrypsin. The serine proteases of blood clotting include the activated forms of factors II, VII, IX, X, XI, and XII. *Biochemistry,* p. 494.
9. The answer is B: bleeding time. The bleeding time measures primary hemostasis, or the instantaneous plugging of a hole in a blood vessel wall. Primary hemostasis is achieved by a combination of vasoconstriction and platelet adhesion and aggregation. The formation of a fibrin clot is not required. Bleeding time is elevated in people with von Willebrand disease and with thrombocytopenia. Thrombocytopenia (low platelet count) is a common cause of blood clotting deficiency. People with hemophilia have a normal bleeding time. *Biochemistry,* p. 497.
10. The answer is C: streptokinase. Streptokinase forms a complex with plasminogen to activate its cryptic protease activity without covalently modifying plasminogen. Streptokinase, a bacterial enzyme, can be used in the treatment of thrombotic diseases such as myocardial infarction and pulmonary embolus. α_2-Antiplasmin inhibits plasmin, an enzyme that operates on fibrin, and is thrombostatic and not thrombolytic. Tissue plasminogen activator and urokinase are proteolytic enzymes that also activate plasminogen by hydrolyzing peptide bonds in the substrate. These agents are also used in the treatment of thrombotic diseases. *Biochemistry,* pp. 496–497.
11. The answer is C: factor VIII (antihemophilic factor). Antihemophilic factor is one of the components of the blood clotting cascade that lacks γ-carboxyglutamate. Factors II, VII, IX, and X contain γ-carboxyglutamate. Moreover, protein S and protein C of the anticoagulant system also contain γ-carboxyglutamate. *Biochemistry,* p. 495.
12. The answer is C: metabolism of glucose by bacteria. Besides the primary diagnosis of sickle cell anemia, the signs and symptoms of this patient are consistent with a diagnosis of bacterial meningitis. The indicators that point to a diagnosis of bacterial meningitis include fever, headache, and elevated white blood count (these can occur, however, with any bacterial infection). Nuchal rigidity and a positive Brudzinski sign are suggestive of meningitis. The presence of a large number of white cells and a positive Gram stain of the cerebrospinal fluid establish the diagnosis. Bacteria use glucose as a source of energy, and this contributes to the decrease in the cerebrospinal fluid glucose concentration. Of course, brain also uses glucose as a source of energy, accounting in large part for the decreased glucose in the cerebrospinal fluid. In a febrile patient with increased energy expenditure as a result of elevated temperature (biochemical reaction rates increase by a factor of about two with each 10°C increase in temperature), neuronal glucose metabolism increases so that more glucose is used, not less. The low concentration of cerebrospinal fluid glucose is not related to hypoglycemia. The serum glucose was 92 mg/dL in this patient, and this is within the normal range. Meningitis decreases the integrity of the blood-brain barrier, which would increase, not decrease, the ability of glucose to cross the blood-brain barrier, thus allowing more rapid equilibration with the normal serum glucose concentration. *Biochemistry,* p. 102; *Nelson,* p. 664.
13. The answer is C: inhibition of bacterial cell wall synthesis. The β-lactam antibiotics including penicillin and ceftriaxone inhibit bacterial cell wall synthesis by forming a covalent bond with the enzyme that adds dipeptidyl D-Ala-D-Ala to nascent peptidoglycan. Streptomycin and other aminoglycoside antibiotics inhibit the initiation of bacterial protein synthesis and cause misreading of the

genetic code. Tetracycline inhibits the introduction of aminoacyl-tRNA into the A site. Chloramphenicol, which inhibits the bacterial peptidyltransferase reaction, is a good alternative choice in the treatment of bacterial meningitis. Because bacterial meningitis is a serious infection that can kill rapidly, antibiotic treatment is initiated immediately after diagnosis. *Biochemistry,* p. 357.

14. The answer is D: the patient's sister has sickle cell trait. The patient's sister, mother, and father all have sickle cell trait, as indicated by the presence of both hemoglobin A and hemoglobin S. Individuals with sickle cell trait suffer no ill effects and have a normal life span. These individuals are more resistant to malaria than are people with hemoglobin A. This resistance accounts for the widespread prevalence of sickle cell trait in the population and is the basis for the so-called heterozygote advantage of the sickle cell gene. The patient's brother is not a carrier of the sickle cell gene, as indicated by the lack of hemoglobin S.
15. The answer is E: lysine. Hemoglobin A contains glutamate (a negatively charged residue) at position 6 of the β-chain, and hemoglobin S contains valine (a neutral amino acid) in this position. Based upon the direction of migration in an electric field, hemoglobin C must be even less negative (more positive). Lysine is the only amino acid in the list that bears a positive charge at neutral pH values (hemoglobin electrophoresis is usually performed at pH 8.6). *Biochemistry,* p. 43.
16. The answer is B: sickle cell aggregation and hemolysis. Deoxyhemoglobin S forms aggregates and causes erythrocytes to form sickle-shaped cells that undergo hemolysis. The spleen participates in metabolizing lysed red blood cells and becomes enlarged during a variety of hemolytic disorders. Sometimes overactivity of the spleen (hypersplenism) aggravates the anemia and produces thrombocytopenia. Aggregation of sickle cells occludes vessels and can lead to tissue infarction (ischemic necrosis or tissue death due to inadequate oxygen supply). Patients with sickle cell anemia commonly develop splenic infarcts, strokes, and other sequelae as a result of vascular occlusion. Moreover, acute painful vasoocclusive episodes represent the most frequent and prominent manifestation of sickle cell disease. Although this patient is anemic, red cell production in the bone marrow is increased in a compensatory fashion. *Biochemistry,* pp. 488–489; *Nelson,* p. 1247.
17. The answer is A: prehepatic. As a result of hemolysis of red cells, heme is released and converted prehepatically to bilirubin. The liver is responsible for the conversion of bilirubin (indirect bilirubin seen in excess in this patient) to bilirubin diglucuronide (direct bilirubin, only slightly elevated in this patient); jaundice is due to the excessive production of bilirubin and not to liver inflammation, posthepatic obstruction, or decreased bilirubin catabolism. *Biochemistry,* p. 491.
18. The answer is C: red cell hemolysis. Red cells contain the enzymes of the glycolytic pathway. As a result of hemolysis, lactate dehydrogenase is released into the serum. Elevated lactate dehydrogenase can also occur with primary liver disease and after a myocardial infarction, but there is no indication of these diseases in this patient. *Biochemistry,* p. 102.

REFERENCES

Roskoski, R., Jr. *Biochemistry.* Philadelphia, W. B. Saunders Company, 1996.

Behrman, R. E. *Nelson Textbook of Pediatrics,* 14th ed. Philadelphia, W. B. Saunders Company, 1992.

CHAPTER TWENTY-FIVE

INTEGRATION OF METABOLISM

SYNOPSIS

OBJECTIVES

1. To explain the regulation of mainstream metabolic pathways.
2. To describe the metabolic interrelationships of various organs of the body.
3. To outline the major consequences of diabetes mellitus.
4. To describe the metabolism of ethanol.

Objective 1: To explain the regulation of mainstream metabolic pathways.

I. General principles of metabolic regulation
   A. Biochemical reactions and pathways can be regulated by allosteric regulators, protein phosphorylation, enzyme induction, and the availability of substrates
   B. Controlling reactions in a metabolic pathway usually possess several common features
      1. The controlling reaction is at or near the beginning of the pathway and is exergonic
      2. The reaction represents a committed step, and the product of the reaction cannot be diverted to another major pathway
      3. Metabolic regulation follows the molecular logic of the cell (PRINCIPLE 9 OF BIOCHEMISTRY)

II. Control of the flux of metabolites in mainstream metabolic pathways
   A. Glycolysis and gluconeogenesis (Tables 25–1 and 25–2) are regulated reciprocally
      1. Phosphofructokinase catalyzes the rate-limiting step of glycolysis and is activated by fructose 2,6-bisphosphate
      2. The regulation of gluconeogenesis is complex
         a. All four enzymes that are required for gluconeogenesis (but not for glycolysis)—pyruvate carboxylase, PEP carboxykinase, fructose-1,6-bisphosphatase, and glucose-6-phosphatase—are induced by the cyclic AMP cascade and by glucocorticoids
         b. The pyruvate carboxylase reaction occurs at a crossroad of metabolism
            (1) The product of the reaction, oxaloacetate, is a substrate for gluconeogenesis and is an intermediate of the Krebs cycle
            (2) The enzyme requires acetyl-CoA for expression of its activity, and the acetyl-CoA/CoA ratio is regulatory
         c. PEP carboxykinase, which catalyzes the committed step, is the controlling enzyme
         d. Fructose-1,6-bisphosphatase is inhibited by fructose 2,6-bisphosphate, and it is thus regulated reciprocally with phosphofructose-1-kinase
   B. Glycogenesis and glycogenolysis (Tables 25–1 and 25–2) are regulated reciprocally
      1. Glycogen synthase is the enzyme controlling glycogenesis, and it is inhibited following phosphorylation by protein kinase A
      2. Glycogen phosphorylase is the enzyme controlling glycogenolysis
   C. The main regulatory enzyme of the Krebs cycle is isocitrate dehydrogenase, which is activated allosterically by ADP
   D. Regulation of lipogenesis and lipolysis involves reactions in different organs
      1. Acetyl-CoA carboxylase is the controlling enzyme of fatty acid biosynthesis
      2. Activation of adipocyte hormone-sensitive lipase by the cyclic AMP cascade liberates free fatty acids into the circulation, and this promotes β-oxidation in most cells (excluding brain and erythrocytes)
      3. Carnitine acyltransferase I is the controlling enzyme of β-oxidation
         a. This enzyme is inhibited by malonyl-CoA, the product of the acetyl-CoA carboxylase reaction
         b. Fatty acid synthesis and β-oxidation are thus regulated reciprocally
   E. Control of nitrogen metabolism (Table 25–3) involves diverse pathways
      1. Carbamoyl-phosphate synthetase I, which is activated by *N*-acetylglutamate, is the controlling enzyme of the urea cycle
      2. Carbamoyl-phosphate synthetase II, which is inhibited by UTP and UDP, is the controlling enzyme of pyrimidine synthesis in humans; aspartate transcarbamoylase catalyzes the rate-limiting step in *Escherichia coli*
      3. PRPP amidotransferase catalyzes the rate-limiting reaction in purine synthesis

TABLE 25–1. Sites of Control of Mainstream Metabolic Pathways

Pathway	Major Regulatory Enzymes	Activators	Inhibitors	Hormonal Effects	Comment
Glycolysis	Phosphofructokinase	Fructose 2,6-bisphosphate, AMP	Citrate (except liver), ATP	Glucagon cascade ↓ [fructose 2,6-bisphosphate]	Insulin cascade induces and glucagon cascade represses synthesis of enzymes catalyzing unidirectional reactions of this pathway in liver.
	Hexokinase		Glucose 6-phosphate		
	Glucokinase		Regulatory protein-fructose 6-phosphate		
	Pyruvate kinase	Fructose 1,6-bisphosphate	Alanine, ATP, fatty acids	Glucagon cascade ↓ enzyme activity (liver only)	
Gluconeogenesis	Pyruvate carboxylase	Acetyl-CoA			Glucagon, glucocorticoids, and epinephrine induce and insulin represses synthesis of enzymes catalyzing unidirectional reactions of this pathway in liver.
	PEP carboxykinase				
	Fructose-1,6-bisphosphatase		Fructose 2,6-bisphosphate, AMP	Glucagon cascade ↓ [fructose 2,6-bisphosphate]	
	Glucose-6-phosphatase				
Glycogenesis	Glycogen synthase	High glucose 6-phosphate (not physiological)		Insulin cascade ↑; glucagon (liver) and epinephrine (muscle) cascades ↓	Insulin cascade induces.
Glycogenolysis	Phosphorylase	AMP (muscle), Ca^{2+}	Glucose, ATP, glucose 6-phosphate (liver)	Glucagon cascade ↑; insulin cascade ↓	
Pentose phosphate pathway	Glucose-6-phosphate dehydrogenase				Insulin cascade induces; $NADP^+$ availability may be regulatory.
Pyruvate dehydrogenase activity	Pyruvate dehydrogenase kinase		Kinase is activated by acetyl-CoA and NADH, and kinase action inhibits dehydrogenase		Phosphorylation of pyruvate dehydrogenase is inhibitory.
Krebs cycle	Isocitrate dehydrogenase	ADP			
Lipogenesis	Acetyl-CoA carboxylase	Citrate	Fatty acyl–CoA	Insulin cascade ↑ (adipocyte); glucagon cascade ↓	Insulin cascade induces.
Lipolysis	Hormone-sensitive lipase			Glucagon, epinephrine cascades ↑; insulin cascade ↓	
β-Oxidation	Carnitine acyltransferase–I		Malonyl-CoA		

TABLE 25-2. Covalent Modification of Regulatory Enzymes*

Kinase Substrate	Kinase/Phosphatase	Effect on Substrate Activity	Comment
Acetyl-CoA carboxylase	AMP-dependent protein kinase	↓	Kinase activated by decreased adenylate charge
Branched-chain keto acid dehydrogenase†	Branched-chain keto acid dehydrogenase kinase	↓	Kinase activated by CoA products and NADH
Glycogen synthase	Protein kinase A and glycogen synthase kinase	↓ ↓	
Glycogen synthase kinase	AMP-dependent protein kinase	↓	Kinase activated by decreased adenylate charge
HMG-CoA reductase	AMP-dependent protein kinase	↓	Kinase activated by decreased adenylate charge
Hormone-sensitive lipase	Protein kinase A	↑	
Pyruvate kinase (liver)	Protein kinase A	↓	
Phosphofructo-2-kinase/ fructose-2,6-bisphosphatase (liver)	Protein kinase A	↓ ↑	
Pyruvate dehydrogenase†	Pyruvate dehydrogenase kinase	↓	Kinase activated by acetyl-CoA and NADH
Pyruvate dehydrogenase†	Pyruvate dehydrogenase phosphatase	↑	Phosphatase activated by calcium and insulin action
Phosphorylase	Phosphorylase kinase	↑	
Phosphorylase kinase	Protein kinase A	↑	

* Actions mediated by protein kinase A are antagonized by the insulin cascade.
† Mitochondrial.

Objective 2: To describe the metabolic interrelationships of various organs of the body.

III. Metabolic interrelationships of the various organs
  A. The brain relies on glucose as a metabolic fuel; after a few days of fasting, brain can obtain up to 50% of its energy from ketone bodies
  B. Red blood cells rely exclusively on glucose as a metabolic fuel
  C. Muscle can oxidize fatty acids, ketone bodies, and glucose as fuels
  D. The kidney can perform gluconeogenesis after fasting (>24 hours), and it can generate ammonium ion during the production of acidic urine
  E. The liver is the most diversified organ of fuel homeostasis
    1. The liver maintains blood glucose, essential for red

TABLE 25-3. Sites of Control of Auxiliary Metabolic Pathways

Pathway	Regulatory Enzyme	Activator	Inhibitor	Hormonal Effects	Comment
Branched-chain keto acid dehydrogenase	Branched-chain keto acid dehydrogenase kinase		Kinase is activated by NADH and acyl-CoA, and kinase inhibits dehydrogenase	Insulin stimulates branched-chain amino acid transport into muscle.	Phosphorylation by kinase is inhibitory.
Cholesterol synthesis	HMG-CoA reductase			Glucagon cascade decreases activity via AMP-dependent protein kinase.	Cholesterol represses enzyme synthesis.
Deoxynucleotide synthesis	Ribonucleotide reductase	ATP	dATP		Regulation by nucleotides is complex; enzyme induced prior to S phase of cell cycle.
Heme synthesis	δ-Aminolevulinate synthase		Heme		Heme represses enzyme synthesis.
Purine nucleotide synthesis	PRPP amidotransferase	PRPP	AMP, GMP, IMP, allopurinol ribonucleotide		
	IMP dehydrogenase		GMP		
	Adenylosuccinate synthetase		AMP		
Pyrimidine synthesis	Carbamoyl-phosphate synthetase II		UTP, UDP		
Urea cycle	Carbamoyl-phosphate synthetase I	*N*-Acetylglutamate			*N*-Acetylglutamate synthase is activated by arginine.

blood cells and brain, via glycogenolysis and gluconeogenesis
2. The generation of lactate by red blood cells and muscle and the reconversion of lactate into glucose by the liver is called the Cori cycle
3. During fasting, the liver converts metabolites generated by fatty acid oxidation to ketone bodies that are exported to extrahepatic cells for fuel
4. The liver synthesizes urea to rid the body of excess nitrogen
5. The liver synthesizes triglyceride, cholesterol, and bile acids
6. The liver releases about 180 g of glucose, 100 g of fat, and 14 g of albumin into the circulation daily

Objective 3: To outline the major consequences of diabetes mellitus.

IV. Diabetes is due to an absolute or relative lack of insulin
  A. There are two types of diabetes mellitus
    1. Type I, which is the result of destruction of the β-cells, develops in childhood and must be treated by insulin injection
    2. Type II develops in adulthood and is often related to insensitivity to insulin
      a. It is most common in obese individuals, and weight loss results in increased insulin sensitivity
      b. Type II diabetes is sometimes treated with sulfonylurea drugs that increase the secretion of endogenous insulin
  B. Decreased transport of glucose into cells, decreased glycogen synthesis, and increased gluconeogenesis lead to hyperglycemia
    1. Elevated glucose levels can result in the chemical modification of proteins
    2. Modification of cellular proteins by nonenzymatic glycosylation may contribute to processes that lead to retinopathy, nephropathy, neuropathy, and altered lipoprotein metabolism characteristic of diabetes
    3. Production of sorbitol in nerve cells may lead to the observed neuropathy of diabetes mellitus
  C. Of the glucose translocases, GLUT4 is activated by insulin
    1. Insulin recruits intracellular translocases to the plasma membrane, and this is responsible for the greater ability of responsive cells to transport more glucose
    2. Although the liver has insulin receptors and responds to insulin, liver lacks GLUT4 receptors; as a result, insulin action does not increase the rate of glucose transport into liver cells
    3. Exercise and other physical activity drive glucose into cells by unknown mechanisms and decrease a diabetic's insulin requirement
  D. Besides carbohydrate metabolism, altered lipid metabolism occurs in diabetes mellitus
    1. Ketosis and ketoacidosis occur in type I diabetes but are rare in type II diabetes; the reason for this discrepancy is a mystery
      a. Elevated glucagon/insulin activates hormone-sensitive lipase, which releases fatty acids from adipocytes
      b. Increased availability of fatty acids in liver leads to increased ketone body synthesis, a process driven by excess acetyl-CoA
    2. At least two mechanisms are responsible for the hypertriglyceridemia often observed in diabetes mellitus
      a. Diminished lipoprotein lipase activity leads to hypertriglyceridemia by decreasing the liberation of triglyceride from chylomicrons and VLDL
      b. Increased availability of fatty acids as a result of enhanced activity of hormone-sensitive lipase in adipocytes can drive hepatic triglyceride and VLDL formation
    3. A broad spectrum of hyperlipoproteinemias can occur in diabetes
      a. Type IV hyperlipoproteinemia (pre-β hyperlipoproteinemia) is the result of increased production of VLDL and decreased catabolism due to impaired lipoprotein lipase
      b. Type V hyperlipoproteinemia, which is a combination of type I (hyperchylomicronemia) and type IV (increased VLDL), occurs as a result of impaired lipoprotein lipase activity; saturation of the enzyme by VLDL results in hyperchylomicronemia
  E. Insulin deficiency decreases amino acid transport into cells and decreases protein synthesis
    1. Amino acids are catabolized at an increased rate, providing substrates for gluconeogenesis and ketone body production
    2. Negative nitrogen balance and protein wasting result

Objective 4: To describe the metabolism of ethanol.

V. Ethanol is metabolized in two steps
  A. Alcohol dehydrogenase in liver catalyzes the oxidation of ethanol to acetaldehyde with the concomitant formation of NADH + H^+
    1. The enzyme, which contains ionic zinc as a cofactor, catalyzes a simple oxidation-reduction reaction and is reversible in accordance with PRINCIPLE 7 OF BIOENERGETICS
    2. The enzyme is saturated after moderate ethanol (30 mL, or 1 oz) intake
  B. A cytochrome P-450 oxidase can also convert ethanol to acetaldehyde
    1. This process involves an endoplasmic reticulum electron transport chain
    2. It also involves the reduction of oxygen to water by NADPH and is exergonic and irreversible in accordance with PRINCIPLE 8 OF BIOENERGETICS
  C. Acetaldehyde is oxidized to acetate, in a reaction catalyzed by aldehyde dehydrogenase, with the concomitant formation of NADH + H^+
    1. Although this process represents a simple oxidation-reduction reaction, the ionization of acetic acid to acetate makes the overall process unidirectional
    2. Some acetate is metabolized by the liver, and the remainder is exported for metabolism by extrahepatic cells
      a. Acetate is converted to the coenzyme A thioester for its metabolism

b. Hepatic acetate may provide a substrate for lipogenesis and the production of a fatty liver
3. Ethanol is a reduced substance, and it provides 7 kcal (Calories) of metabolic energy per gram

D. Ethanol can adversely affect metabolism
1. Increasing the NADH/NAD^+ can decrease gluconeogenesis and produce hypoglycemia by promoting the conversion of pyruvate, a gluconeogenic substrate, to lactate
2. Acetaldehyde is reactive, and it can modify proteins to produce pathological sequelae
3. Malnutrition is common in people who abuse ethanol
a. The most common deficiencies are those of thiamine, folate, and pyridoxine
b. Thiamine deficiency and Wernicke encephalopathy occur frequently in people with alcoholism

QUESTIONS

DIRECTIONS. (Items 1–8): Each set of matching questions in this section consists of a list of several lettered options followed by several numbered items. For each numbered item, select the ONE lettered option that is most closely associated with it. To avoid spending too much time on matching sets with large numbers of options, it is generally advisable to begin each set by reading the list of options. Then, for each item in the list, try to generate the correct answer and locate it in the option list, rather than evaluating each option individually. Each lettered option may be selected once, more than once, or not at all. Correct answers and explanations are given at the end of the chapter.

Items 1–6

(A) Acetyl-CoA carboxylase
(B) Alcohol dehydrogenase
(C) Carnitine acyltransferase I
(D) Citrate synthase
(E) Fructose-1,6-bisphosphatase
(F) Glucokinase
(G) Glucose-6-phosphatase
(H) Glucose-6-phosphate dehydrogenase
(I) Glycogen phosphorylase
(J) Glycogen synthase
(K) Hexokinase
(L) Hormone-sensitive lipase
(M) Isocitrate dehydrogenase
(N) Malate dehydrogenase
(O) Phosphofructokinase
(P) Pyruvate carboxylase
(Q) Pyruvate dehydrogenase
(R) Pyruvate kinase

For each description given, select the correct enzyme.

1. This enzyme catalyzes the rate-controlling step of the Embden-Meyerhof glycolytic pathway
2. This enzyme is inhibited by fructose 2,6-bisphosphate
3. This enzyme is inhibited by regulatory protein-fructose 6-phosphate
4. A deficiency of this enzyme, which requires acetyl-CoA as an allosteric activator, leads to lactic acidosis
5. A deficiency of this enzyme, which requires $NADP^+$ as a substrate, is a common cause of drug-induced hemolytic anemias
6. This enzyme is inhibited by malonyl-CoA

Items 7–8

(A) AMP-dependent protein kinase
(B) Fructose-6-phosphate 2-kinase/fructose-2,6-bisphosphatase
(C) Insulin receptor
(D) Pyruvate dehydrogenase kinase
(E) Phosphorylase kinase

For each characteristic given, select the correct regulatory protein.

7. Protein kinase A catalyzes the phosphorylation of this protein and thus decreases glycolysis and enhances gluconeogenesis
8. This protein contains calmodulin as one of its subunits

DIRECTIONS. (Items 9–18): Each of the numbered items or incomplete statements in this section is followed by answers or by completions of the statement. Select the ONE lettered answer or completion that is BEST in each case.

9. The rate-limiting enzyme of the urea cycle is
(A) arginase
(B) argininosuccinate lyase
(C) carbamoyl-phosphate synthetase I
(D) citrulline synthetase
(E) ornithine transcarbamoylase

10. All of the following tissues are able to use circulating fatty acids as a metabolic fuel EXCEPT
(A) adipocytes
(B) brain
(C) kidney
(D) liver
(E) striated muscle

11. Which one of the following tissues or organs plays a significant role in gluconeogenesis after 4 days of fasting but not after an overnight fast?
(A) Adrenal cortex
(B) Liver
(C) Kidney
(D) Spleen
(E) Striated muscle

12. Which one of the following compounds directly stimulates both insulin and glucagon release from the pancreas?
    (A) Alanine
    (B) Arginine
    (C) Glucose
    (D) Lysine
    (E) Somatostatin

13. Which one of the following amino acids is catabolized preferentially by the liver when compared with skeletal muscle?
    (A) Alanine
    (B) Isoleucine
    (C) Leucine
    (D) Valine

14. The caloric value of one gram of triglyceride is about
    (A) 3 kcal
    (B) 4 kcal
    (C) 7 kcal
    (D) 9 kcal
    (E) 4 Cal

Items 15–18

History

The patient is a 52-year-old male automobile technician with a chief complaint of chronic fatigue. He has suffered from headaches, dizziness, and blurred vision intermittently for a few years. There was no history of polydipsia, polyuria, or loss of consciousness. There was also no history of symptoms of hypothyroidism, pancreatitis, or drug or alcohol abuse. There was no family history of diabetes or hypertension.

Physical Examination

The patient, who is 178 cm (5 ft, 10 in.), weighs 96 kg (212 lb) and has increased abdominal girth. The pulse rate is 82/min; respiratory rate, 14/min; and blood pressure, 134/86 mm Hg. Ophthalmic examination revealed microaneurysms, dilated retinal veins, and white waxy exudates. Results of examination of the chest and heart were normal. Pulses in the extremities, deep tendon reflexes, and sensitivity to touch and pinprick were all normal. His skin texture is normal.

Laboratory

Red and white cell counts and differential, normal
Electrolytes, normal
Blood urea nitrogen (BUN), 24 mg/dL (normal, 7–18 mg/dL)
Creatinine, 1.7 mg/dL (normal, 0.7–1.3 mg/dL)
Serum glucose, 224 mg/dL (normal, 70–105 mg/dL)
Hemoglobin A_{1c}, 11% (normal, 5.6–7.5%)
Total cholesterol, 286 mg/dL (recommended, <200 mg/dL)
LDL cholesterol, 224 mg/dL (recommended, <130 mg/dL)
HDL cholesterol, 38 mg/dL (desirable, >50 mg/dL)
Serum triglyceride, 340 mg/dL (recommended, <150 mg/dL)
Aspartate aminotransferase (AST, SGOT), 14 U/L (normal, 10–30 U/L)
γ-Glutamyl transpeptidase, 19 U/L (normal, 9–50 U/L)
Creatine phosphokinase (CPK), 44 U/L (normal ♂, 38–174 U/L)
Lactate dehydrogenase (LDH), 295 U/L (normal, 208–378 U/L)
Albumin, 4.3 g/dL (normal, 3.5–5.0 g/dL)
Globulins, 2.6 g/dL (normal, 2.2–4.0 g/dL)
T_3, 136 ng/dL (normal, 100–200 ng/dL)
T_4, 7 μg/dL (normal, 5–12 μg/dL)
Plasma insulin, 136 pmol/L or 18.9 μIU/mL (normal, 42–167 pmol/L or 6–24 μIU/mL)

Urinalysis revealed glucosuria (1+) but no proteinuria or ketonuria. A second analysis of a fasting serum sample gave values of glucose, cholesterol, and triglyceride that were within 5% of the initial results.

15. A diagnosis of diabetes mellitus in this patient is based on the hyperglycemia and the elevated levels of hemoglobin A_{1c}. Each of the following accounts in part for the hyperglycemia EXCEPT
    (A) decreased transport of glucose into the liver
    (B) decreased transport of glucose into adipocytes
    (C) decreased transport of glucose into muscle
    (D) increased provision of alanine by skeletal muscle
    (E) increased hepatic gluconeogenesis

16. This patient's disorder results from which one of the following metabolic abnormalities?
    (A) Destruction of the β-cells of the pancreas
    (B) Failure to synthesize insulin
    (C) Failure to process insulin
    (D) Insulin resistance
    (E) Production of antibodies that stimulate the insulin receptor

17. Analysis of the patient's serum revealed an elevated VLDL (pre-β hyperlipoproteinemia). Which one of the following mechanisms accounts, in part, for this process?
    (A) Decreased activity of hormone-sensitive lipase
    (B) Decreased activity of heparin-sensitive lipase
    (C) Increased activity of acid lipase
    (D) Increased activity of hepatic lipase

18. One of the mechanisms for the development of the patient's aberrant lipoprotein levels involves
    (A) intracellular production of sorbitol
    (B) failure to synthesize adequate apo-B-100
    (C) nonenzymatic glycosylation of HDL ("good" cholesterol), leading to increased receptor-mediated uptake and a decrease in HDL
    (D) increased lipoprotein lipase activity and the release of decreased amounts of fatty acids from adipocytes
    (E) increased transport of potassium into cells from the extracellular space

ANSWERS AND EXPLANATIONS

1. The answer is O: phosphofructokinase. Phosphofructokinase catalyzes the rate-controlling step of glycolysis. The reaction proceeds with the loss of a high-energy bond and is exergonic (PRINCIPLE 2 OF BIOENERGETICS). The rate of glucose transport into cells and the rate of the hexokinase reaction can play a secondary regulatory role. Glucose 6-phosphate, the product of the hexokinase reaction, can be metabolized to glycogen or by the pentose phosphate pathway; the hexokinase reaction does not represent a committed step in glycolysis, but the phosphofructokinase reaction is a committed step. *Biochemistry,* p. 501.
2. The answer is E: fructose-1,6-bisphosphatase. Fructose-1,6-bisphosphatase, a gluconeogenic enzyme, catalyzes the reaction, bypassing the unidirectional phosphofructokinase reaction of glycolysis. This reaction involves a hydrolysis and is exergonic (PRINCIPLE 5 OF BIOENERGETICS). These steps are regulated reciprocally by fructose 2,6-bisphosphate; phosphofructokinase is activated and fructose-1,6-bisphosphatase is inhibited. *Biochemistry,* p. 503.
3. The answer is F: glucokinase. Glucokinase, which is present in liver, has a high K_m for glucose ($\approx$10 mM) and is not saturated by the concentration of glucose that is delivered by the hepatic portal vein. Glucokinase is inhibited by a complex consisting of fructose 6-phosphate and regulatory protein. Hexokinase, which is present in all cells including liver, has a low K_m for glucose ($\approx$30 μM), operates at near saturating conditions, and is inhibited by its product, glucose 6-phosphate. Glucokinase is not directly inhibited by glucose 6-phosphate. *Biochemistry,* p. 503.
4. The answer is P: pyruvate carboxylase. Pyruvate carboxylase catalyzes the ATP-dependent conversion of pyruvate to oxaloacetate, accounting for the anaplerotic production (buildup) of Krebs cycle intermediates and providing oxaloacetate for gluconeogenesis. Pyruvate carboxylase requires acetyl-CoA for the expression of its activity. A deficiency of this enzyme results in decreased Krebs cycle function, and pyruvate cannot be oxidized and is converted to lactic acid. Pyruvate carboxylase deficiency also leads to fasting hypoglycemia because of diminished production of substrates for gluconeogenesis. *Biochemistry,* p. 505; *Nelson,* p. 363.
5. The answer is H: glucose-6-phosphate dehydrogenase. Glucose-6-phosphate dehydrogenase catalyzes the first reaction in the pentose phosphate pathway, and the functions of the pathway are to generate NADPH for reductive biosynthesis and to generate pentoses that occur in nucleotides. The 6-phosphogluconate dehydrogenase reaction, also in the pentose phosphate pathway, also generates NADPH. These two reactions are important in providing reducing equivalents for lipid synthesis in liver. Malic enzyme, which catalyzes the oxidative decarboxylation of malate to pyruvate and carbon dioxide, is a third source of NADPH for reductive biosynthetic reactions (PRINCIPLE 16 OF BIOCHEMISTRY). Fatty acid production in adipose tissue relies on both the pentose phosphate pathway and malic enzyme for the production of NADPH. A deficiency of glucose-6-phosphate dehydrogenase is a common cause of drug-induced hemolytic anemia. *Biochemistry,* p. 103.
6. The answer is C: carnitine acyltransferase I. Carnitine acyltransferase I is required to translocate fatty acyl groups from the cytosol into the mitochondrion before β-oxidation occurs. This step and the translocation process are rate-limiting. Carnitine acyltransferase I is inhibited by malonyl-CoA, a precursor for fatty acid biosynthesis. Thus, malonyl-CoA is at a crossroad of metabolism. Metabolic conditions that generate a precursor for fatty acid biosynthesis generate an inhibitor of fatty acid oxidation, and these pathways are reciprocally regulated (PRINCIPLE 9 OF BIOCHEMISTRY). *Biochemistry,* p. 502.
7. The answer is B: fructose-6-phosphate 2-kinase/fructose-2,6-bisphosphatase. This is a single protein with more than one activity and is called a polyprotein. This polyprotein catalyzes both the synthesis and degradation of fructose 2,6-bisphosphate, an important regulator of glycolysis and gluconeogenesis. In response to glucagon in liver, adenylyl cyclase is activated and the cyclic AMP that is produced activates protein kinase A. Protein kinase A catalyzes the phosphorylation of the kinase/phosphatase and inhibits kinase activity and increases phosphatase activity. As a result, an activator of glycolysis and an inhibitor of gluconeogenesis is destroyed. The net result is to increase gluconeogenesis. *Biochemistry,* p. 503.
8. The answer is E: phosphorylase kinase. Phosphorylase kinase is a protein with the following subunit structure: $(\alpha\beta\gamma\delta)_4$; the δ-subunits are calmodulin. This protein is activated by calcium through its association with calmodulin. Muscle contraction is activated by calcium. The simultaneous activation of muscle contraction and glycogen degradation represents a coordinate physiological response. *Biochemistry,* p. 504.
9. The answer is C: carbamoyl-phosphate synthetase I. Carbamoyl-phosphate synthetase I is a mitochondrial enzyme that catalyzes the reaction involving two ATP, bicarbonate, and ammonium ion to produce carbamoyl phosphate. This enzyme, which is activated by *N*-acetylglutamate, catalyzes the rate-controlling reaction of the urea cycle. *Biochemistry,* p. 506.
10. The answer is B: brain. Brain is NOT able to use fatty acids as a fuel. It is for this reason that gluconeogenesis by the liver and kidney during starvation must continue to provide fuels for these cells. After a few days without food, the brain can use ketone bodies, but not fatty acids, for some of its metabolic fuel, but glucose is still required. Red blood cells lack mitochondria and cannot metabolize fatty acids, lacking the enzymes of β-oxidation and the Krebs cycle. Muscle, kidney, liver, and adipocytes can use fatty acids as a metabolic fuel. *Biochemistry,* p. 506.
11. The answer is C: kidney. The two main organs of gluconeogenesis are the liver and kidney; the liver plays the predominant role in glucose production after an overnight fast and during the first few days without food. After 3 or 4 days, the kidney accounts for about half the glucose produced, and this is derived from glutamine. This compound provides carbon atoms for glucose and ammonium ions for excretion in the urine. The excretion of a proton as part of ammonium ion counteracts the acidotic condition that occurs with ketosis. *Biochemistry,* p. 508.

12. The answer is B: arginine. Protein meals promote both insulin and glucagon release, and arginine is responsible for stimulating both insulin and glucagon release from the β-cells and α-cells of the pancreas, respectively. Glucose promotes insulin release following a carbohydrate-containing meal. Glucose, however, inhibits glucagon release. Lysine promotes glucagon but not insulin release. Somatostatin inhibits release of both glucagon and insulin from the pancreas. Balanced meals containing protein and carbohydrate increase insulin release but do not shut off glucagon release. With a carbohydrate-rich, protein-poor meal, glucagon secretion decreases. *Biochemistry,* p. 508.
13. The answer is A: alanine. Alanine is the major amino acid that is released by skeletal muscle during fasting and starvation. It serves as a substrate for gluconeogenesis in the liver. Most amino acids released into the portal vein are metabolized preferentially by the liver, with the exception of the branched-chain amino acids (valine, leucine, and isoleucine). These three amino acids account for 60% of the amino acids entering the circulation from the gut despite their 20% contribution to the total amino acids in a protein meal consisting of lean beef. These amino acids contribute only 20% of the skeletal muscle protein, and excess amounts of branched-chain keto acid metabolites, derived by transamination, can be oxidized by muscle or transported to other cells. *Biochemistry,* p. 511.
14. The answer is D: 9 kcal. The caloric content of carbohydrate and protein is about 4 kcal/g, and the caloric content of alcohol is about 7 kcal/g. Lipid, which contains 9 kcal/g, is the major form of energy storage in the body. With a content of total body fat of about 16%, energy reserves can last for several weeks. *Biochemistry,* p. 34.
15. The answer is A: hyperglycemia is NOT due to decreased transport of glucose into the liver. Insulin increases glucose transport in target cells by recruiting GLUT4 receptors from inside the cell to the plasma membrane. As a result of this recruitment, cells exhibit an increase in the V_{max} but no change in the K_m for glucose transport. Responsive cells include muscle, adipocytes, and most cells in the body except red cells, brain, and liver. Increased gluconeogenesis by the liver, caused by the induction of pyruvate carboxylase, PEP carboxykinase, fructose-1,6-bisphosphatase, and glucose-6-phosphatase by glucagon, accounts in part for the hyperglycemia. Decreased protein synthesis and muscle wasting provide increased alanine that serves as a precursor for gluconeogenesis. *Biochemistry,* p. 508.
16. The answer is D: insulin resistance. The presence of insulin in the serum indicates that the β-cells are functional and can synthesize and process insulin. Antibodies that stimulate the insulin receptor lead to hypoglycemia, not to hyperglycemia. Most (>80%) of type II diabetics (non-insulin-dependent) are obese, as is this patient. The first line of treatment is weight reduction. Weight reduction decreases insulin resistance and can lead to normal serum glucose and lipid levels. Caloric restriction, decreased fat intake, and increased intake of complex carbohydrates are recommended. The success rate for weight reduction is not great, and oral hypoglycemic agents can be prescribed. The long-term safety of such medications, however, is in doubt. Perhaps 2% of the adult population suffers from type II diabetes, and some authorities suggest that the percentage is even higher. Besides primary diabetes, hyperglycemia may be secondary to other conditions. Cushing syndrome (hyperadrenocorticism), for example, is a cause of secondary diabetes and hyperglycemia. Patients with this syndrome have a characteristic obesity (buffalo hump obesity) with characteristic skin striations (striae) that are not mentioned in this clinical description. People with Cushing syndrome often have an elevated serum sodium and decreased serum potassium, but the electrolytes in this patient are reported as normal. *Biochemistry,* p. 512; *Cecil,* p. 1291.
17. The answer is B: decreased activity of heparin-sensitive lipase. The mechanism for increased circulating VLDL in diabetes mellitus is complex and may involve both decreased catabolism and increased production. Heparin-sensitive lipase is a synonym for lipoprotein lipase, and this enzyme is responsible for hydrolyzing the triglyceride of chylomicrons and VLDL at the capillary bed and providing fatty acids for tissues. Lipoprotein lipase can be released from its loose attachment to cells in the capillaries by heparin injection. Hormone-sensitive lipase is antagonized by the action of insulin, and its activity is increased in diabetes as a result of the elevated glucagon/insulin ratio. Increased VLDL can result from augmented production because increased provision of fatty acids to the liver from adipose tissue promotes VLDL production. Increased acid lipase and hepatic lipase activities would result in increased lipoprotein catabolism, and they do not seem to be directly affected by insulin. Other causes of hyperlipemia include hypothyroidism, the nephrotic syndrome, alcoholism, and liver disease. Normal deep tendon reflexes, normal skin texture, and normal serum T_4 and T_3 rule out hypothyroidism as a cause of the hypertriglyceridemia. Although the urea nitrogen and creatinine are somewhat elevated, suggestive of kidney disease, there is no proteinuria, the *sine qua non* for the nephrotic syndrome. End-stage renal disease in diabetes can result in the nephrotic syndrome. Besides kidney disease, the slightly elevated urea nitrogen may reflect increased amino acid catabolism that is common in diabetes. There is no history of alcoholism, and the serum γ-glutamyl transpeptidase activity (a sensitive indicator of alcohol abuse) is normal. Aspartate aminotransferase and lactate dehydrogenase levels are also normal, thereby ruling liver disease unlikely. *Biochemistry,* p. 512; *Cecil,* p. 1291.
18. The answer is C: nonenzymatic glycosylation of HDL leading to increased receptor-mediated uptake. It is postulated that the neuropathy, retinopathy, and nephropathy that accompany diabetes mellitus are the result of nonenzymatic glycosylation of proteins that produces dysfunctional proteins. Glycosylation of HDL has been reported to lead to increased receptor-mediated uptake, and this process may contribute to atherogenesis by decreasing the amount of "good" cholesterol. Increased sorbitol production is implicated in the production of neuropathy but not in abnormal lipoprotein metabolism. Insulin deficiency is associated with decreased, and not increased, lipoprotein lipase activity. Increased hormone-sensitive lipase activity as a result of glucagon action leads to the release of increased amounts of fatty acids from adipocytes. Insulin action leads to increased potassium into entry cells, and a deficiency of insulin action leads to decreased potassium transport. Besides a decrease in "good" cholesterol, this patient exhibits an increase in LDL, or "bad," cholesterol. This finding occurs in many, although not all, diabetic patients. The mechanism is obscure; normal insulin action may play a role in the

normal catabolism of HDL. *Biochemistry,* pp. 512–513; *Robbins,* p. 909.

REFERENCES

Behrman, R. E. *Nelson Textbook of Pediatrics,* 14th ed. Philadelphia, W. B. Saunders Company, 1992.

Cotran, R. S., V. Kumar, S. L. Robbins. *Robbins Pathologic Basis of Disease,* 5th ed. Philadelphia, W. B. Saunders Company, 1994.

Roskoski, R., Jr. *Biochemistry.* Philadelphia, W. B. Saunders Company, 1996.

Wyngaarden, J. B., L. H. Smith, Jr., and J. C. Bennett (eds.). *Cecil Textbook of Medicine,* 19th ed. Philadelphia, W. B. Saunders Company, 1992.

COMPREHENSIVE EXAMINATION

DIRECTIONS (Items 1–90): Each of the numbered items or incomplete statements in this section is followed by answers or by completions of the statement. Select the ONE lettered answer or completion that is BEST in each case. Correct answers and explanations are given at the end.

1. Patients with end-stage renal disease often have altered serum calcium, resulting, in part, from aberrant vitamin D metabolism. A patient undergoing hemodialysis for the treatment of renal failure might be expected to be deficient in which one of the following reactions in the conversion of 7-dehydrocholesterol to calcitriol, the active vitamin D metabolite?

   (A) Photoactivation by ultraviolet light
   (B) 1-Hydroxylation
   (C) 17-Hydroxylation
   (D) 21-Hydroxylation
   (E) 24-Hydroxylation

2. The most serious form of galactosemia in humans is due to deficiency of

   (A) galactokinase
   (B) galactose-1-phosphate uridyltransferase
   (C) galactosidase
   (D) lactase
   (E) UDP-galactose epimerase

3. The transmission of sickle cell anemia from one generation to the next is mediated by

   (A) carbohydrate
   (B) protein
   (C) mitochondrial DNA
   (D) nuclear DNA
   (E) RNA

4. All of the following disorders are accompanied by metabolic acidosis EXCEPT

   (A) maple syrup urine disease
   (B) methylmalonic acidemia
   (C) ornithine transcarbamoylase deficiency
   (D) pyruvate dehydrogenase deficiency
   (E) type I glycogen storage disease

5. Removal of the chief metabolite of cholesterol from the body is used in the treatment of hypercholesterolemia. Therapy is directed toward the elimination of

   (A) neutral sterols
   (B) cortisol
   (C) progesterone
   (D) bile salts
   (E) carbon dioxide

6. Infants with lethargy, hypotonia, metabolic acidosis without ketosis, and very high levels of urinary β-hydroxy-β-methylglutarate in the urine suffer from

   (A) HMG-CoA lyase deficiency
   (B) β-ketothiolase deficiency
   (C) maple syrup urine disease
   (D) medium-chain acyl-CoA dehydrogenase deficiency
   (E) propionyl-CoA carboxylase deficiency

7. Inadequate absorption of which of the following metabolites, as occurs in Hartnup disease, leads to negative nitrogen balance?

   (A) Cobalamin
   (B) Glutathione
   (C) Linoleic acid
   (D) Phenylalanine
   (E) Serine

8. The enzyme that catalyzes replication of human mitochondrial DNA is

   (A) DNA polymerase α
   (B) DNA polymerase β
   (C) DNA polymerase γ
   (D) DNA polymerase δ
   (E) DNA polymerase ε

9. A serving of chicken tostadas contains the following components: carbohydrate, 40 g; protein, 30 g; cholesterol, 50 mg; sodium, 750 mg; fiber, 3 g; fat, 10 g. What percentage of total nutritional Calories, or kcal, of this serving is derived from fat?

   (A) 5%
   (B) 10%
   (C) 15%
   (D) 20%
   (E) 25%

10. The primary regulatory step in pyrimidine synthesis in *E. coli* is catalyzed by which one of the following enzymes?

    (A) Carbamoyl-phosphate synthetase
    (B) Aspartate transcarbamoylase
    (C) Thymidylate synthase
    (D) Ornithine transcarbamoylase
    (E) Dihydroorotate dehydrogenase

11. Using pyruvate dehydrogenase, the Krebs cycle, and oxidative phosphorylation, what does the catabolism of one mole of pyruvate to carbon dioxide and water yield? Assume 1 NADH yields 2.5 ATP and 1 $FADH_2$ yields 1.5 ATP.

    (A) 1 mole of carbon dioxide and 2.5 moles of ATP (or equivalent such as GTP)
    (B) 2 moles of carbon dioxide and 10 moles of ATP (or equivalent such as GTP)
    (C) 3 moles of carbon dioxide and 10 moles of ATP (or equivalent such as GTP)
    (D) 3 moles of carbon dioxide and 12.5 moles of ATP (or equivalent such as GTP)
    (E) 6 moles of carbon dioxide and 25 moles of ATP (or equivalent such as GTP)

12. Failure to digest dietary lipids leads to steatorrhea. All of the following substances are required for digestion of dietary lipid EXCEPT
    (A) bile pigments
    (B) bile salts
    (C) colipase
    (D) pancreatic lipase
    (E) pancreatic phospholipase

13. Which one of the following drugs has little or no effect on the metabolism of normal human cells?
    (A) Actinomycin D
    (B) Azidothymidine (AZT)
    (C) Dideoxyinosine (ddI)
    (D) Dideoxycytidine (ddC)
    (E) Rifamycin

14. The elevated blood glucose seen in diabetes mellitus is a consequence of
    (A) a failure of glucose to enter liver cells
    (B) increased glycolytic activity in liver
    (C) increased activity of gluconeogenic enzymes due to enzyme induction by glucagon
    (D) increased liver glycogenesis as a result of augmented formation of glycogen synthase in response to glucagon
    (E) conversion of fatty acids to glucose

15. A deficiency of which one of the following enzymes results in hypermethioninemia and homocystinuria?
    (A) Methionine aminopeptidase
    (B) *S*-Adenosylhomocysteine hydrolase
    (C) *S*-Adenosylmethionine hydrolase
    (D) Cystathionine lyase
    (E) Cystathionine synthase

16. Which one of the following DNA molecules contains hundreds of origins of replication?
    (A) Human mitochondrial DNA
    (B) *E. coli* DNA
    (C) Plasmid pBR322 DNA
    (D) Human chromosome 22 DNA
    (E) Human immunodeficiency virus (HIV) proviral DNA

17. Actinomycin D, a peptide antibiotic used in the treatment of Kaposi sarcoma and other neoplastic diseases, inhibits
    (A) bacterial DNA polymerase
    (B) human DNA polymerase
    (C) initiation of bacterial RNA synthesis
    (D) human and bacterial gene transcription
    (E) capping of hnRNA

18. G-proteins that alter the activity of adenylyl cyclase are defective in one type of pseudohypoparathyroidism (Albright disease). Which one of the following is a true statement regarding normal G-proteins?
    (A) They are pentamers composed of four different kinds of subunits
    (B) They contain an α-subunit that binds and hydrolyzes GTP
    (C) They are inhibited by d-tubocurarine
    (D) They contain seven transmembrane segments
    (E) They form a cation channel

19. The rapid effects of ethanol in humans are due to its uptake into the body and cells by which one of the following mechanisms?
    (A) Antiport
    (B) Facilitated diffusion
    (C) Primary active transport
    (D) Secondary active transport
    (E) Simple diffusion

20. Which one of the following genetic disorders is due to a defect in lysosomal metabolism?
    (A) Ehlers-Danlos syndrome
    (B) Osteogenesis imperfecta
    (C) Hurler disease (type I mucopolysaccharidosis)
    (D) Von Gierke disease
    (E) Muscular dystrophy

21. The circulating form of hemoglobin that is used to assess chronic blood glucose concentrations in diabetes mellitus is
    (A) hemoglobin A
    (B) hemoglobin A_1
    (C) hemoglobin F
    (D) hemoglobin H
    (E) hemoglobin S

22. The most abundant blood clotting protein by mass in the circulation is
    (A) factor I (fibrinogen)
    (B) factor II (prothrombin)
    (C) factor VIII (antihemophilic factor)
    (D) factor XIII (fibrin stabilizing factor)
    (E) von Willebrand factor

23. Which one of the following enzymes is rate limiting for *de novo* purine nucleotide synthesis and is thus a target for drugs used in the treatment of gout?
    (A) Carbamoyl-phosphate synthetase II
    (B) Hypoxanthine-guanine phosphoribosyl transferase (HGPRT)
    (C) Phosphoribosylpyrophosphate-glutamine amidotransferase (PRPP amidotransferase)
    (D) Xanthine dehydrogenase
    (E) Xanthine oxidase

24. Hydrolysis of the amino group of 5-methylcytosine without subsequent repair leads to which one of the following types of mutation?
    (A) Transduction
    (B) Transformation
    (C) Translocation
    (D) Transversion
    (E) Transition

25. The chief excitatory neurotransmitter in brain is
    (A) acetylcholine
    (B) γ-aminobutyric acid (GABA)
    (C) glutamate
    (D) glycine
    (E) norepinephrine

26. A deficiency of which one of the following enzymes leads to diarrhea and failure to thrive in newborns owing to inadequate cleavage of trypsinogen to trypsin in the intestinal lumen?
    (A) Carboxypeptidase A
    (B) Enterokinase (enteropeptidase)
    (C) Furin
    (D) Leucine aminopeptidase
    (E) Pepsin

27. β-Hydroxybutyrate is synthesized during fasting, starvation, and diabetic ketoacidosis. What is the net molar yield of ATP from complete oxidation of one mole of β-hydroxybutyrate to carbon dioxide and water? Assume 1 NADH yields 2.5 ATP and 1 $FADH_2$ yields 1.5 ATP.
    (A) 9
    (B) 19
    (C) 20
    (D) 21.5
    (E) 22.5

28. Cyanide (CN^-), which is one of the most rapidly acting poisons in humans, blocks oxidative phosphorylation by
    (A) dissipating the proton gradient
    (B) binding to the ferrous iron in myoglobin
    (C) inhibiting ATP synthase
    (D) lowering the oxygen-carrying capacity of the blood
    (E) binding to the ferric iron of cytochrome a_3 in cytochrome oxidase

29. Enzyme deficiencies result in the inability to convert substrates into products. The accumulation of precursors and their aberrant metabolism can lead to various maladies. Enzymes perform their catalytic function by
    (A) decreasing the free energy of activation ($\Delta G^{\ddagger}$) of a reaction
    (B) decreasing the standard free energy change (ΔG°) of a reaction
    (C) decreasing the entropy change (ΔS) of a reaction
    (D) increasing the equilibrium constant (K_{eq}) of a reaction
    (E) increasing the total kinetic energy ($1/2\ mv^2$) of the reactants

30. The hydrolysis of G_{M1} ganglioside by β-galactosidase occurs in which stage of metabolism?
    (A) Stage I
    (B) Stage II
    (C) Stage III
    (D) Stage IV
    (E) Stage V

31. All of the following are true statements regarding a deficiency of bile salts EXCEPT
    (A) the deficiency impairs lipid digestion and absorption
    (B) the deficiency impairs the absorption of vitamins A, D, E, and K
    (C) the deficiency leads to steatorrhea (increased lipid in the stool)
    (D) the deficiency promotes cholelithiasis (gallstones)
    (E) the deficiency leads to hypercholesterolemia

32. All of the following are correct statements regarding gluconeogenesis and glycolysis EXCEPT
    (A) both gluconeogenesis and glycolysis require ATP as a reactant in some steps
    (B) both gluconeogenesis and glycolysis are affected by changes in fructose 2,6-bisphosphate concentration
    (C) both gluconeogenesis and glycolysis proceed with the liberation of free energy (i.e., are exergonic)
    (D) both gluconeogenesis and glycolysis result in the net loss of ATP
    (E) both gluconeogenesis and glycolysis involve the interconversion of two triose phosphates and fructose 1,6-bisphosphate

33. Rotenone is used in several commercial rat poisons, and this substance inhibits the functioning of complex I of electron transport. This substance inhibits mitochondrial electron transport and prevents the translocation of hydrogen ions
    (A) from the intermembrane space to the mitochondrial matrix
    (B) from the cytosol to the intermembrane space
    (C) from the mitochondrial matrix to the intermembrane space
    (D) from the intermembrane space to the cytosol
    (E) from the intermembrane space to the outer mitochondrial membrane

34. The shortest phase of the cell cycle is
    (A) G_0
    (B) G_1
    (C) G_2
    (D) S
    (E) M

35. Bacteria that cause urinary tract infections can be treated with nalidixic acid or norfloxacin. The action of these drugs is to inhibit
    (A) DNA polymerase I
    (B) DNA polymerase II
    (C) topoisomerase I
    (D) topoisomerase II
    (E) DNA ligase

36. With the knowledge that citrate is an intermediate in *de novo* fatty acid synthesis from glucose, which of the following conclusions can be deduced?

(A) The primary regulatory step of the Krebs cycle must be downstream from the citrate synthase reaction
(B) The citrate synthase reaction is reversible in order to release acetyl-CoA into the cytosol
(C) The first committed step of the Krebs cycle is catalyzed by aconitase
(D) The citrate synthase reaction is markedly inhibited when the energy charge is high
(E) The reversible α-ketoglutarate dehydrogenase reaction permits four-carbon metabolites to be converted to acetyl-CoA

37. The final product of glycolysis in human cells under anaerobic conditions, or in cells lacking mitochondria, is

(A) carbon dioxide
(B) ethanol
(C) lactate
(D) phosphoenolpyruvate
(E) pyruvate

38. The elevation of blood ketone bodies seen in hyperketotic hypoglycemia results from a deficiency in which of the following enzymes?

(A) β-Ketothiolase
(B) Hydroxymethylglutaryl-CoA synthase
(C) Hydroxymethylglutaryl-CoA lyase
(D) Hydroxymethylglutaryl-CoA reductase
(E) Succinyl-CoA:acetoacetate CoA-transferase

39. What is the first purine nucleotide formed during *de novo* synthesis?

(A) Carbamoyl phosphate
(B) Orotidine monophosphate
(C) Inosine monophosphate
(D) 5-Phosphoribosyl-1-pyrophosphate (PRPP)
(E) 5-Phosphoribosylamine

40. Which one of the following is a true statement regarding α-amylase, an enzyme whose activity in serum is elevated in pancreatitis?

(A) It catalyzes the hydrolysis of α-1,6-glycosidic bonds of amylopectin
(B) It catalyzes the hydrolysis of milk sugar (lactose) to galactose and glucose
(C) It is most active at the pH of the stomach lumen
(D) It is inhibited by chloride
(E) It catalyzes the hydrolysis of α-1,4-glycosidic bonds of amylose

41. All of the following are essential dietary components EXCEPT

(A) fluoride
(B) linoleate
(C) methionine
(D) selenium
(E) water

42. Bovine insulin, which is effective in humans with diabetes mellitus, differs from human insulin at two of 51 amino acid residues. This variation represents a difference in their

(A) primary structures
(B) secondary structures
(C) tertiary structures
(D) quaternary structures

43. Which one of the following is a true statement regarding noncompetitive inhibitors?

(A) They are structural analogues of the substrate
(B) They include captopril, an angiotensin converting enzyme (ACE) inhibitor, that resembles the physiological substrate
(C) They lead to the same *y*-intercept on Lineweaver-Burk plots as does the noninhibited enzyme
(D) Their action can be overcome by increasing the concentration of the varied substrate
(E) They decrease the apparent V_{max} of an enzyme

44. The administration of L-dopa, which is given in the treatment of Parkinson disease, bypasses the rate-limiting enzyme of catecholamine biosynthesis. What is the name of this rate-limiting enzyme?

(A) Dopamine β-hydroxylase
(B) Glutamate decarboxylase
(C) Phenylalanine hydroxylase
(D) Tryptophan hydroxylase
(E) Tyrosine hydroxylase

45. An inborn error of metabolism that is associated with lactic acidosis, secondary carnitine deficiency, and excretion of β-hydroxy dicarboxylic acids is due to a deficiency of which one of the following enzymes?

(A) Medium-chain fatty acyl–CoA dehydrogenase
(B) Succinyl-CoA: acetoacetate CoA-transferase
(C) Carnitine acyltransferase I
(D) β-Ketothiolase
(E) β-Hydroxyacyl-CoA dehydrogenase

46. Dermatan and heparan sulfates accumulate in Hurler syndrome, the type I and most severe mucopolysaccharide storage disease (MPS I). The donor of sulfate for dermatan and heparan sulfate synthesis is

(A) *S*-adenosyl methionine (AdoMet)
(B) oxidized glutathione (GSSG)
(C) 3′-phosphoadenosine 5′-phosphosulfate (PAPS)
(D) taurocholate
(E) taurine

47. Which one of the following can move reducing equivalents either INTO or OUT OF the mitochondrion?

(A) The glycerol phosphate shuttle
(B) The malate-aspartate shuttle
(C) The ATP/ADP shuttle
(D) The dinitrophenol shuttle
(E) The carnitine/acylcarnitine shuttle

48. Protoporphyrin IX is derived from eight molecules of succinyl-CoA and eight molecules of

(A) alanine
(B) valine
(C) glutamate
(D) histidine
(E) glycine

49. The pH corresponding to a hydrogen ion concentration of 1×10^{-1} M is

(A) 1
(B) 7
(C) 11
(D) 13
(E) 15

50. Myoglobin, a monomeric protein, exhibits all of the following types of structure EXCEPT

(A) primary
(B) secondary
(C) tertiary
(D) quaternary

51. Muscle lactate dehydrogenase deficiency is accompanied by fatigue and myoglobinuria. Lactate dehydrogenase (LDH) deficiency is characterized by each of the following properties EXCEPT that

(A) there is a decrease in activity of M subunits of LDH found in muscle
(B) there is little or no change in blood pyruvate levels following exercise
(C) there is little or no change in blood lactate levels following exercise
(D) there is no change in cardiac pyruvate/lactate production because H subunit expression of lactate dehydrogenase is normal

52. Which one of the following is a true statement regarding transketolase, an enzyme that may exhibit diminished activity in people with alcoholism?

(A) It utilizes thiamine pyrophosphate as cofactor in catalyzing the transfer of a two-carbon fragment from one sugar phosphate to another
(B) It catalyzes the oxidative decarboxylation of 6-phosphogluconate
(C) It catalyzes the conversion of ribulose 5-phosphate to ribose 5-phosphate
(D) It catalyzes the conversion of ribulose 5-phosphate to xylulose 5-phosphate
(E) It catalyzes the formation of the ketone bodies that produce ketoacidosis

53. Dinitrophenol uncouples oxidation and phosphorylation in which one of the following ways?

(A) By dissipating the proton gradient between the mitochondrial matrix and the intermembrane space
(B) By inhibiting the translocation of protons across the mitochondrial membrane
(C) By blocking the reduction of oxygen to water
(D) By inhibiting the oxidation of ubiquinone (coenzyme QH_2)
(E) By blocking the transfer of electrons from cytosol to the mitochondrial matrix

54. Each one of the following statements describes both human and bacterial DNA EXCEPT

(A) The DNA occurs physiologically as nucleosome complexes
(B) The DNA contains major and minor grooves
(C) The DNA consists of an antiparallel duplex
(D) The DNA contains equal molar fractions of adenine and thymine
(E) The DNA contains equal molar fractions of guanine and cytosine

55. Sources of dietary cholesterol include each of the following EXCEPT

(A) bacon
(B) potatoes
(C) beef
(D) chicken
(E) eggs

56. Aspirin is an irreversible inhibitor of

(A) cyclooxygenase
(B) lipoxygenase
(C) phospholipase A_1
(D) phospholipase A_2
(E) phospholipase C

57. The most prevalent protein by mass in humans is

(A) actin
(B) albumin
(C) collagen
(D) hemoglobin
(E) myosin

58. When one mole of dietary fructose is catabolized to pyruvate in liver by fructokinase, aldolase B, glyceraldehyde kinase, and appropriate glycolytic enzymes, what is the net molar ATP yield from substrate level phosphorylation?

(A) 0
(B) 1
(C) 2
(D) 3
(E) 5

59. Which one of the following mechanisms explains how ADP regulates the rate of electron transport during oxidative phosphorylation?

(A) Proton translocation across the inner mitochondrial membrane is decreased when ATP synthase lacks bound ADP and P_i, secondarily retarding electron transport
(B) The ATP/ADP antiport system is not functional with low mitochondrial [ADP]
(C) The transmembrane proton gradient is dissipated with low [ADP]
(D) Low [ADP] accelerates Krebs cycle reaction rates, thereby providing more NADH to activate electron transport
(E) AMP concentrations are increased as ADP concentrations fall

60. Replication of all of the following chromosomes involves Okazaki fragments EXCEPT
   (A) *E. coli* DNA
   (B) human autosomes
   (C) human X chromosome
   (D) human Y chromosome
   (E) mitochondrial DNA

61. Immunoglobulin production involves each of the following steps EXCEPT
   (A) somatic DNA rearrangement
   (B) alternative RNA splicing
   (C) DNA template-independent deoxyribonucleotide incorporation
   (D) information transfer from protein to RNA
   (E) deletion of portions of DNA found in germ cells

62. Chaperones are activated during some conditions of cellular stress. What is the function of chaperones?
   (A) They bind to ribosomes and chaperone them to the endoplasmic reticulum
   (B) They catalyze the removal of signal peptides
   (C) They move proteins from the *cis* to *trans* Golgi
   (D) They are ATP-requiring proteins that promote the folding of newly synthesized proteins into their functional state

63. Which one of the following substances is a dangerous poison that reacts irreversibly with acetylcholinesterase?
   (A) Atropine
   (B) Diisopropylfluorophosphate
   (C) Nicotine
   (D) Succinylcholine
   (E) d-Tubocurarine

64. The excessive production of lactate by tumor cells is called the
   (A) Ames effect
   (B) Crabtree effect
   (C) Krebs effect
   (D) Pasteur effect
   (E) Warburg effect

65. Omeprazole, an inhibitor of the proton/potassium-ATPase, is used for the treatment of peptic ulcers. The proton/potassium-ATPase is an example of a class
   (A) F ATPase
   (B) M ATPase
   (C) P ATPase
   (D) V ATPase

66. The direct source of energy for skeletal and smooth muscle contraction is
   (A) ATP
   (B) creatine phosphate
   (C) GTP
   (D) lactic acid
   (E) a proton-motive force

67. Which one of the following tests is used to monitor the effectiveness of vitamin K–antagonist treatment in the treatment of pulmonary emboli and myocardial infarctions?
   (A) Activated partial thromboplastin time (aPTT)
   (B) Prothrombin time
   (C) Bleeding time
   (D) Platelet count
   (E) Vitamin K assay

68. Which one of the following proteins possesses protein-tyrosine kinase activity?
   (A) AMP-dependent protein kinase
   (B) Fructose-6-phosphate 2-kinase/fructose-2,6-bisphosphatase
   (C) Glucagon receptor
   (D) Insulin receptor
   (E) Pyruvate dehydrogenase kinase

69. The conversion of monocarboxylic acids to dicarboxylic acids (e.g., dodecanedioic acid), which is prevalent in medium-chain fatty acyl–CoA dehydrogenase deficiency, is called
   (A) α-oxidation
   (B) β-oxidation
   (C) δ-oxidation
   (D) ω-oxidation
   (E) the final common pathway of metabolism

70. Which one of the following residues is a hallmark of elastin?
   (A) Desmosine
   (B) Glycine
   (C) Hydroxylysine
   (D) Hydroxynorleucine
   (E) Hydroxyproline

71. All of the following are true statements regarding glutamine PRPP amidotransferase EXCEPT
   (A) It is inhibited by allopurinol ribonucleotide
   (B) It is inhibited by AMP
   (C) It is inhibited by GMP
   (D) It is activated by IMP
   (E) It is activated by PRPP

72. For the carbon dioxide/bicarbonate buffer system

$$(pH = 6.1 + \log [HCO_3^-]/[CO_2 + H_2CO_3]),$$

   what is the $[HCO_3^-]$ at pH 7.1 when the $[CO_2 + H_2CO_3]$ is 1.0 mM?
   (A) 0.1 mM
   (B) 1.0 mM
   (C) 1.5 mM
   (D) 10 mM
   (E) 20 mM

73. The major regulatory step of glycolysis in liver can be bypassed in the catabolism of which one of the following sugars?
   (A) Fructose
   (B) Galactose
   (C) Glucose
   (D) Mannose
   (E) Trehalose

74. During mitochondrial electron transport, the iron in cytochrome heme alternates between

(A) Fe-S and 2Fe-2S
(B) Fe^{+2} and Fe^{0}
(C) Fe^{+2} and Fe^{+1}
(D) Fe^{+3} and Fe^{+1}
(E) Fe^{+3} and Fe^{+2}

75. Assume that 1 mole of mitochondrial NADH yields 2.5 moles of ATP and that 1 mole of $FADH_2$ yields 1.5 moles of ATP via oxidative phosphorylation. What is the molar yield of ATP when one mole of glucose is catabolized only to acetyl-CoA, and the malate-aspartate shuttle is functioning?

(A) 2
(B) 5
(C) 7
(D) 12
(E) 32

76. Which one of the following pairs of amino acids binds to the zinc of zinc finger proteins?

(A) Asparagine and glutamine
(B) Aspartate and glutamate
(C) Cysteine and histidine
(D) Methionine and tryptophan
(E) Phenylalanine and tyrosine

77. Which one of the following carbohydrates is a polymer of D-glucosyl units containing exclusively α-1,4-glycosidic bonds?

(A) Amylose
(B) Cellulose
(C) Fructan
(D) Glycogen
(E) Mutan

78. Which one of the following compounds is not an allosteric regulator of phosphofructokinase activity?

(A) AMP
(B) ATP
(C) Citrate
(D) Fructose 6-phosphate
(E) Fructose 2, 6-bisphosphate

79. Which one of the following fatty acids is classified as an essential human nutrient?

(A) Palmitoleate
(B) Palmitate
(C) Oleate
(D) Myristate
(E) Linoleate

80. A deficiency of any one of the following amino acids leads to a negative nitrogen balance in humans EXCEPT

(A) methionine
(B) isoleucine
(C) leucine
(D) ornithine
(E) phenylalanine

81. Which one of the following aspects of bacterial metabolism is inhibited by sulfonamide antibiotics?

(A) dihydrofolate reductase action
(B) adenylosuccinate synthetase and IMP dehydrogenase actions
(C) utilization of *p*-aminobenzoate in folate synthesis
(D) carbamoyl-phosphate synthetase action
(E) cell-wall peptidoglycan synthesis

82. Which one of the following proteins is required specifically for physiological RNA chain initiation in *E. coli*?

(A) α (Alpha)
(B) β (Beta)
(C) β' (Beta prime)
(D) ρ (Rho)
(E) σ (Sigma)

83. Which one of the following factors is responsible for initiating the extrinsic pathway of blood coagulation?

(A) Prothrombin, or factor II
(B) Thromboplastin, or factor III
(C) Antihemophilic factor, or factor VIII
(D) Christmas factor, or factor IX
(E) von Willebrand factor

84. Reversing the effects of the glucagon cascade in the liver involves all of the following processes EXCEPT

(A) cessation of adenylyl cyclase stimulation
(B) conversion of cyclic AMP to 5′-AMP
(C) re-formation of the inactive R_2C_2 form of protein kinase A
(D) dephosphorylation of phosphatase-1 inhibitor, phosphorylase *a,* phosphorylase kinase, glycogen synthase, fructose-6-phosphate-2-kinase/phosphatase, and pyruvate kinase
(E) increased dephosphorylation of fructose 1,6-bisphosphate to form fructose 6-phosphate

85. Which one of the following bonds is vital in establishing the secondary structure of proteins?

(A) Disulfide
(B) Ionic
(C) Hydrogen
(D) Resonance
(E) van der Waals

86. The rate-limiting reaction in prostaglandin biosynthesis is catalyzed by

(A) phospholipase A_1
(B) phospholipase A_2
(C) phospholipase C
(D) phospholipase D

87. A deficiency of which one of the following enzymes is associated with markedly reduced levels of cholesteryl esters in lipoproteins?

(A) Acid lipase
(B) Acyl-CoA: cholesterol acyltransferase (ACAT)
(C) Hepatic lipase
(D) Lecithin: cholesterol acyltransferase (LCAT)
(E) Lipoprotein lipase

88. Platelet activating factor differs from all other glycerophospholipids in that it
   (A) contains an ether bond at *sn*-1
   (B) contains an acetyl group at *sn*-2
   (C) contains phosphocholine at *sn*-3
   (D) is especially prevalent in nervous tissue

89. When most proteins are exposed to the pH of the stomach ($\approx$1), which one of the following events occurs?
   (A) Ingested proteins donate protons to gastric juice
   (B) Proteins become denatured
   (C) Proteins such as myosin assume their physiological conformation
   (D) Peptide bonds form between the A and B chains of insulin
   (E) The R group of lysine becomes unprotonated

90. All of the following are true statements regarding phosphatidylinositol 4,5-bisphosphate EXCEPT
   (A) It is a precursor of two second messenger molecules
   (B) It is metabolized to diglyceride and inositol 1,4,5-trisphosphate by phospholipase C
   (C) Its cleavage leads to activation of protein kinase C
   (D) Its cleavage leads to an increased intracellular calcium ion concentration
   (E) It is formed from diglyceride and CDP-inositol 4,5-bisphosphate

DIRECTIONS. (Items 91–134): Each set of matching questions in this section consists of a list of lettered options followed by several numbered items. For each numbered item, select the ONE lettered option that is most closely associated with it. To avoid spending too much time on matching sets with large numbers of options, it is generally advisable to begin each set by reading the list of options. Then, for each item in the list, try to generate the correct answer and locate it in the option list, rather than evaluating each option individually. Each lettered option may be selected once, more than once, or not at all.

Items 91–96

(A) Acetyl-CoA carboxylase
(B) Alcohol dehydrogenase
(C) Carnitine acyltransferase
(D) Citrate synthase
(E) Fructose-1,6-bisphosphatase
(F) Glucokinase
(G) Glucose-6-phosphatase
(H) Glucose-6-phosphate dehydrogenase
(I) Glycogen phosphorylase
(J) Glycogen synthase
(K) Hexokinase
(L) Hormone-sensitive lipase
(M) Isocitrate dehydrogenase
(N) Malate dehydrogenase
(O) Phosphofructokinase
(P) Phosphoglycerate kinase
(Q) Pyruvate carboxylase
(R) Pyruvate dehydrogenase kinase
(S) Pyruvate kinase
(T) Succinate dehydrogenase

For each property listed below, select the corresponding enzyme.

91. This enzyme's activity occurs only in liver, kidney, and intestine
92. This enzyme catalyzes a reversible glycolytic reaction
93. This enzyme contains pyridoxal phosphate
94. Mutant forms of this enzyme are sensitive to antimalarials such as chloroquine and many other drugs, and administration of these drugs to sensitive people leads to a hemolytic anemia
95. This enzyme contains FAD as a prosthetic group
96. This enzyme is more sensitive to the action of insulin than are insulin-sensitive glucose translocases

Items 97–99

(A) Alkaptonuria
(B) Histidinemia
(C) Homocystinuria and hypermethioninemia
(D) Hyperprolinemia
(E) Maple syrup urine disease
(F) Phenylketonuria
(G) Tyrosinemia
(H) Urocanic aciduria

For each enzyme deficiency listed below, select the corresponding inborn error of metabolism.

97. Results from a deficiency of glutamate-γ-semialdehyde dehydrogenase
98. Results from a deficiency of fumarylacetoacetate hydrolase
99. Results from a deficiency of phenylalanine hydroxylase

Items 100–102

(A) Cytosol
(B) Lysosome
(C) Mitochondrion
(D) Nucleus
(E) Peroxisome
(F) Plasma membrane
(G) Rough endoplasmic reticulum and Golgi
(H) Smooth endoplasmic reticulum

For each description of a biochemical process, select the most appropriate cellular component.

100. Site of protein glycosylation reactions
101. The therapeutic effect of AZT used in the treatment of AIDS occurs at this site
102. A deficiency of α-ketoglutarate dehydrogenase involves this cellular component

Items 103–106

(A) Actinomycin D
(B) Bleomycin
(C) Cisplatin
(D) Cytosine arabinoside
(E) Daunorubicin
(F) Fluorouracil
(G) Hydroxyurea
(H) Mercaptopurine
(I) Methotrexate
(J) Thioguanine

For each process listed below, select the corresponding cancer chemotherapeutic agent.

103. A drug that inhibits dihydrofolate reductase
104. A prodrug that yields a suicide inhibitor of thymidylate synthase
105. A free-radical scavenger that inhibits ribonucleoside diphosphate reductase
106. An antibiotic that inhibits human topoisomerase II

Items 107–110

(A) Adrenocorticotropic hormone (ACTH)
(B) Aldosterone
(C) Angiotensin II
(D) Atrial natriuretic peptide
(E) Glucagon
(F) Insulin
(G) Insulin-like growth factor–1
(H) Melatonin
(I) Prolactin
(J) Renin
(K) Somatomammotropin
(L) Thyrotropin
(M) Thyrotropin-releasing hormone (TRH)
(N) Vasopressin

For each characteristic listed below, select the corresponding agent.

107. This hormone is a tripeptide
108. This hormone activates guanylyl cyclase activity
109. This protein is an enzyme whose secretion is inhibited by β-adrenergic receptor blockers
110. This hormone is responsible for the increased pigmentation observed in patients with Addison disease

Items 111–114

(A) Acetyl-CoA
(B) Adenosine triphosphate
(C) *S*-Adenosylmethionine
(D) CMP-*N*-acetylneuraminate
(E) Farnesyl pyrophosphate
(F) GDP-mannose
(G) N^5-Methyltetrahydrofolate
(H) Myristoyl-CoA
(I) Palmitoyl-CoA
(J) Phosphoadenosylphosphosulfate
(K) UDP-glucose

For each biochemical property listed below, select the corresponding metabolite.

111. Reacts with protein-lysine residues to form a stable derivative
112. A precursor of sphinganine
113. Participates in both cholesterol biosynthesis and posttranslational modification of Ras
114. Failure to form this metabolite is one cause of homocystinuria

Items 115–120

(A) Calcium
(B) Chloride
(C) Cobalt
(D) Copper
(E) Fluoride
(F) Iodide
(G) Iron
(H) Magnesium
(I) Phosphorus
(J) Potassium
(K) Radon
(L) Sodium

For each characteristic listed below, select the most appropriate element or ion.

115. EDTA (ethylene diamine tetraacetate) forms a complex with this ion and prevents blood plasma from clotting
116. It is necessary to include 40 mEq of this substance daily in patients who are maintained on intravenous fluids
117. A deficiency of this ion produces thyroid enlargement (goiter)
118. This ion is found in vitamin B_{12}
119. This radioactive element is a likely cause of lung cancer
120. This ion is a component of cytosolic superoxide dismutase

Items 121–123

(A) Pyruvate → oxaloacetate
(B) Oxaloacetate → phosphoenolpyruvate
(C) Fructose 1,6-bisphosphate → fructose 6-phosphate
(D) Glucose 6-phosphate → glucose
(E) Glycerol → glycerol phosphate

For each characteristic listed below, select the corresponding chemical reaction.

121. This process requires biotin
122. A defect in this process, which occurs in the endoplasmic reticulum, is responsible for glycogen storage disease I (von Gierke disease)
123. Decreased [acetyl-CoA], which occurs in medium-chain acyl-CoA dehydrogenase deficiency, leads to fasting hypoglycemia because of a defect in this metabolic conversion

Items 124–127

(A) Beriberi
(B) Bleeding disorders
(C) Kwashiorkor
(D) Marasmus
(E) Night blindness
(F) Pellagra
(G) Pernicious anemia
(H) Rickets
(I) Scurvy

For each of the characteristics listed below, select the most appropriate disease.

124. Symptoms of this ailment include ecchymosis, petechiae, and gingival swelling
125. Deficient intrinsic factor production causes this ailment
126. Inadequate protein and caloric intake in children can produce this disease
127. Deficient intake of β-carotene produces this symptom

Items 128–129

(A) Acetylcholine
(B) Dopamine
(C) Enkephalin
(D) Epinephrine
(E) GABA (γ-aminobutyrate)
(F) Glutamate
(G) Glycine
(H) Histamine
(I) Nitric oxide
(J) Serotonin

For each action listed below, select the corresponding neurotransmitter.

128. Action related to morphine
129. Unregulated secretion by a pheochromocytoma produces hypertension

Items 130–132

(A) Eukaryotic initiation factor 1 (eIF1)
(B) Eukaryotic initiation factor 2 (eIF2)
(C) Eukaryotic initiation factor 3 (eIF3)
(D) Eukaryotic initiation factor 4E (eIF4E)
(E) Eukaryotic elongation factor 1α (eEF1α)
(F) Eukaryotic elongation factor 1$\beta\gamma$ (eEF1$\beta\gamma$)
(G) Eukaryotic elongation factor 2 (eEF2)
(H) Eukaryotic release factor (eRF)

For each biochemical property listed below, select the corresponding protein synthesis factor.

130. Recognizes methionine-$tRNA_i^{Met}$
131. Promotes the hydrolysis of peptidyl-tRNA
132. Contains diphthamide

Items 133–134

(A) Apoprotein A-I gene
(B) Apoprotein B-100/B-48 gene
(C) Apoprotein C-II gene
(D) Apoprotein E gene
(E) LDL receptor gene

For each biochemical characteristic listed below, select the corresponding gene.

133. Mutations involving this gene can result in an inability to activate lipoprotein lipase and lead to a clinical disorder that closely resembles lipoprotein lipase deficiency
134. Mutations of this gene lead to impaired ability to produce chylomicrons, VLDL, and LDL, thereby leading to fat malabsorption, diarrhea, retinitis pigmentosa, cerebellar ataxia, and acanthocytosis

Items 135–137

Codon	138	139	140	141	142	143	144	145	146	147	148
Normal	UCC	AAA	UAC	CGU	UAA	GCU	GGA	GCC	UCG	GUA	GCU
Mutant A	UCC	AAU ↑	ACC	GUU	AAG	CUG	GAG	CCU	CGG	UAG	CUA
Mutant B	UCC	AAA	UAC	CGU	CAA ↑	GCU	GGA	GCC	UCG	GUA	GCU

The sequences of normal hemoglobin A mRNA and two mutant mRNAs are given below the genetic code. The numbers specify the particular triplet following the initiating codon for methionine, and the arrows point to the single change that is present in each mutant.

The Standard Genetic Code

Second letter

First letter (5')	U	C	A	G	*Third letter (3')*
U	UUU Phe	UCU Ser	UAU Tyr	UGU Cys	U
	UUC Phe	UCC Ser	UAC Tyr	UGC Cys	C
	UUA Leu	UCA Ser	UAA Stop	UGA Stop	A
	UUG Leu	UCG Ser	UAG Stop	UGG Trp	G
C	CUU Leu	CCU Pro	CAU His	CGU Arg	U
	CUC Leu	CCC Pro	CAC His	CGC Arg	C
	CUA Leu	CCA Pro	CAA Gln	CGA Arg	A
	CUG Leu	CCG Pro	CAG Gln	CGG Arg	G
A	AUU Ile	ACU Thr	AAU Asn	AGU Ser	U
	AUC Ile	ACC Thr	AAC Asn	AGC Ser	C
	AUA Ile	ACA Thr	AAA Lys	AGA Arg	A
	AUG Met	ACG Thr	AAG Lys	AGG Arg	G
G	GUU Val	GCU Ala	GAU Asp	GGU Gly	U
	GUC Val	GCC Ala	GAC Asp	GGC Gly	C
	GUA Val	GCA Ala	GAA Glu	GGA Gly	A
	GUG Val	GCG Ala	GAG Glu	GGG Gly	G

135. Counting the initiating methionine as residue 1, mutant A encodes for a polypeptide with the following number of amino acids.

(A) 140
(B) 141
(C) 145
(D) 146
(E) 147

136. What is the nucleotide sequence of the template strand of DNA that encodes the serine residue near the carboxyl terminus of the normal hemoglobin α-chain?

(A) 5' AGC 3'
(B) 5' AGG 3'
(C) 5' GGA 3'
(D) 5' CGA 3'
(E) 5' ATA 3'

137. What type of mutation is observed in mutant B?

(A) nonsense mutation
(B) Frameshift mutation
(C) Transition
(D) Transversion
(E) Deletion

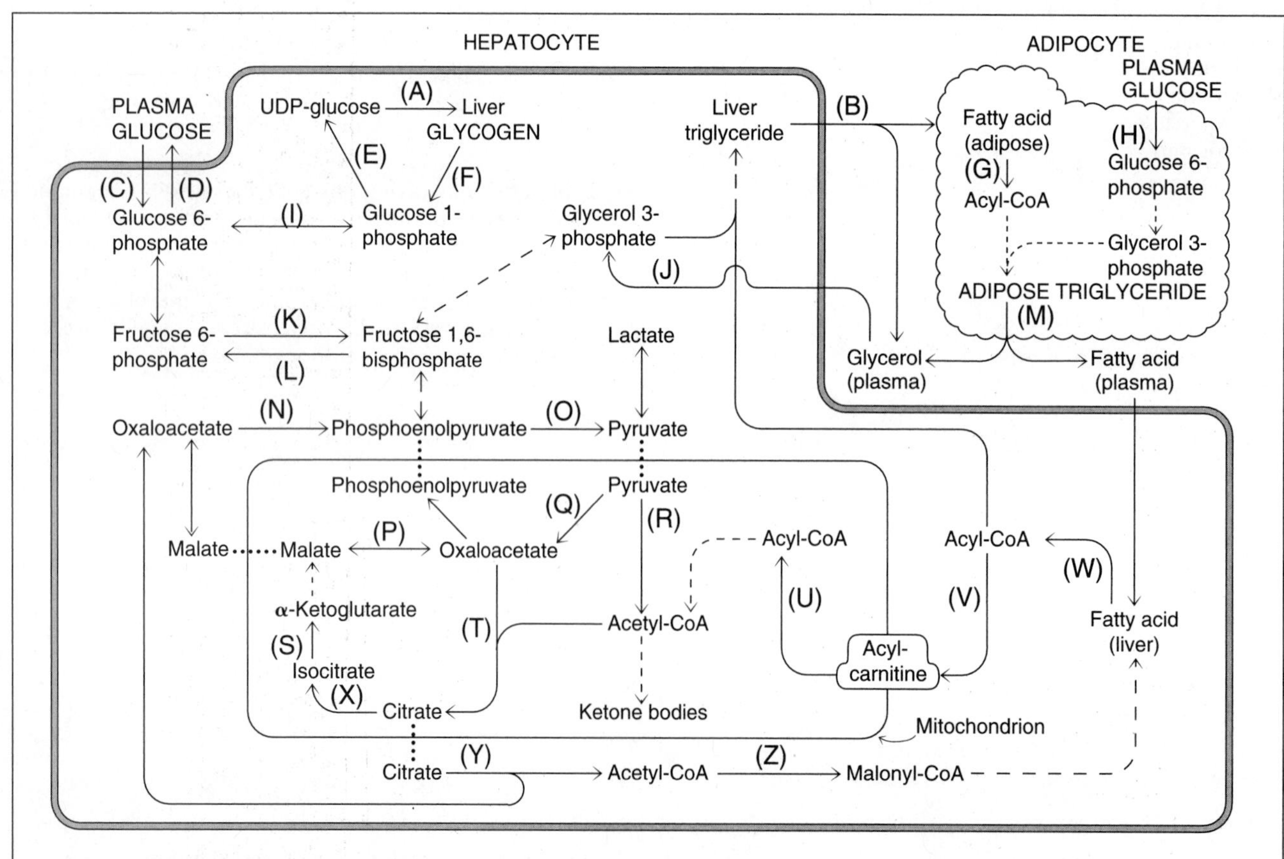

Items 138–148

For each given description of an enzyme, select the correct letter from the accompanying diagram.

138. The enzyme catalyzing this reaction is allosterically activated by acetyl-CoA
139. The enzyme catalyzing this reaction is phosphorylated and INACTIVATED in response to stimulation of its protein kinase by acetyl-CoA
140. The enzyme catalyzing this reaction is allosterically inhibited by malonyl-CoA.
141. The enzyme catalyzing this reaction requires GTP as substrate
142. The enzyme catalyzing this reaction requires UTP as substrate
143. The enzyme catalyzing this reaction is the primary site of regulation of *de novo* fatty acid synthesis
144. The enzyme catalyzing this reaction is the primary site of regulation of glycolysis
145. The enzyme catalyzing this reaction is the primary site of regulation of the Krebs cycle
146. The cytosolic enzyme catalyzing this reaction in gluconeogenesis is regulated allosterically.
147. The enzyme catalyzing this reaction is the primary site of regulation of lipolysis
148. The enzyme catalyzing this reaction is the primary site of regulation of glycogen synthesis

ANSWERS AND EXPLANATIONS

1. The answer is B: 1-hydroxylation. The formation of active vitamin D involves the photoactivation of 7-dehydrocholesterol in the skin, 25-hydroxylation in the liver, and 1-hydroxylation in the kidney. The 24-hydroxylation of vitamin D results in an *inactive* form. 17-Hydroxylation and 21-hydroxylation occur in steroid hormone, but not calcitriol, synthesis. To obviate the inability of these patients to form calcitriol, plasma calcium can be controlled by dialysis. *Biochemistry,* pp. 30, 31.
2. The answer is B: deficiency of galactose-1-phosphate uridyltransferase. Galactose-1-phosphate uridyltransferase deficiency produces classical galactosemia. Biochemical reactions are catalyzed by enzymes (PRINCIPLE 4 OF BIOCHEMISTRY), and in the absence of this enzyme, galactose 1-phosphate accumulates intracellularly. Galactokinase deficiency produces a mild form of galactosemia probably because phosphorylated intermediates do not accumulate intracellularly as they do in classical galactosemia. Galactosidase is a bacterial enzyme that is encoded by the *gal* operon. Lactase deficiency produces milk intolerance but not galactosemia. Epimerase deficiency has not been reported. Galactose and *N*-acetylgalactosamine occur in several glycoproteins, and restricting galactose intake is not detrimental owing to the ability to convert UDP-glucose to UDP-galactose as catalyzed by the epimerase. *Biochemistry,* pp. 106–107; *Nelson,* p. 359.
3. The answer is D: Nuclear DNA is the genetic material of humans and most organisms (PRINCIPLE 22 OF BIOCHEMISTRY), and DNA is responsible for the transmission of normal traits and abnormal traits, such as sickle cell anemia, from one generation to the next. Sickle cell anemia is an autosomal recessive disease, and both males and females are affected. Mitochondrial DNA encodes mitochondrial RNA and a dozen mitochondrial proteins. Mitochondrial DNA is transmitted from the egg to the offspring, and mitochondrial diseases exhibit maternal inheritance; they are transmitted by the mother, and both male and female children can be affected. In X-linked disorders, predominantly male children are affected, and the mutant genes are transmitted by carrier mothers. Some viruses, for example, HIV and poliovirus, use RNA as the genetic material. Although protein is an informational macromolecule (where information is defined as the sequence of amino acids just as the sequence of letters of the alphabet provides information in words), protein does not transmit genetic information. Carbohydrates are not informational macromolecules. *Biochemistry,* p. 7.
4. The answer is C: ornithine transcarbamoylase deficiency. Enzymes are protein catalysts (PRINCIPLE 5 OF BIOCHEMISTRY), and this enzyme catalyzes an early step in urea synthesis, and a deficiency of this enzyme leads to hyperammonemia without acidosis. Moreover, the inability to convert ammonium ion and aspartate into urea as a result of deficiencies of any of the urea cycle enzymes does NOT result in acidosis. Acid metabolites and acidosis, however, occur in maple syrup urine disease (branched-chain keto acid dehydrogenase deficiency) and methylmalonic acidemia (methylmalonate mutase deficiency or defective vitamin B_{12} metabolism). Failure to oxidize pyruvate, because of a deficiency of pyruvate dehydrogenase, results in lactic acidosis, a metabolite of pyruvate. In type I glycogen storage disease (glucose-6-phosphatase deficiency), glucose is not formed from glucose 6-phosphate, and glucose is not released from the liver. Glucose 6-phosphate is converted to lactate, thereby accounting for metabolic acidosis. *Nelson,* p. 327.
5. The answer is D: bile salts. Although cortisol and progesterone are potent hormones, each is present in only small (milligram) amounts in the body. Neutral sterols, which are formed as a result of the action of intestinal bacteria on cholesterol, are not abundant compounds. Animal cells lack the ability to degrade the sterol ring to carbon dioxide; cholesterol thus does not serve as a metabolic fuel. About 0.5 gram of cholesterol is converted to bile salts daily in human adults, and the prescription of oral nonabsorbable ion exchange resins that bind to intestinal bile salts is a common procedure used in treating hypercholesterolemia. *Biochemistry,* p. 190.
6. The answer is A: HMG-CoA lyase deficiency. Acetoacetate is formed in liver mitochondria in a process involving the conversion of β-hydroxy-β-methylglutaryl-CoA (HMG-CoA) to acetoacetate and acetyl-CoA. A deficiency of this enzyme results in an accumulation of HMG-CoA, which is hydrolyzed nonspecifically to β-hydroxy-β-methylglutarate. Ketone bodies cannot be oxidized to carbon dioxide in the liver physiologically because the liver lacks the enzymatic machinery to convert acetoacetate to its coenzyme A derivative, ace-

toacetyl-CoA. β-Hydroxybutyrate is formed by reduction of acetoacetate by NADH, and these two hydrophilic compounds diffuse from liver into the plasma for delivery to extrahepatic tissues. In the peripheral tissues, β-hydroxybutyrate is oxidized to acetoacetate in an NAD^+-dependent reaction, then acetoacetate reacts with succinyl-CoA to form acetoacetyl-CoA and succinate. Acetoacetyl-CoA is converted to two acetyl-CoA molecules in a reaction catalyzed by β-ketothiolase, and the acetyl units are oxidized in the Krebs cycle. Acetone is formed by the nonenzymatic decarboxylation of acetoacetate and is exhaled from the lungs (yielding the "acetone breath" of diabetics) and excreted in the urine. Ketogenesis is increased when plasma free fatty acids are elevated in response to a high glucagon-to-insulin ratio, which accelerates hydrolysis of triglyceride in adipose tissue. HMG-CoA is also an intermediate formed in leucine catabolism in the mitochondrion and in cholesterol synthesis in the endoplasmic reticulum. β-Ketothiolase deficiency, maple syrup urine disease, medium-chain acyl-CoA dehydrogenase deficiency, and propionyl-CoA carboxylase deficiency all lead to the excretion of organic acids in the urine, but there is little or no excretion of urinary hydroxymethylglutarate. *Biochemistry,* p. 169; *Nelson,* p. 320.

7. The answer is D: phenylalanine. Hartnup disease is caused by decreased ability to transport valine, leucine, isoleucine, tryptophan, and phenylalanine. The lack of one or more genetically encoded amino acids impairs protein synthesis, and more nitrogen is excreted than is absorbed (negative nitrogen balance). All the amino acids whose transport is defective in Hartnup disease are essential and cannot be synthesized from endogenous compounds. Inadequate phenylalanine or any other amino acid accounts for a negative nitrogen balance in patients with Hartnup disease. Linoleic acid is an essential fatty acid, but its deficiency would not result directly in negative nitrogen balance. Glutathione is γ-glutamylcysteinylglycine; all three of these amino acids are nonessential, and their decreased absorption would not lead to negative nitrogen balance. Cobalamin, a vitamin, is essential but is not an amino acid, and serine can be synthesized from glycine and methylene-THF. A dietary deficiency of serine is inconsequential. *Biochemistry,* p. 233.
8. The answer is C: DNA polymerase γ. DNA polymerase γ is the mitochondrial replication enzyme. DNA polymerase α catalyzes lagging strand replication, and DNA polymerase δ (with PCNA) catalyzes leading strand replication. DNA polymerases β and ε are repair polymerases. Repair enzymes fill gaps during the combination of Okazaki fragments and during excision repair. *Biochemistry,* p. 281.
9. The answer is E: 25%. The caloric contents of the ingredients of the chicken tostadas are as follows: carbohydrate, 4 kcal/g; protein, 4 kcal/g; cholesterol, 0 kcal/g; sodium, 0 kcal/g; fiber, 0 kcal/g; and fat, 9 kcal/g. The total nutritional value is $40 \times 4 + 30 \times 4 + 10 \times 9 = 160 + 120 + 90 = 370$ kcal. The percentage of the total that is due to fat is $90/370 \times 100 = 24.3\% \approx 25\%$. *Biochemistry,* p. 34.
10. The answer is B: aspartate transcarbamoylase. In *E. coli* and many other bacteria, the site of regulation of pyrimidine synthesis differs from that used in higher animals. Aspartate transcarbamoylase in *E. coli,* a celebrated enzyme, has been extensively studied and considered as the prototype for allosteric enzyme inhibition; this enzyme is allosterically inhibited by CTP. In higher animals, including humans, carbamoyl-phosphate synthetase II is the principal site of regulation, being allosterically inhibited by UDP and UTP, end products of the pyrimidine pathway. Enzymes may be regulated by allosteric agents (PRINCIPLE 8 OF BIOCHEMISTRY), and allosteric effectors follow a pattern that makes physiological sense (PRINCIPLE 9 OF BIOCHEMISTRY). Thymidylate synthase is a frequent target for cancer chemotherapy, but is not a regulatory site for pyrimidine synthesis. Ornithine transcarbamoylase is a urea cycle enzyme and is not used in pyrimidine synthesis. Dihydroorotate dehydrogenase is a mitochondrial membrane enzyme that is on the pathway for pyrimidine synthesis, but it is not a controlling enzyme. Dihydroorotate dehydrogenase, which catalyzes the conversion of dihydroorotate to orotate, resides on the outer surface of the inner mitochondrial membrane and directs reducing equivalents to ubiquinone in the electron transport chain. *Biochemistry,* p. 263.
11. The answer is D: 3 moles of carbon dioxide and 12.5 moles of ATP (or equivalent such as GTP). Catabolism of the three-carbon pyruvate yields 3 CO_2, 4 NADH (yielding 2.5 ATP each via oxidative phosphorylation), 1 $FADH_2$ (yielding 1.5 ATP via oxidative phosphorylation), and 1 GTP (equivalent to 1 ATP). The total amount of ATP produced is $4 \times 2.5 + 1.5 + 1 = 12.5$. *Biochemistry,* p. 115.
12. The answer is A: bile pigments. Bile pigments are breakdown products of heme, are excreted in the bile, and give color to the feces, but they do NOT play a role in digestion. Bile salts, formed in the liver from cholesterol, act as detergents and are required for emulsification of dietary lipid, which allows digestion, and for absorption of fatty acids and monoglycerides. Pancreatic lipase acts in the gut lumen, in the presence of a protein called colipase, to hydrolyze ester bonds involving fatty acyl groups and glycerol at the *sn*-1 and *sn*-3 positions of triglycerides. Pancreatic phospholipase, also acting in the gut lumen, catalyzes the hydrolytic removal of the 2-acyl group of phospholipids. *Biochemistry,* pp. 154, 491.
13. The answer is E: rifamycin. This compound inhibits the initiation of bacterial transcription by interacting with the β-subunit of bacterial RNA polymerase. Rifamycin is commonly used in the treatment of tuberculosis. Actinomycin D inhibits both bacterial and human RNA elongation reactions. AZT, ddI, and ddC cause premature termination of growing DNA chains, and these drugs are used in the treatment of AIDS. *Biochemistry,* p. 337.
14. The answer is C: increased activity of gluconeogenic enzymes due to enzyme induction by glucagon. The increased glucagon/insulin ratio leads to decreased glycolysis and increased glycogenolysis and gluconeogenesis in liver, all of which result in an increased output of glucose from the liver into the extracellular fluid. With increased glucose production and decreased glucose utilization, its concentration in the extracellular fluid, and thus in the blood, is elevated. Without sufficient insulin (or insulin receptor response) glucose is not transported into muscle or adipose tissue cells and it builds up in the extracellular fluid, also contributing to hyperglycemia. The transport of glucose into liver, however, is independent of insulin. Fatty acids cannot be converted to glucose in animals. *Biochemistry,* p. 512.
15. The answer is E: cystathionine synthase. Methionine is normally converted to homocysteine in a sequence of reactions that include formation of *S*-adenosylmethionine, donation of the activated methyl group to an ac-

ceptor with the concomitant formation of *S*-adenosylhomocysteine, and hydrolytic removal of the adenosyl group. Type I homocystinuria is due to a deficiency of cystathionine synthase, the next enzyme in the catabolic sequence, which prevents the usual conversion of homocysteine and serine to cystathionine. The buildup of homocysteine leads to formation of the disulfide homocystine. Homocysteine and its oxidation product, homocystine, cannot be further catabolized and accumulate in body fluids and are excreted in the urine. Inability to catabolize homocysteine decreases the catabolism of methionine and results in hypermethioninemia. Such patients fail to thrive. About 40% respond to high doses of pyridoxine (vitamin B_6), the precursor of the cofactor used by cystathionine synthase. In patients who do not respond to vitamin B_6, betaine (trimethylglycine) is sometimes effective. This compound donates a methyl group to homocysteine to produce methionine. Type II homocystinuria is due to a deficiency in methylcobalamin formation, and type III homocystinuria is due to a deficiency in methylenetetrahydrofolate reductase. Methyltetrahydrofolate and methylcobalamin are required for the regeneration of methionine from homocysteine as catalyzed by methyltetrahydrofolate homocysteine methyltransferase. Patients with type II homocystinuria, who exhibit hypomethioninemia, are treated with large doses of vitamin B_{12}. Patients with type III homocystinuria, who exhibit normal plasma methionine levels, are treated with folate, vitamins B_{12} and B_6, betaine, and methionine. Cystinuria is caused by a different mechanism involving a defect in the transport and thus reabsorption of basic amino acids in the renal tubule. Cystine, which contains two amino groups, is transported by the basic amino acid translocase. Deficiency of methionine aminopeptidase, which catalyzes the removal of the initiating methionine from polypeptide chains, has not been described. Deficiencies of *S*-adenosylmethionine and *S*-adenosylhomocysteine hydrolases, which generate methionine and homocysteine, have also not been reported. A deficiency of cystathionine lyase leads to cystathioninuria. This enzyme also requires pyridoxal phosphate as cofactor, and treatment with pyridoxine is prescribed. Affected individuals have variable symptoms and clinical courses. *Biochemistry,* p. 226; *Nelson,* p. 312.

16. The answer is D: human chromosome 22 contains hundreds of origins of replication. Each origin of replication in eukaryotic nuclear DNA occurs at intervals of about 150,000 nucleotides; based upon this value, chromosome 22 (one of the smallest human chromosomes) contains more than 300 replication origins. The characteristics that define a human origin of replication are unknown. There is a unique origin of replication for each strand of human mitochondrial DNA, and there is a single origin of replication for both strands of bacterial DNA and plasmid DNA. The sequences that constitute the unique origins of replication for these three cases are known. The replication of RNA from the DNA provirus integrated in a chromosome involves a single start site. *Biochemistry,* pp. 227, 360.
17. The answer is D: human and bacterial gene transcription. Actinomycin D, which is used in the treatment of some human neoplasms, is an inhibitor of RNA synthesis, both eukaryotic and prokaryotic. Actinomycin D inhibits RNA elongation but not initiation reactions (rifamycin inhibits bacterial RNA chain initiation). Actinomycin D intercalates between two adjacent GC base pairs of a DNA duplex. Actinomycin D lacks appreciable direct effects on DNA elongation or RNA capping. *Biochemistry,* p. 340.
18. The answer is B: They contain an α-subunit that binds and hydrolyzes GTP. G_s and G_i, proteins that alter adenylyl cyclase activity by stimulation or inhibition, respectively, are heterotrimeric proteins that consist of α-, β-, and γ-subunits. The α-subunit binds and hydrolyzes GTP; the subunit is active when GTP is bound and inactive when GDP is bound. The defective protein in pseudohypoparathyroidism is $G_s\alpha$. Receptors that interact with G-proteins contain seven transmembrane segments. d-Tubocurarine interacts with the nicotinic acetylcholine receptor, which is a pentamer composed of four different subunits. The pentamer forms a cation channel and does not play a direct role in stimulating G-proteins. *Biochemistry,* pp. 401–406; *Nelson,* p. 1434.
19. The answer is E: simple diffusion. Ethanol, carbon dioxide, and oxygen are among the few physiologically active substances that can diffuse across biological membranes. Ethanol can be absorbed from the stomach and distributed rapidly throughout the body. Because it readily diffuses across biological membranes, it bypasses the blood-brain barrier and has rapid central nervous system effects. Primary active transport is energized by ATP; secondary active transport is energized by sodium ion gradients (PRINCIPLE 13 OF BIOCHEMISTRY). Antiport is a process whereby one metabolite crosses a membrane in exchange for a metabolite on the opposite side. The ADP/ATP translocase that is responsible for importing ADP into the mitochondrion in exchange for mitochondrial ATP is an example of an antiport process. Facilitated diffusion refers to protein-mediated translocation across a membrane that is not energy dependent. *Biochemistry,* pp. 458–459.
20. The answer is C: Hurler disease (type I mucopolysaccharidosis) is a genetic disorder due to a defect in iduronidase, a lysosomal enzyme. As a result, iduronate-containing glycosaminoglycans accumulate and lead to disease. Ehlers-Danlos syndrome and osteogenesis imperfecta are characterized by abnormal collagens. Von Gierke disease is a glycogen storage disease due to a deficiency of glucose-6-phosphatase, an endoplasmic reticulum enzyme. Muscular dystrophy results from a defect in dystrophin, a structural protein. Sphingolipidoses are also lysosomal diseases. *Biochemistry,* p. 482; *Nelson,* p. 372.
21. The answer is B: hemoglobin A_1. Hemoglobin A_1 is a glycosylated form of hemoglobin, and it has a distinctive electrophoretic mobility allowing its measurement. Hemoglobin A_1 results from the nonenzymatic glycosylation of hemoglobin via a reaction with the free aldehyde of glucose. In nondiabetics, it accounts for $<6\%$ of total hemoglobin; in individuals with overt diabetes, it accounts for $>6\%$. A reasonable therapeutic goal representing good control of diabetic hyperglycemia is $\leq 9\%$ hemoglobin A_1. In contrast to blood glucose levels, which represent glucose concentrations at a specific time, the levels of hemoglobin A_1 reflect chronic blood glucose values indicative of blood glucose concentrations during the past several weeks. Some clinical laboratories measure a single form of hemoglobin A_1 called A_{1c}. Hemoglobin A_{1c} makes up about two-thirds of hemoglobin A_1, and maintaining the levels of hemoglobin A_{1c} at $<6\%$ in patients with diabetes represents a reasonable therapeutic goal. Hemoglobin A is normal adult hemoglobin ($\alpha_2\beta_2$), and hemoglobin F is normal fetal hemoglobin ($\alpha_2\gamma_2$). Hemoglobin H is the designation for

β_4 hemoglobin, a form that occurs in α-thalassemia. Hemoglobin S, or sickle cell hemoglobin, is $\alpha_2^A\beta_2^S$, where β^S represents the mutant form of the β-chain present in sickle cell anemia. *Biochemistry,* p. 92.

22. The answer is A: factor I (fibrinogen). The early components of the blood clotting cascade are not present in large amounts. The final substrate is fibrinogen, which is present in stoichiometric (200–400 mg/dL) and not catalytic amounts. Thrombin (active factor II) catalyzes the hydrolysis of four specific Arg-Gly bonds in the Aα- and Bβ-subunits (but not γ-subunit) of fibrinogen to form four small fibrinopeptides (two A and two B peptides) and fibrin. Fibrin consists of three different polypeptides found with the following stoichiometry: $\alpha_2\beta_2\gamma_2$ and molecular mass of 340,000 Da. A deficiency of factor VIII leads to hemophilia A, and a deficiency of factor IX leads to hemophilia B. Factor XIII is the transglutaminase that cross-links fibrin together. A deficiency of von Willebrand factor leads to von Willebrand disease, the most common genetic blood-clotting disorder. *Biochemistry,* p. 494.
23. The answer is C: phosphoribosylpyrophosphate-glutamine amidotransferase (PRPP amidotransferase) catalyzes the rate-controlling reaction of purine nucleotide biosynthesis. This enzyme is inhibited by AMP, GMP, and allopurinol ribonucleotide (an active metabolite of allopurinol, a drug that is used in the treatment of gout). Carbamoyl-phosphate synthetase II catalyzes the rate-controlling step in pyrimidine synthesis in humans. Hypoxanthine-guanine phosphoribosyl transferase (HGPRT), the enzyme that is defective in the Lesch-Nyhan syndrome, is in the salvage pathway that converts its substrates into purine nucleotides. Xanthine dehydrogenase and its derivative, xanthine oxidase, catalyze catabolic reactions of purine metabolism. Xanthine dehydrogenase is the physiological enzyme; xanthine oxidase is derived from the dehydrogenase in cells that are oxidatively stressed. *Biochemistry,* p. 263.
24. The answer is E: transition. 5-Methylcytosine, which is derived from cytosine after its incorporation into DNA according to Watson-Crick base pairing with a guanine (PRINCIPLE 23 OF BIOCHEMISTRY), is deaminated by hydrolysis to form thymine, a physiological component of DNA. Thymine directs the incorporation of adenine into the complementary strand. The substitution of a purine for a purine and a pyrimidine for a pyrimidine, as occurs in this example, is called a transition. The substitution of a purine for a pyrimidine is called a transversion. Translocations refer to larger DNA rearrangements such as occur during the formation of the Philadelphia chromosome by reciprocal translocation of portions of chromosomes 9 and 22. Transformation refers to the entry of DNA from outside to inside the cell. Experimentally, this is accomplished by incubating cells with DNA within calcium phosphate precipitates or by exposing cells to high voltages (electroporation). The conversion of a normal cell to a cancerous cell and the conversion of an inactive steroid hormone receptor to the active form following receptor binding to the hormone are also called transformation. Transduction refers to a bacterial virus carrying a segment of bacterial DNA from one bacterial cell to another. *Biochemistry,* p. 290.
25. The answer is C: glutamate. The majority of excitatory cells in the brain use glutamate as neurotransmitter; glutamate is present in large amounts (on the order of 5 mmol/kg). GABA and glycine are the chief inhibitory neurotransmitters in the brain and spinal cord respectively. Acetylcholine and norepinephrine have restricted cellular distribution in brain and are present in small amounts (a few μmol/kg). *Biochemistry,* p. 398.
26. The answer is B: enterokinase (enteropeptidase). This small intestinal enzyme is required to begin the activation of trypsinogen, a zymogen secreted by the pancreas, to trypsin, an active protease operating in the gut lumen. Once active trypsin is formed, it may activate other zymogens including trypsinogen, chymotrypsinogen, and procarboxypeptidase, by hydrolyzing specific peptide bonds. A deficiency of enterokinase thus leads to diminished activity of trypsin, chymotrypsin, and carboxypeptidase. Patients exhibit a severe malnutrition resembling kwashiorkor. Treatment with amino acid hydrolysates and exogenous pancreatic enzymes is prescribed. Furin is an intracellular protease that is involved in the posttranslational processing of proteins which are secreted by cells as part of the constitutive pathway. Carboxypeptidase A, leucine aminopeptidase, and pepsin, also digestive proteases, are not involved in the conversion of trypsinogen to trypsin. *Biochemistry,* p. 213; *Nelson,* p. 382.
27. The answer is D: 21.5 moles of ATP are formed from oxidation of one mole of β-hydroxybutyrate. The conversion of β-hydroxybutyrate to acetoacetate provides one NADH (yielding 2.5 ATP); cleavage of acetoacetyl-CoA yields two acetyl-CoA, each of which yields 10 ATP. However, the activation of acetoacetate to acetoacetyl-CoA costs one ATP equivalent, since the usual Krebs cycle conversion of succinyl-CoA to succinate (ordinarily yielding a GTP) is circumvented. To summarize: $2.5 + (2 \times 10) - 1 = 21.5$. *Biochemistry,* pp. 132, 171.
28. The answer is E: binding to the ferric iron of cytochrome a_3 in cytochrome oxidase. Since the final step of electron transport is blocked by cyanide, all the preceding electron carriers accumulate as reduced intermediates, and no further oxidation-reduction can take place. Without electron transport, proton translocation cannot occur, the proton gradient across the inner mitochondrial membrane cannot be maintained, and there is no further phosphorylation of ADP by ATP synthase. Cyanide does not directly dissipate a proton gradient across the membrane as does 2,4-dinitrophenol, nor does cyanide bind to ferrous iron in myoglobin as does carbon monoxide. Oligomycin, and not cyanide, is an inhibitor of ATP synthase. The oxygen-carrying capacity of the blood is modestly lowered only when a patient is treated with an oxidizing agent such as amyl nitrate, which converts hemoglobin's ferrous iron to the ferric form, thus providing a binding site for cyanide. *Biochemistry,* p. 133.
29. The answer is A: decreasing the free energy of activation ($\Delta G\ddagger$) of a reaction. The free energy of activation, which is the difference in the energy of the reactants and the transition state, is related exponentially to the reaction velocity. A small decrease in the free energy of activation corresponds to a large change in the rate of a reaction, and this is the basis for the enzymatic acceleration of biochemical reactions. Enzymes do not decrease the standard free energy change ($\Delta G°$) or the entropy change (ΔS) of the overall reaction. Enzymes cannot alter the equilibrium constant of a reaction (recall that the standard free energy change and equilibrium constant vary coordinately). The total kinetic energy is determined by the temperature and is not altered by enzymes. *Biochemistry,* p. 54.
30. The answer is A: stage I. Stage I of metabolism, as formulated by Krebs, involves the conversion of complex molecules such as gangliosides (a sphingolipid), carbohy-

drates, and proteins to their monomeric building blocks. The defect in G_{M1} gangliosidosis involves stage I. Stage II represents the conversion of the monomeric building blocks to acetyl-CoA. Stage III represents the oxidation of acetyl-CoA to carbon dioxide and reducing equivalents, and the oxidation of the reducing equivalents to water with the concomitant generation of ATP. Stages IV and V were not formulated by Krebs. *Biochemistry,* pp. 3–4.

31. The answer is E: a deficiency of bile salts does NOT lead to hypercholesterolemia. Bile salts emulsify lipids and promote their hydrolysis by pancreatic lipase. Bile salts also aid in the absorption of fat-soluble substances including β-carotene (provitamin A) and vitamins A, D, E, and K. As a result of impaired fat absorption, there is increased fat in the stool (steatorrhea). Bile salts in the gallbladder help solubilize cholesterol and a deficiency of bile salts can lead to gallstones. A deficiency of bile salts, which can be produced pharmacologically by taking nonabsorbable anion exchange resins (bile-salt binders) orally, promotes conversion of cholesterol to bile salts and decreases serum cholesterol levels. *Biochemistry,* pp. 154, 190.
32. The answer is D: both gluconeogenesis and glycolysis do NOT result in the net loss of ATP. A net loss of ATP occurs during gluconeogenesis but not during glycolysis. A net yield of ATP during glycolysis can fuel muscle contraction under anaerobic conditions and can therefore allow for survival in emergencies. Glycolysis requires ATP at the hexokinase and phosphofructokinase steps, whereas gluconeogenesis uses ATP at the pyruvate carboxylase and phosphoglycerate kinase steps and GTP at the phosphoenolpyruvate carboxykinase step. Fructose 2,6-bisphosphate activates phosphofructokinase (a glycolytic enzyme) and inhibits fructose-1,6-bisphosphatase (a gluconeogenic enzyme), so changes in its concentration affect both pathways. Both pathways proceed with the liberation of free energy (PRINCIPLE 18 OF BIOCHEMISTRY), glycolysis because the free energy content of glucose is considerably higher than that of two pyruvate or two lactate, and gluconeogenesis because glucose synthesis from lactate is linked to cleavage of six high-energy bonds of nucleoside triphosphates (ATP or GTP) per glucose formed. Aldolase, an enzyme used in both pathways, catalyzes the interconversion of two triose phosphates (glyceraldehyde 3-phosphate and dihydroxyacetone phosphate) and fructose 1,6-bisphosphate. *Biochemistry,* p. 137.
33. The answer is C: from the mitochondrial matrix to the intermembrane space. Exergonic electron transport reactions provide the energy required to move protons from the interior of the inner mitochondrial membrane to its exterior. This establishes both an electrical gradient (positive outside) and a chemical gradient (high $[H^+]$ outside) across the inner mitochondrial membrane. It is the energy inherent in this electrochemical gradient that drives ATP synthesis when these protons flow "downhill" through ATP synthase as they return to the mitochondrial matrix (PRINCIPLE 12 OF BIOCHEMISTRY). Electron transport from NADH results in the translocation of 10 protons: four at site 1, two at site 2, and four at site 3. Electron transport from succinate and $FADH_2$ bypasses site 1, and a total of six protons are translocated. Because the number of protons translocated by electron transport is independent of the number of protons required for ATP synthesis, nonintegral values of ATP formed per NADH (2.5) or $FADH_2$ (1.5) oxidized are permitted. *Biochemistry,* p. 127.
34. The answer is E: M. M, or mitosis, requires 1–2 hours. G_1 (gap 1), S (DNA synthesis), and G_2 (gap 2) require several hours each. Quiescent or nondividing cells are said to be in G_0, and G_0 can last for months or years. *Biochemistry,* p. 9.
35. The answer is D: topoisomerase II. Topoisomerase II makes nicks in both strands of a DNA duplex and allows a portion of the intact strand to pass through the discontinuities. Nalidixic acid and norfloxacin interfere with the action of bacterial topoisomerase II at the nick-closing stage. As a result, these compounds produce strand scission. There are no clinically useful drugs that are inhibitors of bacterial DNA polymerases, topoisomerase I, or DNA ligase. *Biochemistry,* p. 284.
36. The answer is A: the primary regulatory step of the Krebs cycle must be downstream from the citrate synthase reaction. Synthesis of fatty acids from dietary carbohydrate involves the cytosolic conversion of glucose to pyruvate, the mitochondrial production of acetyl-CoA from pyruvate, the irreversible production in mitochondria of citrate from acetyl-CoA and oxaloacetate as catalyzed by citrate synthase, transport of citrate to the cytosol, and the ATP-dependent cleavage of citrate catalyzed by ATP-citrate lyase, yielding cytosolic acetyl-CoA and oxaloacetate. The citrate synthase reaction is not significantly inhibited by a high energy charge, since the conversion of carbohydrate to fat takes place when energy is plentiful, and the primary regulatory step of the Krebs cycle is downstream from citrate formation. The interconversion of citrate and isocitrate (catalyzed by aconitase) is isoergonic and reversible, as are most isomerization reactions. Moreover, freely reversible reactions are not generally regulatory steps in a pathway. The participation of the citrate synthase reaction both in fatty acid biosynthesis and in the complete oxidation of acetyl-CoA indicates that the Krebs cycle is amphibolic, i.e., both anabolic and catabolic. The citrate synthase reaction is unidirectional because of the hydrolytic cleavage of coenzyme A from intermediate citryl-CoA (PRINCIPLE 5 OF BIOENERGETICS). The committed step of the oxidative cycle is catalyzed by isocitrate dehydrogenase, and this is the major regulatory step. This oxidative decarboxylation reaction is biochemically reversible; at physiological concentrations of substrates and products, however, the reaction is exergonic and represents a *bona fide* regulatory step. The reaction catalyzed by α-ketoglutarate dehydrogenase is an exergonic and unidirectional reaction. *Biochemistry,* p. 117.
37. The answer is. C: lactate. In cells without mitochondria (erythrocytes) or when oxygen is limiting, NADH cannot be oxidized via the electron transport chain. NAD^+, which is required for glycolysis to continue, is regenerated when NADH reduces pyruvate to lactate, a diffusible substance that can traverse the plasma membrane and enter the circulation. If pyruvate or phosphoenolpyruvate were the final compounds formed under anaerobic conditions, glycolysis would be impaired. Moreover, oxidative generation of carbon dioxide requires the Krebs cycle and mitochondria. *Biochemistry,* p. 102.
38. The answer is E: succinyl-CoA : acetoacetate CoA-transferase. Ketone bodies are synthesized in liver, and fatty acids provide most ketogenic precursors (ketogenic amino acids can provide some substrate). Acetoacetyl-CoA reacts with acetyl-CoA to form hydroxymethylglutaryl-CoA (HMG-CoA) in a reaction catalyzed by liver mitochondrial HMG-CoA synthase. HMG-CoA is cleaved to acetoacetate and acetyl-CoA by liver mitochondrial HMG-CoA lyase. Acetoacetate can be reduced to β-hydroxybutyrate, and these two ketone bodies are re-

leased from the liver into the circulation. Extrahepatic cells (except brain in nonfasting humans and red blood cells) catabolize these substances. β-Hydroxybutyrate is oxidized to acetoacetate, and acetoacetate reacts with succinyl-CoA to form acetoacetyl-CoA and succinate in a reaction catalyzed by succinyl-CoA: acetoacetate CoA-transferase. A deficiency of this enzyme leads to ketoacidosis. The mechanism for the production of hypoglycemia is unclear. Under physiological conditions, acetoacetyl-CoA is converted to two moles of acetyl-CoA in a reaction catalyzed by β-ketothiolase; acetyl-CoA can undergo oxidation by the Krebs cycle. The liver is a ketogenic organ, and extrahepatic tissues are ketolytic. Hydroxymethylglutaryl-CoA reductase is the rate-limiting enzyme for cholesterol biosynthesis, and this cytosolic enzyme is not involved in ketone body metabolism. The ratio of circulating β-hydroxybutyrate/acetoacetate reflects the mitochondrial redox state, and the ratio of circulating lactate/pyruvate reflects the cytosolic redox state. *Biochemistry,* p. 171.

39. The answer is C: inosine monophosphate. Inosine monophosphate (IMP) is the first purine nucleotide formed during *de novo* synthesis. IMP is also the first molecule formed that includes the complete purine ring, since the ring is constructed on a phosphoribosyl foundation. IMP is precursor to both AMP and GMP. Carbamoyl phosphate is a pyrimidine precursor, orotate is the first pyrimidine formed in its pathway, and orotidine 5′-monophosphate (OMP) is the first pyrimidine nucleotide. PRPP furnishes the sugar-phosphate for both purine and pyrimidine nucleotides, and phosphoribosylamine is the first metabolite formed in the pathway of purine synthesis. *Biochemistry,* p. 251.
40. The answer is E: It catalyzes the hydrolysis of α-1,4-glycosidic bonds of amylose. α-Amylase catalyzes the hydrolysis of interior α-1,4 bonds of starch (amylose, amylopectin) and glycogen at neutral pH, but the enzyme is unable to attack α-1,6-glycosidic bonds. α-1,6 Bonds are cleaved by the action of isomaltase. α-Amylase is present in both saliva and pancreatic secretions, and its activity in serum can be elevated because of pancreatitis or mumps. α-Amylase does not catalyze the hydrolysis of either lactose (milk sugar) or sucrose, which are hydrolyzed by lactase and sucrase, respectively. α-Amylase is activated by chloride, an extracellular anion, and this property minimizes enzyme activity within the cell because intracellular chloride concentration is low. *Biochemistry,* p. 96.
41. The answer is A: fluoride. Fluoride, which forms fluorapatite, results in teeth and bones that are stronger than those formed exclusively from hydroxyapatite. Intake of excess fluoride for long periods, however, is toxic and produces fluorosis. The omission of fluoride from the diet is not lethal; hence, while fluoride is NOT essential, it is beneficial. Linoleate is an essential fatty acid, and methionine is an essential amino acid. Selenium, a dietary essential, is a component of glutathione peroxidase. Inadequate water intake or excessive water loss is lethal. *Biochemistry,* p. 33.
42. The answer is A: primary structures. The primary structure refers to the sequence of amino acids in a protein, the position of disulfide bonds, and the structures of attached molecules such as oligosaccharides. The secondary structure refers to patterns of hydrogen bonding, and the tertiary structure describes the three-dimensional disposition of the atoms of the molecule. The quaternary structure describes the interaction of subunits of those proteins that contain two or more subunits. The primary structure of a protein determines its secondary, tertiary, and quaternary structure (PRINCIPLE 6 OF BIOCHEMISTRY). *Biochemistry,* p. 46.
43. The answer is E: noncompetitive inhibitors decrease the apparent V_{max} of an enzyme. Captopril, which contains a proline residue found in *bona fide* substrates, is a competitive inhibitor of angiotensin converting enzyme. Inability to overcome inhibition at high substrate concentrations is manifested by an increase in the *y*-intercept on Lineweaver-Burk plots when compared with the noninhibited enzyme. Noncompetitive inhibitors do not resemble the varied substrate, and inhibition cannot be overcome by increasing substrate concentration. *Biochemistry,* pp. 57, 58.
44. The answer is E: tyrosine hydroxylase. Tyrosine hydroxylase catalyzes the first, rate-limiting, and committed step in the biosynthesis of dopamine, norepinephrine, and epinephrine. Aromatic amino acid decarboxylase, the second enzyme in the catecholamine pathway, and dopamine β-hydroxylase, the third enzyme, have higher activities and are not limiting. Glutamate decarboxylase catalyzes the biosynthesis of GABA from glutamate. Phenylalanine hydroxylase, a hepatic enzyme that is deficient in phenylketonuria, participates in tyrosine synthesis and phenylalanine catabolism, and tryptophan hydroxylase is the rate-limiting enzyme in serotonin biosynthesis. Phenylalanine, tyrosine, and tryptophan hydroxylases require their cognate aromatic amino acid, oxygen, and tetrahydrobiopterin as reductant. These hydroxylation reactions, which involve a reaction of oxygen with organic compounds, are unidirectional (PRINCIPLE 8 OF BIOENERGETICS). *Biochemistry,* p. 398.
45. The answer is E: β-hydroxyacyl-CoA dehydrogenase. As a result of this deficiency, β-hydroxyacyl-CoA cannot be catabolized and β-hydroxyacyl-CoA and β-hydroxyacylcarnitine metabolites accumulate. Depletion of coenzyme A diminishes Krebs cycle activity, leading to diminished pyruvate metabolism and lactic acidosis. β-Hydroxyacyl-CoA is transferred from the mitochondrion (as the acylcarnitine derivative) into the cytosol, where it undergoes ω-oxidation in the endoplasmic reticulum to produce β-hydroxydicarboxyl-CoA derivatives. Hydrolysis of these compounds leads to excretion of urinary β-hydroxydicarboxylates. Medium-chain fatty acyl-CoA dehydrogenase deficiency is similar except that the β-hydroxy derivative cannot form. Medium-chain dicarboxylates are excreted in the urine. Succinyl-CoA:acetoacetate CoA-transferase deficiency leads to ketosis owing to the inability to catabolize ketone bodies. Carnitine acyltransferase I deficiency does not produce dicarboxylic aciduria or secondary carnitine deficiency. β-Ketothiolase deficiency refers to that of α-methylacetoacetyl-CoA β-ketothiolase, and patients with this disorder have acidosis, ketosis, hyperammonemia (secondary to inhibition of carbamoyl-phosphate synthetase I by organic acids), and α-methylacetoacetate excretion in the urine. α-Methylacetoacetyl-CoA thiolase is required for isoleucine and phytanate metabolism (phytanate is a chlorophyll derivative found in the diet). *Biochemistry,* p. 158; *Nelson,* p. 337.
46. The answer is C: 3′-phosphoadenosine 5′-phosphosulfate (PAPS). The mixed acid anhydride linkage between sulfate and the 5′-phosphoryl group is very energy rich, having a standard free energy of hydrolysis of −75 kJ mol^{-1}, and thus possesses a high group-transfer potential. Sulfation involves the formation of an ester between sulfate and an alcohol group, typically one of the alco-

hols of a sugar moiety of heparan or dermatan. *S*-Adenosylmethionine is an activated donor of methyl groups, not of sulfate. Glutathione participates in oxidation-reduction reactions and transpeptidation reactions but does not act as a sulfate donor. Taurine and taurocholate are sulfonic acids, in which the sulfur is bound to a carbon atom, and these compounds do not function as sulfate donors in biosynthesis. *Biochemistry,* p. 183; *Nelson,* p. 372.

47. The answer is B: the malate-aspartate shuttle. The malate-aspartate shuttle can transport reducing equivalents into or out of the mitochondrion, depending on cellular conditions. The components of the shuttle consist of four enzymes (cytosolic and mitochondrial aspartate aminotransferases and malate dehydrogenases) and two inner membrane translocases (malate/α-ketoglutarate and aspartate/glutamate). The glycerol-phosphate shuttle is unidirectional, allowing passage of cytosolic reducing equivalents into the membrane transport chain (but not into the matrix). The ATP/ADP and the carnitine/acylcarnitine antiport systems do not move reducing equivalents, and dinitrophenol allows passage of protons through the membrane, but not reducing equivalents, which are defined as either electrons or hydrogen atoms. *Biochemistry,* p. 122.

48. The answer is E: glycine. Glycine is the source of the nitrogen atoms that occur in heme; one of the carbon atoms contributed by glycine occurs in each protoporphyrin ring. Glycine is also the source of the methylene group that links each ring to the adjacent ring. The first and rate-limiting enzyme of the pathway is δ-aminolevulinate (ALA) synthase, and it catalyzes the reaction between succinyl-CoA and glycine. Porphyrias are caused by a deficiency of any of the eight enzymes required for porphyrin synthesis with the exception of ALA synthase; its deficiency has not been observed. *Biochemistry,* p. 490.

49. The answer is A: 1. pH = $-\log[H^+] = -\log\,[1 \times 10^{-1}] = -[-1] = +1$. This is the approximate pH of gastric juice. *Biochemistry,* p. 38.

50. The answer is D: quaternary structure. The quaternary structure refers to the interactions of subunits. Myoglobin, a monomer, does NOT have quaternary structure. The primary structure refers to the amino acid sequence, location of disulfide bonds, and sites of attachment of nonamino acid components. The secondary structure refers to regular hydrogen-bonding patterns such as α-helix, β-sheet (parallel or antiparallel), or β-bend. The tertiary structure refers to the overall three-dimensional conformation. Myoglobin was the first protein whose three-dimensional structure was determined by x-ray crystallography. The release of myoglobin from myocardial cells following ischemia is under development as a diagnostic aid in the detection of a myocardial infarction. *Biochemistry,* p. 48.

51. The answer is B: lactate dehydrogenase deficiency is NOT characterized by little or no change in blood pyruvate levels following exercise. The metabolic lesion involves lactate dehydrogenase, and pyruvate production in exercising muscle is unimpaired. Since NAD^+ must be continuously regenerated for glycolysis to continue, apparently oxidants other than pyruvate perform this function. Diminished muscle LDH is due to a mutation of the M (muscle) isozyme form, and this accounts for the diminished blood lactate production following exercise. The H (heart) form of the enzyme is normal. The heart, moreover, is an aerobic organ and does not release appreciable pyruvate/lactate under physiological conditions. *Biochemistry,* pp. 63, 102.

52. The answer is A: transketolase utilizes thiamine pyrophosphate as cofactor in catalyzing the transfer of a two-carbon fragment from one sugar phosphate to another. Thiamine pyrophosphate is a cofactor in many oxidative decarboxylations (e.g., pyruvate dehydrogenase) but not in the oxidative decarboxylation of 6-phosphogluconate. Transaldolase, which contains a lysine residue at its active site that reacts with substrate, catalyzes the transfer of three-carbon fragments from one sugar phosphate to another. An isomerase catalyzes the interconversion of ribulose 5-phosphate (a ketone) and ribose 5-phosphate (an aldehyde). An epimerase catalyzes the interconversion of ribulose 5-phosphate and xylulose 5-phosphate. Transketolase is not involved in the pathway for ketone body synthesis or utilization. A deficiency of thiamine, the vitamin precursor of thiamine pyrophosphate, is commonly observed in people with alcoholism. *Biochemistry,* p. 103.

53. The answer is A: by dissipating the proton gradient between the mitochondrial matrix and the intermembrane space. Only by dissipating the proton gradient can electron transport (oxidation) be allowed to proceed in the absence of ATP formation (phosphorylation). Inhibiting proton translocation, blocking oxygen reduction, and inhibiting coenzyme QH_2 oxidation would all block both electron transport and ATP formation. Blocking transfer of electrons from cytosol to matrix might decrease the yield of ATP but would not affect the coupling of electron transport within the membrane and ATP formation by ATP synthase. 2,4-Dinitrophenol was used for the treatment of obesity in the 1930s, but its use was abandoned because it caused several deaths. Brown adipose tissue contains mitochondria with an uncoupling protein that dissipates the proton gradient and generates heat in lieu of ATP. Heat generation by brown adipose tissue is especially important in newborns (and in hibernating animals). *Biochemistry,* pp. 126, 128.

54. The answer is A: Human but NOT bacterial DNA occurs physiologically as nucleosome complexes. Human nuclear DNA forms nucleosomes with histones, but bacteria lack histones. A nucleosome consists of a segment of about 160 base pairs that combines with two molecules each of H2A, H2B, H3, and H4, and a linker region of about 40 base pairs that is associated with histone H1. Both human and bacterial DNA have major and minor grooves, consist of an antiparallel duplex (PRINCIPLE 28 OF BIOCHEMISTRY), contain equal molar fractions of adenine and thymine, and contain equal molar fractions of guanine and cytosine. *Biochemistry,* pp. 272–277.

55. The answer is B: potatoes. Plants lack cholesterol, but animal sources contain varying amounts. Sour cream or butter on a baked potato adds a cholesterol-rich nutrient to one that lacks cholesterol. Beef, red meats, pork, cheese, and other dairy products are rich sources of cholesterol. The cholesterol in egg yolks is highly emulsified and is efficiently absorbed. Egg white, in contrast, is nearly cholesterol free. Bacon is rich in cholesterol and triglyceride. Chicken and other fowl are low in triglyceride and cholesterol. A judicious diet is low in cholesterol ($<$300 mg/d) and fat (fat should provide $<$30% of total calories with $\leq$10% saturated fat and $\leq$10% of polyunsaturated fat). Polyunsaturated fat decreases both HDL and LDL cholesterol. Saturated fat increases LDL cholesterol, and monounsaturated fat decreases LDL cholesterol ("bad" cholesterol) and increases HDL cholesterol ("good" cholesterol). About 15% of calories should be protein, and 55% should be complex carbohydrate (found in potatoes, rice, pasta, bread). *Biochemistry,* p. 187.

56. The answer is A: cyclooxygenase. Cyclooxygenase, which is inhibited by aspirin following modification of an active site serine, catalyzes the initial step in synthesis of the cyclic eicosanoids (prostaglandins, prostacyclins, and thromboxanes), while lipoxygenase catalyzes the initial step in the synthesis of linear eicosanoids, the leukotrienes. Nonsteroidal antiinflammatory drugs such as ibuprofen inhibit cyclooxygenase reversibly and not by covalent modification. *Biochemistry,* p. 57.
57. The answer is C: collagen. Human collagen consists of more than one dozen different types of molecules composed of about two dozen genetically distinct α-chains. The role and function of all collagen types have not been determined. Type I collagen, which forms fibrils, accounts for 90% of all collagen by mass. Type IV collagen, which forms meshes and not fibrils, is important because it forms basement membranes. The most distinguishing property of collagen is that each α-chain forms a **left-handed helix** with three amino acid residues per turn. Three left-handed helical polypeptides combine to form a **right-handed triple helical molecule,** which is a long (300 nm), narrow (1.5 nm), ropelike structure. Hemoglobin, actin, and myosin are major protein constituents, but they are not as prevalent as collagen. Albumin is the major serum protein. *Biochemistry,* p. 475.
58. The answer is C: 2. One ATP is required for the fructokinase reaction, and a second ATP is required for the glyceraldehyde kinase reaction; two ATP molecules are produced by the phosphoglycerate kinase reaction, and two additional ATP molecules are produced by the pyruvate kinase reaction. The net yield of ATP is two by substrate level phosphorylation or under anaerobic conditions. Note that the net yield of ATP for the metabolism of fructose and glucose is the same. *Biochemistry,* p. 106.
59. The answer is A: proton translocation across the inner mitochondrial membrane is decreased when ATP synthase lacks bound ADP and P_i, secondarily retarding electron transport. Without bound ADP and P_i, ATP synthase does not allow passage of protons from the intermembrane space to the matrix. The electrochemical proton gradient thereby remains high, blocking further transport of protons from the matrix to the intermembrane space. Since the reactions of electron transport are coupled to obligatory proton translocation (from matrix to intermembrane space), the failure to transport protons means that electron transport must cease also. If membrane electron transport cannot occur, reduced electron carriers–NADH and $FADH_2$–cannot be oxidized to regenerate NAD^+ and FAD. Without NAD^+ and FAD, the oxidative reactions of the Krebs cycle and β-oxidation cannot occur either. In the presence of an agent capable of dissipating the proton gradient by means other than flow through ATP synthase (e.g., 2,4-dinitrophenol or the inner membrane protein **thermogenin,** found in brown adipose tissue), electron transport can continue in the absence of bound ADP and P_i and the system is said to be "uncoupled." Note that (a) the ATP/ADP antiport system delivers ADP into the mitochondrion in exchange for ATP when cytosolic [ADP] is high and mitochondrial [ADP] is low; (b) the proton gradient is steepened, not dissipated, when mitochondrial [ADP] is low; (c) high [ADP], not low [ADP], accelerates Krebs cycle reactions (by activating isocitrate dehydrogenase); and (d) when [ADP] falls, it is usually because ATP is being formed from ADP and P_i, and under these conditions, [AMP] also falls. The one circumstance in which [ADP] and [AMP] move in opposite directions is when, during anaerobic muscle contraction, an initial increase in [ADP] triggers the myokinase reaction in which 2 ADP $\rightarrow$ 1 ATP + 1 AMP. Here, the initially high [ADP] drops as [AMP] and [ATP] increase. *Biochemistry,* p. 132.
60. The answer is E: mitochondrial DNA synthesis does NOT involve Okazaki fragments. Mitochondrial RNA polymerase initiates DNA replication of the H strand at the H strand promoter region, and primer extension is catalyzed by DNA polymerase γ. When H strand synthesis passes the L strand promoter, RNA polymerase initiates replication of this strand, and primer extension is also catalyzed by DNA polymerase γ. This process, in contrast to *E. coli* and human nuclear DNA replication, does not involve Okazaki fragments. The requirement for Okazaki fragments is necessitated by the antiparallel directions of the two strands of the DNA duplex and the ability of DNA polymerases to extend chains in only the 5′ to 3′ direction (PRINCIPLE 29 OF BIOCHEMISTRY). *Biochemistry,* p. 359.
61. The answer is D: information transfer from protein to RNA does NOT occur. This form of information flow is not included in PRINCIPLE 25 OF BIOCHEMISTRY. Somatic DNA rearrangement occurs during the various joining reactions that occur in both heavy and light chain generation. Alternative RNA splicing occurs during isotype switching to IgD from IgM and the formation of the secretory form of IgM. DNA template–independent DNA synthesis is catalyzed by deoxynucleotidyl terminal transferase which produces a hypervariable region in the immunoglobulin. Deletion of portions of DNA found in germ cells occurs during the various DNA rearrangements. *Biochemistry,* pp. 270, 329.
62. The answer is D: chaperones are ATP-requiring proteins that promote the folding of newly synthesized proteins into their functional state. Chaperones are proteins that bind to hydrophobic regions of proteins and promote proper folding to the thermodynamically most stable conformation. The primary structure of a protein determines the secondary, tertiary, and quaternary structure of a protein (PRINCIPLE 6 OF BIOCHEMISTRY), but chaperones accelerate the attainment of equilibrium. Signal peptidases catalyze the removal of signal peptides. G-proteins such as Rab move proteins from the *cis* to *trans* Golgi. *Biochemistry,* p. 372.
63. The answer is B: diisopropylfluorophosphate. Diisopropylfluorophosphate (DFP) is an irreversible inhibitor of acetylcholinesterase. This volatile compound, used in warfare, is extremely toxic; people exposed to DFP are treated with atropine, a muscarinic acetylcholine antagonist. DFP is alkali labile, and spills of DFP are treated with 1 N sodium or potassium hydroxide to destroy the active agent. Nicotine is a plant alkaloid that first stimulates and then inhibits nicotinic receptors. Succinylcholine is used as a muscle relaxant during anesthesia, and d-tubocurarine is an alkaloid poison that produces muscle paralysis. *Biochemistry,* p. 408.
64. The answer is E: the Warburg effect. Tumor cells produce lactate in greater quantities than their normal counterparts despite the presence of usual amounts of oxygen, mitochondria, Krebs cycle enzymes, and electron transport chains. The mechanism for this effect involves the expression of a fetal form of phosphofructokinase in tumor cells that is not regulated allosterically like the adult enzyme. The Pasteur effect refers to the inhibition of glycolysis by oxygen and aerobic metabolism. The mechanism of this effect is related to the energy charge. Owing to the generation of ATP dur-

ing aerobic metabolism, phosphofructokinase is inhibited. As a result, fructose 6-phosphate and glucose 6-phosphate accumulate. Glucose 6-phosphate is an inhibitor of hexokinase, and inhibition of this enzyme inhibits the entire Embden-Myerhof glycolytic pathway. In the transition to anaerobic metabolism (e.g., in muscle during a 100-m sprint), oxidative metabolism cannot generate adequate ATP. Anaerobic metabolism results in increased ADP and then AMP. AMP activates glycolysis, decreases the concentration of glucose 6-phosphate, and removes an inhibitor of hexokinase. Removal of an inhibitor of hexokinase results in increased glucose consumption. The Ames test is used for screening for potential carcinogens. Krebs is the eponym of the famous tricarboxylic acid cycle and not an effect. The Crabtree effect refers to the suppression of oxidative metabolism by high glycolytic activity. *Biochemistry,* p. 437.

65. The answer is C: P ATPase. The proton/potassium-ATPase possesses a phosphorylated protein-aspartate intermediate and is an example of a class P enzyme. F ATPases are mitochondrial (in humans) or plasma membrane (in bacteria) ATP synthases that are powered by a proton gradient. V ATPases generate proton gradients in vesicles such as lysosomes or secretory granules. M ATPases have not been described. *Biochemistry,* p. 363.

66. The answer is A: ATP. The protein that converts chemical energy to mechanical energy is myosin, and ATP is the substrate for myosin. When high-energy metabolites are measured in exercising skeletal muscle, creatine phosphate levels are decreased and lactate is produced. Earlier theories of muscle contraction were based upon creatine phosphate or lactate as the source of chemical energy that produced motion. After the discovery of the ATPase activity of myosin, these theories were discarded. The discovery of myosin ATPase was an important observation that led to the law of the universality of ATP as the common currency of energy exchange (PRINCIPLE 10 OF BIOCHEMISTRY). *Biochemistry,* p. 471.

67. The answer is B: prothrombin time. The prothrombin time reflects the functional state of both extrinsic and intrinsic pathways of blood clotting. A normal prothrombin time requires adequate fibrinogen, factor X, factor VII, factor V, and prothrombin. Because the production of factors II, VII, IX, and X require vitamin K for the carboxylation of protein-glutamate, the prothrombin time is employed to monitor anticoagulant therapy with vitamin K antagonists such as warfarin and coumarin. The activated partial thromboplastin time (aPTT) is used to monitor the therapeutic effects of heparin, also used in the treatment of acute pulmonary emboli and myocardial infarctions. People with hemophilia A or B also have elevated aPTT values. Platelets are required in the early phase of blood clotting, and thrombocytopenia (low platelet count) can lead to bleeding episodes. *Biochemistry,* p. 497.

68. The answer is D: insulin receptor. The insulin receptor is a tetramer that consists of a dimer of $\alpha\beta$ subunits that are bound in β-α-α-β linkage by three disulfide bonds. The α-subunits, which are extracellular, bind insulin. As a result of ligand binding, the intracellular β-subunits, which possess protein-tyrosine kinase activity, are activated. This kinase undergoes self-phosphorylation and interacts with proteins that contain SH2 domains (src homology 2 domains that recognize protein-tyrosine phosphate) and alters their activity. The insulin receptor also phosphorylates other proteins including IRS-1 (insulin receptor substrate–1), which binds to proteins with SH2 domains to trigger regulatory cascades. Some adaptor proteins also contain SH3 domains that recognize a proline-containing motif called Src-homology domain 3. As a result of downstream events, serine/threonine protein phosphorylation also occurs in response to insulin. Important components of this signal transduction cascade include Ras and the Raf-Mek-Erk kinase system. AMP-dependent protein kinase, fructose-6-phosphate-2-kinase, and pyruvate dehydrogenase kinase are protein-serine/threonine kinases. The glucagon receptor is a seven-transmembrane-segment protein that interacts with G-proteins, but it lacks protein kinase activity. *Biochemistry,* p. 426.

69. The answer is D: ω-oxidation. ω-Oxidation occurs in the endoplasmic reticulum, uses NADPH, oxygen, and cytochrome P-450, and converts the ω-methyl group of a free fatty acid to a carboxylate, thus forming a dicarboxylic acid. Because medium-chain fatty acyl-CoA dehydrogenase deficiency results in the accumulation of medium-chain fatty acyl-CoA, alternative routes of metabolism such as ω-oxidation become more prevalent. α-Oxidation, which occurs in the peroxisome, is initiated by reactions that oxidize the α-carbon of a free fatty acid, requires NADPH, molecular oxygen and cytochromes, and results in the formation of a free fatty acid with one fewer carbon atom following the release of carbon dioxide. This pathway is required for the degradation of phytanic acid, formed from the phytol side chain of chlorophyll. β-Oxidation, which occurs in the mitochondrion and in the peroxisome, involves oxidation of the β-carbon of the acyl chain to a keto group prior to thiolytic cleavage by coenzyme A. Peroxisomes initiate the degradation of fatty acids longer than 18 carbons, which does not occur readily in the mitochondrion, by a β-oxidation process in which the initial step uses molecular oxygen and produces hydrogen peroxide. There is no common biochemical process called δ-oxidation, and the final common pathway of metabolism is the Krebs cycle. *Biochemistry,* p. 161.

70. The answer is A: desmosine. Desmosine, which is a hallmark of elastin, is formed by cross-linking different elastin chains; the participants in the cross-linking include three aldehyde groups derived from lysine and one unmodified lysine. Glycine at every third residue is a hallmark of collagen. Hydroxyproline occurs in collagen and elastin; hydroxylysine occurs in collagen. Hydroxynorleucine is a cross-linking residue that occurs in collagen. *Biochemistry,* p. 479.

71. The answer is D: glutamine PRPP amidotransferase is inhibited, NOT activated, by IMP. All the common purine nucleoside monophosphates, plus the drug derivative, allopurinol ribonucleotide, allosterically inhibit this regulatory enzyme, which catalyzes the first committed step in *de novo* purine nucleotide synthesis. PRPP is both a substrate and an allosteric activator of the enzyme. *Biochemistry,* p. 506.

72. The answer is D: 10 mM.

$$\begin{aligned} pH &= 6.1 + \log [HCO_3^-]/[CO_2 + H_2CO_3] \\ 7.1 &= 6.1 + \log [HCO_3^-]/[CO_2 + H_2CO_3] \\ 1.0 &= \log [HCO_3^-]/[CO_2 + H_2CO_3] \\ 1.0 &= \log [HCO_3^-]/1.0 \text{ mM} \\ 10 &= [HCO_3^-]/1.0 \text{ mM} \\ [HCO_3^-] &= 10 \text{ mM} \end{aligned}$$

This pH, which can be normal in saliva, represents a severe acidic condition when it occurs in the general circulation. *Biochemistry,* pp. 38–39.

73. The answer is A: fructose. The metabolism of fructose in liver via reactions catalyzed by fructokinase, aldolase B, and glyceraldehyde kinase, bypasses the phosphofructokinase reaction, the primary regulatory step of glycolysis. These reactions occur in liver and allow this organ to metabolize fructose despite the presence of large amounts of glucose. Fructose is an abundant sugar in the diet (as free fructose in fruit and as a constituent of sucrose), and dietary intake of 100 g daily is not unusual. Galactose is converted to glucose 6-phosphate in three steps and is metabolized by glycolysis. Mannose is converted to fructose 6-phosphate in two steps, and mannose metabolism does not bypass the phosphofructokinase reaction. Trehalose, which is a nonreducing disaccharide found in mushrooms, is hydrolyzed to produce two molecules of glucose, which are metabolized by glycolysis. *Biochemistry,* p. 106.
74. The answer is E: Fe^{+3} and Fe^{+2}. Heme iron in the cytochromes of electron transport alternates between the oxidized ferric (Fe^{+3}) and reduced ferrous (Fe^{+2}) states. The heme of hemoglobin and myoglobin, in contrast, remains in the ferrous state (Fe^{+2}) after binding oxygen. *Biochemistry,* p. 69.
75. The answer is D: 12. Recall that conversion of one glucose to two pyruvate yields two ATP (by substrate level phosphorylation) and two cytosolic NADH. Transport of electrons from two NADH by the malate-aspartate shuttle yields two NADH in the mitochondrion. Conversion of two pyruvate to two acetyl-CoA yields two more mitochondrial NADH (for a total of four). Ten ATP derived from NADH oxidation (2.5 ATP per NADH), added to the two from glycolysis, yields 12. This calculation corresponds to the energy yield during preparatory reactions for fatty acid synthesis. When dietary carbohydrate is converted to fat in the liver, glucose is converted to acetyl-CoA, which is not further oxidized but is transported to the cytosol for subsequent fatty acid synthesis. *Biochemistry,* p. 132.
76. The answer is C: cysteine and histidine. Each zinc finger domain contains about 30 residues, including two cysteines, two histidines, and several hydrophobic amino acid residues. The zinc atom is bound to the two cysteine and two histidine residues. Zinc finger proteins often bind to DNA. Examples of zinc finger proteins include the glucocorticoid and estrogen steroid hormone receptors and transcription factor TFIIIA. The nitrogen of histidine is a good metal-binding substance. In some proteins, however, all four zinc binding amino acids are cysteine, and a second class of zinc finger protein results. *Biochemistry,* p. 50.
77. The answer is A: amylose. Amylose, a component of plant starch, is a straight-chain polymer of D-glucosyl units in α-1,4 linkage. Cellulose contains D-glucosyl units linked by β-1,4 glycosidic bonds. Glycogen consists of D-glucosyl units in α-1,4 linkage with α-1,6 branch points. Fructan is a bacterially produced polymer made of D-fructosyl units containing β-1,2-furanoside bonds, and mutan is a bacterially produced polymer of D-glucosyl units containing α-1,3 and α-1,6 linkages. *Biochemistry,* p. 95.
78. The answer is D: fructose 6-phosphate. Fructose 6-phosphate is a substrate for phosphofructokinase, but it is not an allosteric regulator. ATP is both a substrate and allosteric inhibitor. Citrate allosterically inhibits while AMP and fructose 2,6-bisphosphate allosterically activate phosphofructokinase. The actions of ATP and AMP reflect regulation by the energy charge. Citrate is elevated in cells that are using fatty acids as a fuel, which decreases the need for glycolysis. Fructose 2,6-bisphosphate, which is a specialized regulatory molecule whose concentration is decreased as a result of the action of cyclic AMP, is the most important regulator of phosphofructokinase. *Biochemistry,* p. 502.
79. The answer is E: linoleate. An essential nutrient is one that is required for life and must be provided in the diet because of the inability of humans to synthesize it in adequate amounts, if at all. Linoleate is elongated and desaturated to produce arachidonate, a precursor of prostaglandins, prostacyclins, and thromboxane. Myristate (14:0), palmitate (16:0), oleate (18:1), and palmitoleate (16:1) can be synthesized by humans. *Biochemistry,* p. 33.
80. The answer is D: ornithine. Ornithine is an important intermediate in urea synthesis. It is a noncoded amino acid, and it is NOT incorporated into proteins. In order for protein synthesis to occur, all 20 of the coded amino acids found in proteins must be available, derived either from the diet or from endogenous sources. A deficiency of a single amino acid interrupts protein synthesis by failure to provide a required precursor. Methionine, isoleucine, leucine, and phenylalanine are essential amino acids in humans, and the elimination of any of them from the diet eliminates a required component of protein synthesis. During normal protein turnover, some of the liberated amino acids are metabolized before they can be incorporated into new protein. Failure to replenish even a single amino acid retards protein synthesis and results in the catabolism of the remaining amino acids as well. Excretion of more nitrogen than is taken in, which can occur as a result of the deficiency of a single amino acid, represents negative nitrogen balance. The production of asparagine deficiency by asparaginase accounts for the antitumorigenic effect of this treatment. Asparaginase catalyzes the hydrolysis of asparagine, and by decreasing the concentration of this amino acid in the serum, tumor cells that cannot synthesize adequate asparagine are unable to synthesize their full complement of protein. *Biochemistry,* p. 33.
81. The answer is C: utilization of *p*-aminobenzoate in folate synthesis. Sulfonamides block *p*-aminobenzoate utilization in sensitive bacteria. Some bacteria cannot import preformed folate and must synthesize their own, using *p*-aminobenzoate as an intermediate substrate. The sulfonamides resemble *p*-aminobenzoate in structure and act as competitive inhibitors in the synthetic pathway. Without folate the bacteria cannot form purines and pyrimidines and thus cannot proliferate. Dihydrofolate reductase, adenylosuccinate synthetase, IMP dehydrogenase, carbamoyl-phosphate synthetase, and cell-wall peptidoglycan biosynthesis are not directly inhibited by sulfonamides. Dihydrofolate reductase, however, is inhibited by methotrexate in humans and by trimethoprim in bacteria. Adenylosuccinate synthetase and IMP dehydrogenase are inhibited by 6-thioinosine 5'-monophosphate, which is formed in the body after administration of 6-mercaptopurine, a hypoxanthine analogue. Cell-wall peptidoglycan synthesis is inhibited by penicillin. Although experimental compounds are available, carbamoyl-phosphate synthetase inhibitors are not used clinically. *Biochemistry,* p. 265.
82. The answer is E: σ (sigma) factor. The protein subunit structure of the *E. coli* RNA polymerase holoenzyme is $\alpha_2\beta\beta'\sigma$. The β and β' subunits are unrelated despite the similarity of the designations. *E. coli* RNA polymerase with a sigma (σ) subunit recognizes and binds to special sequences of DNA (promoters) that direct the initiation of gene transcription. Promoters include

about 50 nucleotides on the 5′ side of the transcription unit and extend about 20 nucleotides into the transcription unit. ρ (Rho) is a transcription termination factor. *Biochemistry,* p. 308.

83. The answer is B: thromboplastin or factor III. Thromboplastin is the tissue factor that initiates the extrinsic pathway of blood coagulation. The intrinsic pathway does not require an extrinsic factor and is initiated by an abnormal surface. There is a complex interplay between the two pathways *in vivo* that is obscured by the designation of the separate pathways. Activation of the intrinsic pathway involves prekallikrein, factor XII, and high molecular mass kininogen. The intrinsic and extrinsic pathways converge to form the common pathway. *Biochemistry,* p. 495.
84. The answer is E: reversal of glucagon effects does NOT involve increased dephosphorylation of fructose 1,6-bisphosphate to form fructose 6-phosphate. This gluconeogenic reaction is stimulated (indirectly) by the glucagon cascade, so reversal would decrease this activity. As glucagon levels fall in the blood, the hormone dissociates from its plasma membrane receptor in the liver. G_s hydrolyzes GTP to GDP, so that adenylyl cyclase is no longer stimulated, and no more cyclic AMP is formed. The cyclic AMP already present is hydrolyzed to 5′-AMP by phosphodiesterase, allowing the active C subunits of protein kinase A to rejoin the (inhibitory) R or regulatory subunits to deactivate the kinase. At this point, the proteins, previously phosphorylated by the various relevant kinases, lose their phosphoryl groups in exergonic hydrolytic reactions (PRINCIPLE 5 OF BIOENERGETICS) catalyzed by protein phosphatase–1. The final result is a return to the original state, in which glycogen is not being degraded and gluconeogenisis is less active. Whether or not glycogen synthesis or glycolysis will occur at greatly increased rates is determined by the metabolic needs of the cell at the moment. *Biochemistry,* pp. 143–146.
85. The answer is C: hydrogen. The hydrogen bonds in the α-helix connect the carbonyl oxygen of residue n with the amino group of residue n + 4. The hydrogen bonds of the β-sheet connect residues that are far apart. β-Pleated sheets whose chains extend in the same direction are parallel; β-sheets whose chains extend in opposite directions are antiparallel. Hydrogen bonds, ionic bonds, and van der Waals bonds are weak, whereas covalent bonds are strong. Hydrogen bonding in nucleic acids is also called secondary structure. Disulfide bonds that result from the oxidation of two cysteine residues represent part of the primary structure of a protein. Resonance refers to the representation of a molecule that cannot be portrayed by a single valence structure but can be embodied as a hybrid of two or more structures where all of the atomic nuclei remain in the same position. *Biochemistry,* p. 203.
86. The answer is B: phospholipase A_2. The ester bond at the *sn*-2 position of phospholipids is hydrolyzed in a reaction catalyzed by phospholipase A_2; fatty acids esterified at this position are generally unsaturated and serve as precursors of the eicosanoids including prostaglandins, prostacyclins, thromboxanes, and leukotrienes. The ester bond at *sn*-1 is hydrolyzed by phospholipase A_1, and the ester bond between phosphatidate and the polar substituent is catalyzed by phospholipase D. Phospholipase C cleaves glycerophospholipids between diglyceride and the phosphorylated polar substituent. Phospholipase C, operating on phosphatidylinositol bisphosphate, generates diglyceride and inositol trisphosphate, two second messengers. *Biochemistry,* p. 203.
87. The answer is D: lecithin-cholesterol acyltransferase (LCAT). This enzyme is responsible for converting cholesterol, released from cells to HDL, to cholesterol ester. In the absence of this enzyme, cholesterol ester cannot be formed, and this results in decreased cholesteryl ester in plasma lipoproteins. Moreover, a deficiency of LCAT results in alterations of virtually all of the plasma lipoproteins: HDL and LDL cholesterol levels are low; triglycerides are generally high, and lipoproteins have abnormal electrophoretic mobility. There is no specific treatment for this very rare inborn error of metabolism, and dietary management includes stringent fat restriction. A similar clinical picture can result from a mutation in the apoprotein A-I gene. This apoprotein is synthesized by both liver and intestine, is found in chylomicrons, and is the major apoprotein in HDL. Its function is to activate LCAT, the cholesteryl ester–forming enzyme. The genes for apo-A-I and apo-C-III are next to each other on chromosome 11, but they are in opposite orientations. An inversion of 5.5 kb of DNA containing portions of the A-I and C-III genes results in the loss of both proteins. Acid lipase is a lysosomal enzyme that catalyzes the conversions of cholesteryl ester in cells to free cholesterol. This liberated cholesterol is converted to cholesteryl ester by ACAT (acyl-CoA: cholesterol acyltransferase), a cytosolic enzyme. Hepatic lipase is an extracellular enzyme that catalyzes the hydrolysis of triglyceride and phospholipids in high-density lipoprotein (HDL) and intermediate-density lipoprotein (IDL). The enzyme is located in liver sinusoids and plays a role in the metabolic degradation of these two classes of lipoprotein. The fatty acids are taken up by the liver. Lipoprotein lipase catalyzes the hydrolysis of triglyceride in very low density lipoprotein (VLDL) and chylomicrons. This enzyme is located at the capillary surface throughout the body, where it is bound to heparin. Lipoprotein lipase is responsible for generating fatty acids and glycerol at the tissue level, where the fatty acid will be taken up by the surrounding cells. *Biochemistry,* p. 191.
88. The answer is B: contains an acetyl group at *sn*-2. Platelet activating factor (PAF) was named because it causes platelet degranulation. Platelet activating factor, however, functions in vascular epithelium, blood cells, brain, kidney, liver, and muscle. Other glycerophospholipids contain a long-chain acyl group, usually unsaturated, at *sn*-2. Plasmalogens contain an ether bond at *sn*-1, and phosphatidylcholine contains phosphocholine at *sn*-3. Plasmalogens, in which the alkyl group at *sn*-1 is unsaturated, are especially prevalent in nervous tissue. *Biochemistry,* p. 155.
89. The answer is B: proteins become denatured. pH 1 is very acidic and denatures most proteins. Exceptions include pepsin (a gastric peptidase) and gastric lipase. These enzymes function in gastric juice and are not denatured at this acidic pH. As a result of the acidic conditions, ingested proteins become protonated; the carboxylate side chains are converted to uncharged carboxylic acids, and essentially all lysines and histidines become positively charged. Although some microbes and viruses survive the acid pH, acid gastric juice is an unfavorable environment for most microbes (because of the acidity). *Biochemistry,* p. 49.
90. The answer is E: Phosphatidyl 4,5-bisphosphate is NOT formed from diglyceride and CDP-inositol 4,5-bisphosphate. The biosynthetic pathway involves a reaction between CDP-diglyceride and inositol (forming phosphatidylinositol), followed by two successive phosphorylations of the inositol moiety. Phosphatidylinosi-

tol 4,5-bisphosphate is hydrolyzed by phospholipase C to diglyceride and inositol 1,4,5-trisphosphate, each of which serves as a second messenger within the cell. Diglyceride activates protein kinase C, which then phosphorylates various intracellular proteins and alters their activities. Many protein kinase C isoforms also require ionic calcium. The interaction of inositol 1,4,5-trisphosphate with intracellular receptors leads to the release of calcium from storage sites within the endoplasmic reticulum. *Biochemistry,* p. 181.

91. The answer is G: glucose-6-phosphatase. Glucose-6-phosphatase, which catalyzes the hydrolysis of glucose 6-phosphate, is present only in liver, kidney, and intestine. This enzyme liberates glucose from the liver and kidney, which are active in gluconeogenesis, to maintain blood glucose. The intestinal enzyme participates in the translocation of glucose from the gut lumen to the portal blood. *Biochemistry,* p. 136.
92. The answer is P: phosphoglycerate kinase. Phosphoglycerate kinase catalyzes the isoergonic and bidirectional interconversion of 1,3-bisphosphoglycerate and ADP to 3-phosphoglycerate and ATP according to PRINCIPLE 1 OF BIOENERGETICS. The reactions catalyzed by hexokinase, glucokinase (an isozyme of hexokinase), and phosphofructokinase are exergonic and unidirectional according to PRINCIPLE 2 OF BIOENERGETICS. The pyruvate kinase reaction, which is the sole exception to PRINCIPLE 1 OF BIOENERGETICS, is exergonic and unidirectional despite the lack of difference in the number of high energy bonds in reactants and products. *Biochemistry,* p. 99.
93. The answer is I: glycogen phosphorylase. Pyridoxal phosphate is a cofactor for all human transaminase enzymes, for serine/threonine dehydratase, for glutamate decarboxylase, and for several other enzymes where it combines initially with an amino group of the substrate to form a Schiff base. Pyridoxal phosphate is bound covalently to glycogen phosphorylase as a Schiff base, but it functions as an acid during catalysis and does not form a Schiff base with the glycogen substrate. It is this exceptional behavior that accounts for the frequent appearance of this question on biochemistry examinations. *Biochemistry,* p. 142.
94. The answer is H: glucose-6-phosphate dehydrogenase. Mutant forms of this enzyme are sensitive to the oxidative stress produced by antimalarials such as chloroquine. Administration of such drugs to sensitive people produces dramatic hemolytic anemia accompanied by the excretion of hemoglobin in the urine, which gives rise to dark urine. *Biochemistry,* p. 103.
95. The answer is T: succinate dehydrogenase. This enzyme, which is an integral membrane protein found in the inner mitochondrial membrane, contains a covalently bound FAD that accepts reducing equivalents from succinate. Succinate dehydrogenase reduces coenzyme Q. This electron transport pathway generates 1.5 moles of ATP per mole of succinate by oxidative phosphorylation. Succinate dehydrogenase is inhibited by malonate, and this inhibition aided Krebs in his elucidation of the celebrated metabolic cycle bearing his name. *Biochemistry,* p. 113.
96. The answer is L: hormone-sensitive lipase. Hormone-sensitive lipase in adipocytes is activated by glucagon and epinephrine, hence its designation as hormone sensitive. These hormones promote release of fatty acids from adipocytes into the circulation, and these fatty acids serve as a source of fuel for most tissues. During the anabolic phase of metabolism, such as occurs after eating, insulin decreases the activity of this enzyme and thereby inhibits fatty acid release and utilization. Of physiological importance, the concentrations of insulin that diminish hormone-sensitive lipase activity are lower than those required to recruit GLUT4 insulin-responsive glucose transporters to the plasma membrane in target cells. Hormone-sensitive lipase is important in providing fatty acid substrates for oxidative metabolism by most cells (except red blood cells and brain), and this enzyme is important during exercise, during overnight and prolonged fasts, and during starvation. Unopposed activation of hormone-sensitive lipase during diabetes mellitus drives ketosis. *Biochemistry,* p. 512.
97. The answer is D: hyperprolinemia. Glutamate γ-semialdehyde spontaneously forms Δ1-pyrroline-5-carboxylate, a compound in the pathway in the degradation of proline. A defect in the dehydrogenase that catalyzes the oxidation of glutamate γ-semialdehyde to glutamate is responsible for type II hyperprolinemia. Type I hyperprolinemia is due to a deficiency of proline dehydrogenase, the first enzyme of the catabolic pathway for proline. Both disorders are benign and do not require treatment. Histidinemia and urocanic aciduria, due to deficiencies of histidine ammonia lyase and urocanase, respectively, are also benign inborn errors of metabolism that do not require treatment. *Nelson,* p. 325.
98. The answer is G: tyrosinemia. A deficiency of fumarylacetoacetate hydrolase, which produces tyrosinemia (type I), results in a moderate elevation of serum tyrosine that results in malfunction of the liver, kidney, and nervous system. The pathology is thought to be due to the accumulation of tyrosine metabolites such as succinylacetone. Death from the acute form occurs before 2 years of age and from a chronic form by 10 years. Diagnosis of this autosomal recessive disease is made by enzyme assay of liver biopsy specimens or fibroblasts in culture. Prenatal diagnosis has been made by assaying succinylacetone in the amniotic fluid. Type II tyrosinemia, also an autosomal recessive disease, is due to a deficiency of hepatic cytosolic tyrosine aminotransferase. Significant hypertyrosinemia and tyrosinuria are present. In contrast to type I tyrosinemia, liver and kidney function is normal. Dietary restriction of phenylalanine and tyrosine is the recommended treatment. *Nelson,* p. 310.
99. The answer is F: phenylketonuria. A defect in phenylalanine hydroxylase, or in enzymes associated with tetrahydrobiopterin metabolism, diminishes the conversion of phenylalanine to tyrosine. Alternative routes of phenylalanine disposal are used; these involve transamination to form phenylpyruvate (a phenylketone), with subsequent conversion to phenyllactate, phenylacetate, and phenylacetylglutamine, which appear in the urine. The accumulation of phenylalanine and these catabolites has severe effects on growth and mental development, and since these defects are comparatively common, nearly all infants in the United States are screened at birth for the disease. Early intervention and dietary control can greatly decrease the severity of the symptoms. *Biochemistry,* p. 231.
100. The answer is G: rough endoplasmic reticulum and Golgi. The intracellular (endoplasmic) membrane network (reticulum) is divided into smooth and rough portions based upon their electron microscopic appearance. The rough endoplasmic reticulum, which received its name because the ribosomes attached to the membrane give it a "rough" appearance, is the site for initiating posttranslational modification of proteins including glycosylation. Proteins are translocated to the Golgi, where further glycosylation reactions occur

prior to insertion into the plasma membrane or secretion from the cell. *Biochemistry,* p. 385.

101. The answer is A: cytosol. After invasion of target cells, reverse transcriptase synthesizes complementary DNA from the RNA template in the cytosol. Since AZT inhibits reverse transcriptase function, the site of its therapeutic effect is the cytosol. Integration of the double-stranded DNA provirus occurs subsequently in the nucleus. *Biochemistry,* p. 336.

102. The answer is C: mitochondrion. The mitochondrion contains the enzymes of the energy-generating Krebs cycle including α-ketoglutarate dehydrogenase, which catalyzes a unidirectional reaction. The Krebs cycle enzymes are found in the matrix, except for succinate dehydrogenase, which occurs in the inner mitochondrial membrane. ATP synthase and the components of the electron transport chain occur in the inner mitochondrial membrane. The enzymes of the Krebs cycle are encoded by nuclear DNA. A few polypeptide components of ATP synthase and the electron transport chain are encoded by mitochondrial DNA. *Biochemistry,* p. 110.

103. The answer is I: methotrexate. Methotrexate is an inhibitor of dihydrofolate reductase, which catalyzes the conversion of dietary folate to di- and tetrahydrofolate. Dihydrofolate is also generated in the thymidylate synthase reaction, where methylenetetrahydrofolate acts as a reductant and methyl group donor. Methotrexate prevents the regeneration of tetrahydrofolate from dihydrofolate, accounting for the effectiveness of this medication. *Biochemistry,* p. 257.

104. The answer is F: fluorouracil. 5-Fluorouracil (FU) must be converted to a nucleoside monophosphate before any effect on cellular metabolism occurs. Orotate phosphoribosyltransferase, one of the two activities of the UMP synthase complex of pyrimidine synthesis, catalyzes the reaction of PRPP with fluorouracil. Fluorouridine monophosphate can be converted to the diphosphate in a reaction involving ATP. Fluorouridine diphosphate can be converted to fluorodeoxyuridine diphosphate as catalyzed by ribonucleotide reductase. Fluorodeoxyuridine monophosphate, derived from precursors, is a suicide inhibitor of thymidylate synthase. Suicide inhibition requires the generation of an active species, during an abortive catalytic cycle, that reacts with and inactivates the enzyme. Fluorouridine triphosphate can also be incorporated into RNA, and this incorporation diminishes the posttranscriptional processing and physiological activity of RNA. The clinical efficacy of fluorouracil is due to its incorporation into RNA and to inhibition of thymidylate synthase. *Biochemistry,* p. 256.

105. The answer is G: hydroxyurea. Hydroxyurea, which is a chemical scavenger that destroys an active site protein-tyrosyl free radical intermediate, is an inhibitor of the ribonucleoside diphosphate reductase. Hydroxyurea decreases the formation of deoxyribonucleoside precursors of DNA. *Biochemistry,* p. 453.

106. The answer is E: daunorubicin. Daunorubicin and doxorubicin produce breaks in DNA in a process that involves topoisomerase II. Topoisomerase II forms phosphodiesters through protein-tyrosine residues with the backbone of DNA during the catalytic cycle. Topoisomerase II thereby creates discontinuities in DNA during its catalytic cycle, and daunorubicin and doxorubicin abort complete catalysis and thereby produce aberrant DNA cleavage. Etoposide and teniposide also cause topoisomerase II to cleave DNA in an aberrant reaction. *Biochemistry,* p. 453.

107. The answer is M: thyrotropin-releasing hormone. This substance, with the structure pyroglutamylhistidylprolinamide, is a tripeptide that is synthesized by an mRNA-dependent ribosomal mechanism and posttranslational processing. The pyroglutamyl group is derived from a glutamine residue by cyclization, and the amide group is derived from glycine. TRH can be used in the diagnosis of thyroid dysfunction, but it is not used therapeutically. *Biochemistry,* p. 421.

108. The answer is D: atrial natriuretic peptide. This hormone is synthesized and secreted by the atrium and interacts with plasma membrane receptors with intrinsic guanylyl cyclase activity. The receptor consists of a single polypeptide chain with an extracellular hormonal recognition domain, a single transmembrane segment, and an intracellular catalytic domain. The action of cyclic GMP is to activate protein kinase G, its cognate protein kinase. The physiological substrates for protein kinase G are uncertain. *Biochemistry,* p. 431.

109. The answer is J: renin. Renin, which is produced by the juxtaglomerular cells of the kidney, is released in response to β-adrenergic receptor activation by the postganglionic sympathetic nervous system. Renin catalyzes the hydrolytic release of angiotensin I from renin substrate, a protein produced by the liver. Inhibition of renin release may contribute to the therapeutic effects of β-blockers used in the treatment of cardiovascular diseases. *Biochemistry,* p. 431.

110. The answer is A: adrenocorticotropic hormone (ACTH). Addison disease, or hypoadrenocorticism, is accompanied by elevated levels of ACTH as part of a feedback loop of reciprocal hormone regulation. This polypeptide hormone, which contains 39 amino acids, includes an amino acid sequence homologous to melanocyte-stimulating hormone (MSH), and elevated levels of ACTH activate MSH receptors and lead to the increased skin pigmentation observed in these patients. *Biochemistry,* p. 243.

111. The answer is C: *S*-adenosylmethionine. *S*-Adenosylmethionine transfers its activated methyl group to specific lysine residues in acceptor proteins in accordance with PRINCIPLE 17 OF BIOCHEMISTRY. Monomethyl- and dimethyllysine occur in cytochrome *c,* and trimethyllysine occurs in calmodulin. Proteolysis of calmodulin and other proteins yields trimethyllysine, a precursor of carnitine. Trimethyllysine is transported to the liver and kidney, where carnitine synthesis occurs. In a reaction involving oxygen, α-ketoglutarate, and ascorbate, trimethyllysine is converted to β-hydroxy-*N*-trimethyllysine, succinate, carbon dioxide, and dehydroascorbate. A lyase converts the β-hydroxy derivative to glycine and butyrobetaine aldehyde, which is oxidized by NAD^+ to yield butyrobetaine. Butyrobetaine reacts with oxygen, α-ketoglutarate, and ascorbate to form carnitine, succinate, carbon dioxide, and dehydroascorbate. Carnitine is transported from liver and kidney to other cells that require carnitine. *Biochemistry,* p. 375.

112. The answer is I: palmitoyl-CoA. Sphinganine, a precursor of sphingosine, is a C_{18} alcohol that is derived from palmitoyl-CoA (C_{16}) and serine (C_3); the products are dihydrosphinganine, carbon dioxide, and coenzyme A. *Biochemistry,* p. 180.

113. The answer is E: farnesyl pyrophosphate. Farnesyl pyrophosphate is a C_{10} isoprenoid that is on the pathway of cholesterol synthesis. This compound also reacts with Ras, a G-protein that occurs in a mutated form in 25% of all human cancers, to form a thioether with a protein cysteine four residues from the carboxyterminal end. This modification of Ras is required for its biological activity. Drugs that inhibit the farnesylation of Ras rep-

resent a potential therapy for several forms of neoplasia. *Biochemistry,* pp. 189, 387.

114. The answer is G: N^5-methyltetrahydrofolate. A deficiency of methylenetetrahydrofolate reductase results in the failure to synthesize N^5-methyltetrahydrofolate, a substrate for homocysteine methyltransferase. As a result of reductase deficiency, homocysteine is not converted to methionine, and homocystinuria results. Other causes of homocystinuria include a deficiency of cystathionine synthase (which produces classical homocystinuria) and aberrations of methylcobalamin formation from cobalamin. *Biochemistry,* p. 242; *Nelson,* p. 314.
115. The answer is A: calcium. Calcium, which binds to γ-carboxyglutamate residues present in blood clotting factors II, VII, IX, and X, is required for blood clotting. Inclusion of EDTA in test tubes, which chelates calcium, prevents the conversion of blood plasma to serum. Calcium, moreover, is a chief constituent of bone and teeth, and a 70-kg human contains about 1 kg of calcium. *Biochemistry,* p. 495.
116. The answer is J: potassium. When potassium intake is restricted, unavoidable potassium loss (about 40 mEq/d) in the urine occurs, and intravenous fluids must include this amount to prevent potassium depletion. One ampule of KCl contains 20 mEq, and two ampules are given per day. When sodium intake is restricted, sodium can be conserved and only trace amounts are lost. The intracellular concentration of potassium is about 100 mM and that in the blood plasma and the interstitial fluid is about 4 mM. The chief extracellular cation is sodium; its concentration is about 140 mM in the blood plasma and about 10 mM intracellularly. *Biochemistry,* p. 15.
117. The answer is F: iodide. Iodide is incorporated into thyroglobulin by a process mediated by thyroid peroxidase; cathepsins catalyze the degradation of thyroglobulin to T_3 and T_4 (thyroid hormones). Oceans contain appreciable iodide, but some inland lakes and streams lack iodide. Iodide is added to table salt (sodium chloride) in many parts of the world to prevent the development of goiter. *Biochemistry,* p. 391.
118. The answer is C: cobalt. The only known role of cobalt in biology is as a component of vitamin B_{12}. In humans, this vitamin participates in the methylmalonyl-CoA mutase reaction during the metabolism of propionyl-CoA and in the N^5-methyl-THF homocysteine methyltransferase reaction resulting in methionine formation. *Biochemistry,* p. 15.
119. The answer is K: radon. Radon is a gas that is derived from the fission of uranium. This element escapes from the ground into dwellings and exposes inhabitants to high-energy radiation. *Biochemistry,* p. 17.
120. The answer is D: copper. The cytosolic superoxide dismutase contains both copper and zinc. There is a suggestion that abnormal cytosolic superoxide dismutase is involved in the pathogenesis of amyotrophic lateral sclerosis. Mitochondrial and bacterial superoxide dismutase contains magnesium. *Biochemistry,* p. 15.
121. The answer is A: pyruvate $\rightarrow$ oxaloacetate. This reaction, catalyzed by pyruvate carboxylase, involves the ATP- and biotin-dependent carboxylation of pyruvate. Biotin, which is covalently attached to a lysyl residue of pyruvate carboxylase, serves as an intermediate carrier of activated carbon dioxide. Biotin and the lysyl side chain form a long mobile carrier of about 1.3 nm that is capable of accepting bicarbonate at one active site of the enzyme and transferring it to another active site of the same enzyme for further reaction. The pyruvate carboxylase reaction maintains adequate levels of Krebs cycle intermediates and is the first step in the conversion of pyruvate to phosphoenolpyruvate (the second step, which is catalyzed by phosphoenolpyruvate carboxykinase, involves the reaction of oxaloacetate with GTP to produce phosphoenolpyruvate, GDP, and carbon dioxide). *Biochemistry,* p. 116.
122. The answer is D: glucose 6-phosphate $\rightarrow$ glucose. Glucose-6-phosphatase catalyzes this reaction after transport of the substrate to the endoplasmic reticulum. Many substances destined for secretion or release from the cell into the extracellular fluid pass first into the endoplasmic reticulum. Besides a decrease in enzyme activity, the inability to transport glucose 6-phosphate into the endoplasmic reticulum results in type I glycogen storage disease. The enzyme deficiency is more common than the translocase deficiency. The inability to release glucose into the circulation leads to hypoglycemia, increased glycogen synthesis (the glycogen possesses a normal structure), and to increased glycolysis and lactic acidosis. *Biochemistry,* pp. 136, 147; *Nelson,* p. 362.
123. The answer is A: pyruvate $\rightarrow$ oxaloacetate. As a result of a deficiency of acyl-CoA dehydrogenase, coenzyme A is trapped in the form of fatty acyl–CoA, whose catabolism is blocked as a result of this enzyme deficiency. This produces a shortage of coenzyme A, which in turn leads to a decrease in acetyl-CoA, an allosteric activator of the pyruvate carboxylase reaction. Decreased pyruvate carboxylase activity results in fasting hypoglycemia owing to decreased conversion of pyruvate to oxaloacetate and thus to decreased gluconeogenesis. Decreased oxaloacetate availability prevents normal catabolism of acetyl-CoA and its precursor, pyruvate, thus leading to lactic acidosis. *Biochemistry,* p. 116; *Nelson,* p. 336.
124. The answer is I: scurvy. The symptoms of ecchymosis, petechiae, and gingival swelling pinpoint the disorder as vitamin C deficiency. Ascorbate participates in the posttranslational modification of collagen, and these symptoms reflect abnormalities in connective tissue. Scurvy can occur in elderly individuals who omit fresh fruits and vegetables (good sources of vitamin C) from their diet. Vitamin C is heat labile, and it is destroyed by excessive cooking. *Biochemistry,* p. 28.
125. The answer is G: pernicious anemia. Intrinsic factor is a glycoprotein, produced by the stomach, which is required for the absorption of extrinsic factor (vitamin B_{12}) in the terminal ileum. A deficiency in intrinsic factor production can occur after partial or complete gastrectomy. Besides anemia, B_{12} deficiency results in a peripheral neuropathy, dorsal and lateral column degeneration, and central nervous system deficits. *Biochemistry,* p. 27.
126. The answer is D: marasmus. Marasmus, which has a distinctive clinical picture, is due to both protein and calorie deficiency. Kwashiorkor, also with a distinctive clinical picture, is due to inadequate protein intake but adequate caloric intake. *Biochemistry,* p. 32; *Nelson,* p. 131.
127. The answer is E: night blindness. β-Carotene is converted to vitamin A by an oxidation reaction. 11 *cis*-Retinal is the vitamin A form that combines with opsin to produce rhodopsin, the light-sensitive pigment of rod cells. *Biochemistry,* pp. 28–29.
128. The answer is C: enkephalin. Enkephalin, dynorphin, and β-endorphin are endogenous opioid peptides that mimic morphine. *Biochemistry,* p. 412.
129. The answer is D: epinephrine. Pheochromocytomas are tumors of the adrenal medulla. These tumors can se-

crete epinephrine and norepinephrine, hormones of the adrenal medulla. This can lead to hypertension, palpitations, hyperglycemia, and other signs and symptoms suggestive of excessive catecholamine secretion. Such tumors represent a curable cause of hypertension, and the disease is treated by surgical removal. The diagnosis is aided by the measurement of total metanephrine, VMA (vanillylmandelic acid), and norepinephrine in a 24-hour urine collection; norepinephrine distinguishes better between affected and unaffected hypertensive individuals. The measurement of plasma catecholamines (norepinephrine and epinephrine) is also used in the diagnosis of pheochromocytoma. Carcinoid tumors arise from enterochromaffin cells of the intestine. These tumors result in overproduction of serotonin, which leads to cutaneous flushing, hypotension, and tachycardia (increased heart rate). There is increased urinary excretion of 5-hydroxyindoleacetic acid, the major metabolite of serotonin. *Biochemistry,* p. 401; *Cecil,* pp. 1391 and 1394.

130. The answer is B: eukaryotic initiation factor 2 (eIF2). eIF2 is the cytosolic protein that recognizes methionine-$tRNA_I^{Met}$ and GTP; this initiation factor delivers methionine-$tRNA_I^{Met}$ to the P site to initiate protein synthesis. eIF2 does not recognize methionine-$tRNA^{Met}$ or other aminoacyl-tRNAs, accounting for the specific placement of the initiating tRNA in the P site. eEF1 recognizes all aminoacyl-tRNAs, except for methionine-$tRNA_I^{Met}$, and delivers them to the A (aminoacyl-tRNA) site in preparation for the elongation process. *Biochemistry,* p. 351.

131. The answer is H: eukaryotic release factor (eRF). Three of the 64 codons code for chain termination: UAA, UAG, and UGA. When one of these codons occupies the A site of the ribosome, it is recognized by eRF-GTP; this converts peptidyltransferase activity to hydrolase activity, and peptidyl-tRNA is hydrolyzed and released from the ribosome. *Biochemistry,* p. 351.

132. The answer is G: eukaryotic elongation factor 2 (eEF2). Diphthamide is a posttranslationally modified histidine residue in eEF2 and is the site of ADP-ribosylation that occurs in the presence of diphtheria toxin. *C. diphtheriae,* the causative agent of diphtheria, contain a bacteriophage that encodes the gene for diphtheria toxin. The toxin binds to host cells and undergoes proteolytic cleavage to form an A and B chain. The A chain enters the cell by a process that requires the aid of the B chain. The A fragment catalyzes the ADP-ribosylation of eEF2 (NAD^+ is the donor). Following chemical modification, the elongation factor is inactivated. One molecule of diphtheria toxin is sufficient to kill a cell. *Biochemistry,* p. 357.

133. The answer is C: apoprotein C-II gene. Apoprotein C-II is an activator of lipoprotein lipase, and a defect in apo-C-II leads to a hypertriglyceridemia that resembles that of lipoprotein lipase deficiency. As a result of apo-C-II or lipoprotein lipase deficiency, there is a prominent hyperchylomicronemia that is due to the inability to release triglyceride from chylomicrons. These patients are treated with medium-chain fatty acids, which are absorbed directly into the portal vein and transported to the liver without requiring chylomicron formation. *Biochemistry,* p. 195; *Nelson,* p. 357.

134. The answer is B: apoprotein B-100/B-48 gene. Apoproteins B-100 and B-48, which are products of the same gene, are synthesized in the intestine (B-48) and liver (B-100) and play a role in the formation of chylomicrons and VLDL, respectively. The intestinal B-48 and the hepatic B-100 differ in size because of differences in the processing of the RNA transcript. As a result of a defect in this gene, all forms of apo-B are absent from plasma, resulting in abetalipoproteinemia, a rare autosomal recessive disease. Consequently, plasma cholesterol and triglyceride levels are extremely low (usually less than 30 mg/dL). This disorder is accompanied by hypocholesterolemia, hypotriglyceridemia, retinopathy, fat malabsorption, progressive neurological disease, and high fatty acid content in the stool. There can be impaired fat-soluble vitamin absorption, and symptoms of vitamin A, E, and K deficiency can develop. There is a decrease in circulating chylomicrons, VLDL, and LDL. There is a deficiency of both exogenous and endogenous lipid transport. Treatment is symptomatic. Affected people are treated with medium-chain-length fatty acids that are transported from the gut independently of chylomicrons. Hydrophilic vitamin A derivatives are also given to alleviate night blindness, and hydrophilic vitamin K derivatives are given to alleviate bleeding. Heterozygotes have no known clinical abnormalities. *Biochemistry,* p. 195; *Nelson,* p. 358.

135. The answer is D: 146. Mutant A is the result of a deletion of a single nucleotide. Because mRNAs are translated triplet by triplet (PRINCIPLE 26 OF BIOCHEMISTRY), all the following codons differ from that of the wild type, resulting in a frameshift mutation that throws the reading frame out of phase and generates a completely new sequence. Not only is amino acid 139 changed from lysine to asparagine, amino acid 140 is converted from tyrosine to threonine. The normal termination codon at position 142 now encodes lysine. A termination codon, UAG, occurs at position 147, and the polypeptide contains 146 amino acids. The resulting hemoglobin is called hemoglobin Wayne, and this mutation is not clinically significant. *Biochemistry,* p. 343.

136. The answer is C: 5′ GGA 3′. Starting from codon 138, the amino acid sequence is Ser-Lys-Tyr-Arg, ending with a termination codon. Although codon 146 corresponds to serine, it occurs after a termination codon and is not incorporated into a polypeptide chain. Codon 138, 5′ UCC 3′, corresponds to serine. The RNA product is antiparallel to the DNA template, and the corresponding DNA has the sequence 5′ GGA 3′ according to Watson-Crick base-pairing rules (PRINCIPLE 23 OF BIOCHEMISTRY) with G pairing with C and A pairing with U.

RNA codon	5′ UCC 3′
DNA template	3′ AGG 5′

Biochemistry, pp. 272, 343.

137. The answer is C: transition. The conversion of uracil to cytosine at the RNA level corresponds to the conversion of a purine to a purine on the DNA template strand and a pyrimidine to a pyrimidine on the opposite (sense) DNA strand. This type of mutation is called a transition. Transversions are mutations involving the conversion of a pyrimidine to a purine or purine to pyrimidine. Deletions refer to the elimination of one or more bases. If one or two bases are eliminated, the triplet reading frame is altered, and this is called a frameshift mutation. Mutant A is an example of a frameshift mutation. If three bases (or multiples of three bases) are eliminated, the reading frame is not disturbed. A nonsense mutation results when a codon corresponding to an amino acid is converted to a stop codon, leading to premature polypeptide chain termination. The conversion of a stop codon to an amino acid codon, as observed in mutant B, leads to the synthesis of hemoglobin Constant Spring, a hemoglobin containing 31 additional residues at the carboxyl terminus. The resulting hemoglo-

bin chain is unstable and leads to a form of α-thalassemia, which is the result of an α-chain deficiency. *Biochemistry,* p. 290; *Nelson,* p. 1254.

138. The answer is Q: the reaction catalyzed by pyruvate carboxylase. This biotin-dependent, ATP-requiring enzyme requires acetyl-CoA for the expression of its activity. *Biochemistry,* p. 116.

139. The answer is R: the reaction catalyzed by pyruvate dehydrogenase. This enzyme is inhibited by phosphorylation, and pyruvate dehydrogenase kinase is allosterically activated by acetyl-CoA (and by NADH, another product of the pyruvate dehydrogenase reaction). Note that this cellular response also makes physiological sense (PRINCIPLE 9 OF BIOCHEMISTRY). If adequate acetyl-CoA is being provided, there is no need to increase its rate of formation from pyruvate. *Biochemistry,* p. 504.

140. The answer is V: the reaction catalyzed by carnitine acyltransferase I. Acylcarnitine, but not acyl-CoA, can be transported into mitochondria. Malonyl-CoA, an intermediate in *de novo* fatty acid synthesis, inhibits carnitine acyltransferase I and thereby diminishes the translocation of acyl groups into mitochondria. By blocking their exit from the cytosol, malonyl-CoA promotes esterification of fatty acids and the formation of triglyceride, first within the liver cell and subsequently within the adipocyte for formation of depot lipid. *Biochemistry,* p. 502.

141. The answer is N: the reaction catalyzed by phosphoenolpyruvate carboxykinase. This enzyme occurs in humans in both a cytosolic and a mitochondrial form, and the molar quantity of enzyme is increased by enzyme induction by glucagon. GTP provides the phosphoryl group forming a high-energy bond in phosphoenolpyruvate. The exergonic decarboxylation of oxaloacetate (PRINCIPLE 6 OF BIOENERGETICS) helps drive the reaction in the direction of phosphoenolpyruvate formation. *Biochemistry,* p. 137.

142. The answer is E: the reaction catalyzed by UDP-glucose pyrophosphorylase. UDP-linked hexoses, amino sugars, and uronic acids are commonly the activated precursors of a wide variety of polysaccharides, of glycosaminoglycans, and of the carbohydrate portion of glycoproteins. The generation of inorganic pyrophosphate and its subsequent hydrolysis serves to pull biochemical reactions forward (PRINCIPLE 14 OF BIOCHEMISTRY). *Biochemistry,* p. 140.

143. The answer is Z: the reaction catalyzed by acetyl-CoA carboxylase. This is another biotin-dependent, ATP-requiring reaction (similar to pyruvate carboxylase), and it is the committed and rate-limiting step in *de novo* fatty acid synthesis. This activity is not part of the multifunction polypeptide known as fatty acid synthase but occurs as an inactive monomer in the presence of long-chain acyl-CoA or following phosphorylation by AMP-dependent protein kinase. Formation of the active, filamentous polymeric enzyme is enhanced by citrate. *Biochemistry,* p. 502.

144. The answer is K: the reaction catalyzed by phosphofructokinase 1. This enzyme is active in the presence of high concentrations of fructose 6-phosphate and, in the presence of more moderate concentrations of fructose 6-phosphate, is activated by fructose 2,6-bisphosphate and AMP and is inhibited by citrate and by ATP, a substrate. *Biochemistry,* p. 502.

145. The answer is S: the reaction catalyzed by isocitrate dehydrogenase. Isocitrate dehydrogenase is the rate-controlling enzyme of the Krebs cycle and is allosterically activated by ADP. This regulation follows the molecular logic of the cell (PRINCIPLE 9 OF BIOCHEMISTRY). The function of the Krebs cycle and oxidative phosphorylation is to generate ATP. When ATP levels fall, there is an accumulation of ADP within the mitochondrion, and this activates the pacemaker enzyme of the Krebs cycle. Citrate synthase is not the chief regulatory enzyme; it does not catalyze the committed step, because citrate can serve as a source of two-carbon fragments for either lipogenesis or for oxidation by the cycle. Isocitrate dehydrogenase catalyzes a bidirectional reaction *in vitro;* the reaction is exergonic at metabolite concentrations *in vivo* and represents a good regulatory step. The α-ketoglutarate dehydrogenase reaction, like the pyruvate dehydrogenase reaction, is unidirectional and makes the entire cycle operate unidirectionally. Of all the Krebs cycle reactions, citrate synthase (which involves a hydrolysis) and α-ketoglutarate dehydrogenase (which involves a decarboxylation) are unidirectional. The Krebs cycle is called the final common pathway of metabolism (PRINCIPLE 15 OF BIOCHEMISTRY) because it is responsible for the conversion of the reduced carbon atoms of fuel molecules (carbohydrates, lipids, and amino acids), beginning with acetyl-CoA, to carbon dioxide. *Biochemistry,* p. 502.

146. The answer is L: the reaction catalyzed by fructose-1,6-bisphosphatase. This cytosolic enzyme is allosterically inhibited by AMP and by fructose 2,6-bisphosphate. The quantity of enzyme is increased by enzyme induction following stimulation of the hepatocyte by glucagon. Note that glycolysis and gluconeogenesis are reciprocally regulated at the reactions catalyzing the interconversion of fructose 6-phosphate and fructose 1,6-bisphosphate. AMP and fructose 2,6-bisphosphate affect these reactions in opposite ways, accelerating glycolysis and inhibiting gluconeogenesis. The level of fructose 2,6-bisphosphate is controlled by a dual-function kinase/phosphatase polypeptide that is a substrate for phosphorylation by protein kinase A. Phosphorylation of this dual-function protein decreases the concentration of fructose 2,6-bisphosphate by increasing the phosphatase activity and decreasing the kinase activity. *Biochemistry,* p. 502.

147. The answer is M: the reaction catalyzed by hormone-sensitive lipase. Following glucagon binding at the adipocyte plasma membrane, this enzyme is activated by phosphorylation by protein kinase A. Since the rate of fatty acid oxidation is dependent on the availability of fatty acyl groups, this reaction represents the primary control step. *Biochemistry,* p. 502.

148. The answer is A: the reaction catalyzed by glycogen synthase. Phosphorylation of this enzyme by protein kinase A results in inactivation, a physiological response that is reasonable considering the simultaneous activation of the glycogenolytic pathway that results from the protein kinase A phosphorylation of phosphorylase kinase and the subsequent phosphorylation (and activation) of glycogen phosphorylase. *Biochemistry,* p. 504.

REFERENCES

Behrman, R. E. *Nelson Textbook of Pediatrics,* 14th ed. Philadelphia, W. B. Saunders Company, 1992.

Roskoski, R., Jr. *Biochemistry.* Philadelphia, W. B. Saunders Company, 1996.

Wyngaarden, J. B., L. H. Smith, Jr., and J. C. Bennett (eds.). *Cecil Textbook of Medicine,* 19th ed. Philadelphia, W. B. Saunders Company, 1992.

BIOCHEMICAL AND MEDICAL GLOSSARY

A site: Site on the ribosome that accommodates *a*minoacyl-tRNA. *Compare* P site.

ABO hemolytic disease: Increased red blood cell breakdown in babies with blood types A or B and mothers with blood type O; due to maternal anti-A or anti-B antibodies.

Abscess: Localized accumulation of pus in a tissue or organ.

Absolute configuration: Steric pattern of the four different substituent groups bound to a chiral (asymmetric) carbon atom in relation to D- and L-glyceraldehyde, the primary standards.

Acceptor control: Regulation of the rate of electron transport by the availability of ADP as phosphate acceptor; also called respiratory control.

Acid: Proton donor.

Acid anhydride: Chemical combination of two acid molecules with the removal of the elements of water.

Acidosis: Disturbance in the acid-base balance of the body in which fluids have a pH less than normal (≤ 7.35).

Acromegaly: Chronic disease in adults resulting from excessive secretion of growth hormone and characterized by enlargement of many parts of the skeleton, especially the distal portions.

Actin: Abundant cytoskeletal protein that occurs in nonmuscle and muscle cells. The interaction of actin and myosin in muscle is responsible for force generation; actin also forms the thin filaments of the cytoskeleton.

Activated partial thromboplastin time (aPTT): Test that measures the overall efficiency of the intrinsic pathway of blood coagulation; elevated in hemophilia, in Christmas disease, and after heparin treatment.

Activation: Conversion of a metabolite into an energy-rich compound so that the metabolite can react with another compound exergonically; also called group activation.

Activation energy: Energy difference between reactants and their transition state ($\Delta G\ddagger$) as they undergo a chemical reaction to form products.

Active site: Portion of an enzyme to which the substrates bind and where they undergo chemical transformation.

Active transport: Movement of a metabolite across a membrane that is coupled to energy expenditure; *see also* Primary active transport and Secondary active transport.

Adapter: Something that accommodates or facilitates the interaction of one substance with another.

Addison disease: Disease due to adrenocortical hypofunction that is characterized by hypotension, weight loss, anorexia, weakness, and bronze-like hyperpigmentation of the skin.

Adenoma: Benign tumor arising from a gland.

Adenosine triphosphate (ATP): High-energy phosphate compound that liberates energy to power numerous cellular metabolic processes; life's most important molecule.

Adjuvant chemotherapy: Anticancer drugs administered after surgical resection of a tumor in an attempt to destroy any undetected foci of metastatic tumor before they become clinically detectable.

Adrenogenital syndrome: Clinical disorder of adrenal function characterized by overproduction of adrenal sex hormones, most commonly due to progesterone 21-hydroxylase deficiency.

Aerobe: Organism that uses oxygen as a reactant in the production of chemical energy.

Aerobic: Exposed to oxygen.

AIDS: Infection called acquired immunodeficiency syndrome caused by a human immunodeficiency virus (HIV-1 or HIV-2). The virus attacks and destroys CD4-expressing helper T lymphocytes, compromising cell-mediated immunity and leading to increased susceptibility to infection and some tumors such as Kaposi sarcoma.

Aldose: Polyhydroxyaldehyde.

Alkalosis: Disturbance in acid-base balance in which the pH of the extracellular fluids is shifted toward the alkaline side of normal (pH ≥ 7.45).

Alkylating agent: Anticancer drug that disrupts cell function by forming a covalent bond with DNA.

Allele: One of several related genes that may occupy the same locus on a homologous chromosome.

Allosteric enzyme: Enzyme whose catalytic activity is modulated by the noncovalent binding of a specific metabolite (allosteric effector) at a site other than the catalytic site.

Allosteric site: Location on an allosteric protein to which the modulator or effector molecule binds. *Compare* Active site.

Alzheimer disease: Degenerative disease of the nervous system with characteristic structural abnormalities (tangles and plaques) within neurons.

Amidation: Attachment of an $-NH_2$ group to a carboxyl ($-COO^-$) group to form an amide ($-CONH_2$).

Amino acid: α-Amino-substituted carboxylic acid, the monomeric building block of protein.

Amino acid activation: ATP-dependent reaction of the carboxyl group of an amino acid with the hydroxyl group at the 3′-end of its cognate or corresponding transfer RNA to form a high-energy ester bond; a carboxyl group can also be activated as an acylphosphate.

Aminoacyl-tRNA: Combination of an amino acid with tRNA through an energy-rich ester bond.

Aminoacyl-tRNA synthetase: Enzyme that catalyzes the formation of an aminoacyl-tRNA at the expense of ATP (ATP $\rightarrow$ AMP + PP_i); a ligase.

Aminotransferase: Enzyme that catalyzes transfer of an amino group from an amino acid to a keto acid; also called transaminase.

Amniocentesis: Removal of amnionic fluid, usually accomplished by inserting a needle through the mother's abdominal and uterine walls into the amnionic cavity.

Amnion: Thin, transparent inner membrane that surrounds the embryo in the uterus during pregnancy.

Amphibolic pathway: Metabolic pathway used in both synthetic and degradative reactions, e.g., the Krebs cycle.

Amphipathic compound: Compound that contains both polar and nonpolar components; an example is cholesterol, which contains both a polar hydroxyl group and the nonpolar steroid ring.

Anabolism: Phase of metabolism concerned with the energy-requiring biosynthesis of cell components from smaller precursor molecules.

Anaerobe: Organism that does not require oxygen for energy production; some anaerobes are killed by oxygen.

Anaerobic: In the absence of oxygen.

Anaplerotic reaction: Enzyme-catalyzed reaction that can furnish intermediates of the citric acid cycle, e.g., the pyruvate carboxylase reaction.

Anemia: Decrease in circulating red blood cells.

Aneurysm: Dilatation of a structure such as the aorta or cerebral artery.

Angina pectoris: Precordial chest pain experienced on exertion owing to inadequate blood supply to the heart muscle.

Angiogram: *See* Arteriogram.

Angstrom (Å): Unit of length (10^{-10} m) used to indicate molecular dimensions: 10 Å = 1 nm.

Anion: Negatively charged ion.

Anion gap: Difference in the sum of plasma sodium plus potassium minus chloride and bicarbonate: anion gap = $([Na^+] + [K^+]) - ([Cl^-] + [HCO_3^-])$; in diabetic ketoacidosis, the anion gap increases above the normal 15 mEq/L because of increased acetoacetate and β-hydroxybutyrate.

Anisotropic: Property of a substance that varies with the direction of observation or measurement. *Compare* Isotropic.

Anomeric carbon: Carbon atom of the carbonyl group (aldehyde or ketone) in a carbohydrate.

Anomers: Pair of cyclic diastereomers of a sugar or glycoside that differ only in the configuration at the point of asymmetry created by ring formation, e.g., α-D-glucose and β-D-glucose. In α-D-glucose, the hydroxyl group is below the plane of the ring in the usual Haworth formula, and in β-D-glucose, the hydroxyl group is above the plane of the ring.

Antibiotic: One of many different organic compounds that are formed and secreted by various species of microorganisms and plants that are toxic to other species.

Antibody: Immunoglobulin protein that is synthesized by lymphocytes in response to a specific foreign molecular stimulus called an antigen. *See also* Immunoglobulin.

Anticoagulant: Compound that inhibits blood clotting; examples are dicumarol, warfarin, and heparin.

Anticodon: Specific sequence of three bases in a transfer RNA complementary to a codon for an amino acid in a messenger RNA; found in the anticodon loop.

Antigen: Substance that elicits antibody formation; usually a foreign or exogenous macromolecule that may contain several antigenic determinants or epitopes.

Antimetabolite: Substance that competes with or replaces another substance (metabolite) required for cell growth or replication.

Antiparallel: Term describing side-by-side objects with polarities running in opposite directions.

Antiport: Obligatory transport of substances in opposite directions across a membrane; an exchange process.

Aplastic anemia: Anemia due to bone marrow failure.

Apoptosis: Programmed cell death, with distinctive morphologic changes that differ from necrosis, that occurs during embryogenesis and hormone-dependent involution, e.g., in the endometrium. *Compare* Necrosis.

Arrhythmia: Irregularity of the heartbeat.

Arteriogram: X-ray technique for studying the caliber of blood vessels by injection of radiopaque material into the vessel.

Arthritis: Inflammation and degeneration of a joint.

Ascites: Accumulation of fluid in the abdominal cavity.

Asterixis: Type of tremor, sometimes called liver flap.

Astrocyte: Star-shaped glial cell.

Asymmetric carbon atom: *See* Chiral carbon atom.

Ataxia: Inability to maintain one's balance.

Atelectasis: Collapse of the lung or a part of the lung.

Atheroma: Lipid accumulation in the intimal lining of an artery that narrows its lumen.

Atherosclerosis: Thickening of the lining (intima) of blood vessels due to accumulation of lipids, with secondary scarring and calcification.

ATP (adenosine triphosphate): Ribonucleoside 5′-triphosphate functioning as the common currency of energy exchange; the most important of all biomolecules.

ATPase: Enzyme that hydrolyzes ATP to yield ADP and phosphate; this reaction is usually coupled to an energy-requiring process.

ATP synthase: Membrane-associated enzyme complex composed of F_oF_1 subunits that forms ATP from ADP and phosphate during oxidative phosphorylation.

Atrophy: Reduction in size of an organ due to decreased function, inadequate hormonal stimulation, or reduced blood supply.

Autoimmune disease: Disease associated with formation of cell-mediated or humoral immunity against the body's own cells or tissue components.

Autosome: Chromosome other than a sex chromosome.

B lymphocyte: White blood cell that differentiates into plasma cells that produce the antibodies of humoral immunity; B refers to *b*one marrow.

Babinski reflex: Dorsiflexion (upward movement) of the big toe on stimulating the sole of the foot; a sign of a lesion of the central nervous system, particularly in the pyramidal tract, of adults, but the reflex can occur normally in infants.

Bacterial endocarditis: Inflammation of the endocardium; usually refers to an inflammation of the heart valves.

Barr body: Inactivated X chromosome in the nuclei of somatic cells of females.

Base pair: Two nucleotides whose purine and pyrimidine interact by hydrogen bonding, e.g., adenine with thymine or guanine with cytosine.

Basement membrane: Thin layer of acellular material containing type IV collagen upon which epithelium rests.

Basophil: White blood cell that stains with basic dyes. It is the least prevalent leukocyte, contains a receptor for immunoglobulin G, and secretes histamine during inflammatory reactions. *See also* Eosinophil and Neutrophil.

Benign tumor: Tumor that lacks the ability to invade locally or spread to distant sites.

Bilayer: Double layer of amphipathic lipid molecules; the hydrocarbon tails face inward to form a continuous nonpolar phase, and the polar heads face the surrounding aqueous phase.

Bile: Secretion of the liver containing bile salts, cholesterol, and other substances.

Bile salt: Derivatives of cholesterol in bile that act as emulsifiers to promote fat digestion and absorption.

Bilirubin: One of the bile pigments derived from breakdown of hemoglobin; reacts slowly in the van den Bergh reaction. Also called indirect bilirubin.

Bioenergetics: Study of energy changes in biochemical systems.

Biopsy: Removal of a small sample of tissue for examination and diagnosis.

Bond energy: Energy required to break a chemical bond. *See* High-energy compound and Low-energy compound for the definition of a different concept.

Bradycardia: Subnormal heart rate.

Bradykinin: Chemical mediator of inflammation derived from components in the blood plasma; can participate in the initiation of blood clotting.

Bruit: Abnormal sound heard in auscultation (pronounced "brew ee").

Buffer: Substance that minimizes change in pH of a solution when an acid or base is added.

Calculus: Stone formed within the body, as in the kidney or gallbladder.

Calorie: The calorie of the physicist and biochemist is the amount of heat energy required to raise the temperature of 1 g of water from 14.5 to 15.5 °C; the calorie of the nutritionist, which equals 1 kcal (1000 calories) and is sometimes written with a capital C (Calorie), corresponds to the energy required to raise the temperature of 1 kg of water from 14.5 to 15.5 °C.

cAMP: *See* Cyclic AMP.

Cancer: Malignant tumor.

Cap: 5′ Terminus of eukaryotic mRNA blocked by a methylated guanosine group linked to the primary transcript in 5′ → 5′ linkage.

Capsid: Protein covering the central nucleic acid core of a virus.

Carbohydrate: Organic compound containing an aldehyde or ketone and at least two hydroxyl groups.

Carboxyl group: Acid group (—COOH) found in organic molecules.

Carcinoma: Malignant tumor derived from epithelial cells.

Cardiomegaly: Enlarged heart.

Cardiomyopathy: General term for any noninflammatory disease of heart muscle.

Caries: Localized destruction of the tooth surface, leading to cavity formation.

Catabolism: Phase of metabolism involved in the energy-yielding degradation of nutrient molecules with the concomitant generation of ATP.

Catalytic site: Site on an enzyme involved in the chemical conversion of reactants to products.

Catecholamine: Derivative of catechol (1,2-dihydroxybenzene) containing an alkyl side chain with an amino group; epinephrine is an example.

Cathepsin: One of a family of lysosomal proteolytic enzymes.

Cation: Positively charged ion.

Cavity (dental): Loss of tooth structure due to the combined action of bacteria and organic acids derived from bacterial fermentation of food.

α-Cell: Glucagon-secreting cell of the pancreatic islets.

β-Cell: Insulin-secreting cell of the pancreatic islets.

δ-Cell: Somatostatin-secreting cell of the pancreatic islets.

Cell wall: Molecular sheet that surrounds the plasma membrane of a cell; found in bacteria and in plants.

Cell-mediated immunity: Reaction of cytotoxic (killer) T cells against virally infected cells and foreign histocompatibility antigens.

Central dogma: Crick's dogma: genetic information flows from DNA to DNA and from DNA to RNA to protein.

Central thiol: Thiol group of acyl carrier protein contributed by 4′-phosphopantetheine. Acyl carrier protein functions as a swinging arm to translocate acyl groups from active site to active site during fatty acid biosynthesis. *Compare* Peripheral thiol.

Centriole: Short cylindrical structure located next to the nucleus that participates in the formation of spindle fibers during nuclear division.

Centromere: Structure that joins each pair of chromatids formed by chromosome duplication.

Centrosome: Region of the cell cytoplasm that contains two centrioles.

Cheilitis: Inflammation of the lips.

Chemical energy: Energy expended in or derived from a chemical reaction.

Chemical reaction: Process of converting one or more substances into different substances.

Chemiosmotic coupling: Coupling of ATP synthesis to electron transport via an electrochemical H^+ gradient across a membrane.

Chemiosmotic theory: Theoretical rationale supporting the idea that a proton-motive force across a membrane provides energy for processes such as ATP biosynthesis, solute transport, and movement of bacterial flagella. Combines a vectorial process with a scaler chemical reaction; also called the Mitchell theory.

Chemistry: Study of the interconversion of substances; a diagram or pictorial representation of the interconversion of substances.

Chiral carbon atom: Carbon atom that is covalently bonded to four different groups. A compound containing a chiral carbon atom may be represented as either of two different tetrahedral configurations that are nonsuperimposable mirror images. Also called asymmetric carbon atom. *See also* Absolute configuration.

Chlorophyll: Family of pigments, which consist of magnesium-tetrapyrroles, that function as acceptors of light energy in photosynthesis.

Cholecystitis: Inflammation of the gallbladder.

Cholelithiasis: Formation of gallstones.

Cholesterol: Lipid containing four fused rings (A, B, C, and D), 27 carbon atoms, and a hydroxyl group. *See also* Steroid.

Chorion: Layer of trophoblast and associated mesoderm that surrounds the developing embryo.

Chorionic villi: Finger-like columns of cells extending from the chorion that anchor the chorionic vesicle in the endometrium.

Chromatid: One of two newly formed chromosomes held together by the centromere.

Chromatin: Complex of DNA, RNA, histones, and other proteins forming eukaryotic chromosomes.

Cirrhosis of the liver: Disease characterized by diffuse intrahepatic scarring and liver cell degeneration.

Citric acid cycle: *See* Krebs cycle.

Clearance test: Test of renal function that measures the ability of kidneys to remove (clear) a substance from the blood and excrete it in the urine.

Codon: Sequence of three adjacent bases in a nucleic acid that codes for a specific amino acid or for chain termination. The genetic code consists of 64 codons: 61 correspond to amino acids and three are termination codons (UAA, UAG, UGA).

Coenzyme: Organic cofactor that serves as a substrate or that plays a role in the catalytic action of certain enzymes; often contains a vitamin as a component.

Coenzyme A (CoA): Pantothenic acid-containing coenzyme serving as an acyl-group carrier (discovered by Fritz Lipmann); the coenzyme of *a*cetylation or *a*cylation.

Cofactor: Low-molecular-weight, heat-stable inorganic or organic substance required for the action of an enzyme.

Cohesive end: Single-stranded loose end of duplex DNA complementary to a single-stranded end of the same or another DNA molecule.

Colitis: Inflammation of the colon.

Coma: State of unconsciousness from which an individual cannot be aroused, even by powerful stimulation.

Common intermediate: Chemical compound common to two chemical reactions as a product of one and a reactant in the other.

Complementary (Watson-Crick) base pairing: Specific base pairing by hydrogen bonds between adenine with thymine (DNA) or uracil (RNA), and guanine with cytosine.

Complementary DNA (cDNA): DNA, usually made by a reaction catalyzed by reverse transcriptase, that is complementary to messenger RNA in the Watson-Crick sense.

Computed tomographic (CT) scan: X-ray technique producing detailed cross-sectional images of the body by means of an x-ray tube and detectors.

Condensation reaction: Process of joining two molecules together, sometimes with the liberation of a small molecule such as water.

Confabulation: Making up tales to give a fluent answer without regard to facts.

Configuration: Steric arrangement of substituent groups around a chiral carbon atom.

Conformation: Three-dimensional or steric structure of a molecule.

Congenital: Present at birth.

Conjugated bilirubin: Bilirubin diglucuronide. Also called direct bilirubin.

Constitutive enzyme: Enzyme that is present in cells whatever the nutritional or hormonal status of the cell or organism. *Compare* Inducible enzymes.

Cori cycle: Transport of lactate from the muscle to the liver, conversion of the lactate to glucose by gluconeogenesis, and the transport of glucose from liver to muscle; discovered by Carl and Gerty Cori.

Coronary thrombosis: *See* Myocardial infarction.

Cortex: Outer layer of an organ. *Compare* Medulla.

Covalent bond: Chemical bond involving the sharing of electron pairs between two atoms.

Creatinine: Nitrogenous waste product derived from the breakdown of muscle phosphocreatine; excreted in urine.

Creatinine clearance: Renal clearance of endogenous creatinine; closely approximates the glomerular filtration rate.

Cretinism: Hypothyroidism in infants and children characterized by arrested physical and mental development. *Compare* Myxedema, in adults.

Crossing-over: Interchange of genetic material between homologous chromosomes during synapse and meiosis.

Cyanosis: Blue tinge of the skin and mucous membranes that results from an excessively large amount of unoxygenated hemoglobin in the blood.

Cyclic AMP: Second messenger within cells; its formation by adenylyl cyclase is stimulated by certain hormones such as glucagon and epinephrine. Also abbreviated cAMP.

Cystic fibrosis: Hereditary disease characterized by glandular dysfunction due to a defect of the cystic fibrosis transmembrane conductance regulator (CFTR), eventually leading to serious disturbances of pulmonary and pancreatic function.

Cystitis: Inflammation of the bladder.

Cytochrome: Family of heme proteins that serve as one-electron carriers.

Cytokinesis: Process dividing the cytoplasm of eukaryotic cells after nuclear division or mitosis.

Cytoplasm: Portion of a cell's contents outside the nucleus or nucleoid.

Cytoskeleton: Filamentous skeleton in cytoplasm; composed of microfilaments, intermediate filaments, and microtubules.

Cytosol: Continuous aqueous phase of cytoplasm with its dissolved solutes; defined operationally as the supernatant of a cell extract following a centrifugation at 100,000 times the force of gravity.

Cytotoxic: Producing cell necrosis or destruction.

Dalton: Mass of a single hydrogen atom (1.66049×10^{-24} g). One dalton is abbreviated Da, and one thousand daltons, or one kilodalton, is abbreviated kDa.

Daughter cell: Cell resulting from division of a single cell (called the parent cell).

Deamination: Removal of amino groups from an organic compound.

Decarboxylation: Removal of carbon dioxide from an organic compound.

Decidua: Endometrium of pregnancy.

Dehydrogenase: Enzyme catalyzing the transfer of hydrogen atoms from one substrate to another.

Denaturation: Loss of activity of a protein or nucleic acid because of partial or complete unfolding of its native conformation.

Dentine: Bony structure of the tooth.

Deoxyribonucleic acid: *See* DNA.

Deoxyribonucleotide: Nucleotide (base-sugar-phosphate) containing 2′-deoxyribose as the pentose or sugar component.

Dermatitis: Inflammation of the skin.

Dextrorotary isomer: An optical isomer, which is designated by a lowercase d, that rotates the plane of polarized light to the right. The isomer denoted by a small capital D has the same steric or absolute configuration as D-glyceraldehyde. The D-isomer does not necessarily rotate the plane of polarized light to the right. *Compare* Levorotory isomer.

Diabetes insipidus: Condition resulting from a deficiency of antidiuretic hormone (also called vasopressin) and characterized by excretion of a large volume of very dilute urine.

Diabetes mellitus: Metabolic disease characterized by hyperglycemia and caused by insufficient insulin secretion or inefficient insulin action (insulin resistance).

Diagnosis: Determination of the nature and cause of a condition.

Dialysis: Diffusion of dissolved substances and water across a semipermeable membrane.

Diastereomers: Stereoisomers that are not mirror images (enantiomers) of one another, e.g., D-glucose and D-galactose.

Differential centrifugation: Separation of cell organelles by their different rates of sedimentation in a centrifugal field.

Differential leukocyte count: Percentages of the total white blood cell count that are neutrophils, lymphocytes, monocytes, eosinophils, and basophils.

Diffusion: Tendency for molecules to move in the direction of lower concentration.

Diphosphopyridine nucleotide (DPN$^+$): *See* NAD$^+$.

Diplopia: Perception of two images of a single object.

Direct bilirubin: Soluble form of bilirubin produced by the addition of two molecules of glucuronic acid to the bilirubin molecule; reacts rapidly in the van den Bergh reaction. Also called conjugated bilirubin.

Disaccharide: Carbohydrate containing two covalently joined monosaccharide units.

Dissociation constant (K_d): Equilibrium constant for the dissociation of a compound or a protein and a ligand into its components. The dissociation constant is expressed as the concentration of the free ligand at which half the protein is free and half contains the bound ligand.

Distributive control of metabolism: Regulation of a pathway or process at several reactions or steps.

Disulfide bond: Covalent cross-link formed between two oxidized polypeptidic cysteines forming a cystine residue; disulfide bonds may be intramolecular or intermolecular, and they are more common in proteins that occur extracellularly.

DNA: Chromosomal nucleic acid that carries genetic information; a polynucleotide that contains 2′-deoxyribose in the repeating sugar-phosphate backbone.

DNA chimera: *See* Recombinant DNA.

DNA ligase: Enzyme that catalyzes the formation of a phosphodiester bond between the 3′-hydroxyl end of one DNA segment and the 5′-phosphate end of another, while they are base-paired to a template strand.

DNA polymerase: Enzyme catalyzing template-dependent synthesis of DNA from deoxyribonucleoside 5′-triphosphate precursors.

DNA repair: Conversion of DNA with a structural abnormality to the normal state.

Dominant gene: Gene that expresses a trait in the heterozygous state.

Double helix: Coiled conformation of two complementary, antiparallel DNA chains associated by complementary base pairing.

Down syndrome: Congenital syndrome usually caused by an extra chromosome 21 (trisomy 21).

Downstream: Toward (1) the 3′-end of a nucleic acid or (2) the carboxyl terminus of a protein.

DPN$^+$ (diphosphopyridine nucleotide): *See* NAD$^+$.

Dysplasia: Abnormal size, shape, or organization of cells.

Dyspnea: Difficult or labored breathing.

Dystrophy: Disorder that results from defective or faulty growth of a structure or organ.

Dysuria: Painful urination.

Ecchymosis: Small black-and-blue spot caused by extravasation of blood into the skin (plural, ecchymoses).

Eclampsia: Edema, hypertension, proteinuria, and possible convulsions during pregnancy.

Ectoderm: Outer germ layer of the embryo.

Ectopic: Out of normal position.

Ectopic pregnancy: Pregnancy occurring outside the endometrial cavity.

Edema: Accumulation of an excess of fluid in the interstitial tissues.

Editing function: *See* Proofreading function.

Effector: Metabolite or allosteric effector that, when bound to the allosteric site of a regulatory enzyme, alters enzyme activity.

Effusion: Escape of fluid into a part or tissue.

Electrocardiogram (ECG or EKG): Technique for measuring the serial changes in the electrical activity of the heart during the various phases of the cardiac cycle.

Electrochemical gradient: Sum of the gradients of concentration and electric charge of an ion across a membrane.

Electrogenic: Process that produces, or results from, an electrical potential across a membrane.

Electrolyte: Positive or negative ion.

Electron acceptor: Oxidant; a substance that receives electrons in an oxidation-reduction reaction.

Electron carrier: Substances such as flavoproteins, cytochromes, or quinones that can gain and lose electrons reversibly and function to transfer electrons from donors to acceptors.

Electron donor: Reductant; a donor of electrons in an oxidation-reduction reaction.

Electron transport: Movement of electrons from donor to acceptor substances via a specific pathway, usually in a membrane-associated system.

Electron transport phosphorylation: Conversion of ADP and P_i to ATP mediated by an F_oF_1 ATP synthase sustained by the transport of electrons along an electron transport chain.

Elongation factor: Specific proteins that transiently associate with the ribosome and are required in polypeptide chain biosynthesis.

Embden-Meyerhof pathway: *See* Glycolytic pathway.

Embolism: Condition in which a detached clot or other mass (embolus) occludes a blood vessel.

Embryo: Developing human organism from the third through the seventh weeks of gestation. *Compare* Fetus.

Emphysema: Disease characterized by enlargement and distention of the pulmonary air spaces distal to the terminal bronchioles.

Enamel: Dense outer covering of the exposed surface of a tooth.

Enantiomers: Stereoisomers that are nonsuperimposable mirror images of each other, e.g., D-glyceraldehyde and L-glyceraldehyde.

Encephalitis: Inflammation of the brain.

Endergonic reaction: Chemical reaction with a positive standard free energy change; one that does not occur without an input of energy.

Endocytosis: Uptake of large molecules, such as proteins, by a cell.

Endoplasmic reticulum: Mass of hollow tubular channels within the cytoplasm of the cell, frequently bordered by ribosomes.

Endothelium: Internal lining of the blood vessels and interior of heart.

Energy: Ability to perform useful work, produce heat, or move a general capacity against a general force, e.g., current against a voltage, or mass against gravity.

Energy charge: Fractional degree to which the ATP-ADP-AMP system is filled with high-energy phosphate groups; the energy charge is ([ATP] + 1/2 [ADP])/([ATP] + [ADP] + [AMP]) and ranges from zero to one.

Energy coupling: Transfer of energy from one process to another; also called energy transduction.

Energy-poor compound: *See* Low-energy compound.

Energy-rich compound: *See* High-energy compound.

Enhancer: DNA segment that increases the rate of transcription of a gene.

Enteritis: Inflammation of the intestine.

Enthalpy: Heat content of a system.

Entoderm: Inner germ layer of the embryo.

Entropy: State of randomness or disorder of a system; heat absorbed divided by the absolute temperature.

Enzyme: Protein catalyst.

Eosinophil: White blood cell that stains with eosin; it helps destroy parasites and modulates allergic responses. *See also* Basophil and Neutrophil.

Epimerase: Enzyme capable of catalyzing the interconversion of two epimers.

Epimers: Two diastereomers differing in configuration at one chiral center in a compound having two or more chiral centers, e.g., D-glucose and D-galactose.

Epstein-Barr virus: Virus that causes Burkitt lymphoma in Africa and infectious mononucleosis.

Equilibrium: State of a system at which no net change is occurring and its free energy is at a minimum.

Equilibrium constant: Constant characteristic for each chemical reaction; relates the specific concentrations (or activities) of all reactants and products at equilibrium at a given temperature, pressure, ionic strength, and pH.

Erythroblast: Precursor cell in the bone marrow that gives rise to red blood cells.

Erythropoiesis: Production of red blood cells.

Erythropoietin: Protein that sustains hematopoiesis and is made by the kidney.

Escherichia coli (E. coli): Common gram-negative bacterium found in the large intestine of vertebrates.

Esophageal varices: Dilated (varicose) veins of the esophagus, which often occur in patients with cirrhosis of the liver.

Essential amino acid: Amino acid that cannot be synthesized by the organism and must be obtained from the diet or environment.

Essential fatty acid: Fatty acid that cannot be synthesized by the organism and must be obtained from the diet or environment. The polyunsaturated fatty acids required by humans are linoleate and linolenate.

Etiology: Cause, especially of a disease.

Eubacteria: Evolutionarily distinct branch of prokaryotes that differ from archaebacteria as determined by rRNA sequence analysis. *E. coli* is a eubacterium.

Eukaryote: Family of organisms having a membrane-surrounded nucleus, multiple chromosomes, and internal organelles. Eukaryotes include animals, plants, fungi (yeast), and protozoa. *Compare* Prokaryote.

Exchange transfusion: Partial replacement of blood of newborns with hemolytic disease with blood lacking the antigen responsible for hemolytic disease, as when transfusing Rh-negative blood to an Rh-positive infant. Performed to reduce hemolysis and jaundice.

Excinuclease: Enzyme that excises a segment of DNA containing an abnormality such as a thymine dimer.

Exergonic reaction: Chemical reaction with a negative standard free energy change that corresponds to a favorable reaction; a spontaneous reaction that occurs without the input of additional energy.

Exocytosis: Secretion of a substance from a cell.

Exon: Segment of a eukaryotic gene that is represented in mature mRNA.

Exonuclease: Enzyme that catalyzes the hydrolysis of a terminal phosphodiester bond of a nucleic acid.

Exudate: Any protein-rich fluid that has passed out of or oozed from a body structure, often because of inflammation. *Compare* Transudate.

Facilitated diffusion: Transport of a metabolite through a membrane mediated by a protein but not requiring chemical energy.

FAD (flavin adenine dinucleotide): Riboflavin-containing coenzyme of some oxidation-reduction enzymes.

Faraday: Quantity that corresponds to the charge of N_A (Avogadro's number), one "mole," or one equivalent of electrons.

Fatty acid: Aliphatic carbon compound that contains a terminal carboxyl group.

Feedback mechanism: Operation by which the end product of a process controls the initial step.

Fermentation: Energy-yielding anaerobic breakdown of a nutrient, such as glucose, occurring without the net oxidation of other components; e.g., the process by which yeast converts glucose to ethanol and carbon dioxide.

α-Fetoprotein: Protein produced by fetal liver early in gestation and sometimes produced by tumor cells. Its concentration can be elevated in amnionic fluid when the fetus has a neural tube defect.

Fetus: Unborn offspring after 8 weeks' gestation. *Compare* Embryo.

Fibrillation: Uncoordinated quivering of cardiac or other muscle that alters normal contraction.

Fibrin: Meshwork of protein that forms during blood clotting.

Fibrin monomer: Derivative of fibrinogen that polymerizes to form the fibrin clot during blood coagulation.

Fibrinogen: Protein precursor in plasma converted to fibrin by thrombin during blood coagulation.

Flavin nucleotide: Nucleotide coenzymes (FMN and FAD) containing riboflavin.

Flavoprotein: Enzyme containing a flavin nucleotide as a prosthetic group.

Fluorescence: Emission of light by excited molecules as they revert to their ground state.

Fracture: Broken bone or other entity.

Free energy: That portion of the total energy of a system that can do work at constant temperature and pressure.

Free energy of hydrolysis: Free energy liberated during the hydrolysis of a compound into the products.

Frozen section: Method of rapid diagnosis of tumors in which tissue is frozen solid, cut into thin sections, stained, and examined microscopically.

Fun: Study (or better, understanding) of biochemistry.

Functionally isoergonic reaction: Reaction that permits the flux of metabolites in the forward or reverse direction depending upon the physiological concentrations of the reactants and products.

Furanose: Sugar containing a five-membered ring (four carbons and one oxygen) similar to the furan ring.

Futile cycle: Enzyme-catalyzed set of cyclic reactions involving the utilization of ATP in formation of product, followed by hydrolysis of the product to yield the original compound. This process occurs with the indirect but net hydrolysis of ATP; e.g., the combined action of phosphofructokinase and fructose-1,6-bisphosphatase leads to the net conversion of ATP to ADP and P_i.

Gangrene: (1) Infection due to gas-forming anaerobic bacteria (gas gangrene) or (2) necrosis of an extremity due to interruption of its blood supply (ischemic gangrene).

Gene: Unit of heredity at a definite position (locus) on a chromosome; a chromosomal segment that codes for a single polypeptide chain or RNA molecule or plays a role in regulation.

Gene library: Collection of random DNA fragments with overlap so that the collection includes all the genetic information of a given category.

Gene splicing: (1) Enzymatic attachment of one gene or part of a gene to another gene or DNA fragment. (2) The removal of introns and splicing of exons during mRNA synthesis.

Genetic code: Set of triplet code words in RNA coding for the amino acids of proteins.

Genetic information: Hereditary information contained in a sequence of nucleotide bases in chromosomal DNA or RNA.

Genetic map: Diagram showing the relative sequence and position of specific genes along a chromosome or plasmid.

Genome: All the genes that make up an organism.

Glomerulonephritis: Inflammation of the renal glomeruli.

Glomerulosclerosis: Diffuse and nodular thickening of glomerular basement membranes, a common occurrence in patients with long-standing (chronic) diabetes mellitus.

Glucagon: Hormone produced by the α-cells of the pancreatic islets that increases blood glucose.

Glucocorticoid: Adrenocortical steroid hormone that regulates metabolism.

Glucogenic amino acid: Amino acids whose carbon chains can be metabolically converted into glucose or glycogen.

Gluconeogenesis: Biosynthesis of new carbohydrate from noncarbohydrate precursors such as amino acids and glycerol.

Glycogen: Storage form of glucose, present chiefly in liver and muscle.

Glycolytic pathway, or **glycolysis:** Catabolism of glucose into two molecules of pyruvate by a series of ten enzyme-catalyzed reactions including phosphofructokinase and aldolase; also called the Embden-Meyerhof pathway.

Glycoprotein: Protein containing one or more carbohydrate groups.

Glycoside diphosphate: Sugar attached via a glycosidic bond to pyrophosphate; these contain two high-energy bonds and function as energy-rich donors of sugar molecules. Uridine diphosphate glucose and phosphoribosylpyrophosphate are examples.

Goiter: Enlarged thyroid gland.

Golgi apparatus: Group of membrane-lined sacs found in the cytoplasm of the cell near the nucleus.

Gonad: General term referring to either the ovary or testis.

Gout: Disorder of purine metabolism characterized by elevated uric acid and deposition of uric acid in and around joints.

G-protein: Protein that binds guanine nucleotides.

Gram-molecular mass: Mass of a compound in grams numerically equal to its molecular weight; the weight of one mole.

Gram-negative bacteria: Bacteria that are unable to retain the iodide complex of crystal violet.

Gram-positive bacteria: Bacteria that can retain the iodide complex of crystal violet.

Gram stain: Staining following the application of the iodide complex of crystal violet; the presence or absence of staining reflects the structure of the cell wall.

Graves disease: Syndrome characterized by hyperthyroidism, goiter, and oculopathy.

Group activation: Chemical group, next to a high-energy bond, that is energized for a group transfer reaction.

Group transfer potential: Negative of the free energy of hydrolysis of a compound, and a measure of a compound's ability to undergo a transfer reaction.

Group translocation: Chemical modification of a metabolite during transfer (translocation) across a membrane such as the formation of γ-glutamylmethionine from glutathione and methionine during methionine's translocation in the nephron.

Half-reaction: Donor and its conjugate acceptor of one part of an oxidation-reduction reaction.

Haplotype: Set of alleles of a group of closely linked genes, such as the human leukocyte-associated (HLA) complex, that is usually inherited as a unit.

Heart attack: *See* Myocardial infarction.

Heart failure: Inability of the heart to adequately maintain cardiovascular output.

Heat energy: Kinetic energy of molecules.

α-Helix: Coiled helical conformation of the polypeptide chain with maximal intrachain hydrogen bonding.

Hemangioma: Abnormal proliferation of blood vessels.

Hematocrit: Percent of blood volume that is cellular.

Hematoma: Bruise or abnormal collection of blood in a tissue.

Hematuria: Blood in the urine.

Heme: Iron-porphyrin complex that occurs in cytochromes, hemoglobin, and myoglobin.

Hemiacetal: Compound formed by the reaction of an aldehyde and an alcohol.

Hemiplegia: Paralysis of one side of the body.

Hemizygous: Term applied to genes located on the X chromosome in the male.

Hemodialysis: Dialysis procedure by which waste products are removed from the blood of patients in chronic renal failure, usually by means of an artificial kidney machine.

Hemolysis: Destruction of red blood cells with escape of hemoglobin into the circulation.

Hemolytic anemia: Anemia due to increased red blood cell destruction.

Hemophilia: Sex-linked, genetically inherited coagulation disturbance characterized by an elevated activated partial thromboplastin time; hemophilia A (classical hemophilia) is due to a deficiency of blood clotting factor VIII, and hemophilia B (Christmas disease) is due to a deficiency of factor IX.

Hemoptysis: Coughing blood.

Hemosiderin: One storage form of iron.

Heparin: Connective tissue glycosaminoglycan that is isolated from animal tissues and used pharmacologically as an anticoagulant.

Hepatitis: Inflammation of the liver.

Hepatomegaly: Enlarged liver.

Hepatosplenomegaly: Enlarged liver and spleen.

Heterozygous: Possessing different alleles at a given locus on each of a pair of homologous chromosomes.

Hexose: Simple sugar containing six carbon atoms, e.g., glucose.

High group transfer potential: Group transfer potential of a high-energy compound.

High-density lipoprotein (HDL) cholesterol: Fraction of cholesterol carried by high-density lipoprotein; levels ≥60 mg/dL reduce the risk of coronary heart disease, and levels ≤35 mg/dL increase the risk.

High-energy compound: Compound that releases ≥30 kJ/mol of free energy upon hydrolysis under standard conditions. Also called energy-rich compound. *Compare* Low-energy compound.

Histocompatibility complex: Cluster of genes on chromosome 6 that determine glycoprotein antigens on the surface of cells.

Histone: Group of five basic proteins (H1, H2A, H2B, H3, and H4) associated with the nuclear chromosomes of all eukaryotic cells.

Homologous chromosomes: Matched pair of chromosomes, one derived from each parent.

Homologous proteins: Proteins containing similar amino acid sequences encoded by evolutionarily related gene sequences.

Homozygous: Possessing identical alleles at a given locus on each of a pair of homologous chromosomes.

Host: Individual infected with a disease-producing organism.

Humoral immunity: Immunity associated with formation of antibodies produced by plasma cells. *See also* Antibody.

Hydrogen bond: Weak (5–20 kJ/mol) electrostatic attraction between one electronegative atom and a hydrogen atom covalently linked to a second electronegative atom; electronegative atoms include oxygen and nitrogen.

Hydrolysis: Cleavage (lysis) of a molecule into two smaller molecules by reaction with water; an OH is found in the molecule corresponding to one side of the cleaved bond, and an H is found in the molecule corresponding to the other side. *Compare* Phosphorolysis.

Hydrophilic: "Water-loving"; polar or charged molecules or groups that associate with and are soluble in water.

Hydrophobic: "Water-fearing"; nonpolar molecules or groups that are insoluble in water.

Hydrophobic interaction: Association of nonpolar groups with each other in aqueous solution because of the tendency of the surrounding water molecules to seek their most random state.

Hypercholesterolemia: Elevated concentration of cholesterol in the blood; 240 mg/dL is considered high, 200–239 mg/dL is considered borderline high, and less than 200 mg/dL is considered desirable.

Hyperglycemia: Elevated concentration of glucose in the blood.

Hyperplasia: Increase in cell number in a tissue.

Hypertension: Abnormally elevated arterial pressure.

Hypertonic: Having an osmotic pressure (osmolarity) greater than that of body fluids.

Hypertriglyceridemia: Elevated concentration of triglyceride in the blood.

Hypertrophy: Enlargement or overgrowth of an organ due to an increase in size of its constituent cells.

Hypoglycemia: Less than normal concentration of glucose in the blood.

Hypotonic: Having an osmotic pressure (osmolarity) less than that of body fluids.

Icterus: *See* Jaundice.

Immunity: Resistance to disease because of humoral and cellular actions of B and T lymphocytes. *See also* Humoral immunity and Cell-mediated immunity.

Immunoglobulin (Ig): Antibody protein that binds to its antigen. Includes IgA, IgD, IgE, IgG, and IgM isotypes. *See also* Antibody.

Immunotherapy: Treatment given to retard growth of a disseminated malignant tumor by stimulating the body's own immune defenses.

***In situ* carcinoma:** Malignant epithelial tumor that is still confined to the surface epithelium and has not yet invaded deeper tissues.

In vitro: "In glass"; originally, in a glass test tube but now in any inanimate reaction vessel.

In vivo: "In life"; in the cell or organism.

Indirect bilirubin: Free bilirubin that is not conjugated with glucuronide; reacts slowly in the van den Bergh reaction. *Compare* Direct bilirubin and Total bilirubin.

Infarction: Cell death (necrosis) due to interruption of its blood supply.

Infection: Inflammation due to a disease-producing organism.

Inflammation: Reaction produced by an irritant or infectious agent, characterized by swelling of the affected tissue due to vascular congestion and exudation of fluid and white blood cells.

Informational macromolecule: Molecule containing information or data as specific sequences of its different monomeric building blocks; includes proteins and nucleic acids but not carbohydrates and lipids.

Initiation codon: AUG. This triplet codes for the first amino acid in a polypeptide chain; the initiating amino acid is methionine; in prokaryotes and in mitochondria, the methionine is *N*-formylated.

Initiation complex: Complex of a ribosome with an mRNA and the initiating Met-$tRNA_i^{Met}$ (eukaryotes) or *N*-formyl-Met-$tRNA_i^{Met}$ (prokaryotes), poised for the elongation steps.

Initiation factor: Specific proteins that transiently associate with the ribosome and are required to start synthesis of a polypeptide.

Insulin: Anabolic protein hormone made of an A chain and a B chain connected by disulfide bonds that is produced by the β-cells of the pancreas and has many effects including that of lowering blood glucose. *See* Diabetes mellitus.

Interferon: Antiviral protein manufactured by various cells in the body.

Interleukin: Regulatory protein produced by lymphocytes that affects other lymphocytes.

Intermediary metabolism: Term signifying all those reactions occurring between the uptake of foodstuffs and the formation of excretory products.

Internal energy: Energy of a system excluding that resulting from its position in space; the latter is the potential energy.

Interstitial: Pertaining to the space between cells.

Intron: Intervening sequence in a gene. The whole gene is transcribed, but the corresponding intron segment is excised to produce the mature RNA; only exons are expressed in the mature RNA.

Irreversible process: Process in which the entropy of the universe increases; any real process has a degree of irreversibility associated with it.

Irreversible reaction: Unidirectional reaction. Although all reactions are, in principle, reversible, the conversion of the products to reactants of an enzyme-catalyzed irreversible reaction does not proceed at a detectable rate.

Ischemia: Reduced blood flow to a tissue or organ.

Ischemic heart disease: Designates heart disease due to inadequate blood flow through the coronary arteries; also called coronary artery disease.

Islets of Langerhans: Clusters of endocrine cells in the pancreas.

Isoergonic reaction: Reaction at equilibrium. *Compare* Functionally isoergonic reaction.

Isomerase: Enzyme catalyzing the transformation of a compound into a positional isomer.

Isomers: Compounds containing the same atoms but having the atoms attached to one another differently, e.g., glyceraldehyde 3-phosphate and dihydroxyacetone phosphate.

Isoprene: Hydrocarbon 2-methyl-1,3-butadiene, a recurring five-carbon structural unit of the terpenoid biomolecules such as vitamin A, coenzyme Q, and dolichol.

Isoprenoid derivative: Compound derived from isoprene.

Isothermal: Occurring at constant temperature.

Isotonic: Having an osmotic pressure (osmolarity) equal to that of body fluids.

Isotopes: Stable or radioactive forms of an element that differ in atomic weight but have the same atomic number and are chemically identical except perhaps for their rates of chemical reaction.

Isotropic: Property of a substance that does not depend upon its direction of observation.

Isozymes (isoenzymes): Multiple forms of an enzyme that differ from each other in their substrate affinity, in their maximum activity, or in regulatory properties.

Jaundice: Yellow color of the skin resulting from accumulation of bile pigments.

Juxtaglomerular (JG) apparatus: Specialized group of cells at the vascular pole of the renal glomerulus that regulate blood flow.

K_m: *See* Michaelis constant.

Ketone: Any compound having a carbonyl (>CO) group bound to two R groups.

Ketone bodies: Acetoacetate, β-hydroxybutyrate, and acetone.

Ketose: Polyhydroxyketone.

Ketosis: Excess of ketone bodies in the blood.

Kinase: Enzyme that catalyzes the phosphorylation of an acceptor molecule with ATP or other nucleoside triphosphate as the phosphoryl group donor.

Kinetic energy: Energy of a system related to motion.

Kinin: Chemical mediator of inflammation.

Krebs cycle: Pathway for the oxidation of the acetyl group of acetyl-coenzyme A to carbon dioxide with the concomitant generation of reduced coenzymes. Initially described by Hans Krebs in 1937; also called citric acid cycle and tricarboxylic acid cycle (the latter is the name used by Krebs). Citrate and isocitrate are the tricarboxylic acids.

Lagging strand: Strand of DNA that is synthesized discontinuously in the direction away from the replication fork. *Compare* Leading strand.

Latent infection: Microbial disease without clinical symptoms.

Law of mass action: Law stating that the rate of a chemical reaction is proportional to the multiplication product of the concentrations of the reactants.

Leading strand: Strand of DNA that is synthesized continuously in the direction leading into the replication fork. *Compare* Lagging strand.

Lecithin: Phosphatidylcholine.

Lesion: Any structural or pathological abnormality.

Leukemia: Neoplastic proliferation of leukocytes.

Leukocyte: White blood cell.

Leukopenia: Abnormally small number of white blood cells in the peripheral blood.

Leukoplakia: White patch on a mucous membrane.

Levorotary isomer: An optical isomer, which is designated by a lowercase l, that rotates the plane of plane-polarized light to the left. The isomer related to L-glyceraldehyde is designated by a small capital L. The L-isomer describes the absolute steric configuration and not necessarily the direction of rotation of the plane of polarized light. *Compare* Dextrorotory isomer.

Ligand: Molecule or ion that can bind to a protein.

Ligase: Enzyme that catalyzes the connection of two molecules in an ATP-dependent fashion (ligate = to tie together).

Lipid: Biomolecule soluble in organic solvents such as chloroform/methanol and insoluble in water.

Lipmann's law: ATP (adenosine triphosphate) serves as the common currency of energy exchange for all forms of life.

Lipoic acid: Compound containing two sulfur atoms that carries hydrogen atoms and acyl groups in α-keto acid dehydrogenases.

Lipoprotein: Protein that participates in the transport of cholesterol, triglyceride, and phospholipid in the blood.

Locus: Position of a gene on a chromosome. Different forms (alleles) of the same gene are found at the same locus on a chromosome.

Low-density lipoprotein (LDL) cholesterol: Fraction of cholesterol carried by low-density lipoproteins, which is correlated with atherosclerosis.

Low-energy compound: Compound that releases <30 kJ/mol of free energy upon hydrolysis under standard conditions. Also called energy-poor compound. *Compare* High-energy compound.

Lyase: Enzyme that catalyzes the cleavage of a molecule or the removal of a group from a molecule to form two molecules with a net increase in the number of double bonds, or the reverse reaction.

Lymphadenopathy: Any disease process affecting a lymph node.

Lymphocyte: Mononuclear blood cell produced in lymphoid tissue that is concerned with cell-mediated and humoral immunity.

Lymphokine: Regulatory protein liberated by lymphocytes.

Lymphoma: Neoplasm of lymphoid cells.

Lysosome: Membrane-enclosed organelle with an acidic (pH ≈ 5) interior that is found in eukaryotic cells and contains many hydrolytic enzymes.

Macromolecule: Molecule having a molecular weight in the range of a few thousand to many millions; includes DNA, RNA, protein, and large carbohydrates such as glycogen, starch, and cellulose.

Macrophage: Large cell derived from monocytes that can remove dead and damaged cells in many tissues and can ingest large microorganisms such as protozoa. *See also* Monocyte.

Macula: Discolored spot on the skin that is not elevated above the surface.

Magnetic resonance imaging (MRI): Diagnostic procedure that yields computer-generated images of tissues, organs, and masses based on the movement of hydrogen atoms in tissues subjected to a strong magnetic field.

Major histocompatibility complex (MHC): Group of genes on chromosome 6 that determines the antigens on the surface of cells.

Malaise: A feeling of illness.

Malignant tumor: Tumor that has invaded or can invade locally and spread to distant sites.

Mammogram: X-ray of the breast, used to detect tumors and other abnormalities.

Mass action: *See* Law of mass action.

Mast cell: Connective tissue cell containing granules filled with histamine and other chemical mediators. *Compare* Eosinophil.

Matrix: Mitochondrial interior; also, material in which connective tissue cells are embedded.

Medulla: Innermost part of an organ. *Compare* cortex.

Megaloblast: Abnormal red cell precursor resulting from vitamin B_{12} or folate deficiency.

Meiosis: Special type of cell division occurring in gametes (ovum and sperm), in which the number of chromosomes is reduced by one-half.

Meiotic nondisjunction: Failure of two members of a chromosome pair to disjoin during meiosis I, or of two chromatids of a chromosome to disjoin during meiosis II, so that both pass to one daughter cell and the other daughter cell receives neither.

Melanin: Dark pigment found in the skin, in the middle coat of the eye, and in other regions.

Melanocyte: Melanin pigment–producing cell in the epidermis of the skin.

Melanoma: Malignant tumor of pigment-producing cells.

Melena: Dark-colored stool due to the presence of breakdown products of the blood.

Membrane transport: Translocation of an ion or metabolite across a membrane, usually mediated by a specific membrane protein.

Meninges: Membranes covering the brain and spinal cord.

Meningioma: Benign tumor arising from the meninges.

Meningitis: Inflammation of the meninges.

Mesoderm: Middle germ layer of the embryo.

Messenger RNA (mRNA): Class of RNA molecules that carries, from its complementary DNA of the chromosome to ribosomes, genetic information encoded as a sequence of bases.

Metabolism: All the chemical reactions that take place in an organism.

Metabolite: Any chemical produced or consumed in the reactions of metabolism; a biochemical.

Metabolon: Group of associated enzymes that catalyzes a sequential series of reactions; a metabolic unit.

Metalloenzyme: Enzyme having a metal ion as its cofactor.

Metastasis: Spread of cancer cells from the site of origin to a distant site.

Michaelis constant (K_m): Substrate concentration at which an enzyme exhibits one-half its maximum velocity.

Michaelis-Menten equation: Equation relating the velocity (v) and the substrate concentration [S], the maximal velocity (V_{max}), and the Michaelis constant (K_m) of an enzyme: $v = (V_{max} \times [S])/(K_m + [S])$. Leonor Michaelis was a biochemist, and Maude Menten was a pediatrician.

Microcytic hypochromic anemia: Anemia characterized by red cells that are smaller than normal with a reduced hemoglobin concentration, usually due to iron deficiency.

Microfilament: Very thin cytoskeletal filament made of actin.

Microsome: Membranous vesicles formed by fragmentation of the endoplasmic reticulum and recovered by high-speed ($>10^5$ times the force of gravity) differential centrifugation.

Microtubule: Thin tubule assembled from α- and β-tubulin.

Mineralocorticoid: Adrenocortical hormone that regulates salt and water metabolism.

Mitchell theory: Also called Mitchell's law. *See* Chemiosmotic theory.

Mitochondria: Membrane-surrounded cellular organelles that contain the enzymes of the Krebs cycle, β-oxidation, electron transport, and oxidative phosphorylation; powerhouse of the cell.

Mitosis: Cell division in which replicated nuclear chromosomes are distributed to the nuclei of daughter cells. Although mitosis is used interchangeably with cell division, it refers to nuclear division, while cytokinesis refers to division of the cytoplasm. Mitosis is characteristic of cell division for all human cells except for the gametes, which employ meiosis. Mitosis also contrasts with the binary fission of bacteria.

Molar (M) solution: One mole of a substance dissolved in water that occupies a final volume of 1.00 liter (L).

Mole: Avogadro's number of molecules (6.02×10^{23}), or one gram-molecular mass of a compound.

Monocistronic: mRNA that codes for a single polypeptide chain; characteristic of eukaryotes but can also occur in prokaryotes.

Monocyte: Relatively large mononuclear leukocyte that matures into a macrophage. *See also* Macrophage.

Monooxygenase: Enzyme catalyzing simultaneous oxidation of two substrates by oxygen; one atom of oxygen is found in one product and the other atom of oxygen is found in another component; also called mixed-function oxygenase.

Monosaccharide: Carbohydrate consisting of a single sugar unit.

Monosomy: Condition of a cell in which only one chromosome of a homologous pair is present.

Monovalent: Having a valence, charge, or combining power of one.

Morphology: Structure or architecture of a component.

Motor neuron: Neuron that carries nerve impulses from the brain and spinal cord to muscles and glands.

Multienzyme complex: Physical aggregate of related enzymes participating in a given metabolic pathway.

Multiple myeloma: Malignant neoplasm of plasma cells.

Multiple sclerosis: Chronic disease characterized by focal areas of demyelination in the central nervous system, followed by glial scarring.

Murein: *See* Peptidoglycan.

Murmur: Sound heard on auscultation of the heart.

Muscular dystrophy: Hereditary disturbance of skeletal muscle leading to necrosis and degeneration of muscle.

Mutase: Enzyme catalyzing the transposition of a chemical group from one position of a substrate to another.

Mutation: Alteration in the nucleotide sequence of DNA that is transmitted from a parent to a daughter cell.

Myalgia: Muscle pain.

Myasthenia gravis: Autoimmune disease characterized by increased fatigability; due to an autoantibody that damages acetylcholine receptors at myoneural junctions.

Myelin: Fatty insulating material that surrounds nerve fibers and is produced by oligodendrocytes.

Myocardial infarction: Necrosis of heart muscle due to interruption of its blood supply; also called heart attack or coronary thrombosis.

Myofibril: Unit of thick and thin filaments of muscle fibers.

Myoglobinuria: Myoglobin in the urine, resulting in a dark amber–colored urine.

Myoma: Benign smooth muscle tumor such as occurs commonly in the uterus.

Myoneural junction: Specialized structure between motor nerve endings and muscle cells.

Myosin: Muscle protein of high molecular mass (500 kDa) possessing ATPase activity and intimately involved in the transduction of chemical to mechanical energy.

Myositis: Inflammation of muscle.

Myxedema: Hypothyroidism in adults. *Compare* Cretinism, in infants and children.

n: Arbitrary integer or whole number.

NAD^+, $NADP^+$ (nicotinamide adenine dinucleotide, nicotinamide adenine dinucleotide phosphate): Nicotinamide-containing coenzymes functioning as carriers of hydride (one proton and two electrons) in some oxidation-reduction reactions. NAD^+ is also called diphosphopyridine nucleotide (DPN^+), and $NADP^+$ is also called triphosphopyridine nucleotide (TPN^+).

Native structure: (1) Functional conformation of a macromolecule. *Compare* Denaturation. (2) Unmodified molecule that is a substrate for chemical modification such as a phosphorylation reaction.

Necrosis: Morphologic changes that follow cell death. *Compare* Apoptosis.

Neoplasia: Pathologic processes that result in autonomously growing cells.

Nephrotic syndrome: Clinical state characterized by proteinuria, decreased plasma albumin, edema, and usually hypercholesterolemia; due to various types of renal disease.

Neuroglia: Cells that support neurons; also called glia.

Neuron: Nerve cell, including the nerve cell body and its processes, that can propagate electrical potentials called action potentials.

Neurotransmitter: Compound secreted by a neuron that affects its target cell; serves to transmit an impulse from a neuron to another cell.

Neutral fat: Compound resulting from the esterification of the three hydroxyl groups of glycerol by fatty acids; usually called triglyceride (common name) or triacylglycerol (systematic name).

Neutrophil: Leukocyte having a multilobed nucleus whose cytoplasm is not acidophilic or basophilic; it is the most prevalent leukocyte and can phagocytose bacteria. Also called polymorphonuclear leukocyte, or poly. *See also* Basophil and Eosinophil.

Nicked DNA: Duplex DNA with a discontinuity or break in a sugar-phosphate backbone.

Nodule: Small, solid mass or node that can be detected by touch.

Nonheme-iron protein: Protein containing iron but lacking a porphyrin group.

Nonpolar group: Hydrophobic group, usually hydrocarbon in nature.

Nonreducing sugar: Sugar such as sucrose that does not reduce alkaline copper Fehling's or Benedict's solutions. These sugars lack a free aldehyde or ketone group.

Nonsense codon: UAA, UAG, UGA; a codon that does not specify an amino acid, but produces polypeptide chain termination.

Nonsense mutation: Change in the sequence of DNA that produces an in-phase termination codon and results in the premature termination of the encoded polypeptide chain.

Noradrenaline: One of the hormones of the adrenal medulla and also a neurotransmitter in the central nervous system and autonomic nervous system; also called norepinephrine.

Normocytic anemia: Anemia characterized by red cells having normal size and hemoglobin concentrations.

Northern blot: Technique involving resolution of RNA molecules by electrophoresis and transfer and fixation to nitrocellulose or nylon sheets with retention of the relative position of the RNA polynucleotides. RNA is detected with a suitable probe following hybridization.

Nuclear body (nucleoid): Nuclear zone in a prokaryotic cell; it contains the DNA chromosome but lacks a surrounding membrane.

Nuclease: Enzyme that catalyzes the hydrolysis of internucleotide linkages of a nucleic acid.

Nucleic acid: DNA or RNA; polynucleotides in which the nucleotide residues are linked in a specific sequence by phosphodiester bonds.

Nucleolus: Densely staining structure found in the nucleus of eukaryotic cells; involved in rRNA synthesis and ribosome formation.

Nucleophile, or **nucleophilic group:** Electron-rich group with a strong tendency to donate electrons to an electron-deficient atomic nucleus with the formation of a chemical bond; the oxygen of hydroxyl or phosphate groups and the nitrogen of an amino group are examples of nucleophiles.

Nucleoside: Compound consisting of a purine or pyrimidine base covalently linked to ribose or deoxyribose.

Nucleoside diphosphate sugar: *See* Glycoside diphosphate.

Nucleosome: Complex of about 200 DNA base pairs of which 160 base pairs combine with an octomer of histone proteins (two molecules each of H2A, H2B, H3, and H4) and 40 base pairs combine with histone H1; an electron micrograph of several nucleosomes resembles pearls on a necklace.

Nucleotide: Compound consisting of a purine or pyrimidine base covalently linked to ribose or deoxyribose, which is linked to phosphate.

Nucleus: Membrane-enclosed organelle in eukaryotes that contains the chromosomes.

Oligomeric protein: Protein consisting of two or more polypeptide chains.

Oligosaccharide: Three to ten monosaccharide groups joined by glycosidic bonds.

Oncogene: Gene whose function results in cancer.

Operator: Region of bacterial DNA that interacts with a regulatory or repressor protein to control the expression of a gene or group of genes.

Operon: Unit of bacterial genetic expression consisting of one or more genes and the operator and promoter sequences that regulate their transcription.

Ophthalmoplegia: Paralysis of motor nerves to the eye.

Opportunistic infection: Infection in an immunocompromised person caused by a microorganism that is normally nonpathogenic or of limited pathogenicity.

Optical activity: Capacity of a substance to rotate the plane of plane-polarized light; associated with chiral organic molecules.

Optimum pH: pH at which an enzyme or other protein shows maximum activity.

Organ: Macroscopic entity made of a group of cells that perform specific functions.

Organelle: Membrane-enclosed structure in eukaryotic cells, such as the mitochondrion, that contains enzymes and other components required for specialized cellular functions.

Orthophosphate cleavage: Cleavage of ATP to yield ADP and orthophosphate, usually coupled to an energy-requiring process or reaction.

Ossification: Process of forming bone.

Osteoarthritis: "Wear-and-tear" degeneration of the major weight-bearing joints.

Osteogenesis imperfecta: Congenital disturbance of bone formation characterized by excessively thin and brittle bones that are easily broken.

Osteoid: Organic matrix on which mineralization occurs.

Osteomalacia: Demineralization of bone without the loss of osteoid; result of vitamin D deficiency in adults.

Osteomyelitis: Inflammation of bone.

Osteoporosis: Generalized thinning and demineralization of bone with the loss of osteoid that occurs in the elderly, especially postmenopausal women.

Oxyhemoglobin: Compound formed by combination of hemoglobin with molecular oxygen.

Oxidation: Removal of electrons from an element or compound.

β-Oxidation: Repetitive degradation of fatty acids by a spiral of oxidative and thiolytic reactions yielding acetyl–coenzyme A; refers to the addition of oxygen to the β-carbon during this process.

Oxidation-reduction reaction: Reaction in which electrons are transferred from an electron donor or reductant to an electron acceptor or oxidant.

Oxidative decarboxylation: Decarboxylation accompanied by the reduction of an oxidizing agent such as NAD^+ or $NADP^+$.

Oxidative phosphorylation: Enzymatic phosphorylation of ADP to ATP coupled to electron transport from a substrate to molecular oxygen. Identical to respiratory chain phosphorylation and an example of electron-transport phosphorylation.

Oxidizing agent (oxidant): Acceptor of electrons in an oxidation-reduction reaction.

Oxygenase: Enzyme catalyzing a reaction of oxygen with an acceptor molecule.

P site: Site on the ribosome that accommodates *p*eptidyl-tRNA. *Compare* A site.

Palindrome: Segment of duplex DNA in which the base sequence of one strand in the 5′ to 3′ direction is the same as the base sequence on the opposite strand, also in the 5′ to 3′ direction.

Palpitation: Forcible, perceptible pulsation of the heart.

Papilloma: Benign tumor projecting from an epithelial surface.

Papule: Small, circumscribed, solid elevation of the skin.

Parallel: Term describing side-by-side objects with polarities running in the same direction.

Parenchyma: Functional cells of an organ, as contrasted with the connective tissue and supporting cells that form its framework.

Paresthesia: Abnormal sensation, such as burning, prickling, or numbness.

Parkinson disease: Chronic disease of the central nervous system that is characterized by rigidity and tremor resulting from decreased dopamine in the substantia nigra.

Partial pressure: Pressure exerted by a single gas in a mixture of gases, designated by the letter "p" preceding the chemical symbol for the gas (e.g., pCO_2).

Pathogenesis: Mechanism by which a disease develops.

Pathogenic: Disease-causing.

PCR: *See* Polymerase chain reaction.

Pentose: Carbohydrate containing five carbon atoms.

Pentose phosphate pathway: Conversion of glucose 6-phosphate to pentose phosphates with the production of reduced nucleotides and rearrangement of numerous sugar phosphates; also called the phosphogluconate pathway or the Warburg-Dickens pathway.

Peptidase: Enzyme that catalyzes the hydrolysis of a peptide bond; also called a protease.

Peptide: Two or more amino acids covalently joined by peptide bonds.

Peptide bond: Substituted amide linkage between the α-amino group of one amino acid and the α-carboxyl group of another.

Peptidoglycan: Cross-linked peptide-sugar complex forming the inner cell wall of eubacteria; consists of alternating residues of *N*-acetylglucosamine and *N*-acetylmuramic acid with peptide side chains. Also called murein.

Periodontal disease: Inflammation of the gingiva (gums) around the roots of the teeth.

Periosteum: Tough, fibrous membrane that covers a bone except for its articular surfaces.

Peripheral thiol: Sulfhydryl group of a cysteine residue on β-ketoacyl–ACP synthase of fatty acid synthetase. *Compare* Central thiol.

Peritoneum: Membrane that lines the abdominal cavity and also invests the external surfaces of the abdominal organs.

Pernicious anemia: Macrocytic anemia caused by inability to absorb vitamin B_{12} because of inadequate production of intrinsic factor by gastric mucosa.

Petechia: Pinpoint, nonraised, purple-red spot, larger than ecchymosis, due to hemorrhage resulting from decreased platelets, abnormal platelet function, or capillary defect caused by vitamin C deficiency (plural, petechiae).

pH: Negative logarithm to the base 10 of the hydrogen ion concentration of an aqueous solution; $pH = -\log_{10}[H^+]$. pH 7.0 is neutral; pH <7.0 is acid; pH >7.0 is alkaline.

Phagocytosis: Ingestion of particulate or foreign material by cells.

Phenotype: Observable characteristics of an organism.

Pheochromocytoma: Catecholamine-secreting tumor of the adrenal medulla.

Philadelphia chromosome: An abbreviated chromosome 22 that results from the reciprocal translocation of a part of chromosome 9 to chromosome 22; it occurs in patients with chronic granulocytic leukemia.

Phosphagen: Energy-storing compound containing a high-energy phosphoryl group attached to a nitrogen atom, e.g., creatine phosphate; named originally because acid treatment of compounds with a P–N bond gives rise to (*gen*) phosphate (*phospha*).

Phosphate-bond energy: Decrease in free energy as one mole of a phosphorylated compound at 1.0 M concentration undergoes hydrolysis at pH 7.0 and 25 °C.

Phosphoramidate: Compound with a P–N bond; also called phosphagen.

Phosphodiester: Molecule that contains two alcohols esterified to one molecule of phosphoric acid, which thus serves as a bridge between them.

Phosphogluconate pathway: *See* Pentose phosphate pathway.

Phospholipid: Lipid containing one or more phosphate groups.

Phosphorolysis: Cleavage of a compound by phosphate. *Compare* Hydrolysis.

Phosphoryl group, or **phosphorylium ion:** PO_3^{1-}; the group that is transferred during a transphosphorylation or kinase reaction.

Phosphorylation: Formation of a phosphate derivative of a biomolecule usually by enzymatic transfer of a phosphoryl group from ATP.

Phosphorylation potential (ΔG_p): Actual free-energy change of ATP synthesis under cellular and not standard conditions.

Photon: Quantal unit of light energy.

pK: Negative logarithm (p) of an equilibrium constant (K). The pK_a is the negative logarithm for the acid dissociation constant of a group and is the pH at which the concentrations of the protonated species and unprotonated species are equal; the a of pK_a is often omitted.

Plasma: Fluid part of the blood. *Compare* Serum.

Plasma membrane: Lipid bilayer immediately surrounding the cytoplasm of a cell.

Plasmid: Extrachromosomal, independently replicating, small, circular DNA molecule.

Platelet: Small (one-third to one-half the size of an erythrocyte), anucleate corpuscle that occurs in blood and participates in blood coagulation.

Pleura: Mesothelial covering of the lung (visceral pleura) and chest wall (parietal pleura).

Pneumocystis carinii (P. carinii): Protozoan parasite that causes severe pulmonary infection in immunocompromised persons.

Pneumonia: Inflammation of the lung.

Polar group: Hydrophilic, or water-loving, group such as $-OH$ or $-NH_2$.

Polarity: Distinction between the 5′ and 3′ ends of nucleic acids or the amino and carboxyl termini of peptides.

Polycistronic: Term describing mRNA that codes for more than one polypeptide chain; found only in bacteria.

Polycythemia: Increased number of red blood cells.

Polydipsia: Frequent drinking because of extreme thirst.

Polymerase chain reaction (PCR): Method for amplifying segments of DNA by using multiple amplification cycles that involve DNA strand separation at high temperature, annealing oligonucleotide DNA polymerase primers complementary to target DNA at a lower temperature, and elongation reactions at an intermediate temperature.

Polyneuritis: Inflammation of multiple nerves.

Polynucleotide: Covalently linked sequence of nucleotides in which the 5′ position of one nucleotide is joined by a phosphodiester bond to the 3′ position of the next.

Polyp: Benign tumor projecting from an epithelial surface.

Polypeptide: Chain of amino acids linked by peptide bonds; all proteins are polypeptides.

Polyphagia: Excessive eating.

Polyprotein: Protein that contains more than one activity; e.g., the fatty acid synthase complex is a dimer of identical polypeptides, each of which contains all the enzymes for fatty acid synthesis except acetyl-CoA carboxylase.

Polyribosome (polysome): Complex of a messenger RNA molecule and two or more ribosomes.

Polysaccharide: Macromolecule composed of many monosaccharide units linked by glycosidic bonds.

Polyuria: Excessive excretion of urine.

Porphyrin: Complex compound containing four substituted pyrroles covalently joined into a ring and often complexed with a central metal atom; a component of heme.

Posttranslational modification: Enzyme-catalyzed chemical modification of a polypeptide chain after its translation from its mRNA; includes such reactions as glycosylation, hydroxylation, proteolysis, and phosphorylation.

Potential energy: Energy of a system that depends upon its position in space; can be related to gravitational, electrical, or magnetic fields.

Primary active transport: Active transport sustained directly by a source of chemical energy such as ATP.

Primary structure: Sequence of component units of a molecule. The primary structure of protein is its amino acid sequence, its inter- and intrachain disulfide bridges, and covalent modifications such as phosphorylation or glycosylation.

Primasome: Group of components (soma = body) needed to initiate DNA replication.

Primer: Foundation molecule to which components are added, as in a primer DNA strand or a glycogen primer.

Processing: Postsynthetic modification reactions required to produce the final form of a molecule.

Prochiral molecule: Molecule containing a carbon atom with three different substituents that can undergo reaction to produce a chiral molecule.

Product: Final substance resulting from a chemical process; by convention, the substances given on the right side of a chemical equation.

Prognosis: Probable outcome of a disease or a disorder; the outlook for recovery.

Prokaryote: Simple unicellular organisms (e.g., bacteria) having a single chromosome but lacking a nuclear membrane and membrane-bound organelles.

Promoter: Region of chromosomal DNA that directs RNA polymerase binding and defines the transcription start site; enhancers and silencers regulate the rate of transcription.

Proofreading function: Mechanism for correcting a mistake or removing an incorrectly added component; generally refers to the 3′-exonuclease activity of DNA polymerase.

Proptosis: Exophthalmos, abnormal protrusion of the eyeball.

Prosthetic group: Organic cofactor bound tightly or even covalently to a protein that does not diffuse from the protein to perform its function.

Protease: Enzyme catalyzing the hydrolysis of proteins or peptides; also called proteolytic enzyme.

Protein: Macromolecule composed of one or more polypeptide chains, each possessing a characteristic amino acid sequence.

Protein kinase: Enzyme that catalyzes the phosphorylation of certain amino acid residues (serine, threonine, or tyrosine) in substrate proteins.

Proteoglycan: Hybrid macromolecule consisting of a polypeptide joined to a polysaccharide; the polysaccharide (glycan) is the major component. (The major component occurs at the end of the name, e.g., proteoglycan, where carbohydrate is the main constituent, versus glycoprotein, where protein is the main constituent.)

Prothrombin time: Test which measures that segment of the coagulation mechanism occurring after the formation of thromboplastin; used to monitor the effects of vitamin K antagonists such as coumarin.

Proton: (1) Hydrogen ion (H^+). (2) Positively charged particle in the nucleus of an atom.

Proton acceptor: Substance capable of binding to a hydrogen ion.

Proton donor: Acid, or substance capable of liberating a hydrogen ion.

Proton pump: Protein that transports protons across a membrane against an electrochemical gradient. *Compare* Q loop and Redox loop.

Proton-motive force (Δp): Electrochemical gradient across a membrane made up of differences in the electrical voltage ($\Delta\Psi_{i\text{-}o}$) and the proton concentration ($\Delta pH_{i\text{-}o}$). $\Delta p = \Delta\Psi_{i\text{-}o} - 0.059\ \Delta pH_{i\text{-}o}$ (in volts); a concept derived from the chemiosmotic, or Mitchell, theory.

Protooncogene: Gene encoding a normal cellular function, usually associated with cell division or development, that has the potential to undergo mutation or express abnormal amounts of product to produce cancer.

Provirus: Viral reverse-transcribed DNA that is integrated into host DNA.

Ptosis: Drooping of the upper eyelid.

Pulp cavity: Central hollow in a tooth, containing nerves, blood vessels, and lymphatics.

Purine: Nitrogen-containing, heterocyclic compound that consists of fused pyrimidine and imidazole rings. Found in nucleotides and nucleic acids; adenine and guanine are examples.

Purpura: Condition characterized by hemorrhages in the skin and mucous membranes (petechiae and ecchymoses).

Purulent: Consisting of pus, a fluid product of inflammation.

Pyelogram: Means for visualizing the contour of the urinary tract by intravenous injection of radiopaque material or by direct injection of the material into the ureters, followed by x-ray studies.

Pyelonephritis: Bacterial infection of the kidney and renal pelvis.

Pyranose: Simple sugar containing a six-membered ring (five carbons and one oxygen) similar to the pyran ring.

Pyridine nucleotide: Nucleotide coenzyme containing the pyridine derivative nicotinamide, i.e., NAD^+ or $NADP^+$.

Pyridoxal phosphate (PLP): Coenzyme derived from pyridoxine (vitamin B_6) and functioning in reactions involving amino-group transfer, racemization, and some decarboxylation reactions.

Pyrimidine: Nitrogen-containing, heterocyclic base serving as a component of a nucleotide or nucleic acid; uracil, cytosine, and thymine are examples.

Pyrophosphatase: Enzyme that catalyzes the hydrolysis of inorganic pyrophosphate to yield two molecules of (ortho)phosphate.

Pyrophosphate split, or **cleavage:** Cleavage of ATP to yield AMP and pyrophosphate; pyrophosphate cleavage is coupled to the formation of a covalent bond joining two biomolecules.

Pyrophosphorylase: Enzyme catalyzing the reaction of a nucleoside triphosphate and acceptor to produce pyrophosphate and a nucleotidyl acceptor, e.g., UDP-glucose. The reaction is actually named for the reverse process in which the nucleotidyl acceptor undergoes cleavage by pyrophosphate, or pyrophosphorolysis.

Pyuria: Pus in the urine.

Q loop: Scheme for coupling electron transport involving coenzyme Q, ubiquinone, or a related compound with translocation of four protons for each electron pair transported.

Quaternary structure: Three-dimensional structure of an oligomeric protein addressing the way in which the subunit chains interact and fit together.

R group: Distinctive side chain of the α-amino acid or other organic compound.

Racemic mixture: Equimolar mixture of the D- and L-stereoisomers of an optically active compound; the mixture exhibits no net rotation of plane-polarized light.

Radical: (1) Fundamental constituent of a molecule. (2) Group of atoms with a single unbonded electron. (3) Directed to the source of a morbid process, as in a radical mastectomy with complete removal of the breast.

Radioactive isotope: Isotopic form of an element with an unstable nucleus that emits α-particles, β-particles, or γ-rays.

Rales: Abnormal lung sounds heard through a stethoscope.

Reactant: Initial chemical substance that is converted into product; by convention, reactants appear on the left side and products on the right side of a chemical equation.

Recessive gene: Gene that expresses a trait only when present in the homozygous state.

Recombinant DNA: DNA that results from joining disparate DNA segments together.

Redox loop: Protons and electrons are transported from the mitochondrial (or bacterial cell) interior, and only protons are released at the exterior surface.

Reducing agent (reductant): Electron donor in an oxidation-reduction reaction.

Reducing equivalent: General term for an electron or an

electron equivalent in the form of a hydrogen atom or hydride ion that is transferred from donor to acceptor.

Reducing sugar: Sugar such as glucose that is oxidized by alkaline copper solutions such as Fehling's solution or Benedict's solution. These sugars have an aldehyde or ketone carbonyl (anomeric) group that is not involved in forming a glycoside bond.

Reductant: Electron donor in an oxidation-reduction reaction.

Reduction: Gain of electrons by an element or compound.

Regenerating substrate: Compound of a cyclic metabolic pathway that initiates the cyclic process and must be resynthesized to initiate another cycle.

Regulatory enzyme: Enzyme with a controlling or rate-determining function. The activity of a regulatory enzyme can be altered by increased or decreased synthesis or degradation or by its capacity to undergo a change in activity by noncovalent or covalent binding of a metabolite.

Regulatory gene: Gene involved in controlling the expression of another gene.

Regulatory sequence: DNA sequence involved in regulating the expression of a gene; e.g., an enhancer or silencer.

Rejection: Immunologic process characterized by destruction of a transplanted organ.

Releasing factors: Nonribosomal proteins required for releasing a completed polypeptide chain from the ribosome and dissociating the ribosome into its two subunits. Also called termination factors.

Releasing hormone: Hypothalamic hormone that causes release of hormone from the anterior lobe of pituitary, e.g., thyrotropin-releasing hormone.

Renaturation: Refolding of an unfolded (i.e., denatured) globular protein or nucleic acid.

Replication: Synthesis of daughter duplex DNA molecules that are identical to the parental duplex DNA.

Replisome: Body of components (soma = body) that participates in DNA replication.

Resonance: Representation of a molecule that cannot be portrayed by a single valence structure but can be embodied as a hybrid of two or more structures where all the atomic nuclei remain in the same position.

Respiration: (1) Oxidative breakdown and release of energy from nutrient molecules by reaction with oxygen mediated by an electron transport chain; also called aerobic respiration. (2) Rhythmic inflation and deflation of the lungs that facilitate gas exchange (oxygen intake and carbon dioxide expiration).

Respiratory chain: Sequence of electron-carrying proteins that transfer electrons from substrates to molecular oxygen during aerobic respiration; also called electron transport chain.

Respiratory chain phosphorylation: Phosphorylation of ADP mediated by an F_oF_1 ATP synthase coupled to electron transport between a substrate and oxygen and sustained by a proton gradient; also called oxidative phosphorylation.

Respiratory control: *See* Acceptor control.

Reticulocyte: Young red cell that is active in hemoglobin synthesis (mature red cells cannot synthesize hemoglobin, since they lack ribosomes).

Retrovirus: RNA virus that contains reverse transcriptase, e.g., the AIDS virus, or HIV.

Reverse transcriptase: RNA-directed DNA polymerase found in retroviruses; capable of making DNA complementary to an RNA.

Reversible reaction: Chemical reaction that can go from reactants to products or products to reactants depending upon the conditions; a functionally isoergonic, bidirectional process.

Ribonuclease: Enzyme that catalyzes the hydrolysis of internucleotide linkages of RNA.

Ribonucleic acid: *See* RNA.

Ribonucleoside: Nucleoside (base-sugar) containing D-ribose as its pentose component.

Ribonucleotide: Nucleoside attached to a phosphate (base-sugar-phosphate).

Ribosomal RNA (rRNA): Class of RNA molecules serving as components of ribosomes.

Ribosome: Macromolecular assembly of rRNAs and proteins that serves as the site of mRNA-directed protein synthesis.

Ribozyme: RNA that functions as a catalyst.

RNA: Polyribonucleotide of a specific sequence linked by successive 3′,5′-phosphodiester bonds; generally contains adenine, uracil, guanine, and cytosine but lacks thymine.

RNA polymerase: Enzyme that catalyzes the formation of RNA from ribonucleoside 5′- triphosphates using DNA as a template.

Rubella: German measles.

S: *See* Sedimentation coefficient.

Salt bridge: Ionic bond between a positively charged and a negatively charged group.

Sarcoma: Malignant tumor arising from mesodermal muscle or connective tissue.

Sarcomere: Functional and structural unit of muscle.

Sarcoplasmic reticulum: Internal membrane network of a muscle cell; releases and takes up calcium.

Saturated fatty acid: Fatty acid containing a fully saturated alkyl chain and a carboxylate group.

Schilling test: Test for the gastrointestinal absorption of vitamin B_{12}. A measured amount of radioactive cyanocobalamin is given orally, followed by a parenteral dose of nonradioactive compound. Percentage excreted in the urine is measured following various standard treatments.

Schwann cell: Elongated cell surrounding a peripheral nerve fiber that produces myelin which insulates the fiber.

Sclera: White of the eye.

Secondary active transport: Active transport sustained by a source of energy derived from another process. For example, a sodium gradient, produced by an ATP-dependent primary process, energizes a secondary metabolite transport process.

Secondary structure: Specific hydrogen-bonding patterns in proteins (α-helix and parallel and antiparallel β-pleated sheets) and nucleic acids (hydrogen bonds between complementary bases).

Sedimentation coefficient: Physical constant specifying the rate of sedimentation of a particle in a centrifugal field that is denoted by an S value, or Svedberg unit. Svedberg units are not directly proportional to the molecular mass; e.g., the 50S and 30S subunits of the ribosome combine to form a particle with a 70S sedimentation coefficient.

Semiconservative DNA replication: One parent strand is apportioned to each daughter duplex along with a newly synthesized strand of DNA.

Septicemia: Infection in which pathogenic bacteria are present in the bloodstream.

Serum: Fluid, expressed from clotted blood, that differs from plasma chiefly by the lack of fibrinogen and some other plasma proteins that are consumed during clotting.

Sex-linked gene: Gene present on the X chromosome.

SH2 domain: Src-homology-2-domain, a portion of a protein that recognizes and binds to protein-tyrosine phosphate.

SH3 domain: Src-homology-3-domain, a portion of a protein that recognizes a specific protein-proline containing sequence. Some proteins, such as the adaptor protein Grb2, possess both SH2 and SH3 domains; Grb2 binds to receptor protein-tyrosine kinases via its SH2 domain and GEF (guanine nucleotide exchange factor) via its SH3 domain.

Shuttle system: Series of chemical transformations involved in the indirect transport of a substance across a membrane.

Sickle cell hemoglobin: Abnormal hemoglobin that precipitates under reduced oxygen tension; residue 6 of the β-chain of sickle cell hemoglobin contains valine in place of the normal glutamate.

Signal peptidase: Proteolytic enzyme that catalyzes the hydrolytic removal of the hydrophobic leader sequence of a polypeptide.

Signal peptide sequence: Polypeptide amino-terminal hydrophobic leader sequence of about 25 amino acids that targets the newly synthesized protein to its appropriate location; it guides the protein to or through a specific membrane or organelle.

Signal recognition particle: Combination of specific proteins and 7SL RNA that recognizes and interacts with the signal peptide after it emerges from the ribosome; a G-protein that is active with bound GTP and is inactive following GTP hydrolysis.

Silencer: Regulatory DNA nucleotide segment that decreases the rate of transcription of a gene.

Silent mutation: Mutation in a gene that causes no detectable change in the biological characteristics of the phenotype or gene product.

Simple oxidation-reduction: Reaction involving the transfer of electrons that (1) does not involve oxygen directly and (2) occurs without a decarboxylation.

Simple protein: Protein that yields only amino acids on hydrolysis; a protein that lacks a cofactor.

Southern blot: Technique involving resolution of DNA molecules by electrophoresis and transfer and fixation to nitrocellulose or nylon sheets with retention of the relative position of the DNA polynucleotides. DNA is detected with a suitable probe following hybridization.

Splicing: Removal of a portion of the interior of a polymeric molecule, followed by connection of the two ends.

Spontaneous process: Process that, in principle, will occur without any additional input of energy. Thermodynamics gives no information on the rate, so the reaction may require a long time.

Standard free energy change ($\Delta G°'$): Gain or loss of free energy of reactants during the conversion to products under standard conditions of temperature (25 °C), pressure (1 atm), concentration (1 M), and pH (pH 7 is indicated by the prime [′]). One molar is the usual standard concentration except for water and hydrogen ions.

Standard reduction potential ($E°'$): electromotive force exhibited at an electrode by 1 M concentration each of a reducing agent and its oxidized form at 25 °C at pH 7.0 (pH 7 is denoted by the prime [′]); the more negative the standard reduction potential, the greater is the tendency to donate electrons.

State function: Properties of a system at equilibrium.

Steady state: Nonequilibrium state of a system through which matter is flowing and in which all components remain in constant concentration.

Steatorrhea: Passage of fat in large amounts in the feces (Greek *stear* "fat," *rhoia* "flow").

Stereoisomers: Two or more isomers that have the same molecular composition and the same atom-to-atom sequence but differ in the spatial arrangement of the atoms attached to one or more carbon atoms.

Steroid: Type of lipid containing a fused four-membered hydrocarbon ring (cyclopentanoperhydrophenanthrene).

Stoichiometric substrate: Substance that is consumed by a metabolic cycle and must be supplied in net amounts. *Compare* Regenerating substrate.

Stroke: Injury to part of the brain due to a disruption of its blood supply.

Structural gene: Gene coding for a protein or RNA. *Compare* Regulatory gene.

Substrate: Compound acted upon by an enzyme.

Substrate level phosphorylation: Net phosphorylation of ADP or some other nucleoside 5′-diphosphate independent of an electron-transport chain and the F_oF_1 ATP synthase.

Supercoiling: Supertwisted DNA; the coiled double helix is itself coiled.

Symport: Obligatory transport of two substances together in the same direction across a membrane.

Synapse: (1) Pairing of homologous chromosomes during meiosis. (2) Specialized connection between a neuron and its target cell.

System: Isolated collection of matter; all other matter in the universe apart from the system is called the surroundings.

T lymphocyte: White blood cell that kills virus-infected cells and regulates the activities of other white blood cells by cell-mediated immunity; T refers to *t*hymus.

Tachycardia: Rapid heart rate.

Tachypnea: Rapid respiratory rate.

Tautomers: Isomers that differ in the position of a bonded hydrogen atom.

Temperature: Intuitively, the hotness or coldness of an object. Thermodynamically, defined as $T = Q_{rev}/\Delta S$, where T is the temperature, Q_{rev} is the heat absorbed reversibly, and ΔS is the change in entropy (this definition is obscure but correct).

Template: Macromolecular mold or pattern for the synthesis of an informational macromolecule.

Teratoma: Tumor of various cell components.

Terminal transferase: Enzyme capable of adding nucleotide residues to the 3′ end of DNA chains that participates in immunoglobulin gene rearrangement.

Termination codon: One of three codons (UAA, UAG, and UGA) that signal termination of a polypeptide chain.

Termination factors: *See* Releasing factors.

Termination sequence: DNA sequence that appears at the end of a transcriptional unit and signals the end of transcription.

Ternary complex: Aggregate made of three components.

Tertiary structure (of a protein): Three-dimensional conformation of the polypeptide chain in its native folded state.

Tetany: Spasm of skeletal muscles, often due to subnormal level of ionized calcium in the blood.

Thermodynamics: The first law of thermodynamics states that energy cannot be created or destroyed in ordinary chemical and physical processes (excluding thermonuclear reactions). The second law of thermodynamics states that the entropy of the universe increases in any real chemical or physical process.

Thioester: Ester of a carboxylic acid with a thiol, or mercaptan (–SH).

Thiohemiacetal: Bond formed by the reaction of an aldehyde with a thiol (–SH) group.

Thiolysis: Cleavage (lysis) of a molecule into two smaller molecules by reaction with a thiol (RSH) such as coenzyme A; an RS is found in the molecule corresponding to one side of the cleaved bond, and an H is found in the molecule corresponding to the other side.

Thrombin: Coagulation factor with enzyme activity formed by activation of prothrombin during blood coagulation.

Thrombocytopenia: Deficiency of blood platelets.

Thrombosis: Blood clot formed within the vascular system.

Thrush: Candidiasis of the oral mucosa.

Tissue: Group of similar cells joined to perform a specific function.

Tophus: Sandy, gritty deposit (plural, tophi).

Topoisomer: Isomers of DNA that differ only in the supercoiling pattern.

Topoisomerase: Enzymes capable of positive or negative supercoiling of duplex DNA circles.

Total bilirubin: Bilirubin (indirect) plus bilirubin diglucuronide (direct bilirubin).

Toxin: Protein synthesized by some organisms that is toxic to other species.

TPN$^+$ (triphosphopyridine nucleotide): *See* NADP$^+$.

Trace element: Chemical element required by humans in small amounts (milligrams or less) daily.

Transaminase: Enzyme that catalyzes the transfer of amino groups from α-amino to α-keto acids. Also called aminotransferase.

Transamination: Enzymatic transfer of an amino group from an α-amino acid to an α-keto acid.

Transcription: Enzymatic process by which the genetic information contained in one strand of DNA is used to specify a complementary sequence of bases in an RNA chain.

Transcriptional control: Regulation of protein synthesis by regulation of the formation of its mRNA.

Transfer RNA (tRNA): Class of RNA molecules (75–95 nucleotides), each of which combines covalently with a specific amino acid as the first step in protein synthesis.

Transition state: Activated form of a molecule that is capable of undergoing a chemical reaction.

Translation: Process in which the genetic information present in an mRNA molecule directs the sequence of amino acids during protein synthesis; the four-letter alphabet of nucleic acids is translated into the 20-letter alphabet of proteins.

Translational control: Regulation of protein synthesis by the rate of its translation on the ribosome.

Translocase: Membrane protein that transports a substance from one to the other side; also called permease.

Translocation: (1) Transfer of a substance from one site to another. (2) Transfer of a piece of one chromosome to a nonhomologous chromosome.

Transudate: Any protein-poor fluid that has passed out of or oozed from a body structure. *Compare* Exudate.

Triacylglycerol: *See* Triglyceride.

Tricarboxylic acid cycle: *See* Krebs cycle.

Triglyceride: Compound composed of three molecules of fatty acid combined with one molecule of glycerol; also called neutral fat or triacylglycerol.

Triphosphopyridine nucleotide (TPN$^+$): *See* NADP$^+$.

Trisomy: Presence of an extra chromosome within a cell; having three of a given chromosome instead of the usual pair.

Tumor: Swelling.

Tumor-associated antigen: Antigen associated with tumor cells that serves as an indicator of tumor proliferation.

Turnover: Constant, steady-state metabolic destruction and replacement of cell components.

Ulcer: Lesion caused by loss of a portion of a cutaneous or mucous surface, such as a peptic ulcer of the stomach or duodenum.

Ultrasonography: Visualization of structures within the body by recording the reflections of pulses of ultrasonic (>20,000 cycles per second) waves directed into the tissues.

Uncoupling agent: Substance such as 2,4-dinitrophenol that uncouples phosphorylation of ADP from electron transport in the respiratory chain by dissipating the proton gradient.

Unsaturated fatty acid: Fatty acid containing one or more double bonds.

Upstream: Toward the 5′-end of a nucleic acid or the amino terminus of a polypeptide.

Urea: Chief nitrogen end product in humans; excreted in the urine.

Uremia: Excess urea in the body resulting from renal failure.

Urinalysis: Chemical and microscopic analysis of the urine.

V_{max}: Maximum velocity of an enzymatic reaction.

Valence: Number of univalent atoms (such as hydrogen) with which a single atom of another element can combine; also called combining power.

Vasoconstriction: Decrease in the caliber of a blood vessel.

Vasodilatation: Increase in the caliber of a blood vessel.

Vesicle: Small sac filled with fluid or gas.

Virulence: Ability of an organism to cause disease.

Virus: Infectious nucleic acid–protein complex which requires an intact host cell for its replication and which contains a chromosome of either DNA or RNA.

Vitamin: Organic substance, not consumed as food energy, required by humans; most vitamins function as enzyme cofactors or cosubstrates for enzymes.

Warburg-Dickens pathway: *See* Pentose phosphate pathway.

Watson-Crick base pairing: *See* Complementary base pairing.

Wernicke-Korsakoff syndrome: Thiamine deficiency that leads to disturbances in ocular motility, ataxia, and tremors (Wernicke syndrome) plus confusion and memory impairment for recent events (Korsakoff syndrome) for which the patient compensates by confabulation (making up tales to give a fluent answer without regard to facts).

Western blot: Technique involving electrophoresis of protein, followed by transfer to a nitrocellulose matrix and identification with an antibody.

Wheeze: Whistling sound made while breathing.

Wilms tumor: Malignant renal tumor of infants and children.

Wobble: Nonstandard or non–Watson-Crick base pairing between the base at the 3′ end of a codon and the complementary base at the 5′ end of the anticodon.

Work: (1) Movement of a general capacity against a general potential; units are the same as those of energy. (2) The study of biochemistry.

X-ray crystallography: Use of x-ray diffraction by crystals of a compound to determine its three-dimensional structure.

Xerostomia: Decreased salivary flow, or dry mouth.

Zygote: Fertilized ovum.

Zymogen: Inactive precursor of an enzyme, e.g., trypsinogen.

HINTS FOR THE STUDY OF BIOCHEMISTRY

General Strategies for Studying Metabolic Pathways

1. Establish the purpose of the pathway—what is the overall function?
2. What are the names and structures of the molecules going into and coming out of the pathway—what is the stoichiometry of the pathway?
3. How does the pathway relate to other metabolic pathways?
4. What are the general metabolic conditions that increase or decrease the activity of the pathway (e.g., feeding, fasting, glucose availability)?
5. Which steps or enzymes of the pathway are regulated?
6. Identify the regulatory molecules and their effects (whether stimulatory or inhibitory).
7. Identify the steps where ATP is consumed or produced.
8. Identify the steps where NAD(P)H is produced or consumed.
9. Identify the vitamins or cofactors involved in the pathway.
10. Compare biosynthetic and degradative pathways.

Specific Strategies for Studying Biochemistry

1. *Be able to draw the structure of ATP.* Make sure that the phosphates have the correct charge and the appropriate double bonds. Indicate the position of the high-energy bonds.
2. *Be able to recognize the structures of the 20 genetically encoded amino acids.* Indicate the correct electrical charges and the positions of double bonds. Know which side chains of amino acids are charged at physiological pH.
3. Be able to recognize the five principal nucleotides that occur in RNA and DNA.
4. Be able to draw the Haworth (pronounced "how-worth") structure of glucose and show the nature of the bonds present in glycogen.
5. Be able to draw the structures of the compounds found in the Embden-Meyerhof glycolytic pathway and the Krebs citric acid cycle.
6. Be able to draw the structure of linoleic acid. Know the numbering systems.
7. Be able to draw the structure of cholesterol. Know the numbering system.
8. Be able to recognize the intermediates in fatty acid oxidation and fatty acid biosynthesis.
9. Indicate the functions associated with each of the following: cell nucleus, mitochondrion, lysosome, Golgi, peroxisome, endoplasmic reticulum, and cytosol.
10. Name the irreversible steps in glycolysis and the Krebs citric acid cycle. Know the rate-limiting reactions in these two processes. Know the pattern of allosteric regulation of these two pathways. Name the two enzymes of the Krebs cycle that catalyze decarboxylation reactions. Which step of the Krebs cycle is associated with substrate-level phosphorylation? Which step of the Krebs cycle is inhibited by malonate?
11. Calculate the ATP yields from the oxidative metabolism of one mole of glucose using 2.5 ATP from NADH and 1.5 ATP from $FADH_2$.
12. Know the three main tenets of the chemiosmotic hypothesis. Know Lipmann's law.
13. Distinguish between competitive, noncompetitive, and uncompetitive enzyme inhibitors.
14. Contrast purine and pyrimidine biosynthesis.
15. Discuss the primary, secondary, tertiary, and quaternary hierarchical structure of proteins.
16. Define pH, pK_a, acid, salt, and buffer.
17. Define positive cooperativity.
18. Describe the pathway of electron transport from NADH to oxygen. What are complexes I, II, III, and IV? Where are sites 1, 2, and 3 located? Describe the action of (a) cyanide, (b) rotenone, (c) carbon monoxide, and (d) antimycin A.
19. Describe the mechanism for ATP formation in mitochondria.
20. Compare and contrast fatty acid oxidation and fatty acid biosynthesis.
21. Calculate the yield of ATP associated with the complete oxidation of (a) palmitate (16-carbon, saturated) and (b) palmitoleate (16-carbon, 1 double bond).
22. How are intermediates of the citric acid cycle maintained at adequate levels? Define (a) catabolic, (b) anabolic, and (c) amphibolic processes.
23. Specify the configuration of (a) amino acids that occur in proteins and (b) glucose that occurs in glycogen relative to D- and L-glyceraldehyde.
24. Describe the role of GTP in (a) purine biosynthesis, (b) gluconeogenesis, and (c) Krebs cycle function.
25. Describe the role of CTP in lipid biosynthesis.
26. Describe the role of UTP in carbohydrate biosynthesis.
27. Describe the substrate specificity of common proteases, especially trypsin and chymotrypsin.
28. Describe replication, RNA synthesis, and protein synthesis.
29. Describe the functions of G-proteins.
30. Describe the two roles of vitamin B_{12} in metabolism in humans.
31. Describe the pathway for converting galactose to glucose 6-phosphate. What is the enzyme deficiency in galactosemia?
32. Name the five cofactors required for the conversion of pyruvate to acetyl-CoA.
33. Name the two enzymes necessary for glycogen formation and the two enzymes necessary for glycogenolysis. Describe the action of glucagon on glycogenolysis.
34. Define (a) transport, (b) symport, and (c) antiport. Give examples of each.
35. Describe the biosynthesis of ketone bodies in the liver and their utilization in extrahepatic tissues.
36. Contrast the salvage and *de novo* pathways for purine nucleotide synthesis. How is it known that the salvage pathway is operational in human metabolism?
37. Define or describe (a) DNA polymerase, (b) 5′-exonuclease activity, (c) 3′-exonuclease activity, (d) DNA ligase, (e) helicase, (f) topoisomerase, (g) single-strand binding protein, (h) leading strand, (i) lagging strand, (j) template, (k) primer, (l) primase, (m) proofreading or editing function, (n) replication fork, and (o) semiconservative replication.
38. Describe excision repair of DNA.

39. Describe the functions of the five eukaryotic DNA polymerases.
40. Define mRNA, rRNA, 5S RNA, tRNA, snRNA, and hnRNA. Which eukaryotic RNA polymerases are involved in the biosynthesis of each?
41. Describe the ribosome. What are the A site and P site? Where is peptidyltransferase activity located?
42. Describe the mechanism of amino acid activation.
43. Recount the role of the soluble (nonribosomal) factors of protein synthesis. Describe how these factors exclude Met-$tRNA^{Met}$ from the initiation reaction and f-Met-$tRNA_i^{Met}$ (in prokaryotes) or Met-$tRNA_i^{Met}$ (in eukaryotes) from participating in the elongation reactions.
44. Describe the reactants that participate in peptide bond formation. In which direction does chain growth occur? Why is a translocation reaction required?
45. How many high-energy bonds are expended in each polymerization reaction, on the average, in (a) DNA biosynthesis, (b) RNA biosynthesis, and (c) protein biosynthesis?
46. What is the neurochemical basis of (a) myasthenia gravis and (b) Parkinson disease?
47. Give the nutritional caloric value of protein, carbohydrate, fat, and ethanol.
48. What is the importance of the following in humans: (a) cobalt, (b) iodine, (c) fluoride, (d) copper, and (e) iron?
49. Distinguish between marasmus and kwashiorkor.
50. Name the vitamin deficiency associated with (a) rickets, (b) beriberi, (c) scurvy, (d) pernicious anemia, and (e) pellagra.
51. Describe the action of (a) cyanide, (b) tetracycline, (c) rotenone, (d) carbon monoxide, (e) antimycin A, (f) streptomycin, (g) actinomycin D, (h) methotrexate, (i) chloramphenicol, and (j) rifamycin.
52. Describe the defect associated with the following disorders: (a) von Gierke disease, (b) Christmas disease, (c) Pompe disease, (d) Tay-Sachs disease, (e) Gaucher disease, (f) familial hypercholesterolemia, (g) maple syrup urine disease, (h) phenylketonuria, (i) cystic fibrosis, (j) hemophilia, (k) Lesch-Nyhan syndrome, (l) sickle cell anemia, (m) Duchenne muscular dystrophy, and (n) drug-induced hemolytic anemia.